T0185187

Contemporary Debates in Bioethics

Contemporary Debates in Philosophy

In teaching and research, philosophy makes progress through argumentation and debate. Contemporary Debates in Philosophy provides a forum for students and their teachers to follow and participate in the debates that animate philosophy today in the western world. Each volume presents pairs of opposing viewpoints on contested themes and topics in the central subfields of philosophy. Each volume is edited and introduced by an expert in the field, and also includes an index, bibliography, and suggestions for further reading. The opposing essays, commissioned especially for the volumes in the series, are thorough but accessible presentations of opposing points of view.

1. Contemporary Debates in Philosophy of Religion
   edited by Michael L. Peterson and Raymond J. Vanarragon
2. Contemporary Debates in Philosophy of Science
   edited by Christopher Hitchcock
3. Contemporary Debates in Epistemology
   edited by Matthias Steup and Ernest Sosa
4. Contemporary Debates in Applied Ethics
   edited by Andrew I. Cohen and Christopher Heath Wellman
5. Contemporary Debates in Aesthetics and the Philosophy of Art
   edited by Matthew Kieran
6. Contemporary Debates in Moral Theory
   edited by James Dreier
7. Contemporary Debates in Cognitive Science
   edited by Robert Stainton
8. Contemporary Debates in Philosophy of Mind
   edited by Brian McLaughlin and Jonathan Cohen
9. Contemporary Debates in Social Philosophy
   edited by Laurence Thomas
10. Contemporary Debates in Metaphysics
    edited by Theodore Sider, John Hawthorne, and Dean W. Zimmerman
11. Contemporary Debates in Political Philosophy
    edited by Thomas Christiano and John Christman
12. Contemporary Debates in Philosophy of Biology
    edited by Francisco J. Ayala and Robert Arp
13. Contemporary Debates in Bioethics
    edited by Arthur L. Caplan and Robert Arp

Contemporary Debates in Bioethics

Edited by

Arthur L. Caplan and Robert Arp

WILEY Blackwell

This edition first published 2014

Wiley-Blackwell is an imprint of John Wiley & Sons, formed by the merger of Wiley's global Scientific, Technical and Medical business with Blackwell Publishing.

Registered Office
John Wiley & Sons Ltd, The Atrium, Southern Gate, Chichester, West Sussex, PO19 8SQ, UK

Editorial Offices
350 Main Street, Malden, MA 02148-5020, USA
9600 Garsington Road, Oxford, OX4 2DQ, UK
The Atrium, Southern Gate, Chichester, West Sussex, PO19 8SQ, UK

For details of our global editorial offices, for customer services, and for information about how to apply for permission to reuse the copyright material in this book please see our website at www.wiley.com/wiley-blackwell.

Library of Congress Cataloging-in-Publication Data

Contemporary debates in bioethics / edited by Arthur L. Caplan, Robert Arp.
p. ; cm. – (Contemporary debates in philosophy ; 13)
Includes bibliographical references and index.
ISBN 978-1-4443-3713-6 (cloth : alk. paper) – ISBN 978-1-4443-3714-3 (pbk. : alk. paper)
I. Caplan, Arthur L. II. Arp, Robert. III. Series: Contemporary debates in philosophy ; 13.
[DNLM: 1. Bioethical Issues. 2. Biomedical Research–ethics. 3. Genetic Enhancement–ethics.
4. Patient Rights–ethics. 5. Reproductive Techniques–ethics. WB 60]
R724
174.2–dc23

2013006628

A catalogue record for this book is available from the British Library.

Cover design by www.cyandesign.co.uk

Set in 10/12pt Bembo by SPi Publisher Services, Pondicherry, India

1 2014

Contents

Notes on Contributors

Nicholas Agar, Ph.D., is Reader in Philosophy at Victoria University of Wellington, New Zealand. He is interested in ethical issues arising out of human enhancement. His most recent book on this topic is *Humanity's End: Why We Should Reject Radical Enhancement* (2010).

Richard J. Arneson, Ph.D., holds the Valtz Family Chair in Philosophy in the Department of Philosophy at the University of California, San Diego. His recent current research is on distributive justice. Some of this work explores how one might best incorporate a reasonable account of personal responsibility into a broadly egalitarian theory of justice. He also considers how consequentialist morality (one ought always to do an act the consequences of which are no worse than those of any alternative available act) might be developed in a version that is appealing and appropriately responsive to its critics. This latter project involves exploring the structure of moderate deontology to identify the best rival of consequentialism.

Robert Arp, Ph.D., is author of *Scenario Visualization: An Evolutionary Account of Creative Problem Solving* (2008), co-editor with George Terzis of *Information and Living Systems: Philosophical and Scientific Perspectives* (2011), co-editor with Francisco Ayala of *Contemporary Debates in Philosophy of Biology* (Wiley-Blackwell, 2009), and co-editor with Alex Rosenberg of *Philosophy of Biology: An Anthology* (Wiley-Blackwell, 2009), and he has interests in bioethics as well. He works as a data analyst and modeler (see www.robertarp.webs.com).

Tom L. Beauchamp, Ph.D., is Professor of Philosophy and Senior Research Scholar, Kennedy Institute of Ethics, Georgetown University. His research interests are in the ethics of human-subjects research, the ethics of animal-subjects research and human uses of animals, the place of universal principles and rights in biomedical ethics, methods of bioethics, Hume and the history of modern philosophy, and business ethics.

James L. Bernat, M.D., is the Louis and Ruth Frank Professor of Neuroscience, and Professor of Neurology and Medicine at the Geisel School of Medicine at Dartmouth. He is a neurologist at Dartmouth-Hitchcock Medical Center where he directs the program in clinical ethics. bernat@dartmouth.edu.

Edwin Black is the award-winning, *New York Times*-bestselling and international investigative author of 80 award-winning editions in 14 languages in 65 countries, as well as scores of newspaper and magazine articles in the leading publications of the United States, Europe, and Israel. With more than a million books in print, his work focuses on genocide and hate, corporate criminality and corruption, governmental misconduct, academic fraud, philanthropic abuse, oil addiction, alternative energy, and historical investigation. For his award-winning eugenic work, *War Against the Weak: Eugenics and America's Campaign to Create a Master Race*, he has received the Justice for All Award, the International Human Rights Award, and numerous other citations.

Catherine M. Brooks, J.D., is a professor of law at Creighton University in Omaha, Nebraska, specializing in children's and family law. She is the co-founder of the Creighton Center for the Study of Children's Issues and co-editor of the *Nebraska Juvenile Court Procedures Manual*. She has numerous publications in peer-reviewed journals and law reviews. Professor Brooks provides consultations to family law practitioners, child advocacy groups, and other social-service organizations, particularly in matters involving child custody disputes and child protection. She earned her law degree from the University of Virginia and her bachelor's and master's degrees from Thomas More College of Fordham University and the Graduate School of Arts and Sciences of Fordham University. Her current work focuses on the use of mediation and negotiation in resolving disputes within families and between families and state protection agencies.

Arthur L. Caplan, Ph.D., is the Drs William F. and Virginia Connolly Mitty Professor and founding head of the Division of Bioethics at New York University Langone Medical Center in New York City. Prior to coming to NYU, he was the Sidney D. Caplan Professor of Bioethics at the University of Pennsylvania Perelman School of Medicine in Philadelphia where he created the Center for Bioethics and the Department of Medical Ethics. He is the author or editor of 30 books and over 550 papers in refereed journals. His most recent books are *Smart Mice Not So Smart People* (2006) and the *Penn Guide to Bioethics* (2009).

Mark J. Cherry, Ph.D., is the Dr Patricia A. Hayes Professor in Applied Ethics and Professor of Philosophy at St. Edward's University. He earned his undergraduate degree in philosophy from the University of Houston and his doctorate degree in philosophy from Rice University in Houston, Texas. His research compasses ethics and bioethics, together with social and political philosophy. He is author of *Kidney for Sale by Owner: Human Organs, Transplantation and the Market* (2005) as well as editor of *The Journal of Medicine and Philosophy*, associate senior editor of *Christian Bioethics*, Editor-in-Chief of *HealthCare Ethics Committee Forum*, co-editor of the book series *The Annals of Bioethics*, and editor of the book series *Philosophical Studies in Contemporary Culture*.

Winston Chiong, M.D., Ph.D., is a clinical fellow in the University of California, San Francisco Department of Neurology, and is a postdoctoral research fellow in the Helen Wills Neuroscience Institute at the University of California, Berkeley. His current research encompasses neuroscientific and conceptual methods to investigate changes in decision-making, moral agency, and personhood in the context of neurological illness.

Carl Cohen, Ph.D., is Professor of Philosophy at the University of Michigan, and co-author (with Tom Regan) of *The Animal Rights Debate* (2001). He was for years a member of the Animal Care and Use Committee of the Pfizer Corporation, and has served for decades on the Institutional Review Board of the University of Michigan Medical Center in Ann Arbor.

Kevin S. Decker, Ph.D., is Associate Professor of Philosophy and Associate Dean of the College of Arts and Letters at Eastern Washington University near Spokane, Washington. His areas of research interest include American pragmatism, social and political theory, and applied ethics. He is the co-editor of three books on philosophy and popular culture.

Katrien Devolder, Ph.D., is Senior Research Fellow at Bioethics Institute Ghent at Ghent University. Her research interests include medical ethics (in particular, the ethics of cloning), stem-cell research, genetic selection, chemical castration, and medical complicity in others' wrongdoing.

Jason T. Eberl, Ph.D., is Associate Professor and Graduate Director of Philosophy in the Indiana University School of Liberal Arts at Indiana University-Purdue University, Indianapolis. He is also an affiliate faculty member of the IU Center for Bioethics and the IUPUI Medical Humanities & Health Studies program. He has published articles and reviews in *American Journal of Bioethics*, *Bioethics*, *Journal of Medicine and Philosophy*, *National Catholic Bioethics Quarterly*, and *Linacre Quarterly*. His book *Thomistic Principles and Bioethics* was published in 2006.

John Geyman, M.D., is Professor Emeritus of Family Medicine at the University of Washington School of Medicine, where he chaired the Department of Family Medicine from 1976 to 1990. He has also practiced family medicine in rural communities for 13 years, edited family-medicine journals for 30 years, served as president of Physicians for a National Health Program from 2005 to 2007, and is a member of the Institute of Medicine. His books include *The Corporate Transformation of Health Care: Can the Public Interest Still Be Served?* (2004), *The Corrosion of Medicine: Can the Profession Reclaim Its Moral Legacy?* (2008), and *Health Care Wars: How Market Ideology and Corporate Power Are Killing Americans* (2012).

Jean Kazez, Ph.D., is Adjunct Assistant Professor of Philosophy at Southern Methodist University. She is the author of *Animalkind: What We Owe to Animals* (2010) and *The Weight of Things: Philosophy and the Good Life* (2007), both published by Wiley-Blackwell.

David Koepsell, Ph.D., earned his law degree and Ph.D. in philosophy from the University at Buffalo. He teaches ethics in the Philosophy Section, Faculty of Values and Technology, Delft University of Technology, The Netherlands. He has published widely on the philosophy of intellectual property, applied ethics, ontology, and civil rights (see http://davidkoepsell.com).

John Lachs, Ph.D., is Centennial Professor of Philosophy at Vanderbilt University. His latest book, *Stoic Pragmatism* (Indiana University Press), has just appeared.

Patrick Lee, Ph.D., holds the John N. and Jamie D. McAleer Chair of Bioethics, and is the Director of the Institute of Bioethics, at Franciscan University of Steubenville. He has published widely on bioethics, including written articles and books on bioethics, including *Body-Self Dualism in Contemporary Ethics and Politics* (with Robert P. George, 2007), *Abortion and Unborn Human Life* (2010).

Stephen E. Levick, M.D., is a clinical assistant professor of psychiatry at the University of Pennsylvania School of Medicine, where he supervises psychotherapy, and has his own private practice nearby. His book, *Clone Being: Exploring the Psychological and Social Dimensions* (2004), was described by cloning pioneer, Ian Wilmut, as "the first framework for detailed analysis of the ethical, psychological, and social consequences of human reproductive cloning." He employs arguments generated from that framework as both siege engines and battlements in his debate with Dr Devolder on the issue in this volume.

Jane Maienschein, Ph.D., is Regents' Professor, President's Professor, and Parents Association Professor at Arizona State University, where she serves as Director of the Center for Biology and Society. She is also Adjunct Scientist and Director of the History and Philosophy of Science Program at the Marine Biological Laboratory in Woods Hole, Massachusetts. An MBL-ASU/HPS collaboration includes the Embryo Project (embryo.mbl.edu), HPS Repository, and Digital HPS Consortium. She is (co)editor of a dozen books and author of three, including *Whose View of Life? Embryos, Cloning, and Stem Cells* with Harvard University Press.

Bertha Alvarez Manninen, Ph.D., is an associate professor of philosophy at Arizona State University's West campus. Her primary area of research is bioethics with an emphasis on the moral status of embryos and fetuses. Other interests include philosophy of religion, ancient philosophy, social and political philosophy, and philosophy and film.

Don Marquis, Ph.D., is Professor of Philosophy at The University of Kansas. His essay "Why Abortion is Immoral" was published in *The Journal of Philosophy* in 1989 and has been reprinted over 90 times.

Daryl Pullman, Ph.D., is a professor of medical ethics in the Faculty of Medicine, at Memorial University in Newfoundland and Labrador, Canada. He has published widely on issues in clinical and research ethics.

Laura Purdy, Ph.D., is Professor Emerita of Philosophy at Wells College. Her research has focused primarily on issues in reproduction and family.

Jeffrey Reiman, Ph.D., is the William Fraser McDowell Professor of Philosophy at American University in Washington, DC. He is the author of *In Defense of Political Philosophy* (Harper & Row, 1972), *Justice and Modern Moral Philosophy* (1990), *Critical Moral Liberalism: Theory and Practice* (1997), *The Death Penalty: For and Against* (with Louis Pojman, 1998), *Abortion and the Ways We Value Human Life* (1999), *The Rich Get Richer and the Poor Get Prison: Ideology, Class, and Criminal Justice* (with Paul Leighton, 2012), *As Free and As Just as Possible: The Theory of Marxian*

Liberalism (Wiley-Blackwell, 2012), and more than 120 articles in philosophy and criminal justice journals and anthologies.

Lawrence M. Sung, J.D., Ph.D., is a Partner with the law firm of Baker & Hostetler LLP in the Washington, DC office, specializing in biotechnology, pharmaceutical, and medical device patent litigation, counseling, and technology transfer. Dr Sung is also a professor and the Director of the Intellectual Property Law Program at the University of Maryland School of Law in Baltimore, MD. He may be contacted at lsung@bakerlaw.com or lsung@law.umaryland.edu.

Christopher Tollefsen, Ph.D., is Professor of Philosophy at the University of South Carolina; he has twice been a visiting fellow in the James Madison Program at Princeton University. He has published over 60 articles, book chapters, and reviews on bioethics and natural law ethics, and is the author, co-author, or editor of five recent books, including *Biomedical Research and Beyond: Expanding the Ethics of Inquiry* (2012) and, with Robert P. George, *Embryo: A Defense of Human Life* (2011). He has recently completed a book manuscript, provisionally titled *Truth, Lies, and the Natural Law: Why Lying for a Good Cause is Always Wrong*. Tollefsen sits on the editorial board of a number of journals and is the editor of the Springer book series, *Catholic Studies in Bioethics*.

Jamie Carlin Watson, Ph.D., is Assistant Professor of Philosophy at Young Harris College (Young Harris, GA). With Robert Arp, he is the author of *Critical Thinking: An Introduction to Reasoning Well* (2011), *Philosophy DeMYSTiFied* (2011), and *What's Good on TV: Understanding Ethics Through Television* (Wiley-Blackwell, 2011). He is currently working with Peter Fosl and Galen Foresman on *The Critical Thinker's Toolkit* (Wiley-Blackwell).

Glen Whitman, Ph.D., is a professor of economics at California State University, Northridge and an adjunct scholar with the Cato Institute. He received his Ph.D. in economics from New York University in 2000. His research in applied game theory, economic analysis of law, and economic methodology has appeared in the *Journal of Legal Studies*, *UCLA Law Review*, *Journal of Economic Behavior and Organization*, and other scholarly journals. His current research interests include healthcare and paternalistic legislation.

William J. Winslade, J.D., Ph.D., Ph.D., is James Wade Rockwell Professor of Philosophy of Medicine, Professor of Preventive Medicine and Community Health, and Professor of Psychiatry and Behavioral Sciences, and is a member of the Institute for the Medical Humanities at the University of Texas Medical Branch, Galveston, Texas. He is also Distinguished Visiting Professor of Law at the University of Houston Health Law and Policy Institute. Philosophic, legal, and psychoanalytic ideas are applied in his work to the study of human values in science, medicine, technology, and law. His book *Confronting Traumatic Brain Injury: Devastation, Hope and Healing* was published in 1998. He has co-authored three other books: *Clinical Ethics: A Practical Approach to Ethical Decisions in Clinical Medicine, Sixth Edition* (2006), written for health professionals; *The Insanity Plea: The Uses and Abuses of The Insanity Defense* (1983), written for a general audience; and *Choosing Life and Death* (1986), written for patients and their families as well as health professionals about medical–moral–legal–technological topics such as kidney dialysis, organ transplantation, treatment or non-treatment of damaged newborns, termination of life support, genetic screening and counseling, and healthcare costs and policies. In addition, he has written numerous scholarly articles and essays for general readers on topics such as privacy and confidentiality, human rights, death and dying, and legal and ethical aspects of mental-health practice. He is currently working on a book with Stacey Tovino, J.D., Ph.D., tentatively titled *The Birth Life and Death of the Brain: Legal and Ethical Perspectives*.

Acknowledgments

Art wants to acknowledge the support of the New York University Langone Medical Center and its Dean, Robert Grossman, in giving him the opportunity to complete this book. Rob acknowledges the support of Jeff Dean at Wiley-Blackwell, who believed in the project in the first place.

General Introduction

Who Is This Book for?

This book features chapters written by contemporary scholars doing work in the central topics of the branch of applied ethics known as *bioethics*. The chapters are presented in a debate style with *yes* and *no* responses—often qualified—to core contemporary quandaries in the field. The book is intended to provoke discussion and debate for students in ethics, bioethics, and medical ethics classrooms in high school, college, and professional school.

What Is Bioethics?

The English word "bioethics" comes from two Greek words: *bios* (βίος) meaning "life" and *ethikos* (ἠθικός) meaning "displaying moral character." In 1927, Fritz Jahr used the term in an article, "Bio-Ethik: Eine Umschau über die ethischen Beziehungen des Menschen zu Tier und Pflanze," which can be translated as "Bio-Ethics: A Review of the Ethical Relationships of Humans to Animals and Plants" (Jahr, 1927; Sass, 2007; Goldim, 2009). In that article, Jahr wanted to extend a "bioethical imperative" to all forms of life, arguing that we ought to treat other humans and living things with respect as ends in and of themselves (Kant, 1785/1998). In 1971, Van Rensselaer Potter also used the term in his book, *Bioethics: Bridge to the Future* (Potter, 1971). He subsequently wrote *Global Bioethics: Building on the Leopold Legacy*, and in 1995 co-authored the article, "Global Bioethics: Converting Sustainable Development to Global Survival" (Potter, 1971, 1988; Potter & Potter, 1995). For both Jahr and Potter, what they referred to as "bioethics" would be considered today to be the related branch of applied ethics known as *environmental ethics*. This area of ethics explores our relationship to the natural world, our duties to preserve and protect nature, and whether morality extends beyond humans to animals, other living things, and the entire biosphere itself (Attfield, 2003; Keller, 2010).

Bioethics, while keenly aware of the ways in which health is shaped by climate and the environment, is focused today mainly on humans and the issues that emerge in conducting biomedical and clinical research, healthcare, and the policies that ought to govern medicine, nursing, allied health, and the related biomedical sciences (Caplan, 1992b, 1994, 1997, 1998, 2009; Jonsen et al., 2011). So, while the name "bioethics" derives from scholars seeking to create environmental ethics, the history of bioethics is actually rooted in *medical ethics*, a branch of applied ethics concerned with the practice of medicine and healthcare (Ramsey, 1970; Katz, 1984; Veatch, 1989, 2011; Pellegrino, 2008; Kuhse & Singer, 2009; Pence, 2010). Given the close connection between bioethics and medical ethics, some refer to the discipline as *biomedical*

Contemporary Debates in Bioethics, First Edition. Edited by Arthur L. Caplan and Robert Arp.

ethics (Beauchamp & Childress, 1979/2009; also Glannon, 2004; Mappes & DeGrazia, 2005).

The Canon of Bioethics

Bioethics has a subject matter and specific questions that it has developed near the end of the twentieth century, and the topics that comprise this subject matter include:

- abortion;
- contraception;
- cloning;
- genetic engineering and enhancement;
- patenting genes and organisms;
- markets for human organs and tissues;
- physician-assisted suicide;
- stem-cell research and therapies;
- defining death;
- in vitro fertilization and reproductive technologies;
- animal experimentation;
- clinical trials;
- patients' rights and informed consent;
- codes of ethics for healthcare professionals;
- psychosurgery and engineering the human brain;
- healthcare access and reform;
- allocation and rationing of scarce medical resources.

Most of these topics are debated by the contributors to this book. Each core topic is described further in the introductions to each section, including relevant reading material. The reader should consult various other resources in bioethics to get a sense of the scope and breadth of view on the core topics such as:

Edited books and encyclopedias:

- *Encyclopedia of Bioethics*, edited by Warren Reich (Macmillan, 1995);
- *Medical Ethics: Applying Theories and Principles to the Patient Encounter*, edited by Matt Weinberg and Arthur L. Caplan (Humanity Books, 2000);
- *Encyclopedia of Bioethics*, edited by Stephen Post (Macmillan, 2003);
- *Bioethics: An Anthology*, edited by Helga Kuhse and Peter Singer (Wiley-Blackwell, 2006);
- *The Oxford Companion to Bioethics*, edited by Bonnie Steinbock (Oxford University Press, 2007);
- *The Blackwell Guide to Medical Ethics*, edited by Leslie Francis, Anita Silvers, and Rosamond Rhodes (Blackwell, 2007);
- *The Penn Center Guide to Bioethics*, edited by Vardit Ravitsky, Autumn Fiester, and Arthur L. Caplan (Springer, 2009);
- *Case Studies in Bioethics*, edited by Robert Veatch, Amy Haddad, and Dan English (Oxford University Press, 2009);
- *The Ethics of Research Biobanking*, edited by Jan Helge Solbakk, Soren Holm, and Bjorn Hofmann (Springer, 2009);
- *Trust and Integrity in Biomedical Research: The Case of Financial Conflicts of Interest*, edited by Thomas Murray and Josephine Johnston (Johns Hopkins, 2010);
- *Progress in Bioethics: Science, Policy, and Politics*, edited by Jonathan Moreno and Sam Berger (MIT Press, 2010);
- *The Oxford Textbook of Clinical Research Ethics*, edited by Ezekiel Emanuel, Christine Grady, Robert Crouch, Reidar Lie, Franklin Miller, and David Wendler (Oxford University Press, 2011);
- *A Companion to Bioethics*, edited by Helga Kuhse and Peter Singer (Wiley-Blackwell, 2011);
- *Global Justice and Bioethics*, edited by Joseph Millum and Ezekiel Emanuel (Oxford University Press, 2012);
- Also see the books in the Basic Bioethics series, edited by Glenn McGee and Art Caplan (MIT Press, 1999 to present).

Journals:

- *Bioethics*;
- *The Hastings Center Report*;
- *Journal of Medical Ethics*;
- *Journal of Medicine and Philosophy*;
- *American Journal of Bioethics*;
- *Kennedy Institute of Ethics Journal*;
- *Theoretical Medicine and Bioethics*;
- *Cambridge Quarterly of Healthcare Ethics*;
- *Journal of Clinical Ethics*.

Bioethics centers maintain websites with useful information, including:

- Columbia University Center for Bioethics:
  - http://www.bioethicscolumbia.org/
- The Hastings Center:
  - http://www.thehastingscenter.org/

- Kennedy Institute of Ethics at Georgetown University:
    - o http://kennedyinstitute.georgetown.edu/
- The University of Pennsylvania Center for Bioethics:
    - o http://www.bioethics.upenn.edu/
- The Ethox Centre at the University of Oxford:
    - o http://www.publichealth.ox.ac.uk/ethox/
- Centre for Human Bioethics at Monash University:
    - o http://arts.monash.edu.au/bioethics/
- MacLean Center for Clinical Medical Ethics at the University of Chicago
    - o http://medicine.uchicago.edu/centers/ethics/library.html
- The Centre for Bioethics of the Clinical Research at the Institute of Montreal:
    - o http://www.ircm.qc.ca/Pages/IRCMDefault.aspx?PFLG=1036&lan=1036
- Berman Institute of Bioethics at Johns Hopkins University:
    - o http://www.bioethicsinstitute.org/
- The Brocher Foundation:
    - o http://www.brocher.ch/en/publications-1/

Motivations for Topics in Bioethics

The core topics of bioethics oftentimes emerged as a result of the moral outcry elicited by some highly publicized practice, event, or series of events in biomedicine or clinical research that actually (or potentially) harmed people, animals, or even the biosphere. In this respect, the topics in bioethics are no different than any ethical topic that has emerged in the course of human history (Cavalier et al., 1989; MacIntyre, 1998).

For example, the Nazi experimentation on humans that took place between 1939 and 1945, where people were subjected to various hazardous and horrific experiments often designed to assist in the advancement of military medicine and the physician-directed racial euthanasia campaigns of the Nazis, raised many questions about the ethics of those involved (Caplan, 1992a; Conot, 1993; Annas & Grodin, 1995; Lifton, 2000; Spitz, 2005). During and after the Nuremberg trials (1946–1949), where numerous Nazis were tried for a variety of atrocious crimes, the Nuremberg Code was devised and codified in response to the systematic abuse of human subjects in research. The Code, which was in reality the decision in one of the trials of German doctors, includes basic biomedical principles related to human experimentation (clinical research) such as absence of coercion in recruiting subjects, the necessity of informed consent, nonmaleficence toward participants in experiments, and the correct formulation of a scientific protocol (Weindling, 2004; Schmidt & Frewer, 2007; NIH, 2011a).

It would seem that anyone who lived during the middle of the twentieth century and was made aware of the Nazi human experimentation would sympathize with the Jewish slogan that refers to the atrocities of the Holocaust and murder fueled by racism and anti-Semitism: *Never Again!* However, the US and the world were shocked to hear in 1972 that, for 40 years, an experiment monitoring the effects of syphilis upon poor, rural, and illiterate African-American men—who, having been lied to by researchers, *thought* they were being treated for the disease but in fact were not—had been conducted by the US Public Health Service and Centers for Disease Control and Prevention. The Tuskegee Syphilis Experiment—so named because Tuskegee Institute was a willing participant—began as an observational study in 1932 with 600 African-American men, 399 with syphilis and 201 without the disease. In 1972, when the study became known through whistle-blowing in the media, 74 of the 600 men were still alive. Concerning the original 399 men with syphilis, 28 died of syphilis, and 100 died of syphilis-related complications, while 40 of their wives were infected with syphilis, and 19 of their children were born with syphilis (Jones, 1992; Reverby, 2009). What makes this experiment all the more insidious is the fact that, by 1945, penicillin was being mass-produced in the US to treat diseases like syphilis, and the infected men in the experiment easily could have been treated after 1945; and many lives would have been saved as well as much pain and suffering avoided (Katz & Warren, 2011).

In response to the Tuskegee Syphilis Experiment as well as increased public awareness of other unethical experiments conducted in the US and in other countries (Beecher, 1966), in 1974 the National Research Act (Pub. L. 93-348) of the US established the

National Commission for the Protection of Human Subjects of Biomedical and Behavioral Research (1974–1978), and in 1979 the Commission issued a landmark document for biomedicine or clinical research called, "The Belmont Report: Ethical Principles and Guidelines for the Protection of Human Subjects of Research." It was named "The Belmont Report" for the Smithsonian Institution's Belmont Conference Center (Elkridge, MD) where the Commission met in February of 1976 when first drafting the report (Childress et al., 2005; NIH, 2011b). The Belmont Report affirmed all of the basic bioethical principles found in the Nuremberg Code, as well as articulated other principles, including the principle of justice whereby "equals ought to be treated equally." The report called for peer review of all studies to insure that the risk/benefit ratio involved made moral sense and that the informed consent of subjects was adequate. Unfortunately, there are numerous cases of unethical human experimentation documented in the US and other countries throughout the twentieth century, and these cases form the basis for a central topic in bioethics (Moreno, 2000; Dresser, 2001; Goliszek, 2003; Guerrini, 2003; the papers in Hawkins & Emanuel, 2008).

Scandal was not the only driver of bioethics. Controversy plays a key role in the development of the field as well. Although abortion has been practiced by numerous cultures throughout human history and even can be traced to a Chinese medical text from the reign of Shen Nung (2737–2696 BCE), and although it is true that, by 1970, scholars had already been debating the abortion issue as a result of increased recognition of women's reproductive rights, improvement in abortion technology, many ER instances of bungled backroom abortions, and the American Medical Association's call to decriminalize abortion in the US (Noonan, 1970; Thomson, 1971; Warren, 1973), it was the landmark decision by the US Supreme Court to disallow many state and federal restrictions on abortion in *Roe v. Wade* (410 US 113) in 1973 that brought bioethical attention to the abortion issue (Jonsen, 1998; Joffe, 2009). And with that attention, another topic in bioethics was solidified.

Technological innovation has also driven the emergence of bioethics. Although Willem Kolff is credited with inventing the first kidney-dialysis machine (he also helped invent the artificial heart and heart–lung machine, as well as invented an artificial eye and ear, and the intra-aortic balloon pump), it was Belding Scribner who improved upon Kolff's machine and opened the first center devoted to dialysis, the Seattle Artificial Kidney Center, in 1962 (Pietzman, 2007; Brown, 2009). Since there were a limited number of machines in the center and many more patients who needed dialysis in order to live, ethical questions related to who should receive dialysis emerged immediately (Jonsen, 2000, pp. 104–106; also Katz & Capron, 1982; Emanuel, 1991; Elger et al., 2008).

Harvard medical researchers, Philip Drinker and Louis Agassiz Shaw, invented the "iron lung" in 1927 to assist or restart breathing in individuals; but even with John Emerson's improvements on the mechanism in 1931, iron lungs were big, bulky, and expensive to operate. Simple, hand-operated, bag valve mask ventilators began to be used by doctors and others in 1953; but they suffered from the obvious problem of having to be constantly squeezed by someone (Gorman, 1979; Laurie, 2002; Ambu, 2011). In 1971, Siemens introduced the medical world to a small, fairly quiet electronic ventilator—the SERVO 900—and various models soon became a staple in ERs, then in ambulances, too (Maquet Critical Care, 2001, 2005). The electronic ventilator now could be used to assist someone in their breathing, potentially indefinitely, and this occurred regularly for people in comas. The extended use of a ventilator (usually in combination with a feeding tube) has been the source of much debate, and cases of people in persistent vegetative states requiring ventilators and feeding tubes—such as the widely publicized cases of Karen Ann Quinlan, who lived with a feeding tube in a persistent vegetative state from 1975 to 1985, and Terri Schiavo, who lived with a feeding tube in a persistent vegetative state from 1990 to 2005—cause people to think about the extent to which these biomedical technologies are ethically appropriate or not (Armstrong & Colen, 1988; Buchanan & Brock, 1990; Caplan et al., 2006).

By the end of the twentieth century, women were giving birth to so-called "designer babies," which is a negative term really, but refers to babies who have been born after having their embryos screened for genetic diseases through methods of pre-implantation genetic diagnosis (PGD). PGD requires in vitro fertilization (IVF) techniques to obtain the embryos for the screening, and IVF itself is its own bioethical topic surrounded by arguments and controversy (Cook-Deegan, 1996; Buchanan et al., 2000; Skloot, 2010). In 1990, Debbie Edwards gave birth to twin girls in Hammersmith Hospital in London after having been implanted with female embryos that had been screened by Drs Alan Handyside and Norman Winston utilizing methods of PGD. Given Edwards' medical history, there would have been a 50% chance that a baby boy would have developed brain damage and die young, so she turned to Handyside, Winston, and PGD to ensure that she would give birth to a baby girl (Maugh, 1990; Handyside et al., 1992). One can imagine screening embryos so as to "design" the kind of child we want—affecting intelligence, height, eye color, looks, etc.—so it is easy to see how the moniker has been applied (see the papers in Savelescu & Bostrom, 2009; Harris, 2007).

PGD has also been used to screen embryos when a mother wants to give birth to a child who can act as a "savior sibling" by providing a cell transplant to a sibling who suffers from a disease like anemia or leukemia. In 2000, a young girl named Molly Nash received stem cells from the umbilical cord of her newborn brother (whose tissue type had been screened as an embryo), and the stem cells were successful in treating Nash's Fanconi anemia (Wolf et al., 2003; Marcotty, 2010).

Still more fascinating, at the American Society for Reproductive Medicine's 2007 annual meeting, it was announced that researchers used a virus to add a gene, a green fluorescent protein, to an embryo left over from assisted reproduction (Zaninovic et al., 2007; CellNEWS, 2008). Many take this to be the first documented case of genetic modification of a human embryo. The kind of genetic engineering of the traits in these examples fits squarely as a key topic in the realm of bioethics, as a question like, "Are doctors and scientists justified in playing god or altering the course of nature with respect to living things, especially human beings?" becomes front and center (see the papers in Magnus et al., 2002).

Dr Jack Kevorkian died on June 3, 2011 at the age of 83. His actions caused the controversial topic of physician-assisted suicide to be part and parcel of contemporary bioethics. He was a medical doctor with a specialty in pathology who claimed to have assisted over 130 people with their own suicides. He invented and used the Thanatron (named after the Greek god that personifies death, *Thanatos*), a device that allowed one to push a button that released deadly potassium chloride into one's body intravenously, and the Mercitron, a device that employed a gas mask that could be filled with carbon monoxide to let people kill themselves (Kevorkian, 1988; Roscoe et al., 2000; Dowbiggin, 2003; Nicol & Wylie, 2005; Schoifet, 2011).

The Hippocratic Oath is something that every medical school student knows about. The oath specifically asks the new doctor to promise ἐπὶ δηλήσει δὲ καὶ ἀδικίῃ εἴρξειν, "to refrain from doing harm" (AMA, 2001, 2004; Magner, 2005). So, when Kevorkian assisted in the suicide of Janet Adkins in 1990 with the Thanatron—his first assisted suicide—many utilized the ethical obligation to "refrain from doing harm" to condemn his actions (Kass, 1989; Hartmann and & Meyerson, 1998; Somerville, 2001).

Morally, it is one thing to assist in a suicide by providing the person who wishes to do so with instruction and a device that they may activate on their own. It is ethically different if someone administers a lethal injection seeking to kill a person. Kevorkian killed a severely disabled man, Thomas Youk, on September 17, 1998, and taped his behavior for later broadcast on national television. His involvement in homicide resulted in a second-degree murder conviction and over 8 years of prison time (Johnson, 1999). Still, many argue that Kevorkian's lethal injection was a sympathetic action, along the lines of the Scottish doctor, John Gregory's, claim—made in the beginning of the nineteenth century—that a doctor, like any other human being, needs to have a "sensibility of heart which makes us feel for the distresses of our fellow creatures, and which, of consequence, incites in us the most powerful manner to relieve them" (Gregory, 1817, p. 22).

The 1972 play and 1981 movie by the same name, *Whose Life is It Anyway?*, is a fictional story about a man who becomes paralyzed from the neck down after a car accident and wants to end his own life, and he offers several arguments in favor of his position, including the "I have a right to do with my body what I want to" argument (also see Berg et al., 2001; Annas,

2004, 2011). This popular story was solidly planted in the American psyche when Dr Kevorkian assisted in Adkins' suicide in 1990 and, not only did fiction become reality, but a bioethical "hot-button" topic became fodder for discussion, dialogue, and debate.

In this introduction, we could speak about the motivations for all of the topics in bioethics, but because of space limitations, we are unable to do so. Bioethics has a varied and complex history that would take several lifetimes to ingest completely, but a great place to start is with Albert Jonsen's *The Birth of Bioethics* (Jonsen, 1998) and Vincent Barry's *Bioethics in a Cultural Context: Philosophy, Religion, History, Politics* (Barry, 2012).

The Classification of Bioethics

Concerning its classification within the general discipline of Western philosophy, bioethics is usually envisioned as a branch of applied or practical ethics, along with environmental ethics, business ethics, legal ethics, engineering ethics, and cyberethics (there are others). Applied ethics, metaethics, and normative ethics are branches of ethics or moral philosophy, and ethics, political philosophy, metaphysics, epistemology, and logic are understood to be the classical branches of Western philosophy (Copleston, 1994; Jones, 1997; Solomon, 2005). *Metaethics* deals with issues such as the nature of moral knowledge, the proper grounds for justifying moral claims, the metaphysical/ontological status of moral norms and entities, and cultural and ethical relativism (Bok, 2002; Jacobs, 2002; Miller, 2003; for a discussion of relativism in relation to bioethics, see Macklin, 1999). *Normative ethics* deals primarily with the development, investigation, and critique of various ethical/moral theories such as religious-based deontology, ethical egoism, Kantian deontology, utilitarianism, natural rights theory, and virtue ethics (Kagan, 1997; Fieser, 1999; Pojman, 2005; Kamm, 2006; for application of normative ethical theories specifically to bioethics, see Pellegrino & Thomasma, 1981; Powers & Faden, 2006; Veatch, 2011). As the name suggests, *applied ethics* is primarily concerned with the application of ethical/moral theory to practice insofar as the actions and interactions of humans (as well as the interactions of humans with animals and the biosphere) in the realms of professions, institutions, and public policy generate ethical problems and dilemmas that are in need of solutions and resolutions (McGee, 1999; Cohen & Wellman, 2005; LaFollette, 2006).

Figure 0.1 represents a partial taxonomic classification of bioethics, and we are aware that there are many other philosophical disciplines and sub-disciplines not shown, as well as that it is possible to classify the discipline of Western philosophy by historical time periods or major movements. Also, note that the figure attempts to represent the idea that bioethics could also be called biomedical ethics, and that medical ethics could be considered a species of bio(medical)ethics.

A Philosophical Discipline

Although doctors, nurses, clinicians, lawyers, biologists, theologians, and other researchers make valuable contributions to it, bioethics is first and foremost a philosophical discipline concerned with "issues that emerge in conducting biomedical and clinical research, healthcare, and the policies that ought to govern medicine, nursing, allied health, and the related biomedical sciences," as we noted in the definition of bioethics above. And we also saw that bioethics is a branch of applied ethics, which is a branch of ethics, itself a branch of Western philosophy; thus, if the classification is correct, the basic features, properties, and characteristics of Western philosophy should be present in bioethics. This means that the principles of correct reasoning and logic trumpeted and championed by the philosopher—including the formation of sound or cogent arguments, complete with objective evidence that any rational person could assent to—*should* not only act as the primary tool utilized in discussing the topics in bioethics, but also provide thinkers with a level playing field, so to speak, where ideas and arguments can be respectfully explained, analyzed, debated, evaluated, and critiqued. Anyone, regardless of ideology, world view, or perspective, is welcome to play on the field, provided they play by the rules of correct reasoning and logic. Beauchamp and Childress (1979/2009) affirm this philosophical approach in the first chapter of their famous work in bioethics, *Principles of Biomedical Ethics*, as does H. Tristram Engelhardt (1986/1996) in the first two chapters of his book, *The*

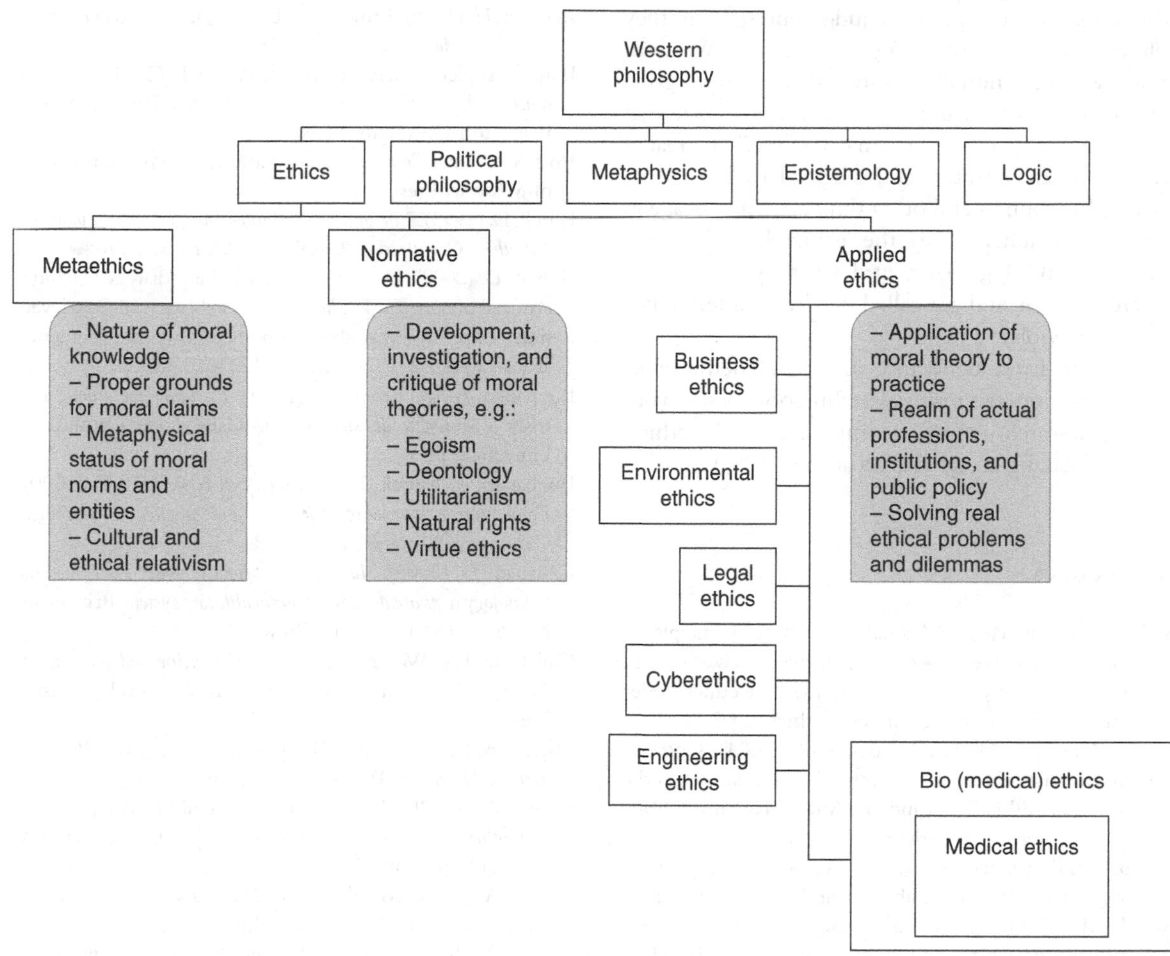

Figure 0.1 Bioethics classified

Foundations of Bioethics. Of course, as Dan Brock (1993, pp. 414–416) notes in the final pages of his book, *Life and Death: Philosophical Essays in Biomedical Ethics*, philosophers have a bad reputation as being "unrealistic, head in the clouds, ivory tower academics;" however, as Brock also notes, philosophers have made important contributions to bioethics and the public policies generated from this important discipline.

Dealing with Hot-Button Issues

The topics discussed in bioethics are some of the most emotionally charged of all of the disciplines in applied ethics—abortion, suicide, stem-cell research, the allocation of scarce vital organs, and socialized medicine, for example, are "hot-button" issues for most Americans (see Steinbock, 1996; Caplan & Coelho, 1998; Meisel & Cerminara, 2004; Angell, 2005; Callahan & Wasunna, 2006; George & Tollefsen, 2008; Callahan, 2009). While it is important to be sensitive to these emotions, the bottom line is that reason motivated by a sincere desire to find common moral ground ought to drive bioethical reflection and discussion. One of the authors in this book, Jeffrey Reiman, puts the point a little differently in his chapter defending abortion: "People's moral beliefs may be influenced by emotions, affections, and fears, which may distort people's judgment so that they believe what is not rationally grounded … We want an answer (to a moral question) that we have good reason to believe is true; and we must recognize that what people actually believe may be false." The reader will see that the chapters of this book have been written by philosophers and other thinkers who engage in the debates adhering to the principles of correct reasoning and logic—or, at least they attempt to adhere to them, and are called out by an interlocutor when they violate a principle.

We hope that students and scholars of bioethics alike will benefit from the material in this book. Best in your reading, research, reflection, thinking, and bioethical decision-making.—Art Caplan and Robert Arp

References

AMA (American Medical Association). (2001). Principles of medical ethics. Retrieved from: http://www.ama-assn.org/ama/pub/physician-resources/medical-ethics/code-medical-ethics/principles-medical-ethics.page?

AMA (American Medical Association). (2004). Code of medical ethics: Current opinions with annotations of the Council on Ethical and Judicial Affairs. Retrieved from: http://www.ama-assn.org/go/ceja

Ambu. (2011). Ambu's history. Retrieved from: http://www.ambu.co.uk/uk/about_ambu_ltd/ambu´s_history.aspx

Angell, M. (2005). *The truth about drug companies: How they deceive us and what to do about it.* New York: Random House.

Annas, G. (2004). *The rights of patients: The authoritative ACLU guide to the rights of patients.* Carbondale, IL: Southern Illinois University Press.

Annas, G. (2011). *Worst case bioethics: Death, disaster, and public health.* Oxford: Oxford University Press.

Annas, G., & Grodin, M. (Eds.). (1995). *The Nazi doctors and the Nuremberg code: Human rights in human experimentation.* Oxford: Oxford University Press.

Armstrong, P., & Colen, B. (1988). From Quinlan to Jobes: The courts and the PVS patient. *The Hastings Center Report, 18*(1), 37–40.

Attfield, R. (2003). *Environmental ethics: An overview for the twenty-first century.* Cambridge: Polity Press.

Barry, V. (2012). *Bioethics in a cultural context: Philosophy, religion, history, politics.* Belmont, CA: Wadsworth.

Beauchamp, T., & Childress, J. (1979/2009). *Principles of biomedical ethics.* Oxford: Oxford University Press.

Beecher, H. (1966). Ethics and clinical research. *New England Journal of Medicine, 274,* 1354–1360.

Berg, J., Applebaum, P., Lidz, C., & Parker, L. (2001). *Informed consent: Legal theory and clinical practice.* Princeton, NJ: Princeton University Press.

Bok, S. (2002). *Common values.* Columbia, MO: University of Missouri Press.

Brock, D. (1993). *Life and death: Philosophical essays in biomedical ethics.* Cambridge: Cambridge University Press.

Brown, D. (2009). Doctor invented kidney dialysis machine, artificial organs. *The Washington Post.* February 13. Retrieved from: http://www.washingtonpost.com/wp-dyn/content/article/2009/02/12/AR2009021203610.html

Buchanan, A., & Brock, D. (1990). *Deciding for others: The ethics of surrogate decision making.* Cambridge: Cambridge University Press.

Buchanan, A., Brock, D., Daniels, N., & Wikler, D. (2000). *From chance to choice: Genetics and justice.* Cambridge: Cambridge University Press.

Callahan, D. (2009). *Taming the beloved beast: How medical technology costs are destroying our health care system.* Princeton, NJ: Princeton University Press.

Callahan, D., & Wasunna, A. (2006). *Medicine and the market: Equity v. choice.* Baltimore, MD: Johns Hopkins University Press.

Caplan, A. (Ed.). (1992a). *When medicine went mad: Bioethics and the Holocaust.* Totowa, NJ: Humana Press.

Caplan, A. (1992b). *If I were a rich man could I buy a pancreas? and other essays on the ethics of health care.* Indianapolis: Indiana University Press.

Caplan, A. (1994). *Moral matters: Ethical issues in medicine and the life sciences.* Hoboken, NJ: John Wiley & Sons.

Caplan, A. (1997). *Due consideration: Controversy in the age of medical miracles.* Hoboken, NJ: John Wiley & Sons.

Caplan, A. (1998). *Am I my brother's keeper? The ethical frontiers of biomedicine.* Indianapolis: Indiana University Press.

Caplan, A. (2009). *Smart mice, not-so-smart people: An interesting and amusing guide to bioethics.* New York: Rowman & Littlefield.

Caplan, A., & Coelho, D. (Eds.). (1998). *The ethics of organ transplants: The current debate.* Amherst, NY: Prometheus Books.

Caplan, A., McCartney, J., & Sisti, D. (Eds.). (2006). *The case of Terri Schiavo: Ethics at the end of life.* Amherst, NY: Prometheus Books.

Cavalier, R., Gouinlock, J., & Sterba, J. (Eds.). (1989). *Ethics in the history of Western philosophy.* New York: Palgrave Macmillan.

CellNEWS (2008). Genetically modified human embryo stirs controversy. *CellNEWS.* May 27. Retrieved from: http://cellnews-blog.blogspot.com/2008/05/genetically-modified-human-embryo-stirs.html

Childress, J., Meslin, E., & Shapiro, H. (Eds.). (2005). *Belmont revisited: Ethical principles for research with human subjects*. Washington, DC: Georgetown University Press.

Cohen, A., & Wellman, C. (Eds.). (2005). *Contemporary debates in practical ethics*. Malden, MA: Wiley-Blackwell.

Conot, R. (1993). *Justice at Nuremberg*. New York: Basic Books.

Cook-Deegan, R. (1996). *The gene wars: Science, politics, and the human genome*. New York: W. W. Norton.

Copleston, F. (1994). *A history of Western philosophy: Volumes I–IX*. New York: Image Books.

Dowbiggin, I. (2003). *A merciful end: The euthanasia movement in modern America*. Oxford: Oxford University Press.

Dresser, R. (2001). *When science offers salvation: Patient advocacy and research ethics*. Oxford: Oxford University Press.

Elger, B., Biller-Andorno, N., & Capron, A. (Ed.). (2008). *Ethical issues in governing biobanks*. New York: Ashgate.

Emanuel, E. (1991). *The ends of human life: Medical ethics in a liberal polity*. Cambridge, MA: Harvard University Press.

Emanuel, E., Grady, C., Crouch, R., Lie, R., Miller, F., & Wendler, D. (Eds.). (2011). *The Oxford textbook of clinical research ethics*. Oxford: Oxford University Press.

Engelhardt, H. T. (1986/1996). *The foundations of bioethics*. Oxford: Oxford University Press.

Fieser, J. (Ed.). (1999). *Metaethics, normative ethics, and applied ethics: Contemporary and historical readings*. Belmont, CA: Wadsworth.

George, R., & Tollefsen, C. (2008). *Embryo: A defense of human life*. New York: Doubleday Books.

Glannon, W. (2004). *Biomedical ethics*. Oxford: Oxford University Press.

Goldim, J. (2009). Revisiting the beginning of bioethics: The contribution of Fritz Jahr (1927). *Perspectives in Biology and Medicine, 52*(3), 377–380.

Goliszek, A. (2003). *In the name of science: A history of secret programs, medical research, and human experimentation*. New York: St. Martin's Press.

Gorman, J. (1979). A medical triumph: The iron lung. *Respiratory Therapy, 9*(1), 71–73.

Gregory, J. (1817). *Lectures on the duties and qualifications of a physician*. Philadelphia: M. Carey & Son.

Guerrini, A. (2003). *Experimenting with humans and animals: From Galen to animal rights*. Baltimore, MD: The Johns Hopkins University Press.

Handyside, A., Lesko, J., Tarín, J., Winston, R., & Hughes, M. (1992). Birth of a normal girl after in vitro fertilization and preimplantation diagnostic testing for cystic fibrosis. *New England Journal of Medicine, 327*(13), 905–909.

Harris, J. (2007). *Enhancing evolution: The ethical case for making better people*. Princeton, NJ: Princeton University Press.

Hartmann, L., & Meyerson, A. (1998). A debate on physician-assisted suicide. *Psychiatric Services, 49*, 1468–1474.

Hawkins J., & Emanuel, E. (Eds.). (2008). *Exploitation and developing countries: The ethics of clinical research*. Princeton, NJ: Princeton University Press.

Jacobs, J. (2002). *Dimensions of moral theory: An introduction to metaethics and moral psychology*. Malden, MA: Wiley-Blackwell.

Jahr, F. (1927). Bio-Ethik: Eine Umschau über die ethischen Beziehungen des Menschen zu Tier und Pflanze. *Kosmos: Handweiser für Naturfreunde, 24*(1), 2–4.

Joffe, C. (2009). Abortion and medicine: A sociopolitical history. In M. Paul, E. Lichtenberg, L. Borgatta, D. Grimes, P. Stubblefield, & M. Creinin (Eds.), *Management of unintended and abnormal pregnancy* (pp. 1–9). Malden, MA: Wiley-Blackwell.

Johnson, D. (1999). Kevorkian sentenced to 10 to 25 years in prison. *The New York Times*. April 14. Retrieved from: http://www.nytimes.com/1999/04/14/us/kevorkian-sentenced-to-10-to-25-years-in-prison.html?ref=thomasyouk

Jones, J. (1992). *Bad blood: The Tuskegee syphilis experiment*. New York: The Free Press.

Jones, W. (1997). *A history of Western philosophy: Volumes I–V*. Belmont, CA: Wadsworth Publishing.

Jonsen, A. (1998). *The birth of bioethics*. Oxford: Oxford University Press.

Jonsen, A. (2000). *A short history of medical ethics*. Oxford: Oxford University Press.

Jonsen, A., Siegler, M., & Winslade, W. (2011). *Clinical ethics: A practical approach to ethical decisions in clinical medicine*. New York: McGraw-Hill.

Kagan, S. (1997). *Normative ethics*. Boulder, CO: Westview Press.

Kamm, F. M. (2006). *Intricate ethics: Rights, responsibilities, and permissable harm*. Oxford: Oxford University Press.

Kant, I. (1785/1998). *Groundwork of the metaphysics of morals*. (M. Gregor, Trans.). (Section I: Transition from common rational to philosophic moral cognition). Cambridge: Cambridge University Press.

Kass, L. (1989). Neither for love nor money: Why doctors must not kill. *National Affairs, 94*, 25–46.

Katz, J. (1984). *The silent world of doctor and patient*. New York: The Free Press.

Katz, J., & Capron, A. (1982). *Catastrophic diseases: Who decides what?* Camden, NJ: Transactions.

Katz, R., & Warren, R. (Eds.). (2011). *The search for the legacy of the USPHS syphilis study at Tuskegee*. Lanham, MD: Lexington Books.

Keller, D. (Ed.). (2010). *Environmental ethics: The big questions*. Malden, MA: Wiley-Blackwell.

Kevorkian, J. (1988). The last fearsome taboo: Medical aspects of planned death. *Medicine and Law*, 7(1), 1–14.

Kuhse, H., & Singer, P. (2009). What is bioethics? A historical introduction. In H. Kuhse & P. Singer (Eds.), *A companion to bioethics* (pp. 3–11). Malden, MA: Wiley-Blackwell.

LaFollette, H. (Ed.). (2006). *Ethics in practice: An anthology.* Malden, MA: Wiley-Blackwell.

Laurie, G. (2002). Ventilator users, home care, and independent living: A historical perspective. In I. Gilgoff, (Ed.), *Breath of life: The role of the ventilator in managing life-threatening illnesses* (pp. 161–201). Lanham, MD: Scarecrow Press.

Lifton, R. (2000). *The Nazi doctors: Medical killing and the psychology of genocide.* New York: Basic Books.

MacIntyre, A. (1998). *A short history of ethics: A history of moral philosophy from the Homeric Age to the Twentieth Century.* London: Routledge.

Macklin, R. (1999). *Against relativism: Cultural diversity and the search for ethical universals in medicine.* Oxford: Oxford University Press.

Magner, L. (2005). *A history of medicine.* Boca Raton, FL: Taylor & Francis.

Magnus, D., Caplan, A., & McGee, G. (Eds.). (2002). *Who owns life?* Amherst, NY: Prometheus Books.

Mappes, T., & DeGrazia, D. (2005). *Biomedical ethics.* New York: McGraw-Hill.

Maugh, T. (1990). Genetic defect screened out; healthy twins born. *Los Angeles Times.* July 31. Retrieved from: http://articles.latimes.com/1990-07-31/news/mn-1192_1_genetic-defect/2

Marcotty, J. (2010). "Savior sibling" raises a decade of life-and-death questions. *Star Tribune.* September 22. Retrieved from: http://www.geneticsandsociety.org/article.php?id= 5388

Maquet Critical Care. (2001). The SERVO story—thirty years of technological innovation evolving with clinical development of ventilator treatment. Retrieved from: http://www.maquet.com/content/Documents/Site_Specific/MAQUETcom/GENERAL_The_Servo_Story.pdf

Maquet Critical Care. (2005). Ventilation interhospital ambulance transport in region Skane, Sweden. Retrieved from: http://www.maquet.com/content/Documents/Application Reports/SERVOI_APPREP_050701_EN_ALL.pdf

McGee, G. (Ed.). (1999). *Pragmatic bioethics.* Cambridge, MA: MIT Press.

Meisel, A., & Cerminara, K. (2004). *The right to die: The law of end-of-life decisionmaking.* New York: Aspen.

Miller, A. (2003). *An introduction to contemporary metaethics.* Cambridge: Polity Press.

Moreno, J. (2000). *Undue risk: Secret state experiments on humans.* London: Routledge.

Nicol, N., & Wylie, H. (2005). *Between the dying and the dead: Dr. Jack Kevorkian's life and the battle to legalize euthanasia.* Madison, WI: University of Wisconsin Press.

NIH (National Institutes of Health). (2011a). *Trials of war criminals before the Nuremberg military tribunals under control council law no. 10, vol. 2,* pp. 181–182. Washington, DC: US Government Printing Office, 1949. Retrieved from: http://ohsr.od.nih.gov/guidelines/nuremberg.html

NIH (National Institutes of Health). (2011b). The Belmont report: Ethical principles and guidelines for the protection of human subjects of research, April 18, 1979. Retrieved from: http://ohsr.od.nih.gov/guidelines/belmont.html

Noonan, J. (1970). An almost absolute value in history. In J. Noonan (Ed.), *The morality of abortion: Legal and historical perspectives* (pp. 51–59). Cambridge, MA: Harvard University Press.

Pellegrino, E. (2008). *The philosophy of medicine reborn.* Notre Dame, IN: University of Notre Dame Press.

Pellegrino, E., & Thomasma, D. (1981). *A philosophical basis of medical practice: Toward a philosophy and ethic of the healing professions.* Oxford: Oxford University Press.

Pence, G. (2010). *Medical ethics: Accounts of ground-breaking cases.* New York: McGraw-Hill.

Pietzman, S. (2007). *Dropsy, dialysis, transplant: A short history of failing kidneys.* Baltimore, MD: The Johns Hopkins University Press.

Pojman, L. (2005). *Ethics: Discovering right and wrong.* Belmont, CA: Wadsworth.

Potter, V. R. (1971). *Bioethics: Bridge to the future.* Englewood Cliffs, NJ: Prentice-Hall.

Potter, V. R. (1988). *Global bioethics: Building on the Leopold legacy.* East Lansing, MI: Michigan State University Press.

Potter, V. R., & Potter, L. (1995). Global bioethics: converting sustainable development to global survival. *Medicine and Global Survival, 2,* 185–190.

Powers, M., & Faden, R. (2006). *Social justice: The moral foundations of public health and health policy.* Oxford: Oxford University Press.

Ramsey, P. (1970). *The patient as person. Explorations in medical ethics.* New Haven, CT: Yale University Press.

Reverby, S. (2009). *Examining Tuskegee: The infamous syphilis study and its legacy.* Chapel Hill: The University of North Carolina Press.

Roscoe, L., Dragovic, L, & Cohen, D. (2000). Dr. Jack Kevorkian and cases of euthanasia in Oakland County, Michigan, 1990–1998. *The New England Journal of Medicine, 343,* 1735–1736.

Sass, H-M. (2007). Fritz Jahr's 1927 concept of bioethics. *Kennedy Institute of Ethics Journal,* 17(4), 279–295.

Savelescu, J., & Bostrom, N. (Eds.). (2009). *Human enhancement.* Oxford: Oxford University Press.

Schoifet, M. (2011). *Bloomberg.* June 3. Retrieved from: http://www.bloomberg.com/news/2011-06-03/jack-kevorkian-assisted-suicide-advocate-dies-at-83.html

Schmidt, U., & Frewer, A. (Eds.). (2007). *History and theory of human experimentation: The Declaration of Helsinki and modern medical ethics.* New York: Franz Steiner.

Skloot, R. (2010). *The immortal life of Henrietta Lacks.* New York: The Crown Publishing Group.

Solomon, R. (2005). *The big questions: A short introduction to philosophy.* Belmont, CA: Wadsworth.

Somerville, M. (2001). *Death talk: The case against euthanasia and physician-assisted suicide.* Montreal: McGill-Queen's University Press.

Spitz, V. (2005). *Doctors from hell: The horrific account of Nazi experiments on humans.* Boulder, CO: Sentient Publications.

Steinbock, B. (1996). *Life before birth: The moral and legal status of embryos and fetuses.* Oxford: Oxford University Press.

Thomson, J. J. (1971). A defense of abortion. *Philosophy and Public Affairs, 1,* 47–66.

Veatch, R. (1989). *Medical ethics.* London: Jones & Bartlett.

Veatch, R. (2011). *The basics of bioethics.* Upper Saddle River, NJ: Prentice-Hall.

Warren, M. A. (1973). On the moral and legal status of abortion. *The Monist, 57,* 43–61.

Weindling, P. (2004). *Nazi medicine and the Nuremberg trials: from medical war crimes to informed consent.* New York: Palgrave Macmillan.

Wolf, S., Kahn, J., & Wagner, J. (2003). Using preimplantation genetic diagnosis to create a stem cell donor: Issues, guidelines & limits. *The Journal of Law, Medicine & Ethics, 17*(4), 279–295.

Zaninovic, N., Hao, J., Pareja, J., James, D., Rafii, S., & Rosenwaks, Z. (2007). Genetic modification of preimplantation embryos and embryonic stem cells (ESC) by recombinant lentiviral vectors: Efficient and stable method for creating transgenic embryos and ESC. *ASRM 2007 Annual Meeting,* Poster session.

Part 1

Are There Universal Ethical Principles That Should Govern the Conduct of Medicine and Research Worldwide?

Introduction

If the question that forms the basis for the debate in this section were "Are there universal ethical principles that *do in fact* (rather than *should*) govern the conduct of medicine and research worldwide?" the answer would prima facie be *no*, and the matter likely settled by appealing to data and facts contrasting the current ethical justifications for the medical practices of one group, culture, or nation with another (or several groups, culture, or nations). For example, female genital mutilation (FGM)—defined by the World Health Organization (WHO) as "all procedures that involve partial or total removal of the external female genitalia, or other injury to the female genital organs for nonmedical reasons"—is not practiced in the mainstream medical communities of the US and many other countries based primarily on ethical reasons pertaining to principles of autonomy, beneficence, and nonmaleficence. By contrast, the WHO estimates that, as of February 2010, between 100 and 140 million girls and women worldwide have had some form of FGM, and in many of the countries where FGM is practiced there are oftentimes *religious*, ethical reasons given as justification for the procedure (Boyle, 2002; Skaine, 2005; WHO, 2010). So, by virtue of the fact that FGM *is* practiced in certain societies around the world, it is apparent that principles of autonomy, beneficence, and nonmaleficence are not governing the conduct of medicine and research worldwide; conversely, by virtue of the fact that FGM *is not* practiced in societies such as the US, it is also apparent that certain religiously based ethical principles also are not governing the conduct of medicine and research worldwide. And there are many other conflicting or

Contemporary Debates in Bioethics, First Edition. Edited by Arthur L. Caplan and Robert Arp.

contradictory medical and biomedical practices worldwide that can be pointed to as examples of the fact that there seem not to be *universal* ethical principles governing these practices (Young, 2006; Unschuld, 2009; Caplan, 2010).

A cultural anthropologist, sociologist, psychologist, or any other researcher can look at medical and biomedical practices worldwide and note *descriptively* that *it is the case* that there are not universal ethical principles governing these practices. Although, we must be cautious here since many thinkers who have argued for one version or another of *soft universalism* have attempted to show that there are in fact a handful of universal ethical principles in existence, but that these principles make themselves manifest in culturally grounded ways, giving the mere appearance of being relative (Foot, 1979/2002; Nussbaum, 1993; Walzer, 1994; Bok, 2002; Miller, 2002). In any event, the bioethician (and any other thinker, for that matter), as philosopher, can look at medical and biomedical practices worldwide and question whether *prescriptively* there *should be* universal ethical principles governing these practices. Consider FGM again. The number of good arguments against FGM that appeal to (ostensibly) universalizable principles of autonomy, beneficence, and nonmaleficence would seem to suggest that practitioners of FGM either are unaware of these principles, knowingly disregarding them, or may be pressured into disregarding them due to cultural or religious factors (Nussbaum, 1999; Cohen, Howard, and Nussbaum, 1999; Gruenbaum, 2001). In other words, it can be argued that these ethical principles (and laws emerging from them) should be guiding medical practice worldwide such that FGM stops occurring altogether, no matter what the culture or social situation.

Immanuel Kant's (1724–1804) deontological moral theory, with its emphasis upon autonomy, respect for persons, and blind justice, as well as John Stuart Mill's (1806–1873) utilitarian moral theory, with its emphasis upon bringing about the most nonharmful (and hence, pleasurable) and beneficial consequences to a person (or sentient being) affected by an action, have acted as the basis for practical moral decision-making since the theories were formulated in the eighteenth and nineteenth centuries (Kant, 1785/1998; Mill, 1861/2001; Korsgaard, 1996; Baron, 1999; Hooker, 2000). And many of the standard philosophical arguments against FGM appeal to Kant and/or Mill, in one form or another (Nussbaum, 1999; Cohen et al., 1999; Wallis, 2005; Bikoo, 2007; Burkhardt and Nathaniel, 2008; cf. Lander, 1999). The principles emerging from these theories were affirmed in the Nuremberg Code (1946–1949), The Belmont Report (1979), and Tom Beauchamp and James Childress' famous work, *Principles of Biomedical Ethics* (NIH, 2011a, 2011b; Beauchamp and Childress, 1979/2009), which has become a standard reference work for medical and other bioethical decisions. Given the wide rational appeal and application of these principles to multiple practical issues—bioethical or otherwise—along with their success in application in terms of conflict resolution and just policy making in numerous countries, it can be argued that they are the types of universal ethical principles that *should* govern the conduct of medicine and research worldwide.

In fact, in the first chapter of this section Daryl Pullman affirms what he calls the *principle of respect for human dignity*, which he argues is present most clearly in Kant's moral philosophy and acts as the foundation for any moral decision. Thus, it is Pullman's contention that not only is a respect for human dignity *actually at* work universally in moral decision-making (descriptively), but also that it *should be at* work universally in moral decision-making (prescriptively) (also see Walzer, 1994; Macklin, 1999; Bok, 2002). "Our concept of morality is predicated on the assumption of the intrinsic moral worth or dignity of humanity," Pullman notes, and the "essence of morality is to guard, protect, and advance this fundamental value." To bolster his position, Pullman appeals to a well-known strategy that has been used against proponents of ethical relativism who think that it is not possible for one group, society, or culture to criticize morally the actions of another group, society, or culture (see Harman, 1975/2000, 1984/2000, 1996), namely, without *at least* the principle of respect for human dignity, there is "no way to measure moral progress or regress, and no basis for judging the actions of other nations, social groups, or even individuals as either morally praiseworthy or blameworthy."

"It might seem surprising to demand of ethical principles that they be universal, given that most moral decision-making will concern those fairly close to us: ourselves, our extended family, plus a relatively small community of friends, work associates, and acquaintances." So claims Kevin Decker in the second chapter of this section. While Decker maintains that he is no ethical relativist, as a pragmatist who thinks that moral judgments and actions are intimately connected and circumstantially grounded, he does subscribe to David Wong's (1993) view that "moral truth and justifiability, if there are any such things, are in some way relative to factors that are culturally and historically contingent" (p. 442). Principles are just "one part of a balanced breakfast" when making a moral decision, claims Decker, along with other factors such as would be considered by the typical utilitarian (consequences) and virtue ethicist (character), among others. And while principles can be appealed to in some group, society, or culture, it seems inaccurate and illegitimate to maintain that principles *are* or *should be universally* binding.

References

Baron, M. (1999). *Kantian ethics almost without apology*. Ithaca, NY: Cornell University Press.

Beauchamp, T., & Childress, J. (1979/2009). *Principles of biomedical ethics*. Oxford: Oxford University Press.

Bikoo, M. (2007). Female genital mutilation: Classification and management. *Nursing Standard, 22*(7), 43–49.

Bok, S. (2002). *Common values*. Columbia, MO: University of Missouri Press.

Boyle, E. (2002). *Female genital cutting: Cultural conflict in the global community*. Baltimore, MD: The Johns Hopkins University Press.

Burkhardt, M., & Nathaniel, A. (2008). *Ethics & issues in contemporary nursing*. Clifton Park, NY: Delmar Cengage Learning.

Caplan, A. (2010). Clinical trials of drugs and vaccines among the desperately poor in poor nations: Ethical challenges and ethical solutions. *Clinical Pharmacology and Therapeutics, 88*, 583–584.

Cohen, J., Howard, M., & Nussbaum, M. (Eds.). (1999). *Is multiculturalism bad for women?* Princeton, NJ: Princeton University Press.

Foot, P. (1979/2002). Moral relativism. In P. Foot (Ed.), *Moral dilemmas and other topics in moral philosophy* (pp. 20–36). Oxford: Clarendon Press.

Gruenbaum, E. (2001). *The female circumcision controversy: An anthropological perspective*. Philadelphia: University of Pennsylvania Press.

Harman, G. (1975/2000). Moral relativism defended. In G. Harman (Ed.), *Explaining value: and other essays in moral philosophy* (pp. 3–19). Oxford: Clarendon Press. Original publication date: 1975.

Harman, G. (1984/2000). Is there a single true morality? In G. Harman (Ed.), *Explaining value and other essays in moral philosophy* (pp. 77–99). Oxford: Clarendon Press.

Harman, G. (1996). Moral relativism. In G. Harman & J. J. Thompson (Eds.), *Moral relativism and moral objectivity* (pp. 3–64). Cambridge MA: Blackwell.

Hooker, B. (2000). *Ideal code, real world: A rule-consequentialist theory of morality*. Oxford: Oxford University Press.

Kant, I. (1785/1998). *Groundwork of the metaphysics of morals* (M. Gregor, Trans.). (Section I: Transition from common rational to philosophic moral cognition). Cambridge: Cambridge University Press.

Korsgaard, C. (1996). *Creating the kingdom of ends*. Cambridge: Cambridge University Press.

Lander, M. (1999). Circumcision and virtue ethics. In G. Denniston, F. Hodges, & M. Milos (Eds.), *Male and female circumcision: medical, legal, and ethical considerations in pediatric practice* (pp. 409–412). New York: Kluwer Academic.

Macklin, R. (1999). *Against relativism: Cultural diversity and the search for ethical universals in medicine*. Oxford: Oxford University Press.

Mill, J. S. (1861/2001). *Utilitarianism*. Indianapolis, IN: Hackett Publishing Company.

Miller, A. (2002). *An introduction to contemporary metaethics*. Cambridge: Polity Press.

NIH (National Institutes of Health). (2011a). *Trials of war criminals before the Nuremberg military tribunals under control council law no. 10, vol. 2*, pp. 181–182. Washington, DC: US Government Printing Office, 1949. Retrieved from: http://ohsr.od.nih.gov/guid lines/nuremberg.html

NIH (National Institutes of Health). (2011b). The Belmont report: Ethical principles and guidelines for the protection of human subjects of research, April 18, 1979. Retrieved from: http://ohsr.od.nih.gov/guidelines/belmont.html

Nussbaum, M. (1993). Non-relative virtues: An Aristotelian approach. In M. Nussbaum & A. Sen (Eds.), *The quality of life* (pp. 242–269). Oxford: Clarendon Press.

Nussbaum, M. (1999). *Sex and social justice*. Oxford: Oxford University Press.

Skaine, R. (2005). *Female genital mutilation: Legal, cultural and medical issues*. Jefferson, NC: McFarland.

Unschuld, P. (2009). *What is medicine? Western and Eastern approaches to healing* (K. Reimers, Trans.). Berkeley: University of California Press.

Wallis, L. (2005). When rites are wrong. *Nursing Standard, 20*(4), 24–26.

Walzer, M. (1994). *Thick and thin: Moral argument at home and abroad.* Notre Dame, IN: University of Notre Dame Press.

WHO (World Health Organization). (2010). Female genital mutilation. Retrieved from: http://www.who.int/mediacentre/factsheets/fs241/en/

Wong, D. (1993). Moral relativism. In P. Singer (Ed.), *A companion to ethics* (pp. 442–450). Malden, MA: Blackwell.

Young, J. (2006). The medical messiahs: A social history of health quackery in twentieth-century America. Retrieved from: http://www.quackwatch.com/13Hx/MM/00.html

Chapter One

There Are Universal Ethical Principles That Should Govern the Conduct of Medicine and Research Worldwide

Daryl Pullman

In this chapter, I defend the claim that the very notion of morality requires the recognition of at least one overarching, universal moral principle that I call the *principle of respect for human dignity*. I begin by placing the contemporary universalist versus particularist debate in historical perspective, demonstrating that the current discussion is a continuation of a long-standing argument in moral philosophy. I then outline the conception of human dignity that underwrites the universal principle defended here, arguing that some such overarching principle is essential to the very notion of morality. Nevertheless, while the principle of respect for human dignity acts to constrain moral discourse in the broad sense, I demonstrate that the notion of human dignity is nevertheless amenable to particularist interpretations and applications.

Introduction

It is fitting that a book dedicated to contemporary debates in bioethics should open with a discussion of one of the most basic and fundamental questions in moral philosophy, namely, whether there are or can be any universal moral principles. How one responds to this question indicates a great deal about what one thinks about the nature of morality, the process or moral reasoning, the goals of moral discourse, and the possibility of moral progress. Indeed, this question has implications for the nature of the relationship between ethics and the law and the rule of law locally, nationally, and internationally.

In this chapter, I will defend the claim that there is at least one universal moral principle that has been described variously in the history of moral philosophy (at least since Kant, 1785/1948) as the *principle of humanity*, *principle of respect for persons*, and *principle of human dignity*. This is not to say that all of these formulations are equivalent; anyone who has read even a little philosophy has discovered that philosophers are wont to make distinctions and to write treatises on the same, even though such distinctions at times make little if any practical difference. Nevertheless, for the purposes of this discussion, these various formulations of what might be termed the *fundamental principle of morality* will be treated as roughly equivalent. I will focus on the concept of human dignity in an attempt to demonstrate both the necessity of some such general principle to our understanding of the nature of morality and the process of moral discourse, as well as

Contemporary Debates in Bioethics, First Edition. Edited by Arthur L. Caplan and Robert Arp.

to outline how such a general moral principle is nevertheless amenable to more particular and local interpretations and applications. Although the concept of human dignity has been much discussed and debated in recent years, it is still invoked widely in various national and international ethical and legal codes, including many that pertain to healthcare and health research. Combining aspects of the various formulations listed above, the universal principle defended here will be called the *principle of respect for human dignity*.

Now, such a general principle is admittedly abstract, and it is not immediately clear what it captures in terms of moral content, or how the principle would be applied to give moral guidance in specific cases. Defenders of principlism, or some version of it, generally argue that more specific action guiding principles are derived from some such fundamental principle. For example, Downie and Telfer (1969) refer to particular principles that deal with such actions as truth-telling and promise-keeping—and the many other specific requirements of morality—as reflecting the existence of moral *rules*, while the general, universal principle (*respect for persons* is their preferred formulation) serves as the "supreme regulative *principle*" for such specific rules (p. 15). A similar taxonomy underlies the famous four principles of bioethics—autonomy, beneficence, nonmaleficence, and justice—popularized in various editions of Beauchamp and Childress' (1979/2009) *Principles of Biomedical Ethics*. However, we cannot simply assume the existence either of some universal moral principle or of any specific requirements of morality per se, for there are those who deny the existence of both (Rorty, 1989; Dancy, 2004).

Particularism is the view that there are no general, universal moral principles that apply to all cultures; neither does moral reasoning consist in looking to such general principles for guidance when deciding on a morally appropriate act in any given situation. "I do not think there are any plain moral facts out there in the world," states Richard Rorty (1989), "nor any truths independent of language, nor any neutral ground on which to stand and argue that either torture or kindness are preferable to the other" (p. 173). According to the particularist, what is "right" or "wrong" is culturally or situationally relative; as such, a reason that might be given to claim that a certain act is right in one situation might, in a different circumstance, serve as a reason to argue that the same action is wrong (Dancy, 2004). This being the case, particularism is akin to one or more species of *ethical* or *moral relativism* (Benbaji & Fisch, 2004; Capps et al., 2008). If the claim we are defending is that there are universal moral principles (at least one, in any case) that apply irrespective of particular context, then arguments must be martialed in support of that claim. The purpose of this chapter is to outline such an argument.

In what follows, I begin by describing the current universalism versus particularism debate in moral philosophy, a debate that has been ongoing in various guises for much of the history of Western philosophy. As Daniel Callahan (2000) has noted: "There are only a limited number of ways of understanding morality, most of them by now historically repetitive. They may be dressed up in new clothes, or have had their hair cut since last year, but in their most naked state they have a familiar looking visage: haven't I seen that face somewhere before?" (p. 37).

Given this rich and somewhat repetitive history, it would be presumptuous to suggest that some original insights on this age-old argument are about to be presented here. Nor will we cover all of the key historical and intellectual moments that have brought us to where we are today. Nevertheless, it will be necessary to touch upon a few historical details, particularly as they relate to the concept of human dignity, in order to appreciate some of the key differences in the understanding of the nature of morality and the process of moral reasoning that underlie the current debate. The latter part of the chapter will elaborate the claim that the very notion of morality requires at least one universal moral principle, which, for present purposes, is labeled the *principle of respect for human dignity*.

The Universalism–Particularism Debate in Historical Perspective

Almost two decades ago, physician-ethicist Edmund Pellegrino (1993) published a short article titled "The metamorphosis of medical ethics," in which he recounted briefly the history of medical ethics and the major changes in theoretical and critical perspectives then occurring that he believed threatened to reshape bioethics in succeeding years. In recounting this metamorphosis, Pellegrino divided the history of medical ethics into four overlapping periods: the quiescent period, the period of principlism, the period of antiprinciplism, and the period of crisis. By far the longest is what he called the *quiescent period* stretching all the way from Hippocrates in ancient Greece until the 1960s in the United States—a period that he believed was enriched over the centuries by contact with Stoic and religious traditions.

The 1960s saw the advent of modern, technologically driven medicine and with it the ethical challenges presented by such developments as artificial ventilation, nutrition, and hydration, the allocation of expensive and scarce resources like kidney dialysis, and many other complex problems. On Pellegrino's reading, the 1960s and 1970s saw the beginnings of a metamorphosis in which the quiescent period of bioethics was subjected to critical philosophical inquiry and when a second period of principle-based ethical theories reshaped the virtue-based ethic of the Hippocratic tradition. This, to use the now familiar terminology, was the rise of the period of *principlism*. However, by the early 1990s, Pellegrino believed this period had already come to an end. Indeed, in his view, modern medical ethics was then at the end of a third period of *antiprinciplism*, in which competing moral theories were challenging the primacy of principles in bioethical decision-making.

According to Pellegrino, the fourth period of this metamorphosis, which he dubbed a period of *crisis*, was just beginning at the time he wrote his article, a period in which "the conceptual conflicts in ethics and the scepticism of moral philosophy challenge the very idea of a universal, normative ethic for medicine" (p. 1158). It is this supposed period of crisis that serves as the backdrop to the present volume of contemporary debates in bioethics, and gives rise to the question of the very existence of universal moral principles discussed here.

The metamorphosis of medical ethics that Pellegrino describes occurred over a period of little more than three decades at the end of the twentieth century. However, this rapid transformation serves as a kind of microcosm for a much larger and longer debate that has animated the history of moral philosophy from ancient times forward, culminating to some extent with the Enlightenment (see MacIntyre, 1981, especially Chapters 1–6). What Pellegrino describes then as a quiescent period for medical ethics, was an often-tumultuous period as far as the broader history of moral philosophy is concerned. The Enlightenment project of establishing morality on a solid rational base thus parallels Pellegrino's period of principlism. Indeed, Kant's (1785/1948) categorical imperative—particularly the practical formulation that requires that we "treat humanity, whether in our own person or in that of any other, never simply as a means, but always at the same time as an end"—is still considered by many as the quintessential moral principle.

However, just as Pellegrino's period of principlism gave rise almost immediately to an antiprinciplist backlash, the post-Enlightment period, beginning in the late eighteenth century and stretching all the way to the post-modern present, has been one of continuous philosophical debate about the nature of knowledge in general, and the possibility of moral knowledge in particular. Thus, Pellegrino's period of crisis for contemporary bioethics, which started a mere two decades ago, has its roots in the previous two centuries of what might be described variously as a post-Enlightenment era of epistemic, existential, and moral turmoil.

Whether we are now in a period of a particularly acute moral crisis is thus a matter of perspective. Antiprinciplists and particularists will not see the current state of moral knowledge, whether in bioethics or otherwise, as a matter of crisis, as this is all there is as far as morality is concerned. To put the point somewhat facetiously, since in principle there are no moral principles, there cannot be a crisis if no principles can be established. Supporters of principism, on the other hand, may or may not see this as a crisis. On the one hand, some like Pellegrino will see the rejection of principlism in bioethics as the loss of a basis of moral authority, opening the door to unbridled relativism and the potential for anarchy and nihilism, as far as ethics is concerned. Others, however, will see the current anti-principlism backlash as just one more skirmish in a larger intellectual debate that has been ongoing since the Enlightenment, if not longer.

Despite such sceptical attacks on knowledge in general, and moral knowledge in particular, science has continued to advance, and even moral sceptics like Rorty (2007) admit that post-Englightenment developments such as the abolition of slavery and the emancipation of women represent genuine moral progress. On this latter view, then, the current period in bioethics does not represent any particular crisis, but is rather one more chapter in an ongoing debate about the nature and possibility of moral knowledge. An equally facetious way of characterizing this latter perspective is that since, in principle, moral thinking requires principles (at least one, in any case), there can be no crisis occasioned by the particularist's supposed rejection of principlism.

The position defended here is that the very idea of morality requires the existence of at least one overarching moral principle that we have called the *principle of respect for human dignity*. In order to appreciate the nature of this claim and the notions of moral knowledge, the process of moral reasoning, and the goals of moral discourse to which it gives rise, we need to touch briefly on some of the key historical developments of the concept of human dignity which culminated in the Enlightenment thinking of Kant and his contemporaries, and which are reflected in subsequent philosophical debates still ongoing today.

Emergence of the Concept of Human Dignity

Although the actual phrase *human dignity* first appears in Renaissance literature only shortly before the Enlightenment, the ideas of human excellence and superiority over the rest of nature have existed since antiquity. Greek and Judeo-Christian notions of human superiority thus represent the roots of the Western concept of human dignity, albeit with decided ethno-centric and religious overtones. Thus, the human excellence mentioned in Hellenistic thought tends to focus on Greek superiority over other barbarous peoples, while the Judeo-Christian variety focused on those who found salvation through the Church. In the early Middle Ages, Christian theology and Greek philosophy merged, first in neo-Platonic interpretations of the gospel such as that of St. Augustine, and later, after the rediscovery of Aristotle in the West, in the philosophical theology of St. Thomas Aquinas. It is this hybrid notion of human superiority and excellence that gave rise to the notion of human dignity that was crystalized eventually in Renaissance humanism (Baker, 1947; Kristeller, 1972).

The exaltation of human beings simply because of their humanity rather than as god-like beings thus has its birth in Renaissance humanist thought, albeit with strong religious overtones. However, with the advance of scientific knowledge during the Enlightenment, there was increasing emphasis on the regularities of nature discoverable by human reason, and a concomitant de-emphasis of the centrality of divine law. Once the idea of Natural Law came to be formulated in terms of subjective rights inherent in individual persons—as it did, for example in the thought of John Locke—it made sense to think of human beings as worthy of respect simply on the basis of their being human.

The challenge for eighteenth century moralists, like Hume, Kant, and their contemporaries, was to reaffirm morality on a nonreligious base. Like his contemporaries, Kant wrote from the perspective of one with access to a rich historical tradition concerning the subject of human dignity, but faced the challenge of a scientific age that both undermined the traditional metaphysical underpinnings of that concept, and with it, seemingly, the very foundations of morality.

Kant (1785/1948) believed that the basis of morality had to apply universally, and as such it could not be discovered in the contingent phenomenal world. Thus, he posited the existence of an ideal noumenal realm that he called the *kingdom of ends*, which is populated by analytic and eternal truths. It is there he purports to discover both the ubiquitous human capacity for autonomous self-legislation of the moral law—the very basis of human dignity in his view—and with this capacity, the supreme principle of morality, namely the *categorical imperative*. In Kant's view, it is this capacity for autonomous choice that gives humanity its dignity.

Human dignity is still invoked in this universal sense, such as when we speak of the basic moral worth possessed by all human beings; it is this notion that underwrites the principle of respect for human dignity that is the focus of this chapter. To refer to dignity in this manner is to invoke a species-referenced conception that *ascribes* worth to human beings simply on the basis of their humanity. When used in this sense, we mean to convey the idea that all human beings have basic moral worth irrespective of any contingent historical, traditional, or cultural circumstance. One does nothing to earn basic dignity, and one can do nothing to lose it. Just being human invests one with this basic moral worth irrespective of rank or station. Although history is replete with examples of moral atrocities in which this basic human dignity has been denied or otherwise violated, no such action can erase this fundamental worth. Indeed, the very notion of "crimes against humanity" presupposes such a fundamental and universal moral norm that can be violated and which we are all responsible to protect.

Our concept of morality is predicated on the assumption of the intrinsic moral worth or dignity of humanity. The essence of morality is to guard, protect, and advance this fundamental value. A crime against humanity thus not only violates the dignity of the individual persons who are subjected to torture, ethnic cleansing, rape, unsanctioned biological experimentation, or whatever other atrocities one might imagine, but violates the very notion of what it is to be human, which we all share. As such, a crime against humanity is a crime against us all. If the human community fails to respond to such atrocities, we lose something of ourselves in the process. In point of fact, the human community has responded by invoking just such a notion of dignity as reflected in the *Preamble to the Universal Declaration of Human Rights* (1948), in the European *Convention for the Protection of Human Rights and Dignity of the Human Being with regard to the Application of Biology and Medicine* (1997), in the Report of the President's Council on Bioethics (2002) titled "Human Cloning and Human Dignity", and in various other national and international charters. The essence of this conception of dignity is not that people have a right to be treated with dignity, but rather that people have rights *because* they have dignity. Some such notion is part and parcel of our contemporary understanding of the very nature of morality itself.

Kant's contribution to our current understanding of human dignity is significant, as he helped to articulate the notion in nontheological language. Nevertheless, his attempt to establish the universal basis of morality on a nonreligious ground ultimately failed. The concept of dignity that he developed and tied to the capacity for rational autonomy required an excursion into speculative metaphysics after all. Although his transcendental deduction of the categorical imperative ostensibly circumvented religious metaphysics, many of his post-Enlightenment critics found it difficult to buy his alternative metaphysical deduction that occurred in the mysterious kingdom of ends. Indeed, Kant himself found it difficult to make the return trip from the transcendental noumenal realm where he ostensibly discovered the supreme principle of morality, to the actual phenomenal world that we all inhabit and in which that principle is supposed to provide practical guidance. Thus, in one infamous essay, he argues that the categorical imperative would require one to tell the truth to a murderer who was searching for the whereabouts of innocent victims, even though doing so would predictably result in the death of these innocent others. In Kant's view, to tell a lie, even to a murderer in an attempt to protect innocent victims, would be to treat the murderer merely as a means rather than as an end, and as such would violate the categorical imperative. It is this kind of inflexible application of principle without any consideration for the contingencies of actual life situations that has vexed particularists who understandably have little patience with such wooden formalism.

As John Arras (2010) notes in his entry from the *Stanford Encyclopedia of Philosophy*, not only is such an insensitive and formalistic approach to ethical decision-making fodder for the particularist, but also it frustrates contemporary principlists: "Blundering into a situation armed with inflexible and invariant moral principles that must hold everywhere and always in the same way, no matter what the facts on the ground, is … a big mistake, although identifying actual theorists who are guilty of such ham-handed blundering might prove to be a challenge."

In fact, Kant himself, the grandfather of contemporary principlist theorists, appears to commit just such a ham-handed blunder, much to the chagrin of many of his principlist posterity. So, while Kant has captured something about the very essence of morality in his formulation of the categorical imperative, he appears to confuse the form of moral discourse with its content in his wooden and inflexible application of that principle. As Arras correctly notes, few contemporary principlists commit this same blunder. Instead it is mainly the particularist critics who confuse the form of moral discourse, the process of moral reasoning, and the content of moral judgments when they reject such Kantian caricatures of principlism.

The Dynamics of Dignity and Moral Particularism

Although appeals to human dignity still figure prominently in various contemporary bioethical documents, conventions, and treatises such as those noted previously, the concept often receives short shrift in contemporary bioethical discussions, especially in the United States. Callahan (1999) notes that the idea of human dignity is "typically scorned by secular minded American bioethicists as too vague to be useful and too weighted with the baggage of religion to be safely used in a pluralistic society" (p. 281). This apparent vagueness has prompted Ruth Macklin (2003) to reject the notion outright as a "useless concept."

Neither Callahan nor Macklin are moral sceptics. Indeed, Callahan (2000) has argued that "an underlying universalism is inescapable" in contemporary morality, and Macklin (1999) has argued forcefully against scepticism and relativism in ethics: "My own view," she says, "is that without ethical principles as part of a framework, there can be no systematic way to justify ethical judgments." She also argues, "the key to rebutting ethical relativism lies in understanding that an ultimate moral principle can be consistent with a variety of specific standards and rules that can be found in the moral codes of different societies" (p. 43).

I share both Callahan's and Macklin's views about the nature or morality and the necessity for some underlying, universal moral principle. However, I do not share their aversion to the concept of human dignity. In various writings (Pullman 1996, 1999, 2002a, 2002b, 2004a, 2004b, 2010), I have explicated a notion of human dignity that can serve as an underlying universal principle for morality but which is nevertheless amenable to a variety of standards, rules, and codes that might arise in different social and cultural contexts. Like Robert Paul Wolff (1973), I believe that in the categorical imperative, Kant "touched the very heart of morality" (p. 175). The principle of respect for human dignity defended here is thus intended to capture the essence of the categorical imperative. Unlike Kant, however, I do not believe we need to wander into speculative metaphysics (religious, secular, or, otherwise) in order to establish the priority of this principle for moral discourse. Instead, I argue that basic dignity functions as a meaning constraint on moral discourse (Pullman, 2004a, 2004b). By this, I mean that the very notion of morality entails a commitment to the fundamental moral worth (i.e., dignity) of all humanity. As such, I follow a tradition in moral philosophy that maintains that the proposition "all human beings *qua* humanity are possessed of dignity" functions as a logical primitive or fundamental axiom in moral discourse (Goodin, 1981, p. 97). It is a postulate of moral experience, albeit a very unique postulate. Writing half a century ago, at about the time Pellegrino identifies as the birth of contemporary principlism, Pepita Haezrahi (1961/1962) sums up the point this way: "moral experience, though it is our only means of discovering this postulate, is not to be treated as though it were the cause or the ground of the postulate. On the contrary, the postulate is to be treated as though it were the cause and the ground of moral experience, on the justification that moral experience can be explained only completely by this postulate" (p. 223). Respect for the fundamental moral worth of all humanity (i.e., respect for human dignity) functions as a presupposition or pre-understanding of our moral experience as expressed in our linguistic communities. It is what Habermas (2003) describes as "a prior ethical self-understanding of the species, which is shared by all moral persons" (p. 40). "It is not merely out of a desire to spread our own way of life that we demand universal acknowledgment of a certain fundamental dignity in all human beings," states Fleischacker (1994), "we cannot avoid believing that those who do not recognize human dignity are *wrong* about something, that they have failed to recognize something about the very nature of morality" (p. 17).

Although it is one thing to claim that the notion of basic human dignity is essential to the very notion of morality as we now understand it, we are nevertheless still faced with the question of how that notion provides moral guidance in particular life situations. How does the principle of respect for human dignity overcome the kind of ham-fisted formalism of which Kant was guilty in his attempt to apply the categorical imperative? How does such a formal principle provide normative direction in the wide variety of particular historical, social, and cultural circumstances that characterize the human situation? Given the focus of this volume, how does the principle of respect for human dignity inform contemporary debates in bioethics?

The beginnings of an answer to such questions can be found in a companion notion of dignity that is also extant in our ordinary moral discourse. Unlike the formal, universal conception that underlies the principle of respect for human dignity defended here, this companion conception is contingent on a variety of historical, social, and cultural perspectives. This is the notion of dignity we have in mind when we speak of living and dying with dignity, of conducting ourselves in a dignified manner, or even the dignity that might be attached to a certain station or office in life such that holding that position might qualify one as a "dignitary." This is a dignity that might be gained or lost through personal effort, failure, or even through good or bad fortune. At times, we speak of a debilitating illness as robbing a person of his or her dignity, while in another situation, we might say that someone else bore the burden of a similar illness with dignity. Health psychologist, Alan Radley (2004), sums up some aspects of this conception of dignity as it arises in the medical context this way: "dignity is something worked out between people, an idea that makes its appearance in the practices of sufferers and observers. It is therefore contingent upon social relationships, both between medical professionals and patients, and between sufferers and carers" (p. 183).

While we have used the term "basic dignity" to identify the formal, universal, noncontingent conception of fundamental moral worth articulated to some degree by Kant, we can refer to this latter, companion, contingent conception under the rubric of *personal dignity*. Two immediate caveats are in order: First, basic and personal dignity as described here are not two different concepts of dignity; rather, they are complementary conceptions of a single unified concept. Basic dignity as such is a formal notion that articulates something fundamental about the nature of morality itself; personal dignity then expresses something of morality's content. To paraphrase something Kant said in a somewhat different context: "Basic dignity without personal dignity is empty; personal dignity without basic dignity is blind."

A second immediate caveat has to do with the term *personal*, for it is important not to confuse it with the term *individual*. Rather, the intent of the notion of personal dignity is to capture the fact that the self is a socially constructed entity. Our understanding of personal dignity is tied to notions of self-respect and self-esteem, and is intimately related to the complex social and psychological processes involved in self-formation and self-expression, not just as individual persons, but also as a society at large. Indeed, depending on the context, it might be appropriate to use the term *social dignity* to describe this socially constructed conception. The point here is that this conception of dignity captures the broad range of complex factors that contribute to our understandings of who we are, both corporately and individually.

Perspectives on personal or social dignity vary with historical, cultural, and traditional experiences and values, as individuals and communities engage in the ongoing process of defining and redefining who they are and the kinds of people they are striving to become. Indeed, our understanding of moral progress is tied to some degree to this process of social construction and individual identity, as various cultures and societies throughout human history have engaged in practices and developed customs that express how they perceive themselves in a different light. To allude to an example mentioned earlier, the abolition of slavery in the United States in the nineteenth century represented an intentional act of the American people to define themselves in a different way. Like any other major social transformation, this change was resisted by many. Indeed, many slave owners were indignant that others would judge them for a practice they believed to be morally acceptable. It took a civil war to effect a social change that the vast majority of contemporary Americans now see as a matter of moral progress. Abolition served to recognize the basic dignity of every human person while at the same time providing the opportunity to enhance the personal and social dignity (i.e., communal self-perception) of all Americans.

The foregoing example illustrates, to some degree, the manner in which the conceptions of basic dignity on the one hand, and social or personal dignity on the other, work together in a kind of dynamic interaction. In nineteenth-century America, there was a certain subset of the population who saw nothing inherently wrong with the practice of slavery. Indeed, for many, there may well have been a sense of personal dignity attached to the social status achieved from being a slave owner. However, given the role that the principle of respect for basic dignity plays in moral discourse, all such particular understandings of social and personal dignity are constrained finally by the presupposition of the basic fundamental moral worth of every human being. It was this basic conception that served to ground and motivate the social change that was eventually effected.

The slavery example illustrates how basic dignity acts as a constraint on the manner in which various social and individual practices expressive of particular self-understandings are manifested in various times and places. However, given that the relationship between basic and social or personal dignity is dynamic, we should expect that at times particular social and personal self-understandings and expressions of dignity might have a reciprocal effect on our understanding of basic dignity. Here we can think of the manner in which the laws on therapeutic abortion have evolved in various Western democracies over much of the past half century. Kant's efforts to distance morality from religious metaphysics notwithstanding, it is a historical fact that the Judeo-Christian faith has continued to play a defining role in many Western democracies, even after the Enlightenment. Hence, the notion of basic dignity that has constrained moral discourse in these broader communities is still often articulated with strong religious overtones. This explains, to some degree, the continuing aversion to the notion of basic dignity within American bioethics. Thus, many Western democracies have prohibited therapeutic abortion on largely religious grounds as a violation of the *sanctity of human life*, where this latter phrase serves as a religiously informed surrogate for the basic conception of dignity. Nevertheless, over time, as the notion of the separation of church and state evolved from a political ideal to a practical social principle, it became evident that on a range of social issues, individual persons should have the liberty to decide for themselves what was expressive of their own particular values on such issues as the moral status of the early-term fetus, and on the permissibility of therapeutic abortion. Here, the right of various individuals or social groups to express their own perceptions of what constituted a dignified life for them has pushed back against what was perceived to be an overly restrictive, inflexible, and religiously based conception of basic dignity; hence many formerly restrictive laws were relaxed accordingly. This is not to say that the notion of basic dignity was lost in the process; only that it was separated to some degree from its historical association with a particular religious tradition. While the principle of respect for basic dignity continued to constrain moral content, it did not dictate specific normative content in the manner it had done so previously when articulated in largely religious terms.

Individual persons in most Western societies now have greater liberty to decide for themselves how to dispose over early-term fetuses. Nevertheless, the vast majority of jurisdictions continue to place some restrictions on what constitutes appropriate actions vis-à-vis later-term and viable fetuses that are for all intents and purposes equivalent in biological status (if not legal status) to newborn infants. The latter is an area of ongoing discussion and debate in contemporary bioethics, and illustrates again the dynamic interaction that takes place within the full concept of human dignity between the formal, basic principle of respect for human dignity, and the particular expressions of that dignity as articulated across various social and cultural circumstances (Pullman, 2010).

Conclusion

Not every contemporary issue in bioethics can or should be reduced to a discussion of the dynamic tension between the basic, universal, principle of respect for human dignity, on the one hand, and the socially and culturally contingent expression of social or personal dignity on the other. The key point for our current discussion of contemporary debates in bioethics is to note that some such universal moral principle is both necessary to the nature of moral discourse in general, while at the same time recognizing that such a principle is amenable to a variety of particularist expressions, depending on social or cultural circumstances. When we consider such contemporary issues as human cloning, patents on human genes and embryos, the buying and selling of human organs, in vitro fertilization, eugenics, and so forth, the nature of moral discourse behoves us to consider how our discussion and responses are informed by our understanding of the common dignity we all share. Indeed, this is essentially what is captured in the various universal declarations of human rights and human dignity mentioned previously. Each such document recognizes the moral imperative to treat all humanity with dignity and respect irrespective of social or cultural circumstance. At the same time, the dynamic flexibility afforded by such a notion allows that not every social or cultural group, let alone every individual, will arrive at the same answers to these questions.

The conversations we have about such questions and the answers we provide will have implications for how we think about our common dignity, and could well open up possibilities for further conversations, while perhaps foreclosing the kinds of conversations we might have on such matters in the future. Given the potential of contemporary reproductive technologies, within the not too distant future we could see the advent of human cloning, the creation of human–nonhuman chimeras, germ-line changes to the human genome, and so forth. What we perceive to be essentially human today could be something quite different tomorrow. How we think about our basic human dignity and its normative consequences could also be affected. It is no small matter as to how we conceive of the nature of morality, and the role of moral principles in such discussions.

The ongoing moral discourse that occurs within and between communities on these and other issues presupposes something like the principle of respect for human dignity. Without some such common understanding, we have no means of articulating a common moral vision as a social group, nation, or broader international community, no way to measure moral progress or regress, and no basis for judging the actions of other nations, social groups, or even individuals as either morally praiseworthy or blameworthy. Ultimately, without such principles, we have no basis on which to sustain the ongoing conversation that defines and articulates our common humanity.

References

Arras, J. (2010). Theory and bioethics. *Stanford Encyclopedia of Philosophy*. Retrieved from: http://plato.stanford.edu/entries/theory-bioethics/

Baker, E. (1947). *The image of man*. New York: Harper & Row.

Beauchamp, T. L., & Childress, J. F. (1979/2009). *Principles of biomedical ethics*. New York: Oxford University Press.

Benbaji, Y., & Fisch, M. (2004). Through thick and thin: A new defense of cultural relativism. *Southern Journal of Philosophy*, *42*, 1–24.

Callahan, D. (1999). The social sciences and the task of bioethics. *Daedalus*, *128*(4), 275–294.

Callahan, D. (2000). Universalism & particularism fighting to a draw. *The Hastings Center Report*, *30*(1), 37–44.

Capps, D., Lynch, M., & Massey, D. (2008). A coherent moral relativism. *Synthese*, *151*, 1–26.

Convention for the Protection of Human Rights and Dignity of the Human Being with regard to the Application of Biology and Medicine: Convention on Human Rights and Biomedicine (1997). Retrieved from: http://conventions.coe.int/Treaty/en/Treaties/html/164.htm

Dancy, J. (2004). *Ethics without principles*. Oxford: Clarendon Press.

Downie, R. S., & Telfer, E. (1969). *Respect for persons*. London: George Allen & Unwin.

Fleischacker, S. (1994). *The ethics of culture*. Ithaca, NY: Cornell University Press.

Goodin, R. E. (1981). The political theories of choice and dignity. *American Philosophical Quarterly*, *18*(2), 91–100.

Habermas, J. (2003). *The future of human nature*. Cambridge: Polity Press.

Haezrahi, P. (1961/1962). The concept of man as end-in-himself. *Kant-Studien*, *53*, 209–224.

Kant, I. (1785/1948). *Groundwork of the Metaphysics of Morals* (H. J. Paton, Trans.) New York: Harper & Row.

Kristeller, P. O. (1972). *Renaissance concepts of man*. New York: Harper & Row.

MacIntyre, A. (1981). *After virtue*. Notre Dame, IN: University of Notre Dame Press.

Macklin, R. (1999). *Against relativism*. New York: Oxford University Press.

Macklin, R. (2003). Dignity is a useless concept. *British Medical Journal, 327*, 1419–1420.

Pellegrino, E. D. (1993). The metamorphosis of medical ethics. *Journal of the American Medical Association, 269*(9), 1158–1162.

President's Council on Bioethics. (2002). *Human cloning and human dignity*. New York: Public Affairs.

Pullman, D. (1996). Dying with dignity and the death of dignity. *Health Law Journal, 4*, 197–219.

Pullman, D. (1999). The ethics of autonomy and dignity in long-term care. *Canadian Journal on Aging, 18*(1), 26–46.

Pullman, D. (2002a). Human dignity and the ethics and aesthetics of pain and suffering. *Theoretical Medicine and Bioethics, 23*, 75–94.

Pullman, D. (2002b). Universalism, particularism and the ethics of dignity. *Christian Bioethics*, 7(3), 333–358.

Pullman, D. (2004a). Death, dignity and moral nonsense. *Journal of Palliative Care, 20*(3), 171–178.

Pullman, D. (2004b). Afterthoughts: Death, dignity, and moral nonsense. *Journal of Palliative Care, 20*(3), 178.

Pullman, D. (2010). Human non-persons, feticide, and the erosion of dignity. *Journal of Bioethical Inquiry*, 7(4), 353–364.

Radley, A. (2004). Pity, modernity and the spectacle of suffering. *Journal of Palliative Care, 20*(3), 179–184.

Rorty, R. (1989). *Contingency, irony and solidarity*. New York: Cambridge University Press.

Rorty, R. (2007) Dewey and Posner on pragmatism and moral progress. *The University of Chicago Law Review*, 74(3), 915–927.

Universal Declaration of Human Rights (1948). Retrieved from: http://www.un.org/en/documents/udhr/index.shtml

Wolff, R. P. (1973). *The autonomy of reason*. New York: Harper & Row.

Chapter Two

There Are No Universal Ethical Principles That Should Govern the Conduct of Medicine and Research Worldwide

Kevin S. Decker

In this chapter, I argue that while there are ethical principles that should guide medical practice and research, there are good reasons to believe that these principles are not universal. First, moral principles in medicine are better understood as tools rather than standards, and we must be careful about what is historically contingent in them. Second, the effort to find universal principles behind divergent practices seems arbitrary, since principles are essentially contested. Third, the normative force of principles that seem universal has diffuse sources, meaning that they are conditioned by the prior existence of relationships between moral agents and patients.

Introduction

Coming to grips with whether or not universal principles can provide guidance in clinical decisions concerning health and welfare, in medical research, and in beginning-of-life and end-of-life situations requires preliminary answers to three questions. First of all, what are ethical principles? Our common experience of the moral life is one in which we often think of ourselves or others as "principled," and areas like art criticism and jurisprudence appeal to norms and principles of their own. So, we should not doubt that there are such things as ethical principles, but the question of whether those principles are *universal* is still an open one.

Second, what would make certain ethical principles universal? There are three distinct senses of *universal* that should concern us. One takes its cue from science in claiming that the extent to which physical laws operate on matter is universal—without exception, these laws determine the course of events. The second sense defines universal in terms of traits of human beings within cultures. In anthropology, human universals "comprise those features of culture, society, language, behavior and psyche for which there are no known exceptions to their existence in all ethnographically or historically recorded human societies" (Shermer, 2004, p. 60). Just a few examples of such human universal traits are attachment, beliefs about death, promise-making, and use of symbolism. Of course, these admit of exceptions, since not every member of a culture will express them. The third meaning of universal is the lynchpin of the discussion in this introduction. It is normative in the sense that

Contemporary Debates in Bioethics, First Edition. Edited by Arthur L. Caplan and Robert Arp.

certain unrealized intentions, actions, or consequences *should be brought about*. This *should* trumps personal self-interest and, as universal, also cuts across ideologies, national boundaries, cultures, and perhaps even time. This sense of universal also admits of exceptions, given that moral freedom allows us to *not* bring about these intentions, actions, or consequences. But we call this a failure to adhere to the universal dictate of morality, and lay blame accordingly.

The third preliminary question, then, is this: what is the *normative force* of universal principles in this third sense mentioned in the previous paragraph? Principles must be able to motivate particular judgments, or they are morally meaningless. The principle that "human beings should not use their telepathic powers to dominate lesser species," for example, may apply to particular judgments in the year 3000, but not today. As James Childress (2001) claims, "most principle-based approaches reject … a strictly deductivist, mechanical method that appears to flounder in cases of conflict" (p. 64). What is a universal principle's normative force if the mere fact that a universal principle applies to a particular situation is not by itself enough to reliably cause us to act according to that principle?

In what follows, answers to these questions will support the claim that there are no universal ethical principles that apply to all medical practice and research. I do not endorse a form of *moral relativism*, leading to the consequence that "it is wrong to pass judgment on others who have substantially different values or to try to make them conform to one's values, for the reason that their values are as valid as one's own" (Wong, 1993, p. 442). In fact, exercising such judgment seems integral to what Kurt Baier (1998) called "the point of view of morality," and part of this prescriptive exercise is exercised in efforts to convince others to share our moral point of view.

A different kind of relativism, *meta-ethical* relativism, accepts that "moral truth and justifiability, if there are any such things, are in some way relative to factors that are culturally and historically contingent" (Wong, 1993, p. 442). I will attempt to show that this form of relativism can both happily coexist with the prescriptive force of moral judgments and indicate how moral problem-solving could be supported by anthropology, cognitive science, and other disciplines. My perspective as a pragmatist emphasizes judgment and action as continuous with each other, and sees ethical deliberation as a phase in problem-solving in concrete, lived experience. It is also pluralist, interested in the diversity of ethical traditions that inform our notions of health, life, and death in our rapidly shrinking world.

Principles: One Part of a Balanced Breakfast

John Rawls (1951/1999) is correct to say that "the principal aim of ethics is the formulation of justifiable principles which may be used in cases wherein there are conflicting interests to determine which one of them should be given preference" (p. 10). There is far more to say about our moral life than can be expressed through principles, though. Although deontological theories of ethics are most commonly identified as "ethics of principles," utilitarianism also relies on its utility principle (and others). Even virtue ethics generates principles of a kind.

The key difference among views of principles is found in theories and ideas of how they are generated in the first place. One such method, which can be traced back to Samuel Clarke's *Discourses concerning the Unchangeable Obligations of Natural Religion* (1706), is well expressed in Immanuel Kant's (1997) dictum that "*duty is the necessity of an action from respect for law*" (p. 13). Kant means that moral obligation originates in thinking through a rule–case–result model, where the moral law (inferred by application of a test for moral maxims) is the *rule*, and a judgment about the ethically relevant features of the particular situation is the *case*. A more inductively flavored method for generating principles can be found in the early work of Rawls (1951/1999) himself: "[Justifiable] principles explicate the considered judgments of competent judges, and since these judgments are more likely than any other judgments to represent the mature convictions of competent men as they have been worked out under the most favorable existing conditions, the invariant in what we call "moral insight," if it exists, is more likely to be approximated by the principles of a successful explication than by the principles which a man might fashion out of his own head" (p. 10).

In bioethics, what Rawls sees as explication of considered judgments typically takes one of two different forms: *specification* and *balancing*. Specified principlism states that the deployment of relevant principles is to be followed by specification of how they fit the situation at hand and, ultimately, what should be done. In applying the principle that "physicians should not lie to their patients," Childress (2001) points out that it is important to specify whether the prohibition on lying in the case at hand has to do with "making an intentionally deceptive statement," on the one hand, or "withholding information from *someone who has the right to the truth*" on the other (p. 64). This makes it possible to determine what further moral considerations we must take: whether we must balance the prohibition on lying against other values or principles, or whether we should be determining who has a right to the truth. "According to specified principlism's advocates, a specification is rationally defensible if it maintains or increases the mutual support among the total set of judgments, norms, and theories" (Strong, 2000, p. 235).

In contradistinction to specification, *balancing* norms assumes that there is a kind of "moral weight" to principles, but balancing would be impossible if principles had *absolute* moral weight. Medical researchers often have to think in terms of rigid constructions of principles of nonmaleficence and beneficence, which are then lexically ordered based on production of good consequences for individuals (Hippocratic individualism) or society (utilitarianism) (Childress, 2001, p. 68).

But such principles, and others like respect for autonomy, justice, and, of course, dignity (Childress, 2001, p. 66; Pullman, 2002), need to be understood not just in terms of their justifiability, but also in terms of their *function* in the context of medicine and society. The pragmatist, John Dewey, continually calls our attention to how myopic efforts to specify or balance abstract principles lead to treating principles as *standards* for judgment, instead of as *tools* for this purpose. We must also take into account the extent to which acting ethically helps achieve significant goods, as well as "the enormous part played in human life by facts of approbation and condemnation, praise and blame, reward and punishment" (Dewey & Tufts, 1932/1989, p. 182). For the pragmatist, principles (along with duties and the value of loyalty) represent the normative models of "law and regulation," only one of at least three such models common to our moral life. The other two models reference good consequences and our concern for choosing ends that serve ethical purposes, and virtue, regarding our felt need for recognition by others. More recent contributions to ethical theory expand this range of normative models to include care, trust, and love (Baier, 1994).

But principles have served a crucial role in bioethics literally from its very beginnings in the Hippocratic Oath. Historically, they have provided a basis for the physician's integration into the social order via professional self-regulation. But they have also tended, over time, to create a picture of patient as a "Hippocratic individual," constructed as the bearer of certain *rights* to which correspond *principles* that specify duties of practitioners, as in the various versions of the American Medical Association's "Principles of Medical Ethics." A notable variant is the American Nursing Association's 1998 "Code of Ethics for Nursing," which specifies that the nurses' primary commitment is to "the patient, whether an individual, family, or community group" (Teays & Purdy, 2001, p. 181). Robert Veatch (1999) suggests that the secularized, neutral construction of the Hippocratic individual occurred even before the profession's reclamation of Hippocrates' Oath in the early nineteenth century (pp. 161–162).

And yet the history of bioethical principles demonstrates that it is difficult to separate what is historically contingent, from what is universal in them. In the AMA's first code of medical ethics in 1847, for example, physicians are sworn to "treat every case with attention and humanity" and acknowledge that, "secrecy and delicacy should be strictly observed." In these days of house calls and paternalism, doctors "should not fail, on proper occasions, to give to the friends of the patient timely notice of danger, when it really occurs, and even to the patient himself, if absolutely necessary" (Teays & Purdy, 2001, p. 177). Patients also have duties not to "weary the physician with tedious details not pertaining to the disease" and, when dismissing their physicians, "common courtesy requires that he should declare his reasons for doing so" (Teays & Purdy, 2001, p. 178). These directives are not merely quaint throwbacks—they demonstrate two important points. First, a significant overlap was still possible in 1847 between professional medical ethics and a small-scale, community-minded "ethics of intimates." As the medical profession and needs of patients have changed, that overlap has been erased and a new, larger one created between professional ethics and the "ethics of strangers," where principles serve par excellence to infuse moral judgments with the qualities of consistency and homogeneity (Toulmin, 1981, p. 35). The other point is that while the 1847 code seems to confuse the boundary between professional ethics and "bourgeois morality," its principles were taken, at the time, as being quite objectively valid. This disconnect suggests adoption of a humble historicism on our part toward the relative authority of principles.

The function and history of principles certainly suggest an important place for them in bioethics as crystallizations of practices that have, on balance, helped preserve the right and the good in questions of health. What about their status as universal rules?

Universalism: Promises and Pitfalls

It might seem surprising to demand of ethical principles that they be universal, given that most moral decision-making will concern those fairly close to us: ourselves, our extended family, plus a relatively small community of friends, work associates, and acquaintances. Early moral codes, even those of Plato and Aristotle, violate the spirit of inclusiveness by unambiguously creating moral distinctions between classes and genders, cultural insiders and "barbarians." The first formulation of ethical universalism is found in the thought of the Stoics, who argued that there was a comprehensive, binding "natural law" that spanned education, social status, and nationality. Cicero (1997), for example, claimed that "law is the highest reason, implanted in Nature, which commands what ought to be done and forbids the opposite. This reason, when firmly fixed and firmly developed in the human mind, is Law" (p. 24). Stoic influence on Immanuel Kant led him to believe that an ultimate moral principle must be universal in the sense that it applies to all rational beings whatever. The quest for such an ultimate principle, free of the historical contingencies of differing religious traditions or educational schemes, produced the hallmark of Kant's (1997) ethical theory, the universalizability thesis, or the *categorical imperative*: "Act only in accordance with that maxim through which you can at the same time will that it become a universal law" (p. 31).

In hindsight, it is less surprising that the question of universal principles should be raised in bioethics within the first years of its germination in the mid-twentieth century, as recorded by Edmund Pellegrino (1993, pp. 1157–1158). For new questions of applied ethics were put to us not merely by advances in life-sustaining technology of the time, but also by the post-colonial internationalization of professional medical training and practice. In this milieu of Cold War rapprochement and fresh third-world cultural paradigms for "morality" and "goodness," the United Nations' Universal Declaration of Human Rights (1948) rose as the epitome of the West's principle-based reaction. Kant, an early defender of a peaceful, international cosmopolitan order, can be seen as the forerunner of such approaches (Bohman & Lutz-Bachmann, 1997). In turn, his thinking provides the basis for a number of principles of bioethics, including autonomy, justice, nonmaleficence, and dignity (Beauchamp & Childress, 1979/2009).

This deontological approach rejects nearly every other ethical theory as merely "conventional," holding to the contrary that "our rights and duties do not depend wholly on the offices we hold, the agreements we have made, the commands addressed to us, or the positive laws that exist" (Nielsen, 1990, p. 43). Furthermore, moral rights and duties do not originate on biological or psychological terms, either; Kant (1997) understands these sciences as reliant on a *deterministic* scheme of explanation that is incompatible with moral freedom. The only principles or laws that can be genuinely moral in character are both (1) compatible with freedom (because an agent follows the law out of their own rational deduction, not external coercion) and (2) universal (because they are not in any way "conventional").

Arguments against moral relativism offer two good reasons to think that there are such principles. One is that "there are some moral rules that all societies will have in common, because those rules are necessary for society to exist" (Rachels, 1998, p. 555). James Rachels offers two universal prohibitions against lying and murder that happen to be key to bioethical discussions of the doctor–patient relationship and physician-assisted euthanasia, respectively. The second reason is that the apparent differences in practices and beliefs between cultures that might lead us to adopt moral relativism are themselves misleading. As Rachels (1998) puts it, "We cannot conclude merely because customs differ, that there is a disagreement about *values*" (p. 553). Ruth Macklin (2006) gives us this example: suppose that a physician's commitment to telling the truth to her patients is dependent upon the principle of respect for autonomy. But in cultures where autonomy is respected at the *familial*, rather than the individual, level, "doctors in [these] other countries do readily honor a family's request not to tell the patient a diagnosis of cancer or other terminal illness" (p. 671). Faced with a similar request, an American doctor might find himself facing a dilemma over patient autonomy versus respecting cultural values. But Macklin claims that a principled approach can prevail in this case by correctly understanding the sense of "autonomy" here. "The principle [of autonomy] does not require inflicting unwanted information on people; rather, it requires first finding out how much and what kind of information they want to know and then respecting that expressed wish" (Macklin, 2006, p. 674).

Rachels' and Macklin's attempts to find cultural commonality that would smooth over the worst intercultural moral interactions are commendable, yet flawed. First, Rachels seems to underestimate how much a culture can differ ethically from his own, and still prevail. Certain societies subsist amid ritual murder or torture, for example, the Aztecs, but also sub-cultures within large-scale industrial societies today (James, 2011, p. 111). Others, like the Dobu of Papua New Guinea, have selective prohibitions on lying. While many other examples could be added, the disappearance of the Aztecs and the continued existence of the Dobu Islanders are evidence that the presence of certain moral rules within a culture is neither a necessary nor a sufficient condition for its livelihood. Second, Rachels' contention that certain moral rules are necessities for society seems to invert the type of justification that a principled approach demands. After all, we want to know *if there are principles worth following for their own sake*, not simply because they ensure the furtherance of our way of life.

Macklin appears to gerrymander the meaning of the term "autonomy" to produce understanding at the theoretical level despite continued intercultural division. In its Kantian beginnings, autonomy's meaning is predicated as against religious, political, or cultural suasion. If family decisions may be autonomous in ways comparable to individual decisions, how would we resolve a conflict between an "autonomous" patient and their dissenting, "autonomous" family? A point against both Macklin and Rachels—if two members of very different societies do not agree in a situation upon the application of a principle, but they *do* agree that the principle applies, what do they really agree on? At best, it seems that something like a dispute over semantics is involved here. At worst, a flaw is exposed in what seem like arbitrary attempts to class certain principles as universal, despite disparities of application. In Macklin's case, being able to trace differing Western and Japanese attitudes about consent back to a "shared" principle of autonomy settles the case, but when we trace both the Muslim practice of female genital mutilation and our revulsion to this practice back to a shared principle of religious liberty, little is settled.

It is far better, I think, to avoid the temptation to gerrymander principles by acknowledging that the content of such rules, far from being universal, is today essentially contested (Furrow, 2009). We should avoid assuming a kind of false consistency in principles that overshadows the relevant differences in particular cases. When Childress (2001) claims, "the requirement of universalizability or generalizability, many philosophers argue, entails that moral agents extend their moral judgment that 'X is wrong' to all relevantly similar 'Xs'" (p. 68), the requirement of consistency here is of heuristic import but does not have clear moral status. Instead, what we are concerned about in the judgment that "X is wrong" is primarily the *reasons* for that judgment. If X is "relevantly similar" to other precedents, this is certainly important in a *juridical* sense (one that Kant was very fond of importing into his view of morality), but not as much in a wider moral sense (Decker, 2002). Consistency as a *formal* characteristic of judgments pairs well in bioethics with the neutral, impartial ideal of the Hippocratic individual, but this ideal itself is not a cultural universal embraced by all patients and practitioners.

Binding Moral Norms and Self-Evidence

A claim that invokes a universal principle becomes part of our deliberations on a course of action for a seriously ill patient. How does that principle affect our ultimate decision? We are not in new territory here, since the "normative force," or moral bindingness of such principles is not unique in ethics, as Hannah Arendt (2003) tells us: "Moral propositions, like all propositions claiming to be true, must be either self-evident or sustained by proofs or demonstrations. If they are self-evident, they are of a coercive nature; the human mind cannot help accepting them, it bows to the dictate of reason. The evidence is compelling and no argument to sustain them is needed, no discourse except elucidation and clarification" (p. 71).

If universal principles were self-evident, their authority would also be *absolute* in any case to which they validly applied. Universal moral principles would be like the logical laws learned by college undergraduates, where no further progress could be made in their area of application until they were accepted. And most defenses of universal principles do not ascribe *this* kind of normative force to them (Donagan, 1977; Childress, 2001).

Embracing the route of "proof or demonstration," then, we still face a stumbling block to why we should acknowledge the authority of universal principles, as Arendt (2003) claims "Does reason then command the will? In that case the will would no longer be free but would stand under the dictate of reason. Reason can only tell the will: this is good, in accordance with reason; if you wish to attain it you ought to act accordingly" (p. 71).

The literature in response to this last point is vast and forbidding, and most bioethicists are less interested in the metaphysics of free will than they are in establishing solid moral ground for making difficult and painful decisions. Considering, then, the most likely explanations for the normative force behind normative principles, we fall upon two: One possibility is that this bindingness is sui generis, not derived from the logical self-evidence of moral rules or through proof, which can be convincing yet ignored. The other is that the authority of principles is actually prima facie, that is, it is such that we are required to consider the principle as determining a course of action in an applicable case, *but* other factors may, in due course, cause us to legitimately reconceive the necessity of acting according to the principle.

Let's deal with prima facie status first. What could cause me, as a health professional, to think that a particular prima facie principle like that which commits me to my patient's autonomy by guaranteeing the confidentiality of her case would not hold in a particular situation? The likely answer is: another principle conflicts with the first. W. D. Ross's (1998) introduction of the idea of prima facie duties is a persuasive rejoinder to conflicts of duties in Kant's ethics and helps answer this question. Suppose my patient has a communicable disease, but I am aware that the patient's right to privacy is limited by state statutes mandating that I report my finding to public-health officials. Here, the original autonomy principle may run up against another prima facie principle, that of reasonable compliance with the law. Now, is there anything about this case that would render my decision easier or better by introducing the idea that either of the principles is *universal*?

The answer, I think, is *no*. The mere fact that a principle is universal does not imply that it is absolute, as we have already seen; the case just described can clearly have more than one outcome. Depending on the particular circumstances, the weight of the other principle could reasonably convince us that the autonomy principle is merely prima facie and should be overridden. In this, there is greater normative force against protecting confidentiality absolutely, and the "universality" of the autonomy principle simply indicates that this situation *cannot be adequately morally analyzed without reference to considerations about autonomy*. But the same necessity for consideration could be true of a number of different factors in the case, including nonmoral ones such as the nature of the communicable disease, the gender and economic class of the patient, etc. We would not pretend, however, that any of these factors were universal simply by admitting that they should not be overlooked in the judgment at hand. Even Ross (1998) recognizes this:

"When I ask what it is that makes me in certain cases sure that I have a prima facie duty to do so and so, I find that it lies in the fact that I have made a promise; when I ask the same question in another case, I find the answer lies in the fact that I have done a wrong. And if on reflection I find (as I think I do) that neither of these reasons is reducible to one another, I must no on any a priori ground assume that such a reduction is possible" (p. 490). We can see that Ross's own subtle view on principles was that they provide a heuristic device for ordering different duties, not that prima facie status settles cases consistently.

If we do not want to admit prima facie principles, then the type of normative force of universal principles must differ radically from logical or empirical validity. This idea is explored in religious morality, as well as in evolutionary ethics (strange bedfellows, indeed!). While I do not have the space to consider religion, it is important to note that "some of the religious traditions which invoke ... rule-based constraints insist that at least some can be justified in purely secular terms" (Gregory, 2001, p. 47), as well as that some religiously justified principles could also be prima facie. Regarding evolutionary ethics, the work of Richard Joyce (2006) may have pinpointed the natural basis for "negative" principles—prohibitions like "do not violate a patient's autonomous right to informed consent." Acknowledging that certain behaviors are prohibited is, for Joyce, a trait that distinguishes genuinely moral creatures from those that merely display empathy or self-sacrificing behavior. What is even more interesting in Joyce's account is that certain desires and emotional states accompany genuinely moral judgments. In the words of one of his interpreters, "Moral judgments are tightly linked to motivation: sincerely judging that some act is wrong appears to entail at least some desire to *refrain from* performing the act" and "moral judgments imply notions of desert: doing what you know to be morally prohibited implies that punishment would be justified" (James, 2011, p. 56). In addition, moral creatures experience emotional responses to their own wrongdoing (e.g., shame) and the perceived wrongdoing of others. This suggests that what we understand as "moral" in judgments, motivations, and emotions is a quality that is *relational* in origin—in other words, that is conditioned by "the prior existence of social or ecological relationships between ourselves" and other moral agents (Warren, 1997, p. 123). The normative force of principles is so difficult to locate because it is so diffuse: it is dependent upon social, economic, educational, and religious influences upon our ideas of proper motivation, desert, and even upon our own reflective understanding of our ethical-emotional states. "It is not as a particular that an action is ethically significant, but as a response to an ethical problem in an individual's life" (Stenlund, 1997, p. 267). Ethical situations are extended in time and social space, and in short, not the sort of things that admit of being "isolated, possible instance[s] of something general" (Stenlund, 1997, p. 268). This relational view does not as much privilege the particularity of moral situations as it undermines the particular versus universal dichotomy of ethical theory itself. But is it possible to hold this view without devolving into merely subjective preferences?

Conclusion

The apparent drawback of the relational approach is that it asserts a connection of reason-giving force between "objective" relations of history and social institutions, and ethical deliberation; as a result, the normative force of principles will be conceived as relative to these objective factors in any case when deliberation proceeds long enough. But this rejection of universal principles depends upon an important fact about ethical deliberation: "it is in every case first-personal," where "the action I decide upon will be mine, and ... its being mine means not just that it will be arrived at by this deliberation, but that it will involve changes in the world of which I shall empirically be the cause, and of which these desires and this deliberation itself will be, in some part, the cause" (Williams, 1985, pp. 68–69).

Yet in bioethical problem-solving, we can avoid charges of subjectivism at the same time as we use principles that are not universal in nature. The pragmatism of Dewey again shows a middle course:

> Only if some rigid form of intutionalism were true, would the state of culture and the growth of ["nonmoral"] knowledge ... be without significance for

> distinctively moral knowledge and judgment. Because the two things are connected, each generation, especially one living in a time like the present, is under the responsibility for overhauling its inherited stock of moral principles and reconsidering them in relation to contemporary conditions and needs. It is stupid to suppose that this signifies that all moral principles are so relative to a particular state of society that they have no binding force in any social condition. The obligation is to discover *what* principles *are* relevant to our own social estate. Since this social condition is a fact, the principles which are related to it are real and significant, even though they be not adapted to some other set and style of social institutions, culture, and scientific knowledge. (Dewey & Tufts, 1932/1989, p. 283)

To get at the implication of Dewey's words, consider Brandt's (1992) comparison between the *moral code* of a society and the rules of its *institutions*. Brandt, a utilitarian, believes that it is important to distinguish between normative enterprise of a moral code and the rules that serve to describe institutions (the latter is not really a concern for ethics). He defines an "institution" as a "set of positions or statuses, with which certain privileges and jobs are associated ... The individuals occupying these positions are a group of cooperating agents in a system which as a whole is thought to have the aim of serving certain ends" (p. 122). What distinguishes a moral code from institutional rules is the scope of morality: it applies across the entire society. By contrast, institutional positions and rules are derived, as Brandt argues, from the *purpose* of the institution—the shared ends of its workers or members. But the moral code of a society is distinctive because society, as a whole, has no such overarching purpose. "There is no specific goal in the achievement of which each position has a designated role to play," he claims (p. 122).

This view seems to ignore the perspective of the individual person about the nature of society in favor of an abstract *theory* about society. Contrary to Brandt's theory, society's members *do* define their collective as serving certain purposes, even if they cannot agree on what those purposes are. Proposed economic, social, or religious purposes can be considered society's "ends-in-view" as reflected in the partial and limited convictions of individuals and groups, even if they are not "*the* ends of society" as established by a social scientist (McDonald, 2004, p. 92ff.). The idea of morality as itself an institution that is distinctive because of its wholesale, if incomplete, permeation of other institutions strengthens the appeal to principles of wide scope without claiming they are universal.

This institutional view takes very seriously the interpretation of the connection between principles and ends-in-view in, say, a health practitioner's or patient's mind, while at the same time allowing ethical analysis to take into account various institutional but "nonmoral" influences on how both principles and ends-in-view are interpreted. It also integrates Veatch's (1999) insight that "medical decisions are made regularly, not only by ordinary citizens, but also by judges, legislatures, educators, and others in many other roles" (p. 163).

In bioethics and other areas of normative discourse, public moral claims that have the greatest degree of *scope*, encompassing particular, "thick" commitments within wider, "thin" principles or "ends-in-view" are very likely to achieve the greatest degree of deliberative acceptance (Walzer, 2006). Examples include interdenominational religious support for joint social justice or public-health projects, or mandating a program of vaccination, albeit one with a degree of selectivity, for the children of educated parents worried about the health risks of vaccines. At the same time, we have to accept that the scope of acceptable principles will invite a wide variety of interpretations of them. When a number of incommensurable interpretations need to be reconciled and action taken, a method of inquiry developed by pragmatists Dewey and Charles S. Peirce shows itself particularly well suited for problem-solving in applied ethics (Fins et al., 2003). This method, which stresses respectful criticism, reconstruction of traditional solutions, fallibilism, experimentation based on hypothetically correct courses of action, and the importance of individual experience, "gives us the wherewithal to explain how our beliefs are rooted in our history and our practices, but nonetheless can be justified" (Misak, 2000, p. 53).

References

Arendt, H. (2003). Some questions of moral philosophy. In J. Kohn (Ed.), *Responsibility and judgment* (pp. 49–146). New York: Random House.

Baier, A. (1994). *Moral prejudices: Essays on ethics*. Cambridge, MA: Harvard University Press.

Baier, K. (1998). The point of view of morality. In S. Cahn & P. Markie (Eds.), *Ethics: History, theory, and contemporary issues* (pp. 514–528). Oxford: Oxford University Press.

Beauchamp, T. L., & Childress, J. F. (1979/2009). *Principles of biomedical ethics*. New York: Oxford University Press.

Bohman, J., & Lutz-Bachmann, M. (Eds.). (1997). *Perpetual peace: Essay on Kant's cosmopolitan ideal*. Cambridge, MA: MIT Press.

Brandt, R. (1992). *Morality, utilitarianism, and rights*. Cambridge: Cambridge University Press.

Childress, J. F. (2001). A principle-based approach. In H. Kuhse & P. Singer (Eds.), *A companion to bioethics* (pp. 67–76). Malden, MA: Blackwell.

Cicero (1997) *The laws*. In M. Ishay (Ed.), *The human rights reader* (pp. 15–25). New York: Routledge.

Decker, K. (2002). Habermas on human rights and cloning: A pragmatist response. *Essays in Philosophy, 3*(2), 1–28.

Dewey, J., & Tufts, J. (1932/1989). *Ethics*. In J Boydston (Ed.), *John Dewey: the later works, 1925–1953*. Carbondale, IL: Southern Illinois University Press.

Donagan, A. (1977). *The theory of morality*. Chicago: University of Chicago Press.

Fins, J., Bacchetta, M., & Miller, F. (2003). Clinical pragmatism: A method of moral problem solving. In G. McGee (Ed.), *Pragmatic bioethics* (pp. 29–44). Cambridge, MA: MIT Press.

Furrow, D. (2009). Of cave dwellers and spirits: The trouble with moral absolutes. In M. Minch & C. Weigel (Eds.), *Living ethics* (pp. 235–247). Belmont, CA: Wadsworth.

Gregory, E. (2001). Religion and bioethics. In H. Kuhse & P. Singer (Eds.), *A companion to bioethics* (pp. 46–55). Malden, MA: Blackwell.

James, S. (2011). *An introduction to evolutionary ethics*. Malden, MA: Wiley-Blackwell.

Joyce, R. (2006). *The evolution of morality*. Cambridge, MA: MIT Press.

Kant, I. (1997). *Groundwork of the metaphysics of morals* (M. Gregor, trans.). Cambridge: Cambridge University Press.

Macklin, R. (2006). The doctor–patient relationship in different cultures. In H. Kuhse & P. Singer (Eds.), *Bioethics: An anthology* (pp. 664–676). Malden, MA: Blackwell.

McDonald, H. (2004). *John Dewey and environmental philosophy*. Albany, NY: State University of New York Press.

Misak, C. (2000). *Truth, politics, morality: Pragmatism and deliberation*. London: Routledge.

Nielsen, K. (1990). *Ethics without god*. Amherst, NY: Prometheus Books.

Pellegrino, E. D. (1993). The metamorphosis of medical ethics. *Journal of the American Medical Association, 269*(9), 1158–1162.

Pullman, D. (2002). Universalism, particularism and the ethics of dignity. *Christian Bioethics*, 7(3), 333–358.

Rachels, J. (1998). The challenge of cultural relativism. In S. Cahn & P. Markie (Eds.), *Ethics: History, theory, and contemporary issues* (pp. 645–652). Oxford: Oxford University Press.

Rawls, J. (1999). Outline of a decision procedure for ethics. In S. Freeman (Ed.), *John Rawls: Collected papers* (pp. 1–19). Cambridge, MA: Harvard University Press.

Ross, W.D. (1998). The right and the good (selections). In S. Cahn & P. Markie (Eds.), *Ethics: History, theory, and contemporary issues* (pp. 477–487). Oxford: Oxford University Press.

Shermer, M. (2004). *The science of good and evil*. New York: Henry Holt.

Stenlund, S. (1997). Ethics, philosophy and language. In L. Alanen, S. Heinämaa, & T. Wallgren (Eds.), *Commonality and particularity in ethics* (pp. 237–250). New York: St. Martin's Press.

Strong, C. (2000). Specified principlism: What is it, and does it really resolve cases better than casuistry? *Journal of Medicine and Philosophy, 25*(3), 323–341.

Teays, W., & Purdy, L. (Eds.). (2001). *Bioethics, justice, and health care*. Belmont, CA: Wadsworth.

Toulmin, S. (1981). The tyranny of principles. *Hastings Center Report, 11*(6), 31–39.

Veatch, R. (1999). Who should control the scope and nature of medical ethics? In R. Baker, A. Caplan, L. Emanuel, & S. Latham (Eds.), *The American medical ethics revolution: How the AMA's code of ethics has transformed physicians' relationships to patients, professionals, and society* (pp. 158–170). Baltimore, MD: The Johns Hopkins University Press.

Walzer, M. (2006). *Thick and thin: Moral agreement at home and abroad*. Notre Dame, IN: University of Notre Dame Press.

Warren, M.A. (1997). *Moral status*. New York: Oxford University Press.

Williams, B. (1985). *Ethics and the limits of philosophy*. Cambridge, MA: Harvard University Press.

Wong, D. (1993). Moral relativism. In P. Singer (Ed.), *A companion to ethics* (pp. 442–450). Malden, MA: Blackwell.

Reply to Decker

Daryl Pullman

Kevin Decker has provided an interesting and engaging critique of universalism that presents a number of challenges that any defender of that view must address. In what follows, I will attempt a response to some of these criticisms and counterclaims.

Before turning to key points at which we disagree, however, I want to note a number of points at which we agree. We agree, for example, that principles play an important role in moral discourse in general, and in ethical decision-making in medicine and medical research in particular. We agree as well that the particulars of any given situation must inform when and how a given principle should apply; nothing about the form of universalism I espouse is incompatible with Decker's pragmatist perspective that "emphasizes judgment and action as continuous with each other, and sees ethical deliberation as a phase in problem-solving in concrete, lived experience." Finally, we both agree that irrespective of one's position on the question of universalism, there are certain kinds of moral relativism one wants to avoid. In particular, we both eschew the view that all moral perspectives are equally valid. Thus, each of us maintains that part of the point of morality is to convince others to share our moral point of view. As such, each of us is committed to some form of moral progress.

It is this last point of agreement, however, that raises the greatest challenge for the particularist. Any robust moral theory aims to prescribe and proscribe certain kinds of actions and activities not only for those within a narrowly circumscribed community, but also for moral agents outside of a particular cultural or historical context. But once any notion of universals is jettisoned, it is difficult to justify why one particular moral perspective should be considered either superior or inferior to any other. Decker accepts a form of moral relativism that states "moral truth and justifiability … are in some ways relative to factors that are culturally and historically contingent" (Wong, 1993, p. 442). I accept this form of relativism as well when it comes to particular moral judgments. However, it is not clear, from the particularist's perspective, how this version of relativism is materially different from that which Decker wants to avoid. That is, if morality is only a matter of contingent historical and cultural values, on what grounds can one argue that slavery was morally wrong in nineteenth-century America, that Nazi medical experiments on hapless prisoners were wrong from *the* moral point of view, or that there is anything morally problematic about a society that practices ritual torture and murder. Indeed, Richard Rorty (1989) admits that on his version of pragmatism, there is no neutral ground (i.e., no moral point of view) from which to distinguish the moral difference between torture and kindness (173). Nevertheless, he holds on to what he calls "ungroundable desires" which includes "hope that suffering will be diminished" and that "the humiliation of human

Contemporary Debates in Bioethics, First Edition. Edited by Arthur L. Caplan and Robert Arp.

beings by other human beings may cease" (p. xv). Rorty's move from an inability to distinguish a moral difference between torture and kindness to a notion of moral progress measured by greater solidarity with humankind does not invoke the language of moral suasion; it is instead tantamount to an existential leap of faith. While Decker does not necessarily endorse Rorty's brand of pragmatism, it is not immediately apparent how he can avoid a similar irrational leap, given his general view of the contingent nature of all moral principles and hence of all morality.

The version of universalism I defend trades on a fundamental distinction between the *form* of moral discourse and the *content* of particular moral judgments. Part of the problem with Decker's critique of universalism comes from a tendency to conflate the two. Decker is right to note that on-the-ground bioethical problem-solving (i.e., the content of moral discourse) relies largely on the notion of social or personal dignity to do much of the work. However, he is wrong to dismiss the universal principle of basic human dignity as morally vacuous. As a formal constraint on moral discourse, the principle of respect for human dignity functions primarily as a meaning constraint on our moral language. In this sense, the principle does have the kind of self-evident and coercive force of which Hannah Arendt spoke (and Decker quoted in his chapter).

Moral discourse does not consist in applying a series of universal rules to particular cases such as "one must never lie," "one must never kill," or "one must never torture another human being." There could well be exceptional circumstances in which a moral case could be made to justify lying, killing, or even torture. What the universal moral principle of respect for human dignity demands of moral agents, however, is that some morally defensible justification for the act of lying, killing, or torture must be forthcoming. That is, we simply cannot say that there is no need to justify such prima facie unethical acts because in some particular historical and cultural circumstance, such acts are considered morally neutral or perhaps even praiseworthy. Indeed, such acts are prima facie unethical precisely because they offend the universal principle that constrains the form of our moral discourse in the first place. To put it bluntly, to argue there is no neutral ground by which to distinguish a moral difference between torture and kindness is to speak moral nonsense; such a position fails to understand what the moral enterprise is all about. That enterprise presupposes a moral epistemology that trades on the general universal principle that all human beings deserve moral consideration. Even Dewey—who argued for the contingency of everyday moral principles and the need to adapt such principles to contemporary conditions and needs—appealed to a higher-order *responsibility* of each generation "to overhaul its inherited stock of moral principles," and an *obligation* to "discover what principles are relevant to our social estate" (Dewey & Tufts, 1906, p. 283, my emphasis). I would submit that the *responsibility* and *obligation* to which Dewey refers are morally binding, and that their moral force is drawn from the universal form of moral discourse for which the inherited stock of particular moral principles serves as content.

I want to conclude with a brief response to one of Kevin Decker's criticisms that appears not in his original essay, but rather in his response to me. I am speaking now of the supposed problem of speciesism that my brand of universalism ostensibly entails. I want to address this issue here because it points to another key distinction that is of material importance to how we think about the nature of morality in general and moral obligation in particular, and also because it may help to explain something of the moral reach of the universal principle of respect for human dignity that I defend.

Now, the supposed problem of speciesism is that it privileges distinctly human traits over those of nonhuman animals and nonhuman nature in general. Inasmuch as I defend the principle of respect for human dignity (not nonhuman dignity), the charge that my position privileges the human over the nonhuman is true. In this sense, I am certainly a speciesist. But here it is important to distinguish moral agents from moral subjects. Humans alone have the capacity for moral agency, and as such they alone are morally praiseworthy or blameworthy. It is this capacity for moral agency that Kant referred to as the autonomous will. Although other species lack the capacity for moral agency, they are nevertheless included in the community of moral subjects, as are ecosystems and a broad variety of other objects, systems, and projects for which human beings bear moral responsibilities.

On the view I am advancing here, failing to treat nonhuman moral subjects appropriately is a moral failing not because it violates their intrinsic dignity, but because to do so fails to express the fundamental dignity of people like us. So, while human beings may raise animals for slaughter, they are morally obligated to treat them humanely. Failing to do so offends our basic dignity and threatens to make us less than what we can be as moral beings. On the other hand, failing to respect the dignity of other human agents such as when prisoners are tortured or otherwise treated inhumanely violates not only the fundamental dignity of those prisoners but also the basic dignity of the perpetrators. Recognizing and responding to these failings constitutes moral progress for us as a species of moral agents, while failing to respond constitutes moral regress. It is worth noting here that in the above examples, the heavy moral lifting is being done by the universal principle of basic dignity. It is such universals that set the moral limits for the particular judgments that are made in our everyday ethical deliberations.

References

Dewey, J., & Tufts, J. H. (1906). *Ethics*. London: Henry Holt and Company.

Rorty, R. (1989). *Contingency, irony and solidarity*. Cambridge: Cambridge University Press.

Wong, D. (1993). Moral relativism. In P. Singer (Ed.), *A companion to ethics* (pp. 442–450). Malden, MA: Blackwell.

Reply to Pullman

Kevin S. Decker

In Daryl Pullman's thoughtful and cogent defense of principlism, he claims, "Our concept of morality is predicated on the intrinsic moral worth or dignity of humanity. The essence of morality is to guard, protect, and advance this fundamental value." Another way of putting this is that "basic dignity functions as a meaning constraint on moral discourse." The appeal to human dignity does have an important role to play in medicine, but its status as a universal principle is dubious. Among the reasons for believing this is the fact that the appeal to dignity, properly understood, is clearly defeasible: it may often be trumped by other moral or even nonmoral attitudes that we value. In many other cases, the principle of preserving dignity may appear vacuous, or may simply not apply. Let's work through these considerations in reverse order.

Human Dignity and Speciesism

There are a number of types of significant bioethical problems that the principle of human dignity leaves unaddressed, including experimentation with nonhuman animals and the genetic manipulation of germ lines of plants and animals, and questions of therapy and enhancement where what is at stake is the very question of what human dignity entails. Given limited space, I can only deal with the first two of these three areas.

Appeals to the principle of human dignity often deal *indirectly* with issues of experimentation and nonhuman genetics by claiming that nonhuman nature has a derivative moral status, or that it has no status at all, and so may be disposed of as we wish. Such appeals typically invoke some form of the Kantian dichotomy between "persons" and "things." While similar pre-Kantian distinctions were ultimately dependent upon theology, Kant's rests on a secular, if speculative, metaphysics. Kant, in his own times, simply confirmed the overwhelmingly accepted underlying wisdom about a special human nature, a view that coexisted with racism, sexism, and outrageous human degradation. And Kant's theory is also increasingly untenable after the 1859 publication of Darwin's *Origin of Species* and the theory of evolution by natural selection presented there (Dewey, 1910; Decker, 2009).

These considerations point the criticism that human dignity implies speciesism. On this view, speciesists privilege distinctively human traits over those of nonhuman animals. The special moral category of "being human" can be qualified by the fact that humans (a) are rational, autonomous, agents, (b) possess language, (c) have the ability to participate in agreements on which morality depends, (d) are more sensitive to harm than other creatures, or any combination of these. Yet all these contrasts are highly arguable (Rachels, 1990, pp. 184–194).

Contemporary Debates in Bioethics, First Edition. Edited by Arthur L. Caplan and Robert Arp.

On the other hand, to *directly* grapple with issues regarding nonhuman nature, bioethics should be guided by reflection on evolutionary theory. Here, the morally significant differences between human and nonhuman animals do not resolve in terms of the differentiation of "species" groups. Instead, moral differences and similarities vary based on the animals concerned, human or nonhuman, and on context. James Rachels (1990) suggests a basic presupposition of equality between living things, supplemented by this principle: "If A is to be treated differently from B, the justification must be in terms of A's individual characteristics and B's individual characteristics. Treating them differently cannot be justified by pointing out that one or the other is a member of some preferred group, not even the 'group' of human beings" (pp. 173–174). Of course, this principle alone will not cover all the bioethical deliberations in which the principle of human dignity says nothing, but that is because no principle is universal.

In his contribution, Pullman also takes the principle of human dignity as "a logical primitive or fundamental axiom in moral discourse." Yet there could be cases in which we are clearly engaged in moral discourse, without this fundamental axiom applying—for example, when we ask about whether it is ethical for farmers to plant genetically engineered seed, which could lead to the contamination of neighboring organic crops. Clearly, there are moral determinations to be made here, but the question of human dignity never arises. Each such example adds to the evidence that human dignity is not definitive of our moral lives.

The Redundancy of Basic Dignity

Pullman (2010) holds that there are really two senses of dignity, a "universal, basic, ascriptive conception of human dignity" and "various particular, personal, and expressivist accounts" (p. 359). The normative force of *basic* dignity is that "any human entity enjoys a *prima facie* claim to moral consideration simply by virtue of being human" (p. 359). On the other hand, socially constructed personal dignity is "tied to notions of self-respect and self-esteem, and is intimately related to the complex social and psychological processes involved in self-formation and self-expression. As such, perspectives on personal dignity will vary with historical, cultural and traditional experiences and values" (p. 359).

While these definitions are clear and cogent, on-the-ground bioethical problem-solving need utilize only personal dignity to do all its work. The notion of "basic" dignity, meanwhile, is morally vacuous. Even Pullman (2001) concedes the limits of basic dignity's practicality: "Consideration of basic dignity does not tell us, for example, how to respond to questions about abortion, euthanasia, human cloning, or anything else among the myriad moral conundrums that face us today … The detailed moral content on these and other issues will have to come from other sources. The notion of personal dignity is one of these other sources" (p. 348). It is only a short step to further claims that the normative force of particular conceptions of dignity is enough.

Basic dignity places an enormous amount of weight on the idea that humans qua humans are due "moral consideration." But the meaning of "moral consideration" varies wildly. Hospital staff extend moral consideration, for example, to a homeless patient in admitting her to the emergency room, but her case may be low priority in triage because of her lack of ability to communicate her symptoms. The Aztecs extended moral consideration to the victims of their conquests by imprisoning them for later sacrifice: in Mesoamerica, being a sacrifice carried far greater moral and religious standing than simply being slaughtered on the field of battle. I am not claiming that the treatment of the sick, impoverished woman or of the Aztecs' victims is morally correct; just that both situations seem to involve basic moral consideration that nonetheless lack correct moral follow-through.

"Thick" examples of personal dignity may be socially constructed, but what is the moral status of basic dignity as a universal principle? It surely cannot be true that "the idea that humanity has intrinsic worth has functioned historically as a kind of logical primitive in moral discourse" (Pullman, 2010, p. 360). Many cultures lack corresponding concepts for "intrinsic worth" and "humanity" (a species concept). Religious history alone—particularly that of the Abrahamic religions—gives us many counterexamples in which the *infinite worth* of a divine being and its commands outweighs moral consideration of the mere "intrinsic worth" of human beings; particularly if they are heretics or infidels. In fact, the construction of the "idea that all human beings have basic moral worth irrespective of any contingent historical, traditional, or cultural circumstance" has its own historical and traditional story (Pullman, 2001, p. 342; Habermas, 2010, pp. 470–475). We can reasonably expect that another story could supersede this one in the near future, with the claim to basic human dignity radically challenged by environmental depredation or identity-altering technological changes.

In fact, to have the kind of normative force that advocates of basic dignity claim for this principle, dignity cannot be merely an empirical generalization from particular senses of personal dignity. It must be the "ground" of personal dignity, an unchanging and solid foundation rationalizing personal dignity. Interpretive studies of elder patient caregivers shows that personal dignity always references either *claims* (by a subject) or *imputations* (on behalf of a subject) to self-esteem and the esteem of others in bodily, intellectual, and/or spiritual ways (Jakobsen & Sørlie, 2010). In such clinical settings, a medical facility's basic commitment to *therapeutic care* and *restoration of health* does not need to be clarified by reference to a transcendental sense of dignity. Similarly, in research, codified commitments to refrain from causing concretely specified forms of harm to subjects also do all the work, leaving none for basic dignity.

Conclusion

The root of "transcendental" approaches to universal principles (like those of Thomas Aquinas and Kant) and the desire to defend a static concept of "basic" dignity is an understandable one: it comes from our psychological discomfort with uncertainty and the desire to make judgments firmly anchored in truth. This has led philosophers, scientists, and medical practitioners to what John Dewey calls a "quest for certainty" that squanders precious intellectual capital on, among other things, the search for universal principles (Dewey, 1929). But implementing the means for forming reasoned judgments based on claims or imputations of particular, personal "dignities," together with the institutional approach to morality that I outlined in my preceding chapter, provide a compelling response to the claims of universalism. While it is sometimes unfortunate that none of us possesses precisely the same moral intuitions as every other, the many commonalities that issue from our shared human condition make the piecemeal work of bioethical deliberation and consensus building possible.

References

Decker, K. S. (2009). Teaching autonomy and emergence through popular culture. *Teaching Philosophy*, *32*(4), 331–343.

Dewey, J. (1910). *The influence of Darwinism on philosophy and other essays in contemporary thought*. New York: Henry Holt and Company.

Dewey, J. (1929). *The quest for certainty: A study of the relation of knowledge and action*. London: George Allen & Unwin.

Habermas, J. (2010). The concept of human dignity and the realistic utopia of human rights. *Metaphilosophy*, *41*(4), 464–480.

Jakobsen, R., & Sørlie, V. (2010). Dignity of older people in a nursing home: Narratives of care providers. *Nursing Ethics*, *17*(3), 289–300.

Pullman, D. (2001). Universalism, particularism and the ethics of dignity. *Christian Bioethics*, 7(3), 333–358.

Pullman, D. (2010). Human non-persons, feticide, and the erosion of dignity. *Bioethical Inquiry*, 7, 353–364.

Rachels, J. (1990). *Created from animals: The moral implications of Darwinism*. Oxford: Oxford University Press.

Part 2

Is It Morally Acceptable to Buy and Sell Organs for Human Transplantation?

Introduction

"While people's lives continue to be put at risk by the dearth of organs available for transplantation, we must give urgent consideration to any option that may make up the shortfall. A market in organs from living donors is one such option. The market should be ethically supportable, and have built into it, for example, safeguards against wrongful exploitation. This can be accomplished by establishing a single purchaser system within a confined marketplace." The preceding is the abstract from a 2003 paper by Charles Erin and John Harris in the *Journal of Medical Ethics* titled, "An Ethical Market in Human Organs" (Erin & Harris, 2003). Depending upon one's perspective, what they say might strike one person as straightforwardly sensible, or another person as downright reprehensible. Interestingly enough, we praise the person who donates one of their organs, but do not ordinarily praise—and may even condemn—the person who wants to sell a body part. This condemnation occurs notwithstanding the fact that there are many more patients who need organ transplants than there are persons who are willing to provide them altruistically. For example, in 2008, in the United States there were an estimated 139,917 patients waiting for organ donations, yet only 27,281 organ transplants occurred (HRSA, 2009). What might be some of the reasons that a market in human organs is considered reprehensible even in the face of extreme shortage?

Someone of a religious bent might claim that the human body is a sacred temple housing some kind of divine or supernatural entity such as a soul, and *both* body and soul may have been given as a gift from God. Thus, although it is true that the human body is extended in space and time, and subject to physical laws of the universe like any other material thing, its specialness and uniqueness as (a) the temple of the

Contemporary Debates in Bioethics, First Edition. Edited by Arthur L. Caplan and Robert Arp.

soul and (b) a gift from some god(s) means that it should not be treated like any other object, and especially not like a commodity to be bought and sold (May, 1977; CBPC, 1991).

One need not be religious, however, to draw the same conclusion regarding not treating the human body like a commodity. Immanuel Kant's (1724–1804) deontological moral theory emphasizes respect for persons, and this respect can be extended to persons' bodies since, after all, a person can be understood as an *embodied* human being who is rational, free, and responsible (Kant, 1775–89/1963, 1785/1998, 1797/1996; LRCC, 1992; Munzer, 1993; Cohen, 1999; Morelli, 1999).

Interestingly enough, Kant's morality has also been used by proponents of a market in human organs. The part of Kant's morality emphasizing the fact that rational beings are seen as *autonomous*—that is, free to make choices for themselves unimpeded by any coercion—is what becomes significant here. Fundamental rights to privacy and the use of one's body as one sees fit, for example, are viewed as elements of this autonomy, and it is arguable that the right to ownership over one's own body in exercising decisions is the most fundamental of these rights. If an *embodied* human being is autonomous in this sense, then surely she can choose to either donate *or sell* parts of her body, if desired. It is her body, and she can do with her body whatever she sees fit to do with it, including offering it or parts of it to the highest bidder (Markowitz, 1990; Schwarzenbach, 1998; Gill & Sade, 2002; cf. Gerrand, 1999; Merle, 2000; Wilkinson, 2010). Ron Brown (1999) summarizes this commonsense Kantian-based position: "Simply stated, the moral justification is this: each adult owns his body and thus has the absolute right to make all decisions regarding it, providing he abstains from using force or fraud on others."

In the first chapter of this section, Mark Cherry puts forward this "It's my body, and I'll do what I want with it" kind of argument: "A person's authority over himself, his freedom of choice over the use of his body and mind, is part-and-parcel of maintaining personal integrity." This autonomy is oftentimes appealed to in cases where one *donates* an organ, so why shouldn't this autonomy extend to the *selling* of organs? As Cherry notes, "Public policy that prohibits consensual organ procurement from persons who are willing to donate, provided that they receive financial payments or other valuable incentives, denies the very authority of persons over themselves that justifies organ procurement in the first place."

Utilitarian and other consequence-based moral reasons figure as much into the debate concerning the market in human organs, as do Kantian and other deontological-based moral reasons. The standard utilitarian reasoning utilized in favor of a market in human organs is fairly simple: if human organs are needed in the transplant community—which they obviously are—and we can supply them by offering a financial incentive to people, and if people are willing to pay and donors are willing to accept the risks involved, then the end result will be plenty more people surviving, which is an obviously beneficial consequence to the transplant community. Thus, the straightforwardly moral thing to do is allow people to buy and sell human organs, which, at present, is illegal in nearly every nation including the United States (NOTA, 1984; Territo & Matteson, 2012). In the midst of dispelling medical myths, offering counterarguments, and reminding us of the fact that medicine, medical procedures and, in many cases, the human body itself all are instrumental goods in the biomedical marketplace—after all, people sell and pay for a myriad of medical procedures and services, as well as for cadavers, all over the world (Callahan & Wasunna, 2006; Rice & Unruh, 2009)—Cherry also endorses a consequence-based moral reason for a market in human organs,: "altruism-based systems of organ donation are not working adequately, whereas a market in human organs and other body parts would efficiently and effectively save lives, reduce human suffering, encourage highly skilled professional medical practice, and respect the authority of persons over their own bodies."

In the second chapter of this section, Art Caplan notes: "selling organs, even in a tightly regulated market, violates the existing bioethical framework of respect for persons since the sale is clearly being driven by profit." Continuing, Caplan maintains that a market in human organs "violates the ethics of medicine itself" since the "creation of commerce in body parts puts medicine in the position of removing body parts from people solely to abet those people's interest in securing compensation as well as to let middle-men profit." Thus, in opposition to Cherry, Caplan is clearly uncomfortable with the fact that medicine and medical procedures exist as marketplace phenomena. But, at least part of this discomfort is well deserved, since money, or the lack thereof, oftentimes determines access to vital medical care (Wong, 1998; Callahan & Wasunna, 2006; Powers & and Faden, 2006; Hansen, 2008). And any market will be rife with exploitation, despite numerous regulations as well as checks and balances (Radin, 1996; Wertheimer, 1996).

In response to the "It's my body, and I'll do what I want with it" kind of argument, Caplan points out the harsh reality that most people who would be willing to sell a body part are poor, so the decision to sell a body part hardly seems rational and free in the robust Kantian sense: "Talk of individual rights and autonomy is hollow if those with no options must 'choose' to sell their organs to purchase life's basic necessities." Especially since those in the medical profession are supposed to uphold the "do no harm" principle, it seems all the more egregious for medical professionals to be engaging in exploitative behavior. In an attempt to sidestep the exploitation that seems to be inherent in any market, at the end of his chapter Caplan favors default to donation programs like those advocated in Spain, Italy, Austria, France, and Belgium. In such a program, an individual is presumed to wish to donate their body or body parts upon death, unless they make the conscious decision to opt out of the program. And Caplan points to data that would seem to indicate that such programs are working.

References

Brown, R. (1999). A free market in human organs. *Freedom Daily*. February 1. Retrieved from: http://www.fff.org/freedom/0296e.asp

Callahan, D., & Wasunna, A. (2006). *Medicine and the market: Equity v. choice*. Baltimore, MD: The Johns Hopkins University Press.

CBPC (Chilean Bishops' Permanent Commission). (1991). On organ transplants. *Catholic International, 15*(30), 374–375.

Cohen, C. (1999). Selling bits and pieces of humans to make babies. *Journal of Medicine and Philosophy, 24*(3), 288–306.

Erin, C., & Harris, J. (2003). An ethical market in human organs. *Journal of Medical Ethics, 29*, 137–138.

Gerrand, N. (1999). The misuse of Kant in the debate about a market for human body parts. *Journal of Applied Philosophy, 16*(1), 59–67.

Gill, M., & Sade R. (2002). Payment for kidneys: The case for repealing prohibition. *Kennedy Institute of Ethics Journal, 12*(1), 17–46.

Hansen, F. (2008). A revolution in healthcare: Medicine meets the marketplace. *Institute of Public Affairs (January), 43–45.*

HRSA (Health Resources and Services Administration) (2009). 2009 annual report. Retrieved from: http://optn.transplant.hrsa.gov/AR2009.exe

Kant, I. (1775–89/1963). *Lectures on ethics* (L. Infield, Trans.). Indianapolis, IN: Hackett Publishing.

Kant, I. (1785/1998). *Groundwork of the metaphysics of morals* (M. Gregor, Trans.). (Section I: Transition from common rational to philosophic moral cognition). Cambridge: Cambridge University Press.

Kant, I. (1797/1996). *Practical philosophy* (M. Gregor, Trans.). Cambridge: Cambridge University Press.

LRCC (Law Reform Commission of Canada). (1992). *Procurement and transfer of human tissues and organs: Working paper 66*. Ottawa, Canada: Communication Group Publishing.

Markowitz, S. (1990). Abortion and feminism. *Social Theory and Practice, 16*, 1–17.

May, W. (1977). *Human existence, medicine and ethics*. Chicago: Franciscan Herald Press.

Merle, J. (2000). A Kantian argument for a duty to donate one's organs: A reply to Nicole Gerrand. *Journal of Applied Philosophy, 17*(1), 93–101.

Morelli, M. (1999). Commerce in organs: A Kantian critique. *Journal of Social Philosophy, 30*(2), 315–324.

Munzer, S. (1993). Kant and property rights in body parts. *Canadian Journal of Law and Jurisprudence, 6*(2), 319–331.

NOTA (National Organ Transplant Act: Public Law 98-507). (1984). Retrieved from: http://history.nih.gov/research/downloads/PL98-507.pdf; also see http://optn.transplant.hrsa.gov/policiesAndBylaws/nota.asp

Powers, M., & Faden, R. (2006). *Social justice: The moral foundations of public health and health policy*. Oxford: Oxford University Press.

Radin, M.J. (1996). *Contested commodities: The trouble with trade in sex, children, body parts, and other things*. Cambridge, MA: Harvard University Press.

Rice, T., & Unruh, L. (2009). *The economics of health reconsidered*. Chicago: Health Administration Press.

Schwarzenbach, S. (1998). On owning the body. In J. Elias, V. Bullough, V. Elias, & G. Brewer (Eds.), *Prostitution: On whores, hustlers, and johns* (pp. 345–351). Amherst, NY: Prometheus Books.

Territo, L., & Matteson, R. (Eds.). (2012). *The international trafficking of human organs.* Boca Raton, FL: Taylor & Francis.

Wertheimer, A. (1996). *Exploitation.* Princeton, NJ: Princeton University Press.

Wilkinson, M. (2010). Sell organs to save lives. *The British Broadcasting Company (BBC) News.* August 27. Retrieved from: http://www.bbc.co.uk/news/health-10786211

Wong, K. (1998). *Medicine and the marketplace: The moral dimensions of managed care.* Notre Dame, IN: University of Notre Dame Press.

Chapter Three

It Is Morally Acceptable to Buy and Sell Organs for Human Transplantation

Moral Puzzles and Policy Failures

Mark J. Cherry

In this chapter, I argue that embracing market-based incentives for organ procurement would save lives and reduce human suffering, while helping to contain economic costs and stretch healthcare budgets. Financial and other valuable incentives would encourage living persons to donate redundant internal organs, while also increasing access to nonredundant organs with donors (or their families) granting permission for organ harvesting after death. Legislating "altruism" on the part of donors (or the donor's family), coerces self-sacrifice in an otherwise commercial setting, where surgeons, nurses, pharmaceutical companies, hospitals, third-party procurement agencies, government bureaucrats, as well as organ recipients openly profit. At stake, however, is not solely the efficiency and effectiveness of transplantation practice, but more fundamentally the recognition of the moral authority of persons over themselves. Openly embracing a market in human organs for transplantation would encourage virtuous tendencies in transplantation, shed light on what is often a hazy and shrouded policy setting, while better addressing the shortage in human organs for transplantation.

Introduction

Alicia and James are living kidney donors. Each has arranged to donate a kidney to save the life of a child of a close acquaintance, who is in need of transplant. Both are aware that kidney donation comes with the attendant risks of surgery; each seeks to minimize the risks by working with a well-known hospital with a good reputation for providing high-quality medical care for organ donors. Alicia and James both enjoy the recognition that they are saving a life and reducing human suffering. Many consider their actions to be heroic: saving the life of another at some risk to oneself. While James is donating his redundant kidney for free, Alicia has asked the mother of her organ recipient for a significant cash reward, which the mother has happily agreed to pay. What is the moral difference, if any, between Anna and James?

Paid rescue workers, who risk their lives to help others, are accepted in many facets of life. Fire fighters, police officers, Coast Guard naval rescuers, as well as ski search and rescue teams, each risk life and personal injury to help others while collecting a salary. While one may work as a volunteer fire fighter, that someone

Contemporary Debates in Bioethics, First Edition. Edited by Arthur L. Caplan and Robert Arp.

chooses to be paid for services does not reduce the honor of the occupation. With regard to Alicia and James, the organ retrieval surgery will be exactly the same—indeed, all of the medical aspects of the two cases are identical. Consequently, it is unclear why there ought to be any moral difference between compensated and uncompensated organ donation. The legal difference between the two cases is startling: James's choice is praised, encouraged, the subject of positive educational propaganda, and legal; Alicia's request for compensation is decried, denounced, and subject to legal punishment almost everywhere in the world. Why?

The prevailing moral viewpoint is that human organs may be donated, but they should not be sold, despite the shortfall in organs available for transplantation and the consequent increase in human suffering and the deaths of otherwise salvageable patients. Commentators opine that human organs should not be viewed as commodities to be sold for private gain, but rather treasured as an altruistic gift, a social resource to be distributed according to medical criteria. Prohibitions on financial incentives for organ donation are often couched in lofty moralistic terms (e.g., "preserve the nobility of organ donation" (Declaration of Istanbul); International Summit on Transplant Tourism and Organ Trafficking, 2008, p. 1227) and manipulative educational campaigns (e.g., "Give the Gift of Life"). Organ transplantation, it is claimed, should transcend commercial practices and rise above marketplace morality. Yet, the urgent public health challenge due to the considerable disparity between the number of patients who could benefit from organ transplantation and the number of organs available for transplant will not be adequately addressed by the vilification of commodification and market transactions. Despite the fact that such assumptions underlie nearly all public policy regarding organ procurement and transplantation, I conclude that each is misguided and illegitimate.

Embracing market-based incentives for organ procurement would save lives and reduce human suffering, while helping to contain economic costs and stretch healthcare budgets. Financial and other valuable incentives (e.g., college scholarships, tax incentives) would encourage living persons to donate redundant internal organs (e.g., a kidney), while also increasing access to nonredundant organs (e.g., the heart) with donors or their families granting permission for organ harvesting after death. Legislating "altruism" on the part of donors or the donor's family coerces self-sacrifice in an otherwise commercial setting, where surgeons, nurses, pharmaceutical companies, hospitals, third-party procurement agencies, government bureaucrats, as well as organ recipients openly profit. At stake, however, is not solely the efficiency and effectiveness of transplantation practice, but more fundamentally the recognition of the moral authority of persons over themselves. Openly embracing a market in human organs for transplantation would encourage virtuous tendencies in transplantation, shed light on what is often a hazy and shrouded policy setting, while better addressing the shortage in human organs for transplantation.

Some Background Numbers

To assess current transplantation policy realistically, one must also consider the background risks involved in organ transplantation bereft of the significant and valuable incentives of the commercial market. The United Network for Organ Sharing (UNOS) documents that, in the United States alone, some 7182 patients died in 2008 while waiting for an organ transplant (UNOS, 2009, table 1.6). Many more patients die each year after being removed from the transplant waiting lists because they have become too ill to transplant. Others endure suffering, often in hospital on life support, or in expensive outpatient treatments, while queuing for available organs. In 2008, in the United States only 27,281 organ transplants occurred despite the 139,917 patients who queued on the waiting list at some point during that year. At the end of 2007, the waiting list was populated with 96,874 candidates for transplant, compared to some 100,597 at the end of 2008; UNOS currently lists 111,776 candidates (as of August 4, 2011). There has been a 56.6% increase in demand for transplantable organs from 1999 to 2007 (UNOS, Chapter 1, p. 1). While demand for organs has risen significantly, organ donation rates in the United States have been relatively stagnant for some time, with the availability of organs declining over the past five years (UNOS,

Chapter 2). Organs are procured primarily from cadaveric sources; however, living donation constitutes a significant portion of kidney donation (5966 out of 16,067), with a growing number of living liver-lobe donations (249 out of 5568) (OPTN, 1999–2004; UNOS, 2009). Altruism-based policies for organ donation have simply not been adequate to meet the medical demand for transplantation.

The usual circumstance of transplant patients without a private donor is an evermore significant wait and risk of death. UNOS reports, for example, that patients in need of a kidney transplant, with blood type O, who registered in 2001/2002, experienced a median wait time of 1833 days; those with blood type B, who registered in 2001/2002, experienced a median wait time of 2033 days. Patients in need of a liver transplant, with blood type O, who registered in 2001/2002, experienced a median wait time of 1228 days (UNOS, 2009). Given increased demand for human organs, and a concurrently increased queuing time, median wait times for patients with less common blood types, and highly sensitized recipients, has become difficult to calculate accurately because fewer patients as a percentage of those queuing have received a transplant since listing (Hippen, 2005; Xue et al., 2005).

As queuing time for organ transplantation has increased, direct and indirect health risks have increased as well. Patients with end-stage renal failure not due to diabetes have a mortality rate of approximately 60% at five years while waiting for organs; morality rates are worse for patients whose renal failure is due to diabetes. Even queuing for less than six months has a long-term negative impact on health risks relative to preemptive transplantation (Meier-Kriesche and Kaplan, 2002; Abou Ayache et al., 2005). Over time, the body becomes more fragile, creating greater likelihood of poor post-transplant outcomes. According to one study, during a 33-month period, 85 transplant candidates on the waiting list at the University of Minnesota died awaiting transplant (63 waiting for kidney transplant, 22 for simultaneous pancreas–kidney transplant). The transplant candidates' mean age at death was 53 (±11) years. Of the 85 patients, 71% were waiting for a first transplant, and 62% had a 0% panel-reactive antibody level at the time of death (see Casingal et al., 2006). As Arthur Matas, Benjamin Hippen, and Sally Satel (2008) comment regarding this study, "it would have been easy to find a kidney for them, if there were a sufficient supply" (p. 380). The median wait time for a donor kidney routinely exceeds the median life expectancy of dialysis-dependent transplant candidates (Matas et al., 2008). If the median wait time for kidney transplantation continues to increase, which seems likely, it will surpass the life expectancy of an evermore significant portion of potential recipients.

Sustaining patients medically while they await transplantation is very expensive. Financial costs to care for the end-stage renal population increased 57% between 1999 and 2004 (Foley & Collins, 2007). Total Medicare costs for end-stage renal disease in 2000 was just over $12 billion; by 2008, Medicare expenditures for end-stage renal disease had increased to over $23 billion. In 2008, the cost per patient for dialysis was $76,587; in comparison, the per-person cost for transplant patients was $26,668, and for patients with a well-functioning graft, the cost was $19,104 (USRDS, 2010, tables K1 K6, K9, and K12). Insofar as wait times for transplantation can be reduced through financial incentives for organ donation, such incentives would save both monetary and medical resources, while decreasing suffering and improving life and health outcomes for patients.

Financial Incentives: Increasing Access to Transplantation

Such suffering is all the more tragic, since much of it could be prevented by legalizing an open market in human organs for transplantation. Creating significant incentives for living-organ donation will multiply the availability of organs, such as kidneys, bone marrow, and liver segments. The financial rewards helped motivate Alicia's decision to donate; it would likely prompt others to do the same. Some persons might be willing to consider a futures contract in which they agree to sell any usable organs upon their death to an organ-procurement agency, and have the money paid as a death benefit to their survivors. Similarly, financial and other valuable incentives would enable families to sell the organs of a decease loved one, rather than just to donate the organs. Incentives for families to make available body parts from recently deceased relatives would increase access to nonredundant organs, such as hearts, as well as bones, cornea, and other useful body parts from deceased donors. Knowing that their families would financially benefit would likely encourage many more potential donors to state their intentions to be organ donors.

Financial and other market-based incentives encourage persons to raise resources to further personal goals and social interests. Such incentives drive technological and medical innovation; they possess significant motivational force independent of civic mindedness, self-sacrifice, and social solidarity. Other incentives for organ donation might include organ entitlements (i.e., higher priority on the waiting list for families whose members have donated organs), payment of funeral expenses, life-insurance contracts, and tax credits. If the thought of the donor's mother paying Alicia in cash for her kidney seems unduly crass, money need not change hands. Imagine instead Alicia being provided with a four-year college scholarship, or funding for graduate studies, such as medical or law school—a valuable incentive indeed! It is highly plausible that such valuable incentives would be successful in motivating the availability of human organs for transplantation. Each case is little different from the current system of organ donation except that donors, or their families, receive financial or other valuable compensation to stimulate donation. Utilizing various incentives creatively to fashion public policy could efficiently and effectively increase the availability of organs, thereby improving access to transplantation, reducing human suffering, and saving lives.

Barter markets (trafficking by exchange of commodities) in organs already exist, are morally praised, and are being expanded. Examples include paired kidney exchanges and "triple swap" kidney donation and transplant operations, in which three patients, who are not tissue compatible with their own willing donors, exchange their donor's kidney for a kidney from another of the three donors. Each willing donor provides a kidney to one of the three transplant patients (Delmonico et al., 2004; Saldman et al., 2006). Surgeons at Johns Hopkins University Hospital performed just such an organ swap in 2003, and since then what is often termed "human organ paired donation" has become more commonplace (Ferrari & De Klerk, 2009; Gumber et al. 2011). Kidney exchanges and triple-swap donation programs are forms of reciprocal directed donation. A similar kidney-exchange program was established in the Netherlands (De Klerk et al., 2005, 2006; Mahendran & Veitch, 2007). Importantly, such "directed donations" typically bring organs into the transplant pool that would otherwise not have been available (Paramesh et al., 2011). Nongovernmental programs, such as MatchingDonors.com, help those in need of transplant to arrange for potential organ exchanges. Soliciting donors in this manner increases access to transplantation. Most exchanges have been swaps among kidney donors, but other types of organ trades are possible: for example, a segment of healthy liver could be exchanged for a healthy kidney.

In 2007, section 301 of the United States National Organ Transplant Act (Public Law 110–144) was specifically revised to permit paired kidney exchanges and other types of organ exchanges for transplantation. The original Act prohibited the transfer of human organs for use in transplantation for any sort of "valuable consideration." It prohibited for-profit commercial harvesting, financial incentives, or other valuable consideration to encourage donation or sale of human organs for transplantation. As amended, "human organ paired donation," i.e., kidney swaps and other organ exchanges, do not violate the prohibition on receiving "valuable consideration." Amendment was necessary because paired organ exchanges were becoming increasingly popular, and receiving an organ in exchange for an organ, with each party thereby saving the life of a loved one, is quite obviously the receipt of "valuable consideration." The practice is straightforwardly a "trafficking by exchange of commodities"—a barter market in human organs for transplantation.

Human Organs Are Instrumental Goods

Critics charge that compensating organ donors, or their families, would reduce the human body to no more than an instrumental good, a thing, a commodity to be bought and sold. Consider, for example, the comments of S. Daniel Davis and Samuel Crowe (2009):

> Embedded within the ethic of generosity is the idea and the hope that individuals may freely, without any form of coercion, choose to give of themselves for the good—in this case, the health—of another ... In deference to the generosity of donors and the health of transplant recipients, physicians may, in good conscience, undertake the necessary surgical and medical interventions, confident that these interventions are consistent with the ends of medicine. If this ethic of generosity, however, gives way to an ethic of buying and selling, then physicians will be willing accomplices to both instrumentalization and commodification—consequences that would harm the profession of medicine. (p. 600)

This criticism, however, is misdirected: it regards not just compensated organ donation but the very practice of organ transplantation itself. One of the key moral issues underlying live organ donation, as highlighted in the examples of Alicia and James mentioned at the very beginning of this chapter, is the recognition that the transplant surgeon harvests a healthy organ from a healthy person so as to benefit some other fully separate person, who is sick and in need of transplant. In the case of deceased donation, which is usually carried out after the determination of death by neurological criteria, judgment is made that the donor no longer needs his organs (see Iltis & Cherry, 2010); consequently, organs can permissibly be surgically removed and placed into some other person. Transplantation demonstrates empirically that organs are manipulable and interchangeable with other organs of the same kind. This is the physical reality that makes transplantation medically viable. The intention is for the harvested organ to cease being a living part of the donor and to become a living part of the recipient, so transplant teams attempt to find a replacement organ that is as similar as possible to the body part they wish to replace. Such considerations underlie the careful histocompatibility testing for tissue-matching donor organs with potential recipients. This testing maps leukocyte antigens on the surface of the body's cells, which help the immune system protect the body against invaders. The immune system also recognizes the histocompatibility antigens from the tissues of other persons and may react against these antigens leading to the rejection of organ grafts. Transplant professionals attempt to match as many of the antigens as possible between the donor organ and the recipient to reduce the change of rejection (UNOS 2009). In short, transplantation medicine relies on the empirical fact that human organs are instrumentally useful things.

All systems of transplantation, including uncompensated organ donation, objectify human organs and utilize them as fungible replaceable objects. As a surgical practice, organ transplantation requires that we appreciate these body parts as exchangeable objects. Organ transplantation demands that we understand body parts as alienable; i.e., that persons can permissibly donate their redundant internal organs to benefit others, and that families can grant permission for organ harvesting after a patient's death. Instrumentalization of body parts does not flow from whether the donor was offered, requested, or received valuable compensation; instrumentalization of body parts is part and parcel of organ transplantation. As the American Medical Association Council on Ethical and Judicial Affairs (1993) noted, organs are a medical resource: "the shortage of organs is the most obvious example of scarcity in medical resources" (p. 1). Donors, surgeons, procurement agencies, and recipients alike objectify organs and treat them as instrumentally useful medical goods.

Indeed, the market in body parts is quite literally a billion-dollar industry, reaching well beyond organ transplantation:

> In the cadaver business, suppliers sell bodies and body parts to brokers, who in turn funnel them to buyers. Suppliers include morgues, medical schools, tissue banks, independent companies, funeral homes, and even, on occasion, crematoria. Brokers, who facilitate the corpse sales, may be independent businessmen or employees in some of the same places. Their clients include medical associations, major US corporations, researchers, doctors, and hospitals. The demand for bodies and parts surpasses the supply, which keeps the prices of human flesh and bones very high. Each corpse that travels through the system can generate anywhere from $10,000 to $100,000, depending on how it is used. (Cheney, 2006, p. 8; see also Waldby & Mitchell, 2006)

Medical research relies extensively on human body parts. Medical students learn financially valuable information and technical skill while working on human bodies and body parts. Human parts are useful for pharmaceutical, cosmetic, and surgical equipment development, and technical practice, to name but a few marketable uses. Museums display preserved bodies (mummies) as well as the plasticized human bodies in the "Body Worlds" exhibits. The reproduction industry buys and sells sperm and ova (Nelson, 2009), the wig industry buys human hair, and there exists potentially profitable research on human embryos, adult and embryonic stem cells, and human DNA. The market in human plasma, a blood component, is booming with private centers in the United States handling some 18.8 million transactions a year (the current rate is about $20.00 a pint; Kimes, 2009, p. 12). Body parts are commodities.

Marketplace Morality

It is fashionable in bioethics to believe that the role of the market in medicine is less than positive. A quasi-social-democratic political vision and ideological orientation functions as part of the taken-for-granted lingua franca of bioethics. This moral framework seeks to place medicine, and thereby transplantation, above what is characterized as the crass morality of the marketplace. Transplantation is to be set firmly within a morality of generosity and altruism, not the market. As an editorial in the *The Lancet* (2009) opined: "Ethical arguments have been made for and against the practice, with the pro side generally contending that legitimizing a market for organs would increase their availability. But human livers and kidneys are not commodities, and hospitals are not just another convenient locale for money to change hands. Trade in human organs is immoral and ought to be outlawed around the world" (p. 1901).

Having failed to appreciate the ways in which medicine treats livers, kidneys, bone marrow, and so forth as medical resources, the editorial leaves conveniently unstated that surgeons, nurses, hospital administrators, and other staff charge significant amounts of money for access to medical goods and services.

Medicine is a commodity: its goods and services are bought and sold, are valued over against other goods and services, are the subject of economic choices, and are given a monetary equivalence. Hospitals, physicians, and other healthcare workers demand payment for services rendered. Consider these statements regarding payment from the University of Pennsylvania Hospital (2011) website:

> The University of Pennsylvania Health System participates with many medical insurance plans. It is important to understand that your insurance policy is an agreement between you and your insurance carrier. We will submit the claim on your behalf, however that is not a guarantee of payment of the claim. Should your claim be rejected or only partially paid, your insurance company should send you an explanation of benefits. Ultimately, the fees are your responsibility. If we do not participate with your insurance plan, payment is expected at the time of service ... Co-pays, deductibles, co-insurances and fees for noncovered services are expected at the time of your service. A $12.00 administrative fee will be assessed if the co-pay is not paid at the time of service. For your convenience we accept cash, personal checks, Visa, MasterCard, American Express, and debit cards.

Even with state-based healthcare systems, citizens purchase medical care through various forms of high taxes. Such financial, billing, and taxing practices straightforwardly place medicine squarely within marketplace morality—that ethic of buying and selling goods and services.

Moreover, there is no good reason to believe that such circumstances are altogether lamentable. Whereas it has become commonplace to remark that medical research and patient care have become a lucrative enterprise, it would be shortsighted not to note the considerable advancements in material well-being and life expectancy that medical innovation has brought to the industrial world, which includes transplantation medicine (see Cherry, 2006). For-profit medical research has played a crucial role in demonstrating that many treatments once thought to be important parts of healthcare are ineffective, or at least less effective than new alternatives (consider, e.g., the development of advanced immunosuppresives to prevent organ graft rejection; see Ponticelli, 2011). Innovation has increased longevity while decreasing morbidity. Within transplantation, the market has led to important pharmaceutical innovation and greater use of "expanded criteria donors" or "marginal donors"; that is, "donors that would not have been considered suitable for donation previously" (Humar, 2004; UNOS, 2009). Such organs include those that in the past were believed to have an unacceptable risk for primary nonfunction or initial poor function. The positive result of such expanded criteria is that more organs are available for transplantation; the negative aspect is that such transplants often have inferior results, such as greater rates of complications or graft rejection. For liver transplantation, for example, there is a clear correlation between post-transplant outcomes and the quality of the organ graft (Mittler et al., 2008; Müllhaupt et al., 2008). Medical innovation requires the significant investment of economic resources. Financial rewards for organ donation would create significant incentives for innovation in many such areas.

Some critics believe that financially compensating organ donors involves an exchange of incommensurable values. The concern is that financial compensation will fail appropriately to weigh and compare economic versus noneconomic values. However, nonmarket-based strategies for procurement and allocation face similar difficulties. Government-based organ-confiscation policies, for example, are often framed to appear altruistic, even when they are in fact coercive. Presumed consent, for example, involves no actual consent from any actual person; instead, organs are simply taken, unless the individual has specifically and officially made his rejection of organ donation known, such as by signing the properly official forms. Similar challenges beset proposals for "routine retrieval" policies. Imagine a policy of "presumed consent to one's house": unless one specifically and officially stated otherwise, the government coercively takes ownership of one's house upon one's death. Even if it served some plausible state use, such a policy would be neither altruistic nor consensual. Estate taxes are confiscatory nonaltruistic contributions to the state. The government simply takes the funds for its own purposes. Normally, unless otherwise specified in a will or other legal document, the deceased's property—house or bodily remains—passes to the ownership of her/his heirs.

Financial transactions and other types of market exchanges do not require that the goods exchanged be precisely commensurable; such a restriction would rule out nearly all consensual transactions. Permissible transactions require that the parties transact voluntarily, that deception or other forms of coercion are not employed, and that each party agrees to the value or product to be received. This means that what is received in return is worth at least as much to the party as that which was given at the time of the transaction. One can buy or sell "priceless" works of art without claiming that its aesthetic or historic value is commensurate with the money that is paid (Wertheimer, 1992, p. 218). A "priceless" Picasso—"Nude, Green Leaves, and Bust"—was sold in May 2010, at auction in Christie's New York for some US$106.5 million. Money equivalence is usually understood in terms of what persons are willing to pay for the transfer of ownership, even in the case of so-called "priceless" objects.

Similar equivalences can be created for organs and other body parts. As a practical matter, if necessary, it should be possible to establish minimum prices with enforceable contractual duties for medical follow-up, so that compensation will be sufficient to have a significant positive impact on the donor's (or the donor's family's) life. For example, the valuable compensation could be framed to include education, vocational, or other training, on the model of the G.I. Bill, which provides tuition benefits for the college education of those who have served in the US armed forces. Although limiting compensation for organ donation to college scholarships seems to be unduly restrictive, they would be, as I have argued elsewhere, at least a step in the right direction (Cherry, 2009b).

Coerced Altruism

The persistent reference to organ donation as an "altruistic gift" framed within an "ethic of generosity" may be more lofty rhetoric than empirical reality. Presumably, many organ donations are fully motivated by altruistic concerns; however, it is difficult to know what percentage falls squarely into this category without any private negotiation for side-benefits, or implicit understandings of a quid pro quo. Human motivations are complex, multifaceted, and not always fully acknowledged. Requiring strict adherence to altruism may cause more harm than benefit. Most living donations are to family members. These donations are plausibly motivated by love or beneficence; however, they are just as plausibly motivated by family loyalty, gratitude, guilt, or avoidance of the shame of failing to donate. If James is the only member of his family who is tissue-compatible to donate a kidney to his niece, there will be a great deal of social pressure on him to donate—especially if the alternative is the niece's continued suffering and death. For these donors, their willingness to donate stems from their relationship with the particular patient and may not be fully altruistically motivated. Perhaps by donating a kidney to his niece, something he has good reason to do anyway, James believes that his uncle will reciprocate by paying for his college education or by providing a generous inheritance. Transplant surgeons also have complex motivations for practicing their profession: desires to do good, to obtain technical skill, to be paid a high salary, to gain reputation and professional recognition, each of which is compatible with providing high-quality surgical care. It holds donors to too high a standard to presume that they ought to be motivated only by an ethic of generosity or altruism. James should be permitted to save his niece's life, even if his motivations are in part self-serving.

Parents have put forth minor children as living donors, with parents consenting on behalf of those children. In *Hart v. Brown* 289 A.2d 386 (Conn. Super. Ct 1972), the court ruled that the parents of twin girls could consent on behalf of one twin to have a kidney procured and transplanted into her sister. As Angela Holder (1990) documents, "Almost all courts have granted these orders, based on the idea that the donor child derives benefit from the continued life of the sick sibling. The courts' theory is that a child derives more benefit from a happy home and the sibling relationship that he or she would from growing up with two kidneys. Other courts have dispensed with this concept of benefit and have simply found that parents are allowed to consent to donation by one healthy child to a sick child on the basis of a familial cost–benefit analysis" (p. 523). Couples have utilized in vitro fertilization with genetic testing so as to select embryos for implantation that, once born, are destined to become tissue donors for an already-living sibling (Sheldon & Wilkinson, 2004). The donor's altruism in such cases is nonexistent; nor is it plausible that the parents involved are acting selflessly through an ethic of generosity. Still, parents, together with transplantation professionals, seem better placed to make such medical and moral decisions than government bureaucrats.

That transplant recipients, surgeons, insurance companies, and organ procurement agencies would prefer to obtain human organs without financially compensating donors is understandable, but this fact does not imply that potential organ donors act wrongly when they seek or require valuable compensation prior to agreeing to donate. Access to organ transplantation is not free: transplant surgeons, hospitals, and organ procurement agencies charge a great deal of money for their services and expertise; pharmaceuticals and access to other medical goods and services are very expensive. Yet, the only party who is legally prohibited from seeking or accepting compensation for his part in this lucrative market is the organ donor (or his family). Forbidding compensated organ donation legislates altruism and self-sacrifice in an otherwise commercial setting. As long as transplantation utilizing human organs continues, these body parts will be appreciated as highly valuable scarce medical resources. What is at stake is not whether organs should be treated as commodities, but rather who should receive the valuable medical resource and who should bear the costs of appropriation and transfer.

That human organs can only be transferred at a price of zero does not reduce the value of the organs to zero. It straightforwardly transfers the value of the organ from the donor to other parties. Consequently, financially compensating donors of organs and other body parts would also be significantly fairer than the current system of prohibition. Insofar as legal statutes prohibit donors from accepting financial compensation, human organs are a highly constrained commodity, where the state requires donors to part with their valuable property without material compensation, whereas others benefit financially, and the recipient of the organ benefits physically, as well as perhaps financially, in terms of being able to return to work, reduced medical bills, and increased quality and quantity of life.

Persons and Their Bodies

An additional conceptual puzzle concerns the authority of persons to grant permission to organ procurement surgery—Alicia and James are each consenting to the same medical procedure. Common law jurisprudence has appreciated a right of persons to be secure against battery, a right not to be touched, which was grounded in the authority of persons over themselves, rather than in any particular view of the best interests of persons. The weight of this moral and legal tradition establishes persons as in authority to make their own judgments regarding acceptable risks and benefits as they collaborate with others through freedoms of association and contract. Persons are appreciated as possessing a dignity that should not be violated by being touched or used without permission, but who may consent to more or less risky activities. Persons may grant permission to be used in ways that, absent their consent, would be profoundly harmful. Permission marks the distinction, for example, of rape versus free love, sexual assault versus welcome seduction, assault, and battery versus kidney removal surgery. Persons may consent to risky activities and lifestyle choices—joining the military, working on oilrigs, engaging in tattooing and body piercings, breast enhancement or other forms of plastic surgery, or participating in promiscuous or risky sex. Individuals routinely set life and health at risk for national patriotism, for career advancement, or to enhance one's attractiveness to potential sex partners. Others need not approve of such choices; they may even decry the consequences as imprudent or deeply unfortunate. However, there is a prima facie lack of moral authority to interfere in the choices of persons who freely choose to act with consenting others.

Despite rhetoric to the contrary, human organs are not a scarce public resource; organs are retrieved from private persons, who have presumptive authority over themselves, their bodies, and the uses to which parts of their bodies will be put. A person's authority over himself, his freedom of choice over the use of his body and mind, is part and parcel of maintaining personal integrity. Absent agreement regarding the demands of God, or the requirements of moral rationality, individuals have been identified within rather broad side-constraints as the best judges of their own best interests and of their own preferred method for attempting to realize such interests. The authority of persons over themselves is core to the respect of persons that lies at the heart of moral and legal reflections on informed consent to medical treatments, which appreciates persons as able to grant permission to (even risky) medical activities—for example, by choosing to donate a kidney while living, or granting permission for one's organs to be donated upon one's death. The very jurisprudential tradition that makes organ donation morally permissible—the authority of persons over themselves, their own bodies and minds—is denied in the case of compensated organ donation, even though all of the medical aspects of the two cases are identical. Public policy that prohibits consensual organ procurement from persons who are willing to donate, provided that they receive financial payments or other valuable incentives, denies the very authority of persons over themselves that justifies organ procurement in the first place.

Moreover, such policy demeans persons, seeking to supplant personal judgment regarding one's own best interests with the judgment of government bureaucrats and academic bioethicists. It is the presumption that one knows what is in the best interests of others, what is most appropriate for their well-being, without even having asked the persons themselves. Such moralistic substituted judgment combined with legal prohibition on compensated donation uses other persons without their permission to achieve a particular view of moral propriety and human dignity. It fails to respect persons as capable of making prudential and moral decisions about their own fates. It denies persons the opportunity to choose on the basis of their own judgments how best to advantage themselves.

Conclusion

The development of a market for the procurement of organs provides no reason to stop asking patients or their families to consider donation. In the United States, extensive charity infrastructures exist side by side with for-profit markets for food, medicine, and housing. Financial incentives do not preclude the liberties of the altruistically inclined to realize their need to take care of others. Unless governmentally prohibited, even within a market system, private individuals could still donate organs out of charity to family members or to others in need. Social and political institutions that support the free choices of persons to interact with free and consenting others are neutral with regard to the expression of charity; market-based liberties include, but are not limited to, profit-seeking interests. Presuming that the willingness to donate body parts is motivated by actual, rather than coerced, altruism, those who are willing to donate should still be willing to donate regardless of the existence of a market. Additional strategies designed to increase organ availability, such as directed donation, should not be seen as exclusive alternatives to the market. Pursuing multiple parallel strategies may lead to the greatest organ availability. It may be, however, as I have argued in more detail elsewhere, that the goals of increasing organ availability, controlling medical costs, and reducing human suffering would be more effectively and honestly secured with the existence of an open market in human organs for transplantation (see Cherry, 2005).

Market incentives encourage persons to raise resources to further personal as well as social interests and goals. Profits from organ sales would allow for the private pursuit of business and educational opportunities, or to further more public agendas. Given that social and personal advantage is often tied to education and business success, such incentives may be significant. Commercialization would create opportunities, which many may view as attractive, to secure resources for pursuing their own educational, business, political, and welfare interests. It is likely that utilizing the market as a procurement strategy would encourage individuals, who would not otherwise donate, to sell their organs, which would increase the availability of organs for transplantation. The market is also very likely to increase access to nonredundant organs and body parts with harvesting authorized by the families of deceased donors. An open market (unlike the black market) would discourage unscrupulous practices and can be tracked and regulated. Successful procurement and transplantation require the skilled services of many professionals. Hospitals and highly skilled transplant surgeons have significant professional incentives to encourage virtuous tendencies in the medical marketplace. In additional to specific contractual obligations, surgeons and other medical personnel would be governed by the usual professional medical standards of practice. Such standards are nearly impossible to enforce on the current black market (see, e.g., Stacey Taylor, 2009).

Treating uncompensated donation and compensated donation as if such practices were inherently different is morally implausible. Prohibiting compensated organ donation forbids competent adults from engaging in a commercial transaction from which both parties expect to benefit. One may not approve of the choices of other persons, but they are the ones in authority to make such decisions regarding their own lives and bodies. The goal of informed consent to medical treatment, for example, is not simply to endorse patient autonomy as a positive value, but to respect personal autonomy as a side constraint—an acknowledgment that the burden of proof on others, including governments, to interfere in the free choices of persons regarding their bodies is indeed significant. In short, altruism-based systems of organ donation are not working adequately, whereas a market in human organs and other body parts would efficiently and effectively save lives, reduce human suffering, encourage highly skilled professional medical practice, and respect the authority of persons over their own bodies. With an open market, the availability of organs would not be limited to acts of altruism, government coercion, or manipulative educational campaigns designed to convince people to donate their organs for free. Failing to acknowledge that human organs are commodities, even while public policy, commercial interests, and transplantation medicine treats them as such, encourages continuation of a dishonest social political fiction. Prohibiting compensated donation denies persons the opportunity to choose freely on the basis of their own judgments regarding how best to advantage themselves, while condemning those waiting for available organs to significant suffering and increased risk of death.

Acknowledgment

Distantly ancestral versions of some of these arguments appeared in Cherry (2009a).

References

Abou Ayache, R., Bridoux, F., Pessione, F., Thierry, A., Belmouaz, M., Leroy, F. ... Touchard, G. (2005). Preemptive renal transplantation in adults. *Transplantation Proceedings, 37*(6), 2817–2818.

American Medical Association Council on Ethical and Judicial Affairs. (1993). *Ethical considerations in the allocation of organs and other scarce medical resources among patients.* CEJA Report K-A-93. Retrieved from: http://www.ama-assn.org/resources/doc/code-medical-ethics/216a.pdf

Casingal, V., Glumac, E., Tan, M., Sturdevant, M., Nguyen, T., & Matas, A. (2006). Death on the kidney waiting list—good candidates or not? *American Journal of Transplantation, 6*, 1953–1956.

Cheney, A. (2006). *Body brokers: Inside America's underground trade in human remains.* New York: Broadway Books.

Cherry, M. J. (2005). *Kidney for sale by owner: Human organs, transplantation and the market.* Washington, DC: Georgetown University Press.

Cherry, M. J. (2006). Medical innovation, collapsing goods, and the moral centrality of the free-market. *The Journal of Value Inquiry, 40*(2–3), 209–226.

Cherry, M. J. (2009a). Why should we compensate organ donors when we can continue to take organs for free? A response to some of my critics. *The Journal of Medicine and Philosophy, 34*, 649–673.

Cherry, M. J. (2009b). Embracing the commodification of human organs: Transplantation and the freedom to sell body parts. *Saint Louis University Journal of Health Law & Policy, 2*, 359–377.

Davis, F. D., & Crowe, S. J. (2009). Organ markets and the ends of medicine. *The Journal of Medicine and Philosophy, 34*(6), 586–605.

De Klerk, M., Keizer, K., Claas, F., Witvliet, M., Haase-Kramwijk, B., & Weimar, W. (2005). The Dutch national living donor kidney exchange program. *American Journal of Transplantation, 5*(9), 2302–2305.

De Klerk, M., Witvliet, M., Haase-Kramwijk, B., Claas, F., & Weimar, W. (2006). A highly efficient living donor kidney exchange program for both blood type and crossmatch incompatible donor–recipient combinations. *Transplantation, 82*(12), 1616–1620.

Delmonico, F., Morrissey, P., Lipkowitz, G., Stoff, J., Himmelfarb, J., Harmon, W. ... Rohrer, A. (2004). Donor kidney exchanges. *American Journal of Transplantation, 4*(10), 1553–1554.

Ferrari, P., & De Klerk, M. (2009). Paired kidney donations to expand the living donor pool. *Journal of Nephrology, 22*(6), 699–707.

Foley, R., & Collins, A. (2007). End-stage renal disease in the United States: An update from the United States renal data system. *Journal of the American Society of Nephrology, 18*, 2644–2648.

Gumber, M., Kute, V., Goplani, K., Shah, P., Patel, H., Vanikar A. ... Trivedi, H. (2011). Transplantation with kidney paired donation to increase the donor pool: a single-center experience. *Transplantation Proceedings, 43*(5), 1412–1414.

Hippen, B. (2005). In defense of a regulated market in kidneys from living vendors. *The Journal of Medicine and Philosophy, 30*(6), 627–642.

Holder, A. (1990). Legal issues in bone marrow transplantation. *The Yale Journal of Biology and Medicine, 63*, 521–525.

Humar, A. (2004). Maximizing the donor pool: Marginal donors, splits, and living donor liver transplants. *Journal of Gastroenterology and Hepatology, 19*, S410–S413.

Iltis, A., & Cherry, M. J. (2010). Revisiting death and the dead donor rule. *The Journal of Medicine and Philosophy, 35*(3), 223–241.

International Summit on Transplant Tourism and Organ Trafficking. (2008). Declaration of Istanbul on organ trafficking and tourism. *Clinical Journal of the American Society of Nephrology, 3*, 1227–1231.

The Lancet. (2009). Editorial: Legal and illegal organ donation. *The Lancet, 369*(9577), 1901.

Kimes, M. (2009). Blood money. *Fortune, 159*(12), 12.

Matas, A., Hippen, B., & Satel, S. (2008). In defense of a regulated system of compensation for living donation. *Current Opinion in Organ Transplantation, 13*, 379–385.

OPTN (Organ Procurement and Transplantation Network). (1999–2004). All Kaplan–Meier median waiting times for registrations listed: 1999–2004. Retrieved from: http://optn.transplant.hrsa.gov/latestData/rptStrat.asp

Paramesh, A., Hanley, K., Slakey, D., Killackey, M., Zhang, R., & Buell, J. (2011). Who's your donor? Bringing about Louisiana's first domino paired exchange transplants. *Journal of the Louisiana State Medical Societ, 163*(2), 102–104.

Ponticelli, C. (2011). Present and future of immunosuppressive therapy in kidney transplantation. *Transplantation Proceedings, 43*(6), 2439–2440.

Mahendran, A., & Veitch, P. (2007). Paired exchange programmes can expand the live kidney donor pool. *British Journal of Surgery, 94*(6), 657–664.

Meier-Kriesche, H., & Kaplan, B. (2002). Waiting time on dialysis as the strongest modifiable risk factor for renal transplant outcomes: a paired donor kidney analysis. *Transplantation, 74*(10), 1377–1381.

Mittler, J., Pascher, A., Neuhaus, P., & Pratschke, J. (2008). The utility of extended criteria donor organs in severely ill liver transplant recipients. *Transplantation, 8*, 895–896.

Müllhaupt, B., Dimitroulis, J., Gerlach, P., & Clavien, A. (2008). Hot topics in liver transplantation: organ allocation—extended criteria donors—living donor liver transplantation. *Journal of Hepatology*, *48*(1), S58–S67.

Nelson, L. (2009). New York State allows payment for egg donations for research. *The New York Times*, June 26. Retrieved from: http://www.nytimes.com/2009/06/26/nyregion/26stemcell.html

Sheldon, S., & Wilkinson, S. (2004). Should selecting saviour siblings be banned? *Journal of Medical Ethics*, *20*, 533–537.

Saldman, S., Roth, A., Sönmez, T., Unver, M., & Delmonico, F. (2006). Increasing the opportunity of live kidney donation by matching for two- and three-way exchanges. *Transplantation*, *81*(5), 773–782.

Stacey Taylor, J. (2009). Autonomy and organ sales, revisited. *Journal of Medicine and Philosophy*, *34*, 632–648.

University of Pennsylvania Hospital. (2011). Retrieved from: http://www.pennmedicine.org/pat_ins/

UNOS (United Network for Organ Sharing). (2009). The 2009 annual report of the OPTN and SRTR: transplant data 1999–2008. Retrieved from: http://www.unos.org/donation/index.php?topic=data

USRDS (United States Renal Data System). (2010). USRDS 2010 annual data report: Atlas of chronic kidney disease and end-stage renal disease in the United States. Retrieved from: http://usrds.org/reference.htm Retrieved from: http://www.usrds.org/reference.htm

Waldby, C., & Mitchell, R. (2006). *Tissue economies*. Durham, NC: Duke University Press.

Xue, J., Ma, J., Louis, T., & Collins, A. (2005). Forecast of the number of patients with end-stage renal disease in the United States to the year 2010. *Journal of the American Society of Nephrology*, *16*(5), 2753–2758.

Wertheimer, A. (1992). Two questions about surrogacy and exploitation. *Philosophy and Public Affairs*, *21*, 211–239.

Chapter Four

It Is Not Morally Acceptable to Buy and Sell Organs for Human Transplantation

A Very Poor Solution to a Very Pressing Problem

Arthur L. Caplan

Proposals to increase the supply of organs must be very carefully weighed against the prevailing ethical framework of voluntary altruism. Those values are widely known and heavily promoted, and have long served to protect the interests of prospective donors. Changes in these values might well alienate the public or healthcare professionals who have grown used to this ethical framework. Major religious groups who support this bioethical framework or healthcare workers, the majority of whom believe that the current bioethical framework is the appropriate one to govern organ procurement, could react very negatively to any major shift in the ethical infrastructure of organ and tissue procurement. Shifting to markets not only risks alienating important segments of the community who support altruism but also makes it difficult to condemn the practice of trafficking in persons and parts for transplant. And a market does nothing to help increase the supply of hearts and livers while making it less likely that these will be donated while those selling their kidneys get paid. The other key ethical problem facing a shift to some form of market is that it asks physicians to do harm to otherwise-healthy patients solely so that they may personally profit by being made sicker through removal of an organ.

The Harsh Reality of Allowing Markets in Organs—Trafficking of the Poor

Levy Izhak Rosenbaum, an Orthodox Rabbi in Brooklyn, New York liked to refer to himself as a "matchmaker." However, he was not arranging dates for his congregants. Rosenbaum was one of five rabbis indicted on July 23, 2009 in New Jersey for brokering the sale of black-market kidneys and, in a few cases, lobes of livers. He is accused of finding poor, Syrian Jews, who spoke little English or Hebrew and were newly immigrated to Israel, and paying them $10,000 to travel to the US to sell a kidney to patients waiting in various US transplant centers.

Rosenbaum was quite a businessman. He pocketed as much as $150,000 per organ from purchasers for serving as the middleman in his organ trafficking scheme. He not only short-changed his organ sources but even charged them for their transportation and room and board (Sherman & Margolin, 2011).

Contemporary Debates in Bioethics, First Edition. Edited by Arthur L. Caplan and Robert Arp.

Rosenbaum knew that buying organs was illegal. So, he was sure to always describe payment to his kidney sources as compensation for their time. Nevertheless, his scheme constituted blatant trafficking in persons for the purpose of obtaining organs.

Those involved were compelled by poverty to think about selling one of their kidneys. A middleman then took advantage of their poverty and illiteracy, duping them into thinking that they would earn a large sum of money free and clear by selling a kidney. Sadly, in most of the world, allowing financial incentives in kidneys means that trafficking, exploitation, disabling the sellers and even killing is the reality (Rothman & Rothman, 2006a, 2006b; Budiani-Saberi & Delmonico, 2008; Foster, 2009).

Trafficking is an all-too-real phenomenon in the world of kidney transplantation. It can take many forms. Sometimes, people are brought to hospitals against their will or with no true informed consent to "sell" a kidney. Sometimes, would-be patients travel to hospitals where they will meet someone, found by a broker or middleman, who, having been paid, will make a kidney available. And, in some instances, the organs themselves are simply forcefully removed, sometimes after an execution in a prison, and then sent, for a fee, to waiting patients, some of whom come from other countries, at nearby hospitals (Sify News, 2011).

Properly preserved kidneys remain viable for transplant for many hours. They can be flown thousands of miles for the right price. Studies estimate that nearly 10% of all kidneys transplanted around the world are trafficked (WHO, 2007; Caplan et al., 2009).

The New Jersey indictments represent the first known instance of trafficked human organs reaching patients in the United States. But, as numerous reports have documented, there are many examples of organ markets that are nothing more than trafficking occurring in many locations around the globe (COE, 1997; Caplan et al., 2009). In the past few years, wealthy persons needing transplants have traveled from the United Arab Emirates to Sri Lanka, from the United States to Azerbaijan, and from many nations around the world to Pakistan, Egypt, China, and Iraq to receive kidneys sold by desperately poor, ill-informed, uneducated persons. The sellers of these organs are only of interest to those trafficking them as sources of income. Once a kidney is removed, the seller's fate in terms of follow-up care and transportation home is of no concern at all to traffickers.

A typical case of selling a kidney involved a 64-year-old American who underwent kidney transplantation in Baku, Azerbaijan at the end of May 2009. The seller was a 31-year-old poor Ukrainian previously unknown to the recipient. Individuals outside of Azerbaijan arranged the transplant, but it was performed in Azerbaijan by an Israeli transplant surgeon. After the transplant, the seller was left to fend for himself including finding the means to return home. The details of this incident were reported to the Israeli and Azeri authorities by the physician who cared for the patient upon his return to the United States post-surgery (Postrel, 2011).

Patients from the United Arab Emirates, Kuwait, Oman, Australia, the Netherlands, Turkey, Kosovo, and India have undergone transplantation at the Kidney Center of Rawalpindi and the Aadil Hospital of Lahore, Pakistan. Trafficked organs obtained from very poor, often illiterate individuals with little capacity for true informed consent and usually deeply in debt were used (Jawaid Attari, 2009).

Not all trafficking involves crossing national borders. The television network, Al Jazeera, reported on July 20, 2009 that organ brokers were arranging for poor Iraqis to sell their kidneys at the Al-Khakal hospital in Baghdad (Al Jazeera, 2009). And, according to numerous press accounts, despite government condemnation, there continues to be a brisk market in organs taken from the very poor in India and from prisoners in China (Fearon, 2007).

Sales can lead to behavior that goes beyond simply taking advantage of poverty to obtain a kidney. The Associated Press reported on July 20, 2009 that a Saudi Arabian man married a Filipino woman as a cover for buying her kidney. This phony marriage was concocted to circumvent a recent law prohibiting foreigners from undergoing transplantation in the Philippines (Mail Online, 2009).

There are few defenders of trafficking as a solution to organ shortage. Forcing, coercing, or duping adults into making an organ available or removing a kidney from a child or a nonconsenting prisoner, alive or dead, is inconsistent with international human rights conventions but also violates the ethical norms of the professional transplant community (SCIS, 2008). Trafficked persons, those who are duped, forced, coerced, or deceived, are being exploited, even if they are paid.

Trafficking has been condemned by all international bodies that have examined the trade (COE, 1997; WMAGA, 2006; SCIS, 2008; Caplan et al., 2009). Trafficking is a reprehensible response to scarcity. So, why does trafficking persist? And is it possible to create systems using financial incentives to obtain kidneys that would not degenerate into trafficking? If not financial incentives, then are there other ideas or strategies that might alleviate the shortage of transplantable kidneys and other organs?

Scarcity—Bad, Underestimated, and Growing Worse

Every day, dozens of people die around the world while waiting for transplants. Many more await bone, cornea, dural matter, tendon, and other tissue transplants, suffering severe disability while they wait. These deaths and lives struggling with disabilities are especially tragic, since many might be prevented if more organs and tissues were available for transplantation. Scarcity means that hard choices have to be made about who will live and who will die. With more than 100,000 people on waiting lists for kidneys, hearts, livers, lungs, and intestines in North America alone, the pressure to find organs is enormous.

Scarcity, however, is growing worse every year. Waiting lists are growing faster than the supply of organs. Physicians are becoming more adept at dealing with harder cases in performing successful transplants (Reese et al., 2010). Aging populations in many nations increase the demand for kidneys. And increases in the rates of obesity, diabetes, and hypertension are driving up the demand for more kidney transplants as well. The capacity to perform transplants is spreading to many nations around the globe, increasing the demand for organs worldwide (WMA, 2011).

Scarcity is actually a worse problem than it appears to be from published data on demand. Demand for transplants is actually underestimated from that shown on public waiting lists in Canada, the US, Europe, Asia, the Middle East, and South America. If there were greater access to primary healthcare, more people might be identified as needing an organ or tissue transplant before becoming too sick to survive a transplant. And if transplant centers were to relax their current admissions standards to include more people—such as the those who lack money or insurance, those who have severe intellectual disabilities, older persons, prisoners, and foreigners who cannot get transplants in their own countries due to a lack of transplant centers and surgeons—then the lists of those waiting in rich nations could easily triple or quadruple (Quinn et al., 2007).

Duties to Those in Need and Duties to Those Who Might Supply an Organ

Those who care for persons dying of renal failure know the terrible toll the shortage of transplantable kidneys takes. Some doctors and nurses are, apparently, willing to remain ignorant of the provenance of the organs they transplant out of the belief that their sole ethical duty is to their dying patients. Transplant teams do, however, have an ethical duty to protect donor interests. Intentional ignorance about how an organ was obtained—from a scheduled execution of a "prisoner" or an organ that has been trafficked—is not an acceptable ethical excuse on the part of transplant teams and hospitals (COE, 1997; Caplan et al., 2009). Need creates moral pressure, but respect for the dignity, autonomy, and health of living donors is important as well, particularly since the integrity of donor procurement systems relies upon the fulfillment of these duties to maintain trust of all involved. Transplant teams are quite simply obligated to protect the interests and health of the sources of organs as well as recipients.

Ultimately, transplant teams and hospitals must be held accountable for knowing the origin and source, or provenance, of the kidneys and any other organs they transplant (Caplan et al., 2009). Trafficking and execution on demand flourish, not because anyone has made a convincing case they are morally or legally defensible but, in part, due to the willful ignorance of transplant centers eager to help their patients or transplant tourists while turning a profit.

In considering the merits of proposals for inducing people to sell organs, which basically amounts to a strategy that is only applicable to kidneys, it is necessary to understand fully the bioethical framework that has guided organ and tissue donation since solid organ transplants' inception in the 1950s (Caplan & Coelho, 1998).

The Prevailing Ethical Framework for Obtaining Organs and Tissues

The existing bioethical framework for obtaining organs and tissues in most parts of the world and exemplified in professional society norms (SCIS, 2008) is grounded on four key values—respect for persons, the autonomy of the individual, voluntary consent, and altruism. The notion that organs or tissues can be removed from a body for the purposes of transplantation, living or dead, without voluntary consent has not been accepted, except in highly unusual circumstances (i.e., unclaimed bodies at morgues under a coroner's jurisdiction; see Bagheri, 2005; Indiana State, 2009). Persons and their families are recognized in law and ethics as having a controlling interest over the disposition of the body upon death. Deceased and living persons are to be treated with dignity and not merely used to serve the needs of others.

Even though someone might well benefit from obtaining my liver or having bone marrow from my body, these organs and tissues ought not be removed from me, whether I am alive or newly dead, without my permission. To remove them after my death, if I have expressed no preference, then the consent of a surrogate (e.g., a family member, partner, or guardian) must be sought. To do otherwise is to commit a battery or assault upon a living person and to desecrate the body of a newly deceased person. The act of treating persons with dignity is exemplified by affording them control over the disposition of their body and its parts in life and upon death (Santiago, 1997; IOM, 2006). Respect is also shown by following the wishes of the newly dead when they were alive.

Another core element of the existing ethical framework governing the procurement of organs and tissues is that the body and its parts not be made the object of commerce. Prohibitions against slavery and trafficking of persons for prostitution are based upon the bioethical principle that respect for the inherent dignity of human beings requires that they not be bought and sold (Lincoln, 1863; UNGA, 1948; COE, 1997; Caplan et al., 2009). The transplant community has incorporated this view into a prohibition against trading in body parts for profit. In part, this position reflects the fundamental dignity of persons that is exemplified by prohibiting their being enslaved, bought, or sold. The emphasis on altruism in the existing values framework, as reflected in the use of the term *donation*, signals the notion of human dignity is respected by putting sale off limits while permitting gifts (Cohen, 2002).

In order to obtain organs and tissues from the living, there is broad agreement that, ethically, one must only seek a kidney from a competent person who is fully informed and who can make a voluntary, uncoerced choice. In the situation where organs and tissues are sought from the recently deceased, the notion of voluntary consent has been extended, in many nations, to the recognition of donor cards as adequate to direct a donation post-mortem with registration of intent to donate while alive in computerized registries. Variants of policies about who bears the duty to consent exist, but voluntary, informed consent is crucial in making organ and tissue procurement ethical (Sperling, 2009).

Proposals to increase the supply of organs must be very carefully weighed against this prevailing ethical framework, since it is widely known, heavily promoted, and has long served to protect the interests of prospective donors. Changes in these values might well alienate the public or healthcare professionals who have grown used to this ethical framework. Major religious groups who support this bioethical framework or healthcare workers, the majority of whom believe that the current bioethical framework is the appropriate one to govern organ procurement, could react very negatively to any major shift in the ethical infrastructure of organ and tissue procurement (Henegan, 2008).

Increasing the Supply

A number of steps have been taken over the years in many nations to try to increase the supply of organs. An early effort in the 1970s was to enact laws permitting the use of organ donor cards that allowed family consent to donate a deceased relative's organs. Some nations began requiring hospitals to ask all patients' families about organ and tissue donation upon death—so-called required request laws (Caplan, 1986, 1988). Some countries require hospitals to honor a patient's donor card, even when a family member opposes donation.

These policies were somewhat effective in gaining more organs from cadaver donors but the gap between supply and demand continued to increase. Therefore, some now argue for a shift away from a reliance on voluntary altruism in organ donation toward a paid market or system that uses financial incentives (Satel, 2008, 2009; Halpern et al., 2010).

Two basic strategies have been proposed to provide incentives for people to sell their organs upon their death. One strategy is simply to permit organ sale by allowing persons to broker contracts while alive with persons interested in selling at prices mutually agreed upon by both parties (Radcliffe-Richards et al., 1998; Satel, 2006; Taylor, 2009). Markets already exist on the Internet between potential live sellers and people in need of organs (Caplan, 2004; Barclay, 2004).

The other strategy is a "regulated" market in which the government would act as the purchaser of organs—setting a fixed price and enforcing conditions of sale (Harris & Erin, 2002; Matas, 2004; Gimbel & Strosberg, 2010). Iran appears to have such a market in operation, although reports on how it is actually being implemented and how well it functions in terms of protecting sellers are not encouraging (Griffin, 2007). Both proposals have drawn deserved ethical criticism.

The Trouble with Markets in Kidneys

One criticism is that only the poor and desperate will want to sell their body parts. If you need money, you might sell your kidney to try and feed your family or to pay back a debt. This may be a "rational" decision, but that does not make it a matter of free, voluntary choice (Hughes, 2006; Caplan et al., 2007).

Watching your child go hungry when you have no job, and a wealthy person waves a wad of bills in your face, is not exactly a scenario that inspires confidence in the "choice" made by those with few options except to sell vital body parts. Talk of individual rights and autonomy is hollow if those with no options must "choose" to sell their organs to purchase life's basic necessities. Choice requires information, options, and some degree of freedom, as well as the ability to reason about risks without being blinded by the prospect of short-term gain (Feinberg, 1986; Beauchamp & Childress, 1979/2009).

It is hard to imagine many people in wealthy countries eager to sell their organs either while alive or upon their death. In fact, even if compensation is relatively high, few will agree to sell (Rid et al., 2009). That has been the experience with markets in human eggs for research purposes and with paid surrogacy in the United States—prices have escalated, but there are still relatively few sellers (Baylis & McLeod, 2007).

Moreover, markets, if successful, would only have an impact on kidneys. It is not clear what the impact would be of creating a market in kidneys from living persons on the rest of the altruistically oriented organ procurement system. The risk of alienating altruistic donors of hearts, lungs, faces, limbs, and livers by creating a narrow market in kidneys is a huge one to take, given the potential loss of life involved for others. Selling organs, even in a tightly regulated market, violates the existing bioethical framework of respect for persons, since the sale is clearly being driven by profit. It also violates, in the case of living persons, the ethics of medicine itself. The core ethical norm of the medical profession is the principle, "Do no harm." The only way that removing an organ from someone seems morally defensible is if the donor chooses to undergo the harm of surgery solely to help another not to make money. The creation of commerce in body parts puts medicine in the position of removing body parts from people solely to abet those people's interest in securing compensation as well as to let middle-men profit (Rothman & Rothman, 2006a, 2006b).

Is this a role that the health professions can ethically countenance? In a market—even a regulated one—doctors and nurses still would be using their skills to help living people harm themselves solely for money. In a cadaver market, they would risk making families and patients uncertain about the degree to which appropriate care was being offered and continued if a person might be deemed by healthcare workers or greedy relatives worth more "dead than alive." The resulting distrust and loss of professional standards is a high price to pay to gamble on the hope that a market may secure more organs and tissues for those in need (Harmon & Delmonico, 2006).

A Better Option—Default to Donation

There is another option for increasing the organ supply that has been tried in Spain, Italy, Austria, France, and Belgium. These nations have enacted laws that create a presumption that individuals wish to donate their organs. Following public opinion polls that show majoritarian support for organ donation, instead of asking people to opt in to the donation of their organs the laws in these nations ask those who do not wish to donate to opt out. In such a system, the presumption is that a deceased person wants to be an organ donor upon their death—basically an ethical default to the desirability of donation (Caplan, 1983, 1994). People who do not want to be organ donors can say so while alive by carrying a card indicating their objection, or by registering their objection in a computerized registry, or by doing both. They may also tell their loved ones and rely on them to object should procurement present itself as an opportunity (BMA, 2010). Any close relative could also act to prohibit donation if they believed that was not the desire of the deceased. A more felicitous description of presumed consent is *default to donation*. Individuals are familiar with such defaults in a way that might make them far more comfortable with this strategy for obtaining more organs (Cass & Thaler, 2009).

What is remarkable about this strategy is that it has worked! Unlike the hypothetical and unsupported assertions of advocates of financial incentives and markets that there will be interest in sale in rich nations or the ability to control trafficking in poor ones, default to donation has produced results. This policy has done so without creating any problems or difficulties in the nations that have enacted such legislation. And it has done so without any significant increase in cost beyond the costs of education, training, and public-health campaigns about the new policy (Abadie & Gay, 2006; Gil-Diaz, 2009; Verheijde et al., 2009).

What is important about this strategy from a bioethical perspective is that it is completely consistent with the existing, longstanding bioethical framework of voluntary altruism governing organ and tissue procurement. Respect for persons and voluntary, altruistic consent remain the moral foundation for making organs available.

Conclusion

The worldwide shortage of transplantable organs has led to a significant degree of trafficking in kidneys. Some of the groups involved in this illicit trafficking are also linked to trafficking in women and children for prostitution. These markets are immoral on their face. Worse, it is unlikely that permitting trade in kidneys could ever be subject to the kind of oversight and policing that would prevent outright trafficking. Given the well-documented horrors of trafficking, there is no plausible case for shifting to markets or regulated markets in poor nations, especially since this removes any incentive nations lacking cadaver donor programs might have to do so and only contributes, possibly, to the supply of kidneys.

Shortage has led some to call for policies that would legitimize the sale of kidneys. But it is difficult to believe that in most parts of the world, sufficient oversight and government authority exist to regulate markets and that they would not quickly deteriorate into trafficking. Even in nations that might be able to regulate a market in kidneys, it is not evident that this would lead to an increase in the overall supply. There is little empirical evidence that money is a key factor in guiding decisions about making kidneys available for transplant. Nor is it likely that any but the most desperately poor or disadvantaged would be drawn to kidney sale, making a mockery of the entire notion of autonomous, free choice to sell a body part. Markets would also create an untenable situation for healthcare workers asking them to use their skills to harm patients solely for the purpose of allowing them a one-time chance to earn money.

There are alternatives to creating markets. Greater efforts can be made to secure all organs including kidneys by enacting presumed consent legislation. This has been done in some nations with notable results. With sufficient training and educational resources, default to donation policies is known to boost the supply of all organ for transplantation. And by outlawing financial systems, those nations that have made little serious effort to build procurement systems using cadaver organs will be led to do so, thereby decreasing the pressures that contribute to exploitative and immoral organ trafficking.

In the long run, bioengineering organs is the answer to shortage (Marcchiarini et al., 2008). In the short run, protecting the viability of the existing system for obtaining organs by not drastically deviating from the core values that have long prescribed what can be done is the best strategy for helping those in need.

References

Abadie, A., & Gay, S. (2006). The impact of presumed consent legislation on cadaveric organ donation: A cross-country study. *Journal of Health Economics, 25*(4), 599–620.

Al Jazeera, (2009). Poverty drives Iraq organ trade. *English Aljazeera.* July 20. Retrieved from: http://english.aljazeera.net/news/middleeast/2009/07/200972052636416787.html

Bagheri, A. (2005). Organ transplantation laws in Asian countries: A comparative study. *Transplantation Proceedings, 37*, 4159–4162.

Barclay, L. (2004). Organ donation via Internet raises ethical concerns: An expert interview with Arthur L. Caplan, Ph.D. *Medscape.com.* October 22. Retrieved from: http://www.med scape.com/viewarticle/491837

Baylis, F., & McLeod, C. (2007). The stem cell debate continues: The buying and selling of eggs for research. *Journal of Medical Ethics, 33*(12), 726–731.

Beauchamp, T., & Childress, J. (1979/2009). *Principles of biomedical ethics.* Oxford: Oxford University Press.

BMA (British Medical Association). (2010). Organ transplantation and donation. Retrieved from: http://www.bma.org.uk/ethics/organ_transplantation_donation/organdonation brief.jsp.

Budiani-Saberi, D., & Delmonico, F. (2008). Organ trafficking and transplant tourism: A commentary on the global realities. *American Journal of Transplantation, 8*, 925–928.

Caplan, A. L. (1983). Organ transplants: The costs of success. *The Hastings Center Report 13*(6), 23–32.

Caplan, A. L. (1986). Requests, gifts, and obligations: The ethics of organ procurement. *Transplantation Proceedings 18*(3), 49–56.

Caplan, A. L. (1988). Professional arrogance and public misunderstanding. *The Hastings Center Report, 18*(2), 34–37.

Caplan, A. L. (1994). Current ethical issues in organ procurement and transplantation. *The Journal of the American Medical Association, 272*(21), 1708–1709.

Caplan, A. L. (2004). Organs.com: New commercially brokered organ transfers raise questions. *The Hastings Center Report, 34*(6), 8.

Caplan, A. L., & Coelho, D. H. (Eds.). (1998). *The ethics of organ transplants: The current debate.* Amherst, NY: Prometheus.

Caplan, A. L., Tan, H., Marcos, A., & Shapiro, R. (Eds.). (2007). *Living Organ Transplantation.* New York: Informa Healthcare USA, Inc.

Caplan, A. L., Dominguez-Gil, B., Matesanz, R., & Prior, C. (2009). Trafficking organs, tissues and cells and trafficking in human beings for the purpose of the removal of organs: Joint Council of Europe/United Nations study. Retrieved from: http://www.coe.int/t/dghl/monitoring/trafficking/docs/news/OrganTrafficking_study.pdf

Cass, R. S., & Thaler, R. H. (2009). *Nudge.* New York: Penguin Group.

COE (Council of Europe). (1997). Convention for the protection of human rights and dignity of the human being with regard to the application of biology and medicine. Retrieved from: http://conventions.coe.int/Treaty/en/Treaties/html/164.htm

Cohen, C. B. (2002). Public policy and the sale of human organs. *Kennedy Institute of Ethics Journal, 12*(1), 47–64.

Fearon, P. (2007). Kidney sales brisk on India's black market. *Newser.com.* May 9. Retrieved from: http://www.newser.com/story/2038/kidney-sales-brisk-on-indias-black-market.html

Feinberg, G. (1986). *Harm to self: The moral limits of the criminal law.* New York: Oxford University Press.

Foster, P. (2009). China admits organs removed from prisoners for transplants. *The Telegraph.* August 26. Retrieved from: http://www.telegraph.co.uk/news/worldnews/asia/china/6094228/China-admits-organs-removed-from-prisoners-for-transplants.html

Gil-Diaz, C. (2009). Spain's record organ donations: Mining moral conviction. *Cambridge Quarterly of Healthcare Ethics, 18*(3), 256–261.

Gimbel, R. W., & Strosberg, M. A. (2010). Kidney donation: When all else fails, try a regulated market. *Journal of the National Medical Association (January).* Retrieved from:

http://findarticles.com/p/articles/mi_7640/is_201001/ai_n49423324/

Griffin, A. (2007). Kidneys on demand. *British Medical Journal, 334*, 502–505.

Halpern, S., Raz, A., Kohn, R., Rey, M., Asch, D., & Reese, P. (2010). Regulated payments for living kidney donation: An empirical assessment of the ethical concerns. *Annals of Internal Medicine, 152*, 358–365.

Harmon, W., & Delmonico, F. (2006). Payment for kidneys: A government-regulated system is not ethically achievable. *Clinical Journal of the American Society of Nephrology, 1*(6), 1146–1147.

Harris, J., & Erin, C. (2002). An ethically defensible market in organs: A single buyer like the NHS is an answer. *British Medical Journal, 325*, 114–115.

Henegan, T. (2008). Pope slams human organ trade, warns on transplants. *Reuters.com*. November 7. Retrieved from: http://www.reuters.com/article/idUSTRE4A658820081107

Hughes, P. (2006) Ambivalence, autonomy, and organ sales. *Southern Journal of Philosophy, 44*, 237–251.

Indiana State. (2009). Indiana state law code IC 36-2-14-19 2009. Retrieved from: http://www.in.gov/legislative/ic/code/title36/ar2/ch14.html

IOM (Institute of Medicine). (2006). *Organ donation: opportunities for action*. Washington, DC: The National Academies Press.

Jawaid Attari, M. (2009). Mr. Shahbaz Sharif, please act. *Urdunews*. June 17. Retrieved from: http://urdunews.wordpress.com/2009/06/17/mr-shahbaz-sharif-please-act/

Lincoln, A. (1863). The emancipation proclamation. *Archives.gov*. Retrieved from: http://www.archives.gov/exhibits/featured_documents/emancipation_proclamation/

Mail Online. (2009). Saudi man marries Filipino as cover to buy one of her kidneys. *Mail Online*. July 21. Retrieved from: http://www.dailymail.co.uk/news/article-1200926/Saudi-man-marries-Filipino-cover-buy-kidneys.html

Marcchiarini, P., Jungebluth, P., Tetsiuhiko, G., Asmaghi A., & Rees, L. (2008). Clinical transplantation of a tissue-engineered airway. *The Lancet, 372*, 2023–2030.

Matas, A. J. (2004). The case for living kidney sales: Rationale, objections and concerns. *American Journal of Transplantation, 4*, 2007–2017.

Postrel, V. (2011). … With functioning kidneys for all. *The Atlantic*. June 8. Retrieved from: http://www.theatlantic.com/doc/200907u/kidney-donation

Quinn, R. R., Manns, B. J., & McLaughlin, K. M. (2007). Restricting cadaveric kidney transplantation based on age: the impact on efficiency and equity. *Transplantation Proceedings, 39*(5), 1362–1367.

Radcliffe-Richards, J., Daar, A., Guttmann, R., Hoffenberg, R., Kennedy, I., Lock, M. … Tilney, N. (1998). The case for allowing kidney sales. *The Lancet, 351*, 1950–1952.

Reese P., Abt, P., Bloom, R., Karlawish, J., & Caplan, A. L. (2010). How should we use age to ration health care? Lessons from the case of kidney transplantation. *Journal of the American Geriatrics Society, 58*(10), 1–7.

Rid, A., Bachmann, L., Wettstein, V., & Biller-Andorno, N. (2009). Would you sell a kidney in a regulated market system? Results of an exploratory study. *Journal of Medical Ethics, 35*(9), 558–564.

Rothman, D. J., & Rothman, S. M. (2006a). *Trust is not enough: Bringing human rights to medicine*. New York: New York Review Books.

Rothman, D. J., & Rothman, S. M. (2006b). The hidden cost of organ sale. *American Journal of Transplantation, 6*, 1524.

Santiago, C. (1997). Asking for the family consent: analysis and refusals. *Transplantation Proceedings, 29*, 1629–1630.

Satel, S. (2006). The kindness of strangers and the cruelty of some medical ethicists. *The Weekly Standard*. May 29. Retrieved from: http://www.weeklystandard.com/Content/Public/Articles/000/000/012/249jxzdt.asp

Satel, S. (2008). *When altruism isn't enough: The case for compensating kidney donors*. Washington, DC: AEI Press.

Satel, S. (2009). The case for paying organ donors. *The Wall Street Journal*. October 18. Retrieved from: http://online.wsj.com/article/SB10001424052748704322004574477840120222788.html

SCIS (Steering Committee of the Istanbul Summit). (2008). Declaration of Istanbul on organ trafficking and transplant tourism and commercialism. *The Lancet, 372*(9632), 372–373.

Sherman, T., & Margolin, J. (2011). *The Jersey sting: A true story of crooked pols, money-laundering rabbis, black market kidneys and the informant who brought it all down*. New York: St. Martin's Press.

Sify News. (2011). Oz kidney buyers giving China's "transplant tourism" a boost. *Sify News*. February 6. Retrieved from: http://www.sify.com/news/oz-kidney-buyers-giving-china-s-transplant-tourism-a-boost-news-international-lcgpOcbgcgj.html

Sperling, D. (2009). Israel's new brain-respiratory death act. *Reviews in Neurosciences, 20*(3–4), 299–306.

Taylor, J. S. (2009). Autonomy and organ sales, revisited. *Journal of Medicine & Philosophy, 34*, 632–648.

UNGA (United Nations General Assembly). (1948). The universal declaration of human rights. *Un.org*. Retrieved from: http://www.un.org/en/documents/udhr/

Verheijde, J., Rady, M., McGregor, J., & Friederich-Murray, J. (2009). Enforcement of presumed-consent policy and willingness to donate organs as identified in the European Union Survey: The role of legislation in reinforcing ideology in pluralistic societies. *Health Policy*, *90*(1), 26–31.

WHO (World Health Organization). (2007). WHO proposes global agenda on transplantation. March 30. Retrieved from: http://www.who.int/mediacentre/news/releases/2007/pr12/en/index.html

WMA (World Medical Association). (2011). WMA statement on human organ donation and transplantation. Retrieved from: http://www.wma.net/en/30publications/10policies/t7/

WMAGA (World Medical Association's General Assembly). (2006). Statement on human organ donation and transplantation. Retrieved from: http://www.wma.net/en/30publications/10policies/t7/

Reply to Caplan

Mark J. Cherry

Art Caplan's evocative critique of market-based incentives for increasing access to organ transplantation, while rhetorically engaging, routinely misses the mark. At key junctures, his argument either fails adequately to distinguish between legal and illegal markets or relies on ambiguous and moralistic terminology, such as human dignity and personal autonomy. Perhaps most puzzling, Caplan endorses nonconsensual state expropriation of human organs for transplantation from the deceased. A chilling thought, indeed!

Compensated and uncompensated organ donation are not morally distinct. Provided that the procedure takes place in a suitably sterile environment, with adequate surgical skill and attention to the health of the donor, all medical aspects of the two practices are identical. The only distinction is that money changes hands, which, in itself, is not intrinsically morally problematic. For example, surgeons routinely insist on payment for performing life-saving transplant surgery. Caplan rightly notes that illegal markets are open to abuse. However, unlike horror stories surrounding black markets in human organs, the open market would discourage unscrupulous practices. Long-term successful transplantation programs require the skilled services of many professionals. Hospitals, highly skilled transplant surgeons, and their dedicated surgical teams have significant professional incentives to encourage virtuous tendencies in the medical marketplace. In addition to contractual obligations, surgeons, other medical personnel, and institutions would be subject to the usual professional medical standards of practice, and liable to both tort and criminal law for breaches of contract, negligence, or malpractice. Such standards are nearly impossible to track, much less enforce, on the black market. Here, the moral challenge is represented not by financial compensation per se, but by shortsighted public policy.

Defense of compensated organ donation need not affirm personal autonomy as a value, much less as an over-ridding value. Rather, autonomy ought to be appreciated as a side-constraint on the permissible behavior of others. Morally authorized action generally requires, except in emergency and exigent circumstances, that persons not be touched or used without their permission. Moreover, persons, not government bureaucrats or bioethicists, are the presumptive judges of their own best interests (Cherry & Engelhardt, 2004). Persons are morally in authority over themselves. This moral and jurisprudential understanding is core to the practice of informed consent in medicine, including informed consent to organ donation.

Here, the conceptual puzzle is that Caplan both affirms and denies this moral authority of persons over themselves—it is affirmed to justify uncompensated organ donation, but denied to condemn compensated organ donation. This contradiction lies at the heart of contemporary transplantation policy.

Contemporary Debates in Bioethics, First Edition. Edited by Arthur L. Caplan and Robert Arp.

Caplan's intuition that financial compensation violates "human dignity" must be further specified and critically defended. Not all agree on the meaning or implications of human dignity; nor is it clear why such dignity would be so fragile as to be harmed by compensated organ donation. In part, one must adjudicate among moral intuitions, distinguishing between justified and unjustified claims to the loss of human dignity, prior to presupposing that such claims ought to play any role in public policy. Many have deep-seated views, for example, regarding the significant violation of human dignity represented by abortion and common, presumably consensual but high-risk, sex acts. Yet, these are practices that society permits and, indeed, in many quarters celebrates. One might, for example, profitably compare the likelihood of personal harm represented by routinely engaging in high-risk sex acts—e.g., sexually transmitted diseases, virally mediated diseases, such as HIV and HPV-related cancers, as well as long-term risks of infertility, especially among women—with the low risk of one-time, living-kidney donation.

More generally, highly paternalistic regulation that treats adult citizens as mere children, unable to make competent judgments in their own best interests, is hardly affirming of one's dignity. One may not approve of the choices of other persons (e.g., engaging in high-risk sex acts, or accepting financial incentives to donate an organ), and individuals ought to bear the full costs of their choices, but they are the ones in authority to make such decisions regarding their own lives and bodies.

Presumed consent, which Caplan endorses, raises further and difficult challenges. First, *presumed consent* is a mere rhetorical euphemism—a legal fiction, as it were. No actual consent has taken place. If the state simply appropriated all of one's wealth upon death, rather than recognizing that one's worldly goods rightly become the property of one's legitimate heirs, unless one specifically opted out, it would be implausible to conclude that such confiscation was consensual. The hue and cry that such state-based theft would engender is easy to anticipate. Presumed consent is inconsistent with altruism-based transplantation policy.

Second, it is unclear how presumed consent would ally Caplan's expressed concerns that "Deceased and living persons are be to be treated with dignity and not merely used to serve the needs of others." Presumed consent policies are specifically designed to instrumentalize and objectify the human body, to take human organs to serve the needs of others. Such policy manipulates the language of "consent" to exploit citizens, treating them as a mere means to the end of organ appropriation to benefit others.

In summary, as I have argued elsewhere (Cherry, 2005), I do not doubt the sincerity or good intentions of those of my colleagues who support the continued prohibition of compensated organ donation. En passant, commentators in favor of financial incentives for organ donation were not invited to participate in the conference that led to the *Declaration of Istanbul.* It is not difficult to issue a consensus statement on the supposed existence of "human rights," when you only invite activists who are already known to agree with the preferred ideological position that the conference organizers expect to endorse. Such circumstances straightforwardly call into question the supposed universality of the *Declaration*'s assertions regarding such human rights.

I continue to be perplexed, however, by the ways in which such prohibitions exploit vulnerable populations to support highly paternalistic views of moral propriety, human dignity, and inappropriate use of one's body, thereby denying persons the opportunity to choose freely on the basis of one's own judgments how best to advantage oneself, as well as condemning those who are waiting for the availability of organs for transplant to continued suffering and increased risk of death.

References

Cherry, M. J. (2005). *Kidney for sale by owner: Human organs, transplantation and the market.* Washington, DC: Georgetown University Press.

Cherry, M. J., & Engelhardt, H. T. (2004). Informed consent in Texas: Theory and practice. *The Journal of Medicine and Philosophy, 29*(2), 237–252.

Reply to Cherry

Arthur L. Caplan

Professor Cherry has made a strong case for permitting markets in kidneys. However, he has not made a persuasive one. Three reasons stand out as to why this is so.

First, Professor Cherry presents us with the idealized hypothetical of Anna and James both making a kidney available to a child—James from altruism, Anna for money. The problem with the case example is that there are likely to be very few Annas selling organs for cash, "aware that kidney donation comes with the attendant risks of surgery … [seeking] to minimize the risks by working with a well-known hospital with a good reputation for providing high-quality medical care for organ donors." Many of the Annas of the real world are likely to be at their wits' end about how to find money to pay overwhelming debts. They are likely to be unemployed. They are likely to be poorly educated. They are likely to have mental- and physical-health issues of their own. In other words, many who might wish to sell will not really be making a *choice*. They will be acting solely out of desperation when they perceive no other options available to them.

The market Professor Cherry idealizes is not selling one's sperm, hair, plasma, or even eggs. It is one requiring undergoing major surgery with real risk of death or disability for cash. Some Annas may meet Cherry's description and thoughtfully choose to sell a kidney. Others—and I would suggest a good number—will be told by their bookie, abusive boyfriend or husband, or loan shark to find a way to come up with some short-term cash and, having no options and thus no real choices, sell a kidney.

Even worse, many Annas will live in other nations who will emulate our decision to permit markets. Those Annas will have even less potential for choice and will simply be coerced, bullied, threatened, or forced into kidney sales. When a market opens in the United States, it also opens in far less lawful and far more impoverished parts of the globe. Since our ability to combat trafficking for organs, sex, baby sales, and indentured slave labor depends on the moral position that incentives in these domains are wrong, it is a bitter price to pay to allow a few Annas in the US to sell what will be forced from many, many more in other parts of the world.

Second, Cherry argues that medicine is a business: "Medicine is a commodity: its goods and services are bought and sold, valued over against other goods and services, are the subject of economic choices, and are given a monetary equivalence. Hospitals, physicians, and other healthcare workers demand payment for services rendered." Therefore, he concludes, we can have doctors paid and patients paid to undergo surgery to take out their organs for no reason other than profits.

Medicine is a business, but it is also a profession—one that relies on trust. If commercial concerns are seen as overwhelming the protection of patient

Contemporary Debates in Bioethics, First Edition. Edited by Arthur L. Caplan and Robert Arp.

interests, then medicine will not long be able to function. If doctors do useless tests on patients solely to make money, then patients come to distrust recommendations for tests. If doctors will remove your kidney, cornea, lobe of liver, or limbs solely so that you and they may turn a buck, patients soon will come to completely distrust their doctors. Transplantation depends upon trust—to obtain organs such as hearts and lungs, people must believe their loved ones are truly dead before removal. Trust in that the surgeon will not give you an inferior or infected organ just to get a paycheck. Trust in that you cannot bribe your way to access to an organ ahead of those in greater need. There is nothing that will destroy trust more in transplant than showing that doctors are quite willing to harm their patients—especially those who are poor or vulnerable—solely and only for money.

Lastly, Cherry believes that markets will work. They will generate more kidneys to transplant. He bases his case on the fact that markets have relieved scarcity in other areas of life. But, markets have also driven up scarcity—a lack of jobs comes to mind in the US as markets ship jobs overseas or permit downsizing in the name of short-term profit. Markets have not done much to improve the credit situation of Americans. Nor have they proven their merit in distributing access to minimal healthcare to all Americans.

There is every reason to believe that markets will not produce a gain in kidneys. Major religious groups such as the Catholic Church vigorously oppose sales in body parts (see, for example, http://www.catholicnewsagency.com/news/pope_condemns_organ_transplant_abuses_as_abominable/). If major religious organizations condemn markets and proscribe participation in any system that tolerates them, then not only will there not be an increase in kidney availability, but also there could well be a drop in the availability of kidneys and of all other organs and tissues used in transplantation. Introducing known and quite zealous major religious opposition to markets in body parts into the realm of transplantation is a far more concrete reason to predict their failure than any of the generalities about markets that Cherry offers in predicting their success.

In the short run, there are other policy strategies, such as default to donation and presumed consent, that truly protect individual choice, which merit trying without turning to markets. In the long run, the solution to shortage in organs is through encouraging more government support for research on artificial organs, xenografting, and stem-cell regeneration. There will be enormous markets for the products that these strategies, if vigorously pursued, will eventually create.

Part 3

Were It Physically Safe, Would Human Reproductive Cloning Be Acceptable?

Introduction

Cloning is the process whereby a genetically identical copy (the clone) of some biological entity is produced, these entities including genes, cells, tissues, and even entire organisms. Cloning occurs naturally, as when certain plants and bacteria reproduce asexually, or when identical twins are born to humans or other animal species (Klotzko, 2003; Brown, 2010). Artificial cloning by researchers has been taking place since at least the mid 1950s. There are three types: *gene cloning* (or DNA cloning) is concerned with producing cloned segments of DNA or copies of genes; *therapeutic cloning* primarily is concerned with producing cloned embryonic stem cells that can be used to create tissues so as to ultimately treat an injury or disease; *reproductive cloning* is concerned with producing a cloned genetic duplicate of an existing organism (Wilmut et al., 2000).

Robert William Briggs and Thomas Joseph King are credited with the first cases of reproductive cloning of animals—northern leopard frogs (*Rana pipiens*), native to Canada and the US—in 1952 (Briggs & King, 1952; Di Berardino & McKinnell, 2004). In 1996, the "world's most famous sheep," named Dolly, was the first mammal to be cloned from an adult somatic cell by Ian Wilmut and colleagues at the Roslin Institute in Scotland (McKie, 1997; Wilmut et al., 1997). Thus far, clones of animals such as mice, rats, cats, dogs, horses, mules, camels, cows, chickens, and rabbits, to name but a few species, have been produced through reproductive cloning (Guardian, 2011). A cloned Pyrenean ibex was born from a domestic goat in 2008, an amazing feat, since this particular ibex species went extinct in 2000 (Gray & Dobson, 2009; Piña-Aguilar et al., 2009). The woolly mammoth may be the next extinct animal to be cloned (Ryall, 2011).

The following is a useful description of the process of the reproductive cloning of an animal from the National Human Genome Research Institute of the National Institutes of Health (NHGRI, 2011):

Contemporary Debates in Bioethics, First Edition. Edited by Arthur L. Caplan and Robert Arp.

To clone an animal, researchers first take mature cells, such as skin cells, from the animal to be cloned. Next, they take an unfertilized egg from an adult female of the same species and remove the nucleus, which is the cell structure that houses the chromosomes that contain an organism's DNA. Researchers then place one of the skin cells next to the nucleus-free egg and apply an electric pulse, which causes the skin cell to fuse with the egg. The fused cell, which contains the skin cell's nucleus, divides and forms an early-stage embryo. This embryo is implanted in the uterus of another female animal, called a surrogate mother, and allowed to develop. The surrogate mother then gives birth to an animal that is genetically identical to the adult that donated the skin cells. This newborn animal is referred to as a clone.

While there are those who are uncomfortable with any kind of human manipulation of nature or natural processes whatsoever (see Verhey, 1995; Michael, 2002), most people have no problem with gene cloning, which consists of placing a gene from an organism into the genetic material of a vector (for example, a virus, bacterium, or yeast cell) and prompting the vector to multiply so that the cloned genes of the original organism are produced. People tend to be more leery of therapeutic cloning and especially reproductive cloning, however. Embryos from animals such as mice and cattle have been used in therapeutic cloning (Yang et al., 2007; Sung et al., 2010). In 2001, researchers from a biotechnology company called Advanced Cell Technologies (ACT) announced that they had cloned a human embryo (Cibelli et al., 2001; Green, 2001) as did a team of Korean scientists led by Hwang Woo-suk in 2004. The former was never verified, while the latter proved to be a complete fraud (Cyranoski, 2006; TNA, 2006). To date, no verified cloning of a human embryo has occurred.

In 2010, ACT was given permission by the US Food and Drug Administration to begin clinical trials using retinal cells derived from human embryonic stem cells to treat patients with Stargardt's Macular Dystrophy (SMD), which causes progressive vision loss usually culminating in legal blindness (ACT, 2010). In February of 2012, researchers from ACT reported in *The Lancet* that two subjects suffering from SMD who had been treated showed improvement in vision with no harmful side effects (Schwartz et al., 2012).

There are those who argue against therapeutic cloning because of the fact that the cloned embryos are destroyed as a result of the stem cells being harvested from them. On religious or even other secular, life-is-sacred grounds, such destruction could then be deemed immoral, with therapeutic cloning of human embryos probably garnering the most moral outrage. For example, the official Catholic Church position is that human life begins at the moment of conception, and that this life is as dignified, valued, and deserving of protection as any other human life, no matter what stage of human development (zygote, embryo, fetus, infant, child, young adult, adult, elderly adult). Given this inherent value, a human embryo should never be harmed, even for the general good of medical and scientific improvements (John Paul II, 2001; DHC, 2004; NCBC, 2009; O'Brien, 2011). One could argue for the same conclusion on secular grounds pertaining to inherent value, too, as when thinkers utilize Immanuel Kant's (1724–1804) deontological moral theory with its emphasis on respect for persons (Kant, 1775–89/1963, 1785/1998, 1797/1996; Dworkin, 1993; Lachmann, 2001; Novak, 2001; cf. Manninen, 2008).

It is important to note that ACT (mentioned above) was awarded a patent from the United States Patent and Trademark Office for what is referred to as *single-blastomere* technology (US Patent # 7893315), a method that:

> uses a one-cell biopsy approach similar to pre-implantation genetic diagnosis (PGD), which is widely used in the in vitro fertilization (IVF) process and does not interfere with the embryo's developmental potential. The stem cells generated using this approach are healthy, completely normal, and differentiate into all the cell types of the human body, including insulin-producing cells, blood cells, beating heart cells, cartilage, and other cell types of therapeutic importance. (ACT, 2011; Lang, 2011)

What is significant about this technology is that the embryos are *not* destroyed as a result of the stem cells being harvested from them (Klimanskaya et al., 2006, 2007). Still, one may argue that single-blastomere technology is nonetheless immoral—one reason being that any kind of human manipulation of nature or natural processes whatsoever is immoral.

While it may be true that the majority of the mainstream scientific community has no moral problem with therapeutic cloning of animal embryos, or with the reproductive cloning of any organism other than a human, a great number of scientific and medical professionals—and others—view reproductive *human* cloning as immoral. Over 30 countries (including Canada, France, Germany, Spain, and Vietnam) have banned reproductive human cloning. Fifteen countries (including Israel, Japan, and the UK) have banned reproductive human cloning but allow therapeutic cloning (Johnson & Williams, 2006; Public Agenda, 2011). There are no *federal* laws in the United States banning reproductive cloning of any kind. However, 15 states have laws banning human cloning, and Arizona, Missouri, and Maryland have laws against using public funds for human cloning (NCSL, 2011). The United Nations, the European Union, and the Council of Europe have published human-cloning policies and recommendations, and in 2005 the United Nations Declaration on Human Cloning was produced calling upon member states "to prohibit all forms of human cloning in as much as they are incompatible with human dignity and the protection of human life" (UNDHC, 2005).

The most common argument against reproductive cloning of animals, one that is used by research professionals, policy-makers, and laypersons alike, is the slippery-slope argument that reproductive cloning of animals will lead directly to the reproductive cloning of humans. In fact, many use similar reasoning to argue against therapeutic cloning, thinking that it will inevitably lead to reproductive human cloning. While it is understandable that one may think this way, given the fact that many medical achievements and advancements (as well as a whole host of other actions in human history) can be viewed as following the slippery-slope pattern, it is nonetheless wholly fallacious and obviously premature to reason from a premise that, "Since scientists are engaging in therapeutic cloning and/or reproductive animal cloning" to a necessary conclusion that, "Therefore, scientists will be engaging in reproductive animal cloning at some point in the future" (de Wert & Mummery, 2003).

The first author in this section, Katrien Devolder, is aware of this slippery slope, noting that "even if one accepts cloning for research and therapy, one can, without being inconsistent, reject reproductive cloning. Moreover, effective legislation which clearly distinguishes between the two types of cloning could prevent us from sliding down the slope. This can simply be achieved by prohibiting the transfer of cloned embryos to the uterus (as in the UK and Belgium)." Nonetheless, Devolder devotes much of her chapter to refuting claims against reproductive human cloning, before arguing that reproductive human cloning should be allowed for the primary reason that "it will allow infertile people to have a genetically related child."

Devolder allays several fears about human cloning and its effects, three of which include: (1) cloning is unsafe, (2) cloning leaves the clone with no true identity, and (3) cloning discourages adoption. Concerning (1), Devolder admits that at present, cloning is unsafe, but "one cannot exclude a future in which its safety and efficiency will be comparable or superior to that of in vitro fertilization (IVF) or even sexual reproduction." Concerning (2), she notes that this "relies on the mistaken belief that who and what we become is entirely determined by our genes," which is a position that is commonsense enough. Concerning (3), she draws an analogy between cloning and in vitro fertilization (IVF), noting that given that there is no evidence indicating that IVF has led to a decrease in adoptions, so too, it is unlikely that human cloning would lead to a decrease in human adoptions.

The second author in this section, Steven Levick, believes that besides the basic bio-physiological safety issues associated with reproductive human cloning, there are legitimate concerns about the psychological and social well-being of a clone. For example, concerning the obviously vulnerable psyche of a child, "knowing vs. not knowing that one is a clone, and the identity of one's progenitor, could powerfully affect the child clone's ability to develop a unique personal identity." And if a child clone is "told that her genes and Mommy's are the same" then she "would be inclined to think of herself and progenitor mother as the same person based on their identical genes." Whereas there exists this "I am identical with my mommy or daddy" thinking on the part of the *clone*, Levick also points out the converse issue of "My clone is identical to me" thinking on the part of the *parent*, such that the clone could be seen as a "mini-me." Again, the result is a hampering of the clone's ability to develop her/his own healthy identity.

Further, if a clone is that of a deceased child and knows it, there is the possibility that not only would the clone feel like a "replacement," but also the parents might treat the clone as such. In Levick's own words, "one would expect parents' perceptions of, attitudes towards and behavior with the child clone to be shaped even more by their previous experiences with the clone's dead progenitor sibling than they might have been if the child were not that dead sibling's clone. Thus, one should expect at least as much, if not more, psychological harm to befall a replacement child clone as a sexually reproduced replacement child."

While agreeing with Devolder that there need not be a slippery slope from therapeutic cloning to reproductive human cloning, Levick nevertheless believes that there is a slippery slope from allowing reproductive human cloning to "finding it preferable to sexual reproduction." And, according to Levick, the "evolution of our species requires the combination and recombination of genes in sexual reproduction," and "evolution of a sexually reproducing species would grind to a halt if it switched to asexual reproduction exclusively." Of course, one can respond to this by saying that there need not be the slippery slope that leads to cloning exclusively, since it is likely that there will always be those people who want to reproduce sexually. When all is said and done, Levick is probably correct in noting that, were a human clone produced who began living their life just like the rest of us noncloned beings, that human clone would likely "encounter difficulties over and above those associated with simply being human."

References

ACT (Advanced Cell Technologies). (2010). Advanced Cell Technology receives FDA clearance for the first clinical trial using embryonic stem cells to treat macular degeneration. Retrieved from: http://www.advancedcell.com/news-and-media/press-releases/advanced-cell-technology-receives-fda-clearance-for-the-first-clinical-trial-using-embryonic-stem-cel/index.asp

ACT (Advanced Cell Technologies). (2011). ACT secures patent to generate embryonic stem cells without embryo destruction. Retrieved from: http://www.advancedcell.com/news-and-media/press-releases/act-secures-patent-to-generate-embryonic-stem-cells-without-embryo-destruction/index.asp

Briggs, R., & King, T. (1952). Transplantation of living nuclei from blastula cells into enucleated frogs' eggs. *Proceedings of the National Academy of Sciences, 38*, 455–463.

Brown, T. A. (2010). *Gene cloning & DNA analysis: An introduction*. Malden, MA: Wiley-Blackwell.

Cibelli, J., Lanza, R., & West, M. (2001). The first human cloned embryo: Cloned early-stage human embryos and human embryos generated only from eggs, in a process called parthenogenesis now put therapeutic cloning within reach. *Scientific American, 21*, 44–51.

Cyranoski, D. (2006). Verdict: Hwang's human stem cells were all fakes. *Nature, 439*, 122–123.

de Wert, G., & Mummery, C. (2003). Human embryonic stem cells: Research, ethics and policy. *Human Reproduction, 18*(4), 672–682.

DHC (Document of the Holy See on Human Cloning). (2004). Retrieved from: http://www.vatican.va/roman_curia/secretariat_state/2004/documents/rc_seg-st_20040927_ cloning_en.html

Di Berardino, M., & McKinnell, R. (2004). The pathway to animal cloning and beyond—Robert Briggs (1911–1983) and Thomas J. King (1921–2000). *Journal of Experimental Zoology: Part A, Comparative Experimental Biology, 301*, 275–279.

Dworkin, R. (1993). *Life's dominion: An argument about abortion, euthanasia, and individual freedom*. New York: Vintage Books.

Gray, R., & Dobson, R. (2009). Extinct ibex is resurrected by cloning: An extinct animal has been brought back to life for the first time after being cloned from frozen tissue. *The Telegraph*. January 31. Retrieved from: http://www.telegraph.co.uk/science/science-news/4409958/Extinct-ibex-is-resurrected-by-cloning.html

Green, R. (2001). *The human embryo research debates: Bioethics in the vortex of controversy*. Oxford: Oxford University Press.

Guardian. (2011). Cloned animals. *The Guardian*. Retrieved from: http://www.guardian.co.uk/gall/0,8542,627251,00.html

John Paul II. (2001). Pope's address to President Bush at Castel Gandolfo, Italy, July 23, 2001. Retrieved from: http://www.americancatholic.org/news/stemcell/pope_to_bush.asp

Johnson, J., & Williams, E. (2006). CRS report for Congress: Human cloning. Retrieved from: http://www.fas.org/sgp/crs/misc/RL31358.pdf

Kant, I. (1775–89/1963). *Lectures on ethics* (L. Infield, Trans.). Indianapolis, IN: Hackett Publishing.

Kant, I. (1785/1998). *Groundwork of the metaphysics of morals* (M. Gregor, Trans.). (Section I: Transition from common rational to philosophic moral cognition). Cambridge: Cambridge University Press.

Kant, I. (1797/1996). *Practical philosophy* (M. Gregor, Trans.). Cambridge: Cambridge University Press.

Klimanskaya, I., Chung, Y., Becker, S., Lu, S-J., & Lanza, R. (2006). Human embryonic stem cell lines derived from single blastomeres. *Nature*, *444*, 481–485.

Klimanskaya, I., Chung, Y., Becker, S., Lu, S-J., & Lanza, R. (2007). Derivation of human embryonic stem cells from single blastomeres. *Nature Protocols*, *2*, 1963–1972.

Klotzko, A. (Ed.). (2003). *The cloning sourcebook*. Oxford: Oxford University Press.

Lachmann, P. (2001). Stem cell research—why is it regarded as a threat? An investigation of the economic and ethical arguments made against research with human embryonic stem cells. *European Molecular Biology Organization (EMBO) Reports*, *2*(3), 165–168.

Lang, M. (2011). ACT awarded patent for stem cell generation technique. *Mass High Tech*, February 25. Retrieved from: http://www.masshightech.com/stories/2011/02/21/daily53-ACT-awarded-patent-for-stem-cell-generation-technique.html

Manninen, B. (2008). Are human embryos Kantian persons? Kantian considerations in favor of embryonic stem cell research. *Philosophy, Ethics, and Humanities in Medicine*, *3*(4). Retrieved from: http://www.peh-med.com/content/3/1/4

McKie, R. (1997). Scientists clone adult sheep: Triumph for UK raises alarm over human use. *The Observer*. February 22. Retrieved from: http://www.guardian.co.uk/uk/1997/feb/23/robinmckie.theobserver

Michael, M. (2002). Why not interfere with nature? *Ethical Theory and Moral Practice*, *5*(1), 89–112.

NCBC (National Catholic Bioethics Center). (2009). *A Catholic guide to ethical clinical research*. Philadelphia: National Catholic Bioethics Center.

NCSL (National Conference of State Legislatures). (2011). Human cloning laws. Retrieved from: http://www.ncsl.org/default.aspx?tabid=14284

NHGRI (National Human Genome Research Institute). (2011). Reproductive cloning. Retrieved from: http://www.genome.gov/multimedia/illustrations/FactSheet_Cloning.pdf

Novak, M. (2001). The stem cell side: Be alert to the beginnings of evil. In M. Ruse & C. Pynes (Eds.), *The stem cell controversy: Debating the issues* (pp. 111–116). Amherst, NY: Prometheus Books.

O'Brien, N. (2011). Science, religion not in conflict, US bishops say in stem-cell document. *AmericanCatholic.Org*. Retrieved from: http://www.americancatholic.org/News/StemCell/stemcelldocument.asp

Piña-Aguilar, R., Lopez-Saucedo, J., Sheffield, R., Ruiz-Galaz, L., Barroso-Padilla, J., & Gutiérrez-Gutiérrez, A. (2009). Revival of extinct species using nuclear transfer: Hope for the mammoth, true for the Pyrenean ibex, but is it time for "conservation cloning"? *Cloning and Stem Cells*, *11*(3), 341–346.

Public Agenda (2011). Countries with bans on human cloning and/or genetic engineering. Retrieved from: http://www.publicagenda.org/charts/countries-bans-human-cloning-andor-genetic-engineering

Ryall, J. (2011). Mammoth "could be reborn in four years": The woolly mammoth, extinct for thousands of years, could be brought back to life in as little as four years thanks to a breakthrough in cloning technology. *The Telegraph*. January 13. Retrieved from: http://www.telegraph.co.uk/science/science-news/8257223/Mammoth-could-be-reborn-in-four-years.html

Schwartz, S., Hubschman, J-P., Heilwell, G., Franco-Cardenas, V., Pan, C., Ostrick, R. … Lanza, R. (2012). Embryonic stem cell trials for macular degeneration: A preliminary report. *The Lancet*, *379*, 713–720.

Sung, L-Y., Chang, C-C., Amano, T., Lin, C-J., Amano, M., Treaster, S. … Tian, X. (2010). Efficient derivation of embryonic stem cells from nuclear transfer and parthenogenetic embryos derived from cryopreserved oocytes. *Cellular Reprogramming*, *12*(2), 203–211.

TNA (*The New Atlantis*). (2006). Human cloning and scientific corruption. *The New Atlantis*, *11*, 113–117.

UNDHC (United Nations Declaration on Human Cloning). (2005). Retrieved from: http://www.bioeticaweb.com/content/view/1267/765/lang,es/

Verhey, A. (1995). "Playing god" and invoking a perspective. *The Journal of Medicine and Philosophy*, *20*(4), 347–364.

Wilmut, I., Campbell, K., & Tudge, C. (2000). *The second creation: The age of biological control*. London: Headline Book Publishing.

Wilmut, I., Schnieke, A., McWhir, J., Kind, A., & Campbell, K. (1997). Viable offspring derived from fetal and adult mammalian cells. *Nature*, *385*, 810–813.

Yang, X., Smith, S., Tian, C., Lewin, H., Renard, J-P., & Wakayama, T. (2007). Nuclear reprogramming of cloned embryos and its implications for therapeutic cloning. *Nature Genetics*, *39*, 295–302.

Chapter Five

Were It Physically Safe, Human Reproductive Cloning Would Be Acceptable

Katrien Devolder

In this chapter, I discuss a range of concerns expressed about human reproductive cloning, and argue that most of these concerns are unjustified, or at least more controversial than is generally assumed. Moreover, to the extent that some concerns are justified, the question remains whether they can support a conclusive argument against human reproductive cloning. This will depend on how strong reasons *for* reproductive cloning are. I conclude that if cloning were physically safe, it may be permissible to use it as a means of reproduction.

Dolly: A Wolf in Sheep's Clothing?

Dolly the sheep—the first mammal cloned from an adult somatic (body) cell—came into the world innocent as a lamb. However, soon after the announcement of her birth in February 1997 (Wilmut et al., 1997) she caused panic and controversy. An important, and for many people troubling question arose: if the cloning of sheep is possible, will scientists soon start cloning humans as well; and if they did, would this be wrong or unwise?

For most people, Dolly was really a wolf in sheep's clothing. She represented a first undesirable and dangerous step to applying reproductive cloning in humans, something that many agreed should never be done. Only a small minority thought it was permissible, or even morally obligatory to conduct further research into human reproductive cloning (see, for example, Fletcher, 1988; Harris, 2004). Some had no strong objections to it, but did not see any reason to promote it either.

Fifteen years after her birth, Dolly is stuffed and set up for display in the National Museum of Scotland. Many countries or jurisdictions have legally banned reproductive cloning or are in the process of doing so. In some countries, including France and Singapore, human reproductive cloning is a crime. The debate on human reproductive cloning seem to have drawn to a close. It is generally agreed that it is a bad idea to do it.

In this chapter, I discuss a range of concerns expressed about human reproductive cloning, and argue that most of these concerns are unjustified, or at least more controversial than is generally assumed. Moreover, to the extent that some concerns are justified, the question remains whether they can support a conclusive argument against human reproductive cloning. This will depend on how strong the reasons *for* reproductive cloning are. I conclude that if cloning were physically safe, it may be permissible to use it as a means of reproduction.

Contemporary Debates in Bioethics, First Edition. Edited by Arthur L. Caplan and Robert Arp.

What Is Reproductive Cloning?

Strictly speaking, cloning is the creation of a genetic copy of a sequence of DNA or of the entire genome of an organism. In the latter sense, cloning occurs naturally in the birth of identical twins and other multiples, but cloning can also be done artificially in the laboratory via embryo twinning or splitting: an early embryo is split in vitro so that both parts, when transferred to a uterus, can develop into individual organisms genetically identical to each other. In the cloning debate, however, the term *cloning* typically refers to a technique called somatic cell nuclear transfer (SCNT).[1] SCNT involves transferring the nucleus of a somatic cell into an oocyte from which the nucleus and thus most of the DNA have been removed. (The mitochondrial DNA in the cytoplasm is, however, still present). The manipulated oocyte is then treated with an electric current in order to stimulate cell division, resulting in the formation of an embryo. The embryo is genetically identical to, and thus a clone of, the somatic cell donor.

Dolly was the first mammal to be brought into the world using SCNT. Dolly is a case of *reproductive* cloning, the aim of which is to create offspring. Reproductive cloning is to be distinguished from cloning for therapy and research, sometimes also referred to as *therapeutic cloning*. This type of cloning also involves the creation of an embryo via SCNT, but instead of transferring the cloned embryo to the uterus in order to generate a pregnancy, it is used to obtain pluripotent stem cells that are genetically identical to the patient. Such patient-matched embryonic stem cells could offer powerful tools for biomedical research and therapy (Cervera & Stojkovic, 2007). Unfortunately, the development of this technology has received considerable opposition.

One common objection holds that cloning for research and therapy represents the first step on a slippery slope to reproductive cloning (Kass, 1998). The idea is that once we accept cloning for research and therapy, this will inevitably result in a situation where we can no longer say "no" to reproductive cloning. There are two questions one should ask when confronted with a slippery-slope argument. The first is whether the slope is really that slippery. Is it true that if we accept cloning for research and therapy, this will automatically result in a society where people will accept and make use of reproductive cloning? It is not clear why this should be the case. Although the basic technique is the same, the intentions and aims differ, and so do the ethical issues. So, even if one accepts cloning for research and therapy, one can, without being inconsistent, reject reproductive cloning. Moreover, effective legislation which clearly distinguishes between the two types of cloning could prevent us from sliding down the slope. This can simply be achieved by prohibiting the transfer of cloned embryos to the uterus (as in the UK and Belgium). The second question one should ask when confronted with a slippery-slope objection is whether it would really be so bad to end up at the bottom of the slope. Would it really be so bad if we ended up in a society where cloning is used as a mode of reproduction? In what follows, I focus on the last question. I argue that it would not be as wrong or unwise to pursue human reproductive cloning as is generally assumed.

The Argument that Reproductive Cloning Is Physically Unsafe

Despite the successful creation of viable offspring via SCNT in various mammalian species, researchers still have limited understanding of how the technique works on the subcellular and molecular level. Although the overall efficiency and safety of reproductive cloning in mammals have significantly increased over the past 15 years, it is not yet a safe process (Whitworth & Prather, 2010). For example, the rate of abortions, stillbirths, and developmental abnormalities remains high. Another source of concern is the risk of premature aging because of shortened telomeres. Telomeres are repetitive DNA sequences at the tip of chromosomes that get shorter as an animal gets older. When the telomeres of a cell get so short that they disappear, the cell dies. The concern is then that cloned animals may inherit the shortened telomeres from their older progenitor, with possibly premature aging and a shortened lifespan as a result.

For many, the fact that reproductive cloning is unsafe provides a sufficient reason not to pursue it.

It has been argued that it would simply be wrong to impose such significant health risks on humans (see, for example, Kass, 1998, p. 693). However, with the actual rate of advancement in cloning, one cannot exclude a future in which its safety and efficiency will be comparable or superior to that of in vitro fertilization (IVF) or even sexual reproduction. A remaining question, then, is: were human reproductive cloning physically safe, might it be an ethically acceptable means of reproduction?

Let us start with considering some reasons *for* having a child through reproductive cloning (henceforth just *cloning*). Why might anyone want to create a child that is a genetic copy of an existing individual, or of an individual that has existed? In what follows, I do not consider all possible reasons. I restrict myself to the most realistic ones.

Reasons *For* Reproductive Cloning

A first reason why people may want to reproduce through cloning is because it may be their only chance to have a genetically related child. Currently, those who want a child but cannot produce an embryo because they are infertile can either use a donor embryo and carry it to term (or have it carried to term by a surrogate), or adopt a child. In neither case, however, will the child be genetically related. Cloning would allow these people to have a genetically related child. Moreover, if a couple uses the female partner's egg in the cloning procedure, then the child could be genetically related to both rearing parents, as it would share his mitochondrial DNA with the woman whose egg was used, and his nuclear DNA with the woman's partner who provided the somatic cell.

Another possible reason to reproduce through cloning is to avoid that one's child shares half of her genetic material, that is, half of her *nuclear* DNA, with a gamete donor. Individuals, same-sex couples, or couples who cannot together produce an embryo need donor gametes to reproduce. If cloning were available, this would no longer be the case (they might still need donor eggs, but these would be enucleated so that only the mitochondrial DNA remains). It would be possible then to avoid that one's child shares half of her nuclear DNA with a gamete donor.

In 2009, Panos Zavos, a controversial fertility doctor in the US, claimed to have created cloned embryos using tissues from three deceased people, one of them a young girl who had died in a car crash (Jones, 2009). He said his intent was to study the cloning procedure, not to create babies. However, he stressed that in the future, cloning could be used to create genetic copies of deceased loved ones. For example, parents whose child had died could create a genetically identical "replacement child." Some private companies already offer to clone dead pets to create replacements pets (Koningsberg, 2008). As will become clear later, this reason for having a cloned child is the weakest, as it is based on a misunderstanding of what cloning is.

Although many object to cloning because it would give prospective parents more control over their child's genome, others think that this is exactly what makes cloning potentially beneficial (Fletcher, 1988; Harris 1997, 2004; Pence, 1998; Tooley, 1998). Cloning would enable parents to have a child with a genome identical to that of a person with good health and/or other desirable characteristics. John Harris (2004, pp. 29–30) stresses the point that cloning allows someone to be provided with a tried-and-tested genome, not one created by the genetic lottery of sexual reproduction and the random combination of chromosomes. If we choose our cell donor wisely, Harris argues, we will be able to protect the clone from many hereditary disorders and many other genetic problems.

An individual created through cloning would be genetically identical to an existing person. I will refer to that person as the progenitor. The progenitor would thus be a perfect tissue match for the younger clone. This may be advantageous in case the younger clone needs donor stem cells or tissues, or a nonvital organ like a kidney. Donor cells, tissues, and organs need to be immunologically compatible with the recipient to avoid rejection by the immune system.

Not only could the clone benefit from the progenitor being a perfect tissue match, but also the progenitor herself could benefit from having a younger tissue match. For example, if the progenitor has a blood disease, the treatment of which requires a hematopoietic stem-cell transplantation, stem cells from the umbilical cord blood collected after the birth of the younger clone could be used for transplantation to the progenitor. The younger clone would then be a so-called *savior sibling*.

Thus, cloning could significantly expand our procreative options. It could offer a new means to satisfy our reproductive desires with potential advantages to the well-being of the parents, the individual created through cloning, and others. So, why do people have strong objections to cloning?

Reasons Against Reproductive Cloning

In what follows, I consider the most commonly expressed concerns about reproductive cloning. Most often, these concerns have been said to provide a conclusive argument against cloning; sometimes they have been said to provide a strong reason against cloning, which could potentially be outweighed by strong reasons *for* cloning. It is then typically argued that since the reasons for cloning are weak, they cannot outweigh the reasons against it, and, therefore, cloning is impermissible.

That cloning is unnatural and therefore wrong is one of the most often heard arguments against cloning (see, for example, the President's Council on Bioethics [PCBE], 2002, chapter 5) but also one of the least convincing. To say that something is *unnatural* can be interpreted in various ways. Perhaps the most obvious sense in which cloning is unnatural is that it is artificial—it is the product of purposeful human activity. It seems implausible, however, that all that is artificial is bad, as this implies we should get rid of mankind to remove "the bad" from the universe. Another sense in which cloning is unnatural is that it is unusual. It is not what we normally do. But why would the *unusualness* of something make it wrong? Many new technologies are unusual. We do not generally think that this provides a good reason not to develop or use them. To determine whether we should develop or use new unusual technologies, we typically look at the expected consequences of doing so.

Many fear that cloning threatens the identity and individuality of the clone, thus reducing her autonomy. This may be bad in itself, or bad because it might reduce the clone's well-being. It may also be bad because it will severely restrict the array of life plans open to the clone, thus violating her "right to an open future" (Feinberg, 1980). In its report "Human Cloning and Human Dignity: An Ethical Inquiry," the President's Council on Bioethics (2002) wrote that being genetically unique is "an emblem of independence and individuality" and allows us to go forward "with a relatively indeterminate future in front of us" (chapter 5, section c). Such concerns have formed the basis of strong opposition to cloning.

The concern that cloning threatens the clone's identity and individuality relies on the mistaken belief that who and what we become is entirely determined by our genes. Such genetic determinism is clearly false. Though genes influence our personal development, so does the complex and irreproducible context in which our lives take place and this to a significant extent. We know this, among others, from studying monozygotic twins. Notwithstanding the fact that such twins are genetically identical to each other and, therefore, sometimes look very similar and often share many character traits, habits, and preferences, they *are* different individuals, with different identities (Segal, 1999). Thus, having a genetic duplicate does not threaten one's individuality, or one's distinct identity.

One could, however, argue that even though individuals created through cloning would be unique individuals with a distinct identity, they might not *experience* it that way. As Brock (2002) pointed out, what is threatened by cloning then is not the individual's identity or individuality, but her *sense* of identity and individuality, and this may reduce her autonomy. So, even if a clone *has* a unique identity, she may nevertheless experience more difficulties in establishing her identity than if she had not been a clone.

But why would this be the case? Let us compare with monozygotic twins again. Each twin not only *has* a distinct identity, but also generally views him or herself as having a distinct identity, as do their relatives and friends. Moreover, an individual created through cloning would likely be of a different age than her progenitor. There may even be several generations between them. A clone would thus in essence be a "delayed" twin. Presumably this would make it even easier for the clone to view herself as distinct from the progenitor than if she had been genetically identical to someone her same age.

The reference to twins as a model to think about reproductive cloning has, however, been criticized, for example, because it fails to reflect important aspects of the parent–child relationship that would incur if the child were a clone of one of the rearing parents (Jonas, 1974; Levick, 2004). Because of the dominance of the progenitor, the risk of reduced autonomy and confused identity may be greater in such a situation than in the case of ordinary twins. Moreover, just *because* the clone would be a *delayed* twin, she may have the feeling that her life has already been lived or that she is predetermined to do the same things as her progenitor. This problem may be exacerbated by others constantly comparing her life with that of the progenitor, and having problematic expectations of the clone based on these comparisons. The clone may feel under constant pressure to live up to these expectations (Kass, 1998; Levick, 2004, p. 101; Sandel, 2007, pp. 57–62), or may have the feeling she leads "a life in the shadow" of the progenitor (PCBE, 2002, chapter 5). This may especially be the case if the clone was created as a "replacement" for a deceased child. The fear is that the "ghost of the dead child" will get more attention and devotion than the replacement child. Parents may expect the clone to be like the lost child, or some idealized image of it, which could hamper the development of her identity and adversely affect her self-esteem (Levick, 2004, pp. 111–132).

Are these concerns justified? First, it is plausible that, through adequate information, we could largely correct mistaken beliefs about the link between genetic and personal identity, and thus reduce the risk of problematic expectations toward the clone. Of course, some people may nevertheless hold on to their mistaken beliefs and, consequently, to their problematic expectations. However, parents often have expectations of their children based on false beliefs. Although this may be problematic in some cases, we typically do not think that this is a sufficient reason to interfere with people's reproductive plans or to prevent people from making use of assisted reproduction techniques. Moreover, having high expectations, even if based on false beliefs, is not necessarily a bad thing. Parents with high expectations often give their children the best chances to lead a happy and successful life (Pence, 1998, p. 138). Parents not only often have high expectations of their children but also constantly restrict the array of available life plans open to them, for example, by selecting their school or by raising them according to certain values. Though this may somewhat restrict the child's autonomy, there will always be enough decisions to take for the child to be autonomous, and to realize this. It is not clear why this should be different in the case of cloning. Indeed, as Dan Brock (2002) has argued: "The different future that would in fact inevitably unfold for the later twin, and the choices that she would necessarily face in that unfolding future, would likely, at least to some degree, force the recognition on her that her future was hers to autonomously construct and create, though within a variety of constraints that include those set by her genome" (p. 316).

Moreover, there may also be advantages to being a delayed twin. For example, one may acquire knowledge about the progenitor's medical history and use this knowledge to live longer, or to increase one's autonomy. One could, for example, use the information to reduce the risk of getting the disease or condition, or to at least postpone its onset, by behavioral changes, an appropriate diet and/or preventive medication. Information about one's predispositions for certain diseases would also allow one to take better-informed reproductive decisions. One could, for example, avoid bringing a child into the world that has a serious genetic disease.

Cloning arouses people's imagination about the clone, but also about those who will choose to have a child through cloning. Often dubious motives are ascribed to them: they would want a child that is "just like so-and-so" causing people to view them as objects or as commodities like a new car or a new house (see, for example, Putnam, 1997, pp. 7–8). They would want an attractive child (a clone of Scarlett Johansson) or a child with tennis talent (a clone of Kim Clijsters) purely to show off. Dictators would want armies of clones to achieve their political goals. People would clone themselves out of vanity. Parents would clone their existing child so that the clone can serve as an organ bank for that child, or would clone their deceased child to have a replacement child. The conclusion is then that cloning is wrong because the clone will be used as a mere means to others' ends.

But do we have good reason to ascribe such dubious motives to those who would like a child through cloning? Most people who have expressed an interest in cloning are infertile people who would like to have a genetically related child. Although one may question the value of these motivations (see, for example, Levy & Lotz, 2005), it is not clear why they involve creating, or treating the child as a mere means. There may, of course, always be individuals or couples who have morally dubious motives to have children through cloning. However, instead of rejecting cloning altogether, a better response would be to correct some of the major misunderstandings about and prejudices against cloning that these dubious motivations rely on.

But suppose some people create a clone for instrumental reasons, for example, as a stem cell donor. This does not imply that the clone will be treated merely as a means. Parents have children for all kinds of instrumental reasons, including the benefit for the husband–wife relationship, continuity of the family name, and the economic and psychological benefits children provide when their parents become old (Fawcett & Arnold, 1973). This is generally not considered problematic as long as the child is also valued in its own right. What is most important in a parent–child relationship is the love and care inherent in that relationship. We judge people on their attitudes toward children, rather than on their motives for having them. Perhaps this is where the problem lies: the concern that the clone will be treated as a means relies on the assumption that there is a strong link between one's intention or motive to have a child, and the way one will treat the child. It is, however, a mistake to presuppose that the desire or the intention to have a child determines the attitudes of the parents toward the child once born. This would, for example, imply that children conceived in order to create a sibling for an already existing child would not be loved or would be loved only insofar they serve as a sibling to the child, which, fortunately, is not the case.

It is up to opponents of cloning to show that there is good reason to think that prospective parents who want to make use of cloning technology will have dubious motives (more dubious than those of other prospective parents) *and* that these are a reliable indicator for the way children will be treated. Moreover, opponents of cloning have to show that there is good reason to assume that if a child created through cloning is treated as a means, this would not have been the case had the child not been created through cloning.

Another concern is that clones may be the victims of unjustified discrimination and will not be respected as persons (Deech, 1999, Levick, 2004, pp. 185–187). Savulescu (2005) has referred to such negative attitudes towards clones as *clonism*: a new form of discrimination against a group of humans who are different in a nonmorally significant way. But does a fear for "clonism" constitute a good reason for rejecting cloning? If so, then we must conclude that racist attitudes and discriminatory behavior towards people with a certain ethnicity provide a good reason for people with that ethnicity not to procreate. This seems a morally objectionable way to solve the problem of racism. Instead of limiting people's procreative liberty, we should combat existing prejudices and discrimination. Likewise, instead of prohibiting cloning out of concern for clonism, we should combat possible prejudices and discrimination against clones.

Moreover, note that by expressing certain concerns about cloning, one may actually reinforce certain prejudices and misguided stereotypes about clones. For example, saying that a clone would not have a personal identity prejudges the clone as inferior or fraudulent (the idea that originals are more valuable than their copies) or even less than human (as individuality is seen as an essential characteristic of human nature).

Another concern is that cloning threatens traditional family structures, a fear that has come up in debates about homosexuals adopting children, IVF, and other assisted reproduction techniques. But in cloning the situation would be more complex, as it may blur generational boundaries. Glen McGee (2000) put it this way:

> In the case of a cloned embryo, it is not at all obvious who are the parents. The person who donates DNA from a somatic cell is the progenitor, in that the child carries that person's DNA. But the mammalian parents of the cloned child are the grandparents, if what one means by parent is that the person contributed 50% of the genes to the recombination process that formed the

> genome of the person in question … If the egg used to raise the clone comes from another person, as it would in the case of a clone of a male, there is in addition an egg parent, a person who contributes mitochondrial DNA and RNA in the egg wall, the collective role of which on an organism is unknown but perhaps significant. If the progenitor of the clone is itself an embryo or aborted fetus, the parent would not only be a virgin, but also a nonconsenting nonperson that itself has no legally established standing apart from the wishes of its own progenitor. (p. 269)

First, it is not clear why the fact that generational boundaries may be blurred that the cloned child will be more confused about his family ties than are some children now. Many have four nurturing parents because of a divorce, never knew their genetic parents, have nurturing parents that are not their genetic parents, or think that their nurturing father is also their genetic father when it turns out they were actually conceived with the sperm of the nurturing mother's lover. While these complex family relationships can be troubling for some children, they are not insurmountable. There are many aspects about the situation one is born and raised in that may be troublesome. As with all children, the most important thing is the relation with people who nurture and educate them, and children usually know very well who these people are. There is no reason to believe that with cloning, this will be any different. But perhaps there is a morally relevant difference. Even though there are children with confused family relationships, it may be different when prospective parents seek such potentially confused relationships for their children from the start (O'Neil, 2002, pp. 67–68).

However, people who decide to have a child via cloning do not generally *seek* such relationships, like parents do not *seek* such relationships when they divorce, or when they conceive with donor gametes, or a surrogate, or when twins have children. Potentially confusing family relationships are a side effect of the decision to get a divorce, or to use a donor gametes, etc. In these scenarios, the advantages of the divorce, of using donor gametes, etc. presumably are large enough to outweigh the risk that the children will be confused about their family ties. Likewise, then, the advantages of cloning may justify the risk that the clone may be somewhat confused about her family ties.

Harm to Others

Other concerns raised by cloning focus on the potential harmful effects of cloning for *others*. Sometimes, these concerns are related to those about the well-being of the clone. For example, Michael Sandel (2007, pp. 52–57) has argued that cloning and enhancement technologies may result in a society in which parents will not accept their child for what it is, reinforcing an already existing trend of heavily managed, high-pressure child-rearing or *hyper-parenting*. McGee's concern about confused family relationships bears not only on the clone but also on society as a whole. However, since I have already argued why I think these concerns are not justified or why not pursuing cloning would be the wrong response to these concerns, I will, in the remainder of this chapter, focus on other arguments.

The strongest reason for why reproductive cloning should be permissible, if safe, is that it will allow infertile people to have a genetically related child. Cloning can then simply be seen as a new assisted reproduction technique. If parents have a cloned child for this reason, we have no reason to believe their views about cloning are misguided, and that the child will have a life in which it will be harmed more than if it had been created through other means of reproduction. However, this position relies on the view that having genetically related children is morally significant and valuable. This is a controversial view. For example, Levy and Lotz (2005) have denied the importance of a genetic link between parents and their children. Moreover, they have argued that claiming that this link is important will give rise to bad consequences, such as reduced adoption rates and diminished resources for improving the life prospects of the disadvantaged, including those waiting to be adopted. Since, according to these authors, these undesirable consequences would be magnified if we allowed human cloning, we have good reason to prohibit it.

These arguments are not new. They have been adduced against offering and funding *in vitro* fertilization (see, for example, Bartholet, 1999). Indeed, if the arguments hold against cloning, they should also hold against IVF.

Whether the genetic link is valuable or not is a complex question I cannot settle here. Levy and Lotz suggest that empirical data do not support this view. However, against this, it can be argued that neither do empirical data support the view that the genetic link is *less* valuable than is generally assumed. But suppose Levy and Lotz are right about the fact that we tend to overestimate the importance of the genetic link between parents and their children. Does it follow from this that it is wrong for individuals to reproduce through cloning? Their principal objection is that offering reproductive cloning will harm children waiting to be adopted, an argument also advanced by Ahlberg & Brighouse (2011). However, the adverse effect of cloning on children waiting to be adopted is uncertain (Strong, 2008). A thorough analysis by Cohen and Chen (2010) shows that there is no strong evidence for the claim that subsidizing IVF via state-level insurance mandates to increase the availability of IVF in the US decreases the adoption rate. These data provide at least some reason to believe that permitting cloning would not decrease adoption rates either.

A second reason for why cloning should not be allowed according to Levy and Lotz is that it will reinforce the misguided idea of the importance of genetic relatedness, and that this in turn will result in less resources to improve the life prospects of the disadvantaged, including those waiting to be adopted. First, it is not clear whether this will result will occur. Second, one may wonder whether it is ethically acceptable to deny infertile people access to cloning because of *indirect* costs to children waiting to be adopted (Cohen & Chen, 2010, p. 514). If providing hip replacements turned out to lead to a diminution in adoptions, should we stop providing them? Moreover, we may wonder why only infertile people should carry the burden to help children waiting for adoption. A more just way to provide help to these children may be to mobilize society as a whole to make sure they are adopted.

Eugenics

The increase in control over what kind of genome we wish to pass on to our children could have beneficial consequences. We could select a tried and tested genome to have a healthy child. However, a major concern is that this shift "from chance to choice" will lead to problematic eugenic practices.

One version of this concern states that cloning would, from the outset, constitute a problematic form of eugenics. However, this is implausible: the best explanations of what was wrong with immoral cases of eugenics, such as the Nazi eugenic programs, are that they involved coercion and were motivated by objectionable moral beliefs or false nonmoral beliefs (Agar, 2004; Buchanan, 2007). This would not necessarily be the case were cloning to be implemented now.

A more plausible version of the eugenics concern points out the risk of a slippery slope: the claim is that cloning will lead to objectionable forms of eugenics—for example, coercive eugenics—in the future. After all, historical cases of immoral eugenics often developed from earlier well-intentioned and less problematic practices.

Given the history of eugenics, concerns about a slippery slope to immoral eugenics should always be taken seriously. However, in most liberal democracies, reproductive autonomy is firmly entrenched in both the law and the prevailing psyche, and it is unlikely that if cloning became available reproductive autonomy would suddenly be severely restricted. Reproductive autonomy has not been restricted since the use of genetic-selection technologies such as preimplantation genetic diagnosis. Nevertheless, steps should always be taken to ensure that reproductive autonomy remains as secure in the future as it is at present.

Human Dignity

Article 11 of UNESCO's Universal Declaration on the Human Genome and Human Rights (1997) states that "practices which are contrary to human dignity, such as reproductive cloning of human beings, shall not be permitted ..." The World Health Organization and the European Parliament also condemn reproductive cloning on the ground that it violates human dignity. One problem with such references to human dignity is it is rarely specified how human dignity is to be understood, whose dignity is at stake, and how exactly dignity is relevant to the ethics of cloning. Is it the copying of a genome that violates human dignity, as Leon Kass (1998) has suggested? If so, then the existence of twins must violate human dignity too, which is implausible. Human dignity is most often related to Kant's second formulation of the Categorical Imperative, namely the idea that we should never use a person merely as a means. I have argued earlier that there is no good reason to believe that cloning will result in parents treating their children as a mere means.

Others have argued that though cloning in itself is not a violation of human dignity, it *can* be under certain circumstances, as, for example, when it would divert scarce resources away from those who lack sufficient health to enable them to exercise basic rights and liberties (Birnbacher, 2005; McDougall, 2008). However, as I have argued earlier, it is not clear why cloning would have to divert resources away from those who lack sufficient health. Other resources, including private resources, could be used instead to fund cloning.

Conclusion

Whether or not cloning is, all things considered, permissible depends on the weight of the reasons *for* doing it, and the weight of the reasons *against* doing it. I have shown that most concerns adduced against cloning are either unjustified or, at least, less serious than is generally assumed. I have identified some reasons to pursue cloning. In the absence of any strong reason against pursuing cloning, and provided that cloning is safe, it may thus be permissible for infertile people to reproduce through cloning.

Note

1 Note that although SCNT has been the most often discussed cloning technique, other techniques, or a combination of techniques may provide alternative means for reproductive cloning, for example, embryo twinning. However, what many people find disturbing is the idea of creating a genetic duplicate of an existing person, or a person who has existed. This goal could be achieved through SCNT, but also by cryopreserving one of two *in vitro* created twin embryos for a long period before using it to generate a pregnancy. Reproductive cloning could also be achieved by combining the induced pluripotent stem-cell technique with tetraploid complementation. Several research teams succeeded in cloning mice this way (Boland et al., 2009; Kang et al., 2009; Zhao et al., 2009).

References

Agar, N. (2004). *Liberal eugenics: in defense of human enhancement.* Oxford: Blackwell.

Ahlberg, J., & Brighouse, H. (2011). An argument against cloning. *Canadian Journal of Philosophy, 40*(4), 539–566.

Bartholet, E. (1999). *Family bonds: adoption, infertility, and the new world of child production.* Boston: Beacon Press.

Birnbacher, D. (2005). Human cloning and human dignity. *Reproductive Biomedicine Online, 10,* 50–55.

Boland M. J., Hazen, J. L., Nazor, K. L., Rodriguez, A. R., Gifford, W. ... Baldwin, K. K. (2009). Adult mice generated from induced pluripotent stem cells. *Nature, 461*(7260), 91–94.

Brock, D. W. (2002). Human cloning and our sense of self. *Science, 296*(5566), 314–316.

Buchanan, A. (2007). Institutions, beliefs and ethics: eugenics as a case study. *Journal of Political Philosophy, 15*(1), 22–45.

Cervera, R. P., & Stojkovic, M. (2007). Human embryonic stem cell derivation and nuclear transfer: Impact on regenerative therapeutics and drug discovery. *Clinical Pharmacology &* Therapeutics, *82*(3), 310–315.

Cohen, I. G., & Chen, D. L. (2010). Trading-off reproductive technology and adoption: Does subsidizing IVF decrease adoption rates and should it matter? *Minnesota Law Review, 95,* 486–574.

Deech, R. (1999). Human cloning and public policy. In J. Burley (Ed.), *The genetic revolution and human rights* (pp. 95–100). Oxford: Oxford University Press.

Fawcett, J. T., & Arnold, F. S. (1973). The value of children: theory and method. *Representative research in social psychology, 4*(3), 23–25.

Feinberg, J. (1980). A child's right to an open future. In W. Aiken (Ed.), *Whose child? Parental rights, parental authority and state power* (pp. 124–153). Totowa, NJ: Rowman & Littlefield.

Fletcher, J. F. (1988). *The ethics of genetic control: Ending reproductive roulette. Artificial insemination, surrogate pregnancy, nonsexual reproduction, genetic control.* New York: Prometheus.

Harris, J. (1997). Goodbye Dolly: The ethics of human cloning. *Journal of Medical Ethics, 23*(6), 353–360.

Harris, J. (2004). *On cloning.* London: Routledge.

Jonas, H. (1974). *Philosophical essays: From ancient creed to technological man*. Englewood Cliffs, NJ: Prentice-Hall.

Jones, D. (24 April 2009). Clones, cowboys and resurrecting the dead. *Guardian*. Retrieved from: http://www.guardian.co.uk/commentisfree/belief/2009/apr/24/religion-ethics-cloning-embryos.

Kang, L., Wang, J., Zhang, Y., Kou, Z., & Gao, S. (2009). iPS cells can support full-term development of tetraploid blastocyst-complemented embryos. *Cell Stem Cell*, *5*(2), 135–138.

Kass, L. R. (1998). The wisdom of repugnance: Why we should ban the cloning of humans? *Valparaiso University Law Review*, *32*(2), 679–705.

Koningsberg, E. (2008). Beloved pets everlasting? *New York Times*, December 31. Retrieved from: http://www.nytimes.com/2009/01/01/garden/01clones.html?pagewanted=all

Levick, S. E. (2004). *Clone being: Exploring the psychological and social dimensions*. Lanham, MD: Rowman & Littlefield Publishers, Inc.

Levy, N., & Lotz, M. (2005). Reproductive cloning and a (kind of) genetic fallacy. *Bioethics*, *19*(3), 232–250.

McDougall, R. (2008). A resource-based version of the argument that cloning is an affront to human dignity. *Journal of Medical Ethics*, *34*(4), 259–261.

McGee, G. (2000). Cloning, sex, and new kinds of families. *Journal of Sex Research*, *37*(3), 266–272.

O'Neil, O. (2002). *Autonomy and trust in bioethics (Gifford Lectures 2001)*. Cambridge: Cambridge University Press.

Pence, G. (1998). *Who's afraid of human cloning?* Lanham, MD: Rowman & Littlefield.

President's Council on Bioethics. (2002). *Human cloning and human dignity: An ethical inquiry*. Washington, DC: The President's Council on Bioethics.

Putnam, H. (1997). Cloning people. In J. Burley (Ed.), *The genetic revolution and human rights* (pp. 1–13). Oxford: Oxford University Press.

Sandel, M. J. (2007). *The case against perfection. Ethics in the age of genetic engineering*. Cambridge, MA: Harvard University Press.

Savulescu, J. (2005). Equality cloning and clonism, why we must clone. *Bionews*, May 16. Retrieved from: http://www.bionews.org.uk/page_37800.asp

Segal, N. L. (1999). *Entwined lives: twins and what they tell us about human behavior*. New York: Plume.

Strong, C. (2008). Cloning and adoption: A reply to Levy and Lotz. *Bioethics*, *22*(2), 130–136.

Tooley, M. (1998). The moral status of the cloning of humans. In J. M. Humber & R. Almeder (Eds.), *Human cloning: Biomedical ethical reviews* (pp. 65–102). Totowa, NJ: Humana Press.

United Nations Educational, Scientific and Cultural Organization (UNESCO). (1997). Universal Declaration on the Human Genome and Human Rights. Retrieved from: http://portal.unesco.org/en/ev.php-URL_ID=13177&URL_DO=DO_TOPIC&URL_SECTION=201.html

Whitworth, K. M., & Prather, R. S. (2010). Somatic cell nuclear transfer efficiency: How can it be improved through nuclear remodeling and reprogramming? *Molecular Reproduction and Development*, 77(12), 1001–1015.

Wilmut I., Schnieke A., McWhir J., Kind A., & Campbell K. (1997). Viable offspring derived from fetal and adult mammalian cells. *Nature*, *385*, 810–813.

Zhao, X., Li, W., Lv, Z., Liu, L., Tong, M., Hai, T … Zhou, Q. (2009). iPS cells produce viable mice through tetraploid complementation. *Nature*, *461*(7260), 86–90.

Chapter Six

Were It Physically Safe, Human Reproductive Cloning Would Not Be Acceptable

Stephen E. Levick

The prospect of human reproductive cloning (HRC) raises terribly important issues and concerns for bioethics. When it comes to medical procedures and interventions, safety is evaluated relative to: (1) not treating the condition that the experimental procedure for which the intervention is intended, and also (2) the success and safety of other interventions already in clinical use to address the condition. Risk is a complex concept, and also a personal one medically. In my view, assessing the relative physical safety of HRC should not even be attempted before *also* considering possible psychological, social, and societal risks it may pose. In this chapter, I hope to demonstrate that, aside from whatever risks of physical harm HRC might pose, it is reasonable to believe that the practice may well present sufficient risk of psychological, social, and societal harms such that it *should not* be acceptable.

Introduction

In Hollywood, Florida, on December 27, 2002, the chief scientist of "Clonaid" made a headline-grabbing public announcement: She claimed that thanks to their efforts, a human clone baby named "Eve" had been born the previous night.

Attorney Bernard Segal doubted this was true, but was also concerned about the welfare of the child, if she existed. He petitioned the local county court to appoint a guardian for the child, arguing that she might be at risk medically or physically as a result of being a clone. Furthermore, Segal's petition specifically stated that "the minor child may undergo emotional stress and have significant psychological risks attendant to being a cloned human being." The court was actively considering the matter, when the group's chief scientist said that the child had been born not in Florida, but in Israel, placing the matter outside the court's jurisdiction. It also made it implicit that the whole thing had been a hoax (Siegel, 2007). The case of fictitious baby "Eve" is instructive in illustrating that a renegade medical scientist may attempt human reproductive cloning with little consideration of its physical and other risks. An unsuccessful attempt has since been reported in the medical literature (Zavos & Illmensee, 2006).

The prospect of human reproductive cloning (HRC) raises terribly important issues and concerns for bioethics. In the preceding chapter, Katrien Devolder explained why she believes HRC would be acceptable. In this chapter, I will explain why I conclude the opposite. Thankfully, Dr Devolder has already explained crucial concepts, defined key terms, and reviewed the most relevant literature.

Contemporary Debates in Bioethics, First Edition. Edited by Arthur L. Caplan and Robert Arp.

Would it be morally acceptable to try to establish the premise of safety for the proposition that Devolder and I debate here? Answering this question would entail entertaining this one: "Is any good claimed for HRC worth the physical risks it may pose?" Most of the same reasons for adjudging HRC unacceptable if it were safe physically are also relevant to answering this question.

When it comes to medical procedures and interventions, safety is evaluated relative to: (1) not treating the condition that the experimental procedure for which the intervention is intended, and also (2) the success and safety of other interventions already in clinical use to address the condition. Risk is a complex concept, and also a personal one medically (e.g., Hartzband & Groopman, 2012). In my view, assessing the relative physical safety of HRC should not even be attempted before *also* considering possible psychological, social, and societal risks it may pose. I hope to demonstrate that, aside from whatever risks of physical harm HRC might pose, it is reasonable to believe that the practice may well present sufficient risk of psychological, social, and societal harms that it *should not* be acceptable.

Dr Devolder considers possible justifications for HRC, as well as several key reasons for opposing it. She anticipates possible motivations of a prospective parent or parents to have a child by cloning. These motives include ones that they might believe would enhance their own well-being, and others they might believe would enhance the well-being of the child clone. She foresees four motivations in the first category, in which prospective parents want: (1) a child genetically related to one of them, (2) a child not genetically related to nonrearing parents, (3) a replacement child, and (4) a child who could be a perfect tissue match to his or her progenitor parent, should the medical need arise. In the second category, Devolder foresees two motivations for prospective parents of a self-clone of one of them. They might want a child through HRC: (1) to give the child a good genetic start, and/or (2) so that the progenitor parent would be a perfect tissue match to his or her self-clone, should the medical need arise.

My counterpart also considers a number of possible harms to the clone, as well as several other concerns for society in general. She highlights issues, alleged advantages, and a number of possible nonphysical risks. On balance, Devolder concludes that the hoped-for benefits of HRC outweigh the risks, and that if it were physically safe, it would be acceptable.

I will show how certain existing situations and phenomena are analogous to one or more aspect(s) of cloning. For each of the eight analogues that I have identified, there is a body of clinical experience, theory, and research in psychology and the social sciences, a portion of which is relevant by analogy to the cloning situation (Levick, 2004, 2006, 2007).

The analogues can inform our thinking about the cloning situation by drawing parallels to situations with which we are already familiar. By doing so, they can help the HRC situation seem less hypothetical and abstract. Moreover, many of us should be able to relate to one or more of the analogues personally, which can help us to engage our empathic imagination. This can help to vivify and humanize what might otherwise seem strange and cold. When it comes to moral reasoning, warm is well done.

Consequently, the analogues can also help redress the empathetic imbalance between: (1) prospective parents wanting to have HRC as an additional assisted reproductive technology (ART) and (2) the as-yet nonexistent hypothetical human clone. In my view, Dr Devolder's analysis favors the former over the latter.

Each HRC analogue has its own conceptual strength(s) and weakness(es), but taken together they point to some of the same conclusions from different directions. I will address many of Devolder's arguments within the analogues' systematic frameworks. I sketch five of the analogues below.

The Identical Twin Analogue

This analogue's conceptual strength lies in the fact that identical twins are true genetic clones of one another by embryo splitting. However, twins are contemporaries. In contrast, the progenitor (or nuclear donor) in cloning by nuclear transfer (NT) or other means outlined by Devolder would have substantial precedence with respect to his or her clone. This analogue's weakness in modeling HRC biologically is actually its greatest strength in modeling it psychologically and socially. Devolder disagrees with my view that by virtue of having a rearing parent as progenitor, the child clone would be at increased risk of psychological harm. But consider that this situation would magnify the already-striking asymmetries in dominance, dependency, knowledge, and strength that characterize the normal parent–child relationship. This analogue is not the only one suggesting this conclusion.

Devolder believes that being a clone of a rearing parent would be advantageous to the clone. Nancy Segal, an expert on the psychology of twins, has thought deeply about cloning, with the clone being, in effect, a "delayed twin" of his or her progenitor (Segal, 1997, 2002, 2006). Devolder believes that the clone's autonomy could be enhanced as a "delayed twin." It is unclear how. She also argues that a delayed twin would have an easier time developing a distinct identity than a same-age twin. If the child's progenitor preceded him by several generations, this might well be true. However, if the progenitor were a rearing parent, there are good reasons to think that this would be more difficult for reasons that I will sketch in other analogues.

Dr Devolder believes that a clone could live a longer and healthier life than her progenitor, due to foreknowledge of medical risks associated with their identical genomes. That might be, but rapidly improving technology and interpretation of total genome scans is likely to obviate this alleged advantage.

The Identical Twin Analogue is relevant to Devolder's claim that HRC could be of mutual benefit to both clone and progenitor, in that each is a perfect tissue match for the other, should a medical need for one arise. Currently, only identical twins can do this for one another. However, progress in the regenerative medicine area of tissue engineering (e.g., Fountain, 2012) is likely to increasingly obviate this alleged advantage of HRC.

It is unclear to me what Devolder might be implying by her assertion that the clone could make better-informed reproductive decisions, like avoiding bringing a child into the world with a serious genetic disorder. Presumably, the clone's progenitor would not have manifested such a disorder before serving as NT donor, and also undergone genetic testing for a not-yet-manifesting serious genetic disorder. Hence, genetic risks of the cloning procedure itself and epigenetic factors aside, the clone should be as medically healthy as his progenitor.

When the individual clone is ready to make a personal reproductive decision, he or she might consider the many possible genetic risks associated with sexual reproduction, learn that prenatal testing could identify many, and learn that pre-implantation genetic diagnosis (PGD) done on an extremely early IVF embryo, could identify even more. However, the individual clone might conclude that the most responsible reproductive decision would be to reproduce him or herself asexually—to self-clone, producing another child with a tried and true genome. Such a "well-informed" reproductive decision would constitute a kind of self-chosen or self-selected eugenics. I wonder if Dr Devolder would view that decision as a well-informed reproductive choice.

The ART Analogue

Overcoming infertility does seem likely to be the most common motivation for HRC, as Devolder states, and HRC would be a new ART. In this regard, sexually infertile heterosexual couples would be joined by the intrinsically infertile—same-sex couples and sole individuals. In terms of sexual reproduction, all humans are intrinsically infertile solo.

Some existing ARTs, such as donor insemination and ovum donation, produce children related genetically to only one rearing parent, though any sexually reproduced child is linked to two parents genetically, even if only one is the rearing parent. Sexual reproduction combines and recombines the genes of two parents. ARTs make sexual reproduction possible, without the genetic parents actually having sex. Cloning is a form of asexual reproduction. A clone would be related genetically to only one progenitor. If the rearing mother's egg was enucleated for NT, her mitochondrial DNA would remain in it and be inherited by the clone. Were a rearing parent also the child clone's progenitor, no other genetic parent or parents would be present anywhere elsewhere.

Devolder lists this fact among the advantages of cloning. We should think carefully about the difference between an existing but missing parent vs. a parent that never existed. In my view, an exclusive genetic tie to one and only one rearing parent and no one else would carry risks of its own for the child clone. This is better illustrated in the Parent–Child Resemblance Analogue.

In some situations resulting from ART, only one or neither rearing parent is a genetic parent to the child. In such cases, the rearing parents may grapple with the question of whether and when to disclose their genetic origins to such a child. ART children, whose genetic origins were not disclosed to them at a developmentally appropriate time, may still come to suspect that she may not truly be a genetic child of one or both of her rearing parents. Swedish law now mandates that an individual conceived by donor insemination is entitled to know the truth of his or her genetic origins on reaching adulthood (Gottlieb et al., 2000). What parents think about disclosing such information to their child (Lindblad et al., 2000) might also be relevant to anticipating the related thought process of parents rearing a child clone.

The possibility suggested earlier, that some couples and individuals might prefer HRC to unassisted sexual reproduction, is apt to be mitigated by the arduous nature of the hormone manipulation and IVF procedures that would be required of women who would want HRC.

It is crucial to note that even if overcoming sexual infertility were the conscious motive to pursue HRC, other motives are also likely to be present. For complex human behaviors, what is called the principle of multiple determination operates (Moore & Fine, 1990).

The Adopted Child Analogue

A nonrelated adopted child is not at all linked genetically to her rearing parents, making adoption, in a sense, the conceptual opposite of cloning. Though it may seem paradoxical, this status makes it relevant by analogy to certain aspects of reproductive cloning. This may include the child having been "chosen" and the issue of disclosure of the adopted child's origins, which has long preceded that issue in ART. Added complexity in family relationships is intrinsic to adoption (Lifton, 1988). Adopted individuals often struggle to develop a secure sense of self-identity when they know little or nothing about their genetic parents.

This suggests another way in which cloning and adoption are conceptual opposites: Though the adoptee often knows too little about his or her origins, the clone could know far too much. Knowing vs. not knowing that one is a clone, and the identity of one's progenitor, could powerfully affect the child clone's ability to develop a unique personal identity. Devolder mentions that such an outcome could arise only from the child clone's rearing parents embracing what has been called the "genetic fallacy." Even though genes and their expression are vitally important, a person's self and genetic identity are not the same. However, even if the clone's rearing parents only weakly believed the genetic fallacy, or believed it not at all, a young child clone would still be vulnerable to it. Individuals with limited capacities for abstract thinking, due to psychosis or simply developmental immaturity, employ a primitive form of logic that can ascribe identity between things on the basis of identical predicates (Von Domarus, 1944). Hence, a child clone told that her genes and Mommy's are the same would be inclined to think of herself and progenitor mother as the same person based on their identical genes. This and much more would put the child at risk for what has been called a "foreclosed" identity (Marcia, 1966).

Of course, parents could decide to not tell the child that he is a clone, and make concerted efforts to not be affected by knowing that he is one. Nevertheless, this knowledge would still likely influence their perception of, attitudes toward, and behavior with the child. Even if he were never told of his clonal status, a clone might still ineffably *sense* the template of parental expectations projected onto him.

Devolder argues that some prospective parents might want a child through cloning to give her a good genetic start, reasoning that she could benefit from knowing the health problems of her same-"gene'd" progenitor. Knowing that she would be at high risk of developing the same problems could motivate her to undergo appropriate medical monitoring, lifestyle, and dietary choices to try to avoid her progenitor's fate.

Presently, sperm and egg donors are often selected for allegedly superior qualities. We could expect the same in the selection of somatic cell donors for NT in HRC. In such instances, if the rearing mother provided an enucleated egg into which the donated nucleus was inserted, her child would inherit her mitochondrial DNA, but in every other respect the child clone would be an adopted embryo.

PGD can give an IVF embryo a good genetic start. PGD can be done on a single cell removed from the eight-cell IVF embryo, and can reveal serious genetic defects, and the decision to not implant it for pregnancy. Cloning pioneer, Ian Wilmut, envisages the possibility of eventually remedying such defects instead, engineering a genetic correction of the defect discovered. The genetically corrected nucleus would be extracted from that cell, and transferred into an enucleated egg from the embryo's mother for HRC. The resulting child would not be a clone of any living person, but rather would be a medically corrected clone of a very early embryo (Wilmut & Highfield, 2006). I do not foresee much risk of adverse psychological consequences for such a child. Though technically reproductive, it is more truly therapeutic cloning.

A clone adoptee would not be an oxymoron, and the Adopted Child Analogue would be doubly relevant to that situation. Some infertile prospective parents might prefer to pay a progenitor of their choice to be the nuclear donor for HRC, rather than adopt an already-existing child. Devolder points to a carefully carried out analysis that was unable to demonstrate that the availability of IVF led to fewer adoptions. However, because individuals presenting to IVF clinics do not typically consider adoption seriously unless IVF fails to result in a viable pregnancy, it only stands to reason that IVF availability would reduce the number of adoptions that would occur, were it unavailable.

It is essential to distinguish between the situations serving as analogues to HRC and the situations themselves. This is especially important in the situation and societal practice of adoption. Theory, research, and clinical experience indicate that there are problems inherent to adoption, but being cared for by adoptive parents is almost always better for a child than the alternatives.

Since adoption is acceptable, despite the problems that may be associated with it, why not HRC, too? The crucial difference in the situations underlying the difference in moral judgment is this: The practice of adoption is justified by the need to provide parental care for children whose own parents were unable or unwilling to care for them. These children already exist, and there will surely be many more in the future. In contrast, the parental motivations for HRC that Devolder construes to be of benefit to a future child clone pale in moral significance to those justifying adoption.

The Parent–Child Resemblance Analogue

The wish for self-resemblance in one's child appears to be normal to a degree, and may be understood as a consequence of the need for kin identification, a key concept in modern evolutionary theory (Hamilton, 1964; Erickson, 2000). Psychological research also demonstrates the power of self-resemblance. In one study, subjects presented with images of young children's faces felt more invested in a child whose face had been computer-morphed, without the subject's awareness, to resemble the subject's own (DeBruine, 2004).

Unfortunately, the wish for parent–child resemblance becomes an insistent demand in the pathologically narcissistic parent. Asexual self-reproduction would likely appeal to narcissists, hoping that a child genetically identical to himself might fulfill his own wish for perfection. The prospect of a "mini-me" that he could mold into his imagined "ideal self" would be irresistible. However, the narcissist can never be adequately reassured about his worth, and is ultimately disappointed in his children. His disappointment in a self-clone could be even greater, as that child was supposed to have been his perfect self-reflection (Levick, 2007). As one might expect, the children of narcissistic parents are harmed by such parenting (Mazzano et al., 1999). Were the prospective progenitor parent not pathologically narcissistic, one should still expect him or her to be at least partially motivated by the wish for a highly self-resembling child.

Devolder considers the pathologically narcissistic motive for parenthood by self-cloning to among those motives she labels "dubious." Regarding such motives, she writes: "It is up to opponents of cloning to show that there is good reason to think that prospective parents who want to make use of cloning technology will have dubious motives (more dubious than those of other prospective parents) *and* that these are a reliable indicator for the way children will be treated. Moreover, opponents of cloning have to show that there is good reason to assume that if a child created through cloning is treated as a means, this would not have been the case had the child not been created through cloning."

However, narcissistic motives are typically not fully conscious, and to the extent that they could be, the parent may not want to admit them to either to self or others. And regardless of other motives, it would be hard to imagine that a person wanting to self-clone would not be hoping for and expecting extreme self-similarity in his child clone. Moreover, even if narcissism were only a minor motivating factor for self-cloning, that could change after the child is born, even for a relatively self-aware progenitor parent, also well aware of the "genetic fallacy." Simply knowing that his child is a self-clone could catalyze the emergence of whatever narcissistic potential that progenitor parent might possess. As the child developed beyond infancy and babyhood, he would become increasingly recognizable to his progenitor parent as a highly self-resembling former physical self. With this, that parent would be at risk to "see" himself in the time-warped mirror of self-reflection represented by this child.

The Replacement Child Analogue

Cloning to try to replace a dead or dying loved one is a plausible cloning scenario. The ache of unresolved parental grief is profound (Klass, 1997). It could well lead bereaved parents to want to "replace" their dead child with a new one. If that child is treated as if he were, as if, or ought to be just like the deceased, such a child may evince signs of the "replacement child" syndrome (Cain & Cain, 1962; Johnson, 1989).

The concept of "replacement child" can be more generally applied to situations in which a child is viewed by a parent as a stand-in, in a sense, for a dead child other than one of their own, such as a parental sibling or childhood friend (Levick, 2004). Moreover, this analogue can be applied even more broadly—to the cloning of elderly, dying, and even dead relatives and friends. In the latter instances, the clone would be not a "replacement child," but rather a child "replacement," beginning life like any other human being, as an infant.

This analogue is limited by the fact that the "replacement child" phenomenon has been little explored in the clinical psychological literature, and also by the fact that most parents do not expect children born subsequent to the death of another to "replace" their predecessor. However, cloning would afford the possibility to do exactly that genetically. Moreover, how could bereaved parents, subsequently choosing to have another child by cloning the dead one, not be hoping at some level to "replace," or even "resurrect" their dead child? Indeed, any child clone's progenitor parent could view their self-clone as a future replacement, successor, or resurrected self. Like the parents of a child sexually conceived expressly to try to replace a dead one, adults wanting to clone for the same purpose are bound to be disappointed in the results. There is no reason to think that the "asexually preconceived" replacement child clone would fare any better.

Beyond infancy, the "replacement" child clone would come to resemble her predecessor, more and more, at least physically. As a result, one would expect parents' perceptions of, attitudes towards, and behavior with the child clone to be shaped even more by their previous experiences with the clone's dead progenitor sibling than they might have been if the child were not that dead sibling's clone. Thus, one should expect at least as much, if not more, psychological harm to befall a replacement child clone as a sexually reproduced replacement child.

Devolder believes that prospective parents seeking to clone a deceased child should be informed that the resulting child would not be "as if" the resurrection of the dead child, and not be viewed or treated as a replacement for that child. Unfortunately, education alone often fails to correct false beliefs whose tenaciousness is strongly motivated personally, and is at least partially subconscious. There is no reason to think that the "genetic fallacy" would be an exception to the phenomenon called "transference."

Transference refers to the transferring onto a person currently in an individual's life, feelings, thoughts, and patterns of behavior that were typically first experienced with significant figures in the person's childhood. However, the significant figure could also be another individual about whom the individual has or had very strong feelings. Transference is universal and, to some degree, is part of every relationship to some degree. But, transference can also overshadow the reality of the other person—unduly and detrimentally playing out in the current relationship. An emotionally secure adult recipient of another's transference projections typically feels quite misunderstood, and perceives the other person as behaving toward him in a way that seems incongruous or inappropriate. However, when a child is the recipient of powerful projections of parental transference, self-doubt, guilt, fear, anger, and confusion typically reign.

I doubt that simply educating the progenitor parent would do enough to prevent complex adverse consequences for the child clone. However, augmenting such education with insight-oriented psychotherapy might help such a parent sufficiently to relatively spare the child much harm.

It is hard to imagine prospective parents of a clone not cloning someone they considered ideal at some level, whether one of them, an admired relative, or a lost loved one. A tremendous risk of the HRC scenario, is that the child clone would not only be expected to "replace" his progenitor, but that he be "as if" that other person—as the clone's rearing parents remember that person in an *ideal* sense.

Devolder appears to conflate high parental expectations with highly specific ones. Though high parental expectations can be beneficial, when such expectations are not only high, but also very specific, negative consequences for the child are not unusual. Such would be the case if the rearing parents of a child clone expected that child to be as accomplished in the same ways as her predecessor/progenitor sibling.

Cloning as "Unnatural"

Like Devolder, I am unconvinced by the usual arguments against cloning on the alleged grounds that it would be "unnatural." However, there are serious scientifically grounded notions of the "natural" that deserve our attention. Because phylogentically advanced organisms, including humans, are not capable of reproducing asexually, one can assert without prejudice that HRC would, in fact, be unnatural biologically. This alone is not a reason to oppose it, but to consider whether there is any deep evolutionary reason for why this might be so.

Though prospective parents through HRC might find the genetic certainty of asexual reproduction comforting, evolution of our species requires the combination and recombination of genes in sexual reproduction. Sexual reproduction yields individuals, some well adapted and others poorly adapted to their environment. Evolution results from the relative reproductive success of the most fit or better-adapted individuals. The evolution of a sexually reproducing species would grind to a halt if it switched to asexual reproduction exclusively. From an evolutionary perspective, our species might well be able to tolerate a tiny percentage of human clone beings, in what Lederberg called "tempered clonality" (Lederberg, 1966), but their presence among us could have far-reaching psychological, social, and societal implications. As I see it, there is a "slippery slope" with cloning, but not so much from the therapeutic to the reproductive. Rather, adjudging HRC as acceptable would put one on a slippery slope to finding it preferable to sexual reproduction.

Lederberg also wondered why asexual reproduction does not occur naturally in vertebrates (Lederberg, 1966). I have speculated that asexual reproduction would be less conducive to the altruistic rearing of a cloned offspring by anyone except his or her progenitor (Levick, 2004). E. O. Wilson opined that "biological constraints exist that define zones of improbable or forbidden access" in the future direction of human history. While he was not referring specifically to cloning, perhaps it lies in such a zone. Wilson also warned that if humans were to try to adopt the social system of a nonprimate species, disastrous consequences could well result (Wilson, 1978). Consider that HRC would be more than just a reproductive practice. To some extent, asexual reproduction would surely reconfigure human social systems in hard-to-predict ways.

Based on Richard Dawkins' "selfish gene" theory (Dawkins, 1976), one would predict that a progenitor parent would favor his self-clone over any sexually reproduced children he might also have, because the former would carry all of his genes; the latter, only half. Admixed with even a modest dose of narcissism, such parents would likely have greater difficulty encouraging the child clone to develop his own personal identity—and be willing to let the child make his own independent life.

HRC as a Means

Devolder seriously considers the argument that a clone would be treated as a means. The wish to enhance the well-being of any person other than that of the child clone would qualify. She recognizes this, but persuasively argues that creating a child for instrumental reasons is not problematic if the child is also valued in his or her own right. I agree that: "What is most important in a parent–child relationship is the love and care inherent in that relationship. We judge people on their attitudes toward children, rather than on their motives for having them." I also concur that one should not assume a strong link between motives for having a child and how that child is treated once born. However, evaluating the strength of such a link is a fundamental question for psychological research. The cloning analogues give us good reasons to believe that at least some likely parental motives would be more likely to persist for rearing parents of a child clone than they would for parents of a sexually conceived child, after the child is born.

Autonomy and Beyond

The commonly held fear that a human clone would be without individual identity or autonomy intrinsically is unfounded, but we can minimally infer from the analogues that a clone would be at risk for having added difficulty in becoming a truly autonomous person with a secure personal identity. In essence, it seems clear that it would not be in a child's best interest to be linked genetically to only one person. Such an exclusive linkage could well put the clone's psychosocial development at risk. This is reason enough to oppose reproductive cloning, even if the purely biological and medical concerns were eventually resolved. Furthermore, there are likely to be new alternative means to address sexual infertility. Another means to overcome infertility currently being researched is the transformation of somatic cells into sperm and eggs. At present, only sexual reproduction combines and recombines the genes of two individuals. In my view, this fact may well be the basis for enough, but not too much parental investment in a sexually reproduced child, and also an essential fundamental basis for the social nexus on which human society rests (Levick, 2004, p. 232; Levick, 2007).

In my view, a clone by HRC would be more likely to encounter additional difficulties, over and above those associated with simply being human, in successfully negotiating most, if not all, of Erik Erikson's eight stages of the human life cycle of psychosocial development (Erikson, 1950, 1968; Levick, 2004). My discussion of five cloning analogues in this chapter focused almost exclusively on identity.

Societal Prejudice and Respect

Though I strongly oppose HRC, criminalizing it would risk pushing it underground and engender prejudice towards clones. Devolder properly condemns reasons to oppose cloning based on claims that a clone would lack a soul, be less than human, or have less intrinsic value than the genetic original. However, she goes too far in stating that "expressing certain concerns about cloning one may actually reinforce certain prejudices and misguided stereotypes about clones." This view comes close to one raised by Savalescu, who coined the term *clonism*, referring to discriminating against human clones because of their origins. To the extent that this coin circulates as an aspersive rhetorical term, it risks dampening needed discussion. I do not consider the risk that clones could face social discrimination to be a reason to oppose HRC, but anticipating this possibility should not risk intellectual opprobrium.

Conclusion

Diverse analogues to various psychological and social aspects of HRC can lead us to reasonably infer that human clone beings would be at risk of encountering difficulties over and above those associated with simply being human. These would be consequent to being a nuclear genetic replica or "replacement" of another individual exclusively and in an ideal sense. The risk of harm would be greatest if the clone's progenitor were also a rearing parent. One can anticipate greater psychosocial difficulties throughout an individual clone's life. The risk of sliding down the slippery slope between HRC as an ART infertility option to preferring asexual over sexual reproduction could pose hard-to-foresee societal risks. ART options other than HRC are likely to be developed that will largely obviate the infertility rationale for HRC. Helping individuals to cope emotionally with their sense of loss and personal limitation could help to reduce the wish to pursue HRC. In my view, HRC is unacceptable.

References

Cain, A. C., & Cain, B. S. (1962). On replacing a child. *Journal of the Academy of Child Psychiatry, 1*, 452.

Dawkins, R. (1976). *The selfish gene.* New York: Oxford University Press.

DeBruine, L. M. (2004). Resemblance to self increases the appeal of child faces to both men and women. *Evolution and Human Behavior, 25*, 142–154.

Erickson, M. T. (2000). The evolution of incest avoidance: Oedipus and the psychopathologies of kinship. In P. Gilbert & K. G. Bailey (Eds.), *Genes on the couch: Explorations in evolutionary psychology* (pp. 211–231). Hove, UK: Brunner-Routledge.

Erikson, E. H. (1950). *Childhood and society.* New York: Norton.

Erikson, E. H. (1968). *Identity: Youth and crisis.* New York: Norton.

Fountain, H. (Sept. 15, 2012). A first: Organs tailor-made with body's own cells. *New York Times*, A1.

Gottlieb, C., Lalos, O., & Lindblad, F. (2000). Disclosure of donor insemination to the child: The impact of Swedish legislation on couples' attitudes. *Human Reproduction, 15*, 2051–2056.

Hamilton, W. D. (1964). The genetical evolution of social behavior. *Journal of Theoretical Biology*, 7, 1–52.

Hartzband, P., & Groopman, J. (2012). There is more to life than death. *New England Journal of Medicine, 367*(11), 987–989.

Johnson, S. E. (1989). Replacement children. In E. Klagsbrun et al. (Eds.), *Preventative psychiatry: Early intervention and situational crisis management* (pp. 115–119). Philadelphia: Charles Press.

Klass, D. (1997). The deceased child in the psychic and social worlds of bereaved parents during the resolution of grief. *Death Studies, 21*, 147–176.

Lederberg, J. (1966). Experimental genetics and human evolutions. *Bulletin of the Atomic Scientists, 22*, 4–11.

Levick, S. E. (2004). *Clone being: Exploring the psychological and social dimensions.* Lanham, MD: Rowman & Littlefield Publishers.

Levick, S. E. (2006). Psychological aspects of human reproductive clones: What can we infer from the clone-like? *Psychiatric Times, 23*(14), 1–14.

Levick, S. E. (2007). From *Xenopus* to *Oedipus*: "Dolly," human cloning, and psychological and social "cloneness." *Cloning and Stem Cells, 9*(1), 33–39.

Lifton, B. J. (1988). *Lost and found: The adoption experience.* New York: Harper & Row.

Lindblad, R., Gottlieb, C., & Lalos, O. (2000). To tell or not to tell—What parents think about telling their children that they were born following donor insemination. *Journal of Psychosomatic Obstetrics and Gynecology, 21*, 193–207.

Marcia, J. (1966). The development and validation of ego identity status. *Journal of Personal and Social Psychology, 3*, 551–558.

Mazzano, J., Palacio, E. F., & Zikha, G. (1999). The narcissistic scenarios of parenthood. *International Journal of Psychoanalysis, 80*, 465–476.

Moore, B. E., & Fine, B. D. (Eds.) (1990). *Psychoanalytic terms and concepts.* New Haven, CT: Yale University Press.

Segal N. L. (1997). Behavioral aspects of intergenerational cloning: what twins tell us. *Jurimetrics, 38*, 57–61.

Segal N. L. (2002). Human cloning: Insights from twins and twin research. *Hastings Law Journal, 53*, 1073–1083.

Segal, N. L. (2006). Psychological features of human reproductive cloning: A twin-based perspective. *Psychiatric Times, 23*(14), 1–13.

Siegel, B. (2007). Reflections on the cloning case. *Cloning and Stem Cells, 9*, 40–46.

Von Domarus, E. (1944). The specific laws of logic in schizophrenia. In J. S. Kasanin (Ed.), *Language and thought in schizophrenia: Collected papers* (pp. 104–114). Berkeley: University of California Press.

Wilmut, I., & Highfield, R. (2006). *After Dolly: The uses and misuses of human cloning.* New York: W. W. Norton.

Wilson, E. O. (1978) *On human nature.* Cambridge, MA: Harvard University Press.

Zavos, P. M., & Illmensee, K. (2006). Possible therapy of male infertility by reproductive cloning: one cloned human 4-cell embryo. *Archives of Andrology, 52*(4), 243–254.

Reply to Levick

Katrien Devolder

In the previous chapter, Stephen Levick presents several reasons for thinking that human reproductive cloning would be unacceptable, even if it were safe. His main concern is that it is likely to have adverse psychological and social consequences.

Levick takes an interesting approach. He discusses five existing situations that are analogous in some respect to human reproductive cloning. In each case, he argues that human reproductive cloning is likely to involve either the same or more serious adverse consequences than those associated with the putatively analogous situation. Using analogies is a common method in applied ethics and philosophy. Analogies allow us to think more clearly about situations that are otherwise difficult to imagine, or about which we do not have any empirical information, as in the case of cloning. I will, however, argue that Levick's analogies do not establish the conclusions he wishes to draw from them.

The Identical Twin Analogy

Twins are contemporaries, whereas clones would typically be from different generations. By stressing that a clone would be a *delayed* twin, Levick reveals a *dis*analogy between twins and clones. According to Levick, it is exactly because the clone would be a *delayed* twin that cloning would be problematic, especially if the rearing parent is the progenitor of the child-clone. Levick fears that the already "striking asymmetries in dominance, dependency, knowledge and strength in a normal child–parent relationship" would be magnified in such a case. The child would thus run an increased risk of psychological harm. I think this concern is unjustified, or at least exaggerated. I am not convinced that the fact that the child is genetically identical to a rearing parent will make that parent feel "even more dominant." If genetic similarity between a parent and child aggravates parental dominance, this would imply that rearing parents of an adopted child, or of a child conceived with donor gametes, feel less dominant than "ordinary" parents. This is implausible.

Levick also questions my claim that cloning would enable people to make informed reproductive decisions, for example, enabling them to avoid bringing a child into the world with a serious genetic disease. He suggests that preimplantation genetic diagnosis (PGD) could be used instead. However, it may be that an individual has genetic predispositions for *several* serious diseases. All embryos created via PGD would then likely be carriers of one or more genes linked to these diseases. The potential parent may then think it better if her child inherits genes only from her much healthier partner, and not from her.

Levick also seems to suggest that individuals who have their genome cloned will have had themselves

Contemporary Debates in Bioethics, First Edition. Edited by Arthur L. Caplan and Robert Arp.

genetically screened and that as a result, only "healthy" individuals would be cloned. My point about a clone deriving a health benefit from the information about her progenitor's health would thus disappear. I think that Levick is being too optimistic here. First, not all genetic predispositions can be diagnosed through genetic testing. The cloned child may thus still inherit a predisposition for a disease that slipped through the cracks in genetic testing technology. Second, no prospective progenitor will be completely healthy. Everyone has genetic predispositions for various diseases and conditions. A person without such dispositions simply does not exist. Thus, prospective progenitors cannot avoid passing on genetic predispositions for certain diseases to their cloned children. Fortunately, most of these diseases are caused by (several) genes *and* the environment. If the clone adapts her behavior, she may, in many cases, prevent, or at least postpone the onset of the disease. Thorough screening of prospective progenitors will thus preserve the health advantage to the clone.

The Assisted Reproduction Analogy

Levick refers to psychological difficulties experienced by children who were created via assisted reproduction, in particular children who were conceived using donor gametes. Some of these children may find it troubling to learn about their genetic origins. For example, to some it may be troubling to find out that their rearing father is not their genetic father. Levick points out that similar difficulties may be experienced by clones. Though this may be true, it is not clear why we should think that these potential difficulties provide a strong reason against cloning, but not against the use of donor gametes to conceive a child. More argument is required to justify drawing a moral line between these two types of assisted reproduction.

The Adoption Analogy

Levick notes that some adopted children know too little about their genetic origins and that this is sometimes problematic for their identity formation. Cloned children, Levick points out, would have the opposite problem—they would know too much about their genetic origins. Even though parents may not make the mistake of thinking that their child's identity is determined by genes only, Levick worries that children, "due to psychosis or simply developmental immaturity" may think of themselves and the progenitor as one and the same person. I believe, however, that it is rather unlikely that a child will think she and her progenitor are the same person because of a shared genome. A small child will probably not even understand what a genome is, let alone think something complicated like "individuals who are genetically identical are in fact one and the same person." Any potential problems with identity formation are more likely to result from others' misunderstanding of the link between genes and identity.

The Parent–Child Resemblance Analogy

I agree with Levick that there is a risk that pathologically narcissist individuals will want to make use of cloning on the ground of the mistaken belief that they will create a copy of "their wonderful selves." We can only hope that psychological screening would single out these individuals and that, as a result, they will not be assisted in their wish to reproduce through cloning. But Levick is also worried that cloning could trigger narcissism in "normal" parents, and that this would adversely affect their perception of and attitudes toward the child. This may be true. However, first, narcissism might be triggered in parents who notice that their (sexually produced) child strongly resembles them (which is often the case). Second, there are many things that affect our perception and attitudes toward our children—more argument is needed to show that such moderate narcissistic feelings are something special to worry about.

The Replacement Child Analogy

Levick argues that I conflate high parental expectations with highly specific parental expectations. He agrees with me that high expectations can be a good thing, but that very specific ones, like those that people may have towards a clone that was created as a replacement child, may be much more problematic. According to Levick, this would be the case "if the rearing parents of a child clone expected that child to be as accomplished in the same ways as her predecessor/progenitor sibling." I agree with Levick that such specific expectations could form a serious burden for the "replacement child." This is equally true for currently existing children who were conceived with the intention of replacing a deceased sibling, but the problem may of course be magnified in the case of clones, as parents may believe that the child-clone will be the same as, or very similar to, the dead child. First, I do think that information and screening of parents may help to prevent such bad consequences. Second, I disagree with Levick that parents who clone their dead child necessarily hope to resurrect or replace it. They may have other reasons—for example, they may be infertile. Cloning the child's genome may be their only possibility to have a genetically related child (or a child only genetically related to them).

Levick concludes that "we can minimally infer from the analogues that a clone would be at risk for having added difficulty in becoming a truly autonomous person with a secure personal identity [...]. This is reason enough to oppose reproductive cloning, even if the purely biological and medical concerns were eventually resolved." I think that Levick's concerns, even if they are justified, do not provide sufficient reason to reject reproductive cloning. Though I agree that for some clones it may be psychologically somewhat more difficult (compared to if they had been created the "ordinary" way), I think that Levick underestimates the extent to which these risks could be diminished through screening of potential progenitors and ensuring that they and the general public are well informed. Moreover, there are many situations in which children are born in circumstances that could increase the risk of psychological difficulties (e.g., when the potential parent has a genetic predisposition for early onset Parkinson's, is very poor, is old, is a member of a victimized racial group, or is a celebrity). Though these difficulties may provide some reason against reproducing, or reproducing in a certain way, they usually do not provide an overriding reason not to have children, or not to have children in a certain way. I think the same is true for human reproductive cloning.

Reply to Devolder

Stephen E. Levick

On Reasoning by Analogy

A close friend's son, Jordan Dworkin, then 10 years old, suggested that my book on human reproductive cloning (HRC) be titled *Clones are Us*. Though too evocative of a certain toy store chain to be used, his suggestion did metaphorically reflect the essence of my analogical method. Each analogue examines "whether there are aspects of life in other families that might be similar to those in which a clone would be born" (Wilmut, 2004).

"Analogy is a device for conveying that two situations or domains share relational structure despite arbitrary degrees of difference in the objects that make up the domains" (Gentner & Markman, 1997). Each analogue is a relational structure between the HRC situation and particular aspects of a given set of extant circumstances. The HRC analogues are relational structures of relationship potentials between and among persons represented by the particular set of circumstances upon which a specific analogue is based. For each analogue, relevant psychological and social data, clinical experience, and theory exist, and can be applied by analogy to HRC.

When considering Devolder's critique, bear in mind that each HRC analogue exists within a larger network of analogues. Relations between and among them variously reinforce, complement, and/or corroborate inferences that may be drawn from a single one (Levick, 2004, pp. 161–182).

The Identical Twin Analogue

Devolder thinks my assessment that the self-clone of a progenitor-parent would be at increased risk for psychological harm is exaggerated, if not unjustified. My argument is based neither on the genetic identicality of progenitor-parent and his self-clone, nor on the highly asymmetric nature of their relationship, *but rather on the coexistence of both conditions*. She believes it implausible that compared to parents, each of whom is genetically linked to their child, parents of an adopted child, or one conceived with donor gametes, would feel less dominant in relation to their child. However, there are many psychological studies that demonstrate seemingly implausible realities, and Devolder's critique implies several excellent questions for research: Does a parent's sense of entitlement to exercise authority with a child relate to the degree to which that parent, (a) believes that he is linked genetically to the child and/or (b) perceives self-resemblance in the child? Only very recently has research even nibbled on the margins of the first question (e.g., Dempsey, 2012).

My counterpart indicates that occasions may arise in which a prospective parent through HRC might believe that her potential child would be better off not inheriting her genes only, but instead, only her partner's. However, she could also exclude her genes, and still allow her child to be linked genetically to his

Contemporary Debates in Bioethics, First Edition. Edited by Arthur L. Caplan and Robert Arp.

father, though not exclusively, by obtaining a donor egg to be inseminated by her partner. If she were in a lesbian relationship, her partner could furnish the egg, and a donor, the sperm for IVF. In either case, the prospective rearing mother might also elect gestational motherhood.

Devolder emphasizes that genetic testing fails to detect all potentially harmful genetic predispositions, many of which are polygenic and act in concert with environmental factors. Despite these limitations, she proposes that any potential progenitor be screened genetically to preserve the health advantages she argues could accrue to a clone. As mentioned earlier, regenerative medicine will likely obviate HRC as means to achieve this benefit. Furthermore, genetic risks intrinsic to HRC itself could undermine Devolder's eminently sensible recommendation of genetic screening of prospective progenitors. Though our chapters are predicated on accepting the hypothetical premise of physical safety for HRC, its medical risks cannot be fully known until it becomes a reality, and individual clones followed medically for years. To reiterate: "… *assessing the relative physical safety of HRC should not even be attempted before also considering possible psychological, social, and societal risks it may pose.*"

The Assisted Reproductive Technology Analogue

Devolder finds that "more argument is required to justify drawing a moral line" between HRC and employing donor gametes to have a child. I agree, but no analogue is intended to stand alone.

The Parent–Child Resemblance Analogue

My conjecture that the very existence of a child self-clone could augment whatever narcissism a parent may possess relates to the untested assumption that making much of one's child's self-resemblance is a mark of parental narcissism, and that parental narcissism is enlarged by even lesser degrees of actual filial self-resemblance. The study in which individuals are willing to invest more in children whose faces are computer-morphed to resemble the adult subject bears indirectly on this. Does parental attachment to and investment in a child relate to the extent to which a given parent (a) believes that he or she is linked genetically to the child and/or (b) perceives self-resemblance in his or her child? These questions are testable empirically.

The Replacement Child Analogue

Devolder gives considerable weight to screening potential parents of a child clone, and to the power of information to change beliefs and attitudes, especially for parents who may wish to clone their dead child. She indicates that some such parents may have become an infertile pair since their child's death, and could turn to HRC as the only way to again have a child genetically linked to them both. That situation would not invalidate my assertion that any parent(s) wishing to clone their dead child would almost surely be doing so with the hope and belief that the clone would be the same or similar to its genetically identical predecessor. The principle of multiple determination of motivation should lead us to expect that the infertility motive to clone a dead child would not exclude the coexistence of the psychologically powerful motive of wanting to recreate that particular child.

Devolder's Conclusions in Her Reply

Though agreeing that some clones may have a more difficult time than a child created through other means, Devolder argues that even if my concerns are justified, they are insufficient to reject HRC. She believes that psychological risk could be mitigated by screening potential progenitors, and providing them and the general public with information about HRC.

Devolder points out that many are born into circumstances that could increase their risk of psychological harm, but that such circumstances are not typically adjudged to be sufficient reason for such individuals to not reproduce in one way or another. But are the advantages she alleges for HRC sufficient to introduce it as a risky new circumstance?

Notably, one circumstance that Devolder mentions is represented in the Child of the Famous Analogue—one of three HRC analogues that space constraints precluded including here.

The Child of the Famous Analogue

In part, a person may desire fame in order to attain a kind of immortality. Some might want to further "immortalize" themselves through self-cloning. Add to the desire for fame, the wish for a child through which to live vicariously, and through whom to live on after death. Combined, these motivational ingredients could motivate an individual or couple to want to parent a clone of a famous person, in order to feel linked to that person. Individuals in the general public not uncommonly relate "parasocially" to celebrities and other famous people, blurring the distinction between the person they think they know and the actual person (Horton & Wohl, 1956; e.g., Nimoy, 1975). It is a phenomenon that can leave such individuals feeling lonely, isolated, and distrustful of even close friends (Giles, 1999). If his clonal status were known, any clone would be at risk to be related to parasocially. If he had a famous progenitor, and others knew it, he would be at even greater risk of risk of harm—specifically, in developing both his own individual identity and trusting relationships.

Conclusion

One can sympathize; even empathize with the motives of those who believe medically "safe" HRC should be an available reproductive option. However, one can reasonably infer from the analogues to the HRC situation that the clone could well be at increased risk of certain psychological and social harms. HRC could also prove indirectly detrimental to others, and society as a whole. Research designed specifically to be analogically relevant to key aspects of HRC could further inform these concerns. Those who would attempt HRC should recall the Hippocratic Oath's dictum to physicians: "*Primum non nocere*" ("Above all, do no harm").

References

Dempsey, D. (2012). More like a donor or more like a father? Gay men's concepts of relatedness to children. *Sexualities, 15*, 156.

Gentner, D., & Markman, A. (1997). Structure mapping in analogy and similarity. *American Psychologist, 52*, 45–56.

Giles, D. (1999). *Illusions of immortality: A psychology of fame and celebrity*. New York: St. Martin's Press.

Horton, D., & Wohl, R. (1956). Mass communication and parasocial interaction. *Psychiatry, 19*, 215–219.

Levick, S. E. (2004). *Clone Being: Exploring the psychological and social dimensions*. Lanham, MD: Rowman & Littlefield Publishers.

Nimoy, L. (1975). *I am not Spock*. New York: Ballantine.

Wilmut, I. W. (2004). The likely effect of being a clone. *Cloning and Stem Cells, 6*, 209–210.

Part 4

Is the Deliberately Induced Abortion of a Human Pregnancy Ethically Justifiable?

Introduction

"In short, the unborn have never been recognized in the law as persons in the whole sense." So claimed Mr Justice Harry Blackmun, speaking for the majority of the US Supreme Court in *Roe v. Wade* (410 US 113), one of the most controversial legal decisions in US history. By 1973, when the *Roe v. Wade* decision was made, abortions had been performed for many years all over the world by both trained physicians and untrained persons. Surgical abortion utilizing vacuum aspiration (with anesthesia) and menstrual extraction had proven to be effective and safe for the mother, drastically cutting down on the number of women who were admitted to the hospital or died due to hemorrhage and/or sepsis as a result of so called "back-alley abortions" (Joffe, 1995, 2009; Paul et al., 1999, pp. 3–10). Data from the US Centers for Disease Control and Prevention and the Alan Guttmacher Institute indicate that more than 50 million abortions have been performed in the US alone since 1973 (GI, 2011; Jones & Koolstra, 2011). While feeling unready to parent and not having enough money rank as two prominent reasons that women have given for having abortions (there are others; see Bankole et al., 1998; Finer et al., 2005; Henshaw & Kost, 2008; Johnston, 2011), it is arguable that the sheer number of abortions in the US and worldwide (some 1 billion since 1973) is in some sense attributed to Blackmun's thinking. After all, there needs to be a strong justification for ending a potential person's life—no matter what the circumstances—in order for the action to be considered morally appropriate. Some contend that unborn humans simply are not persons (Tooley, 1972). Judith Jarvis Thomson (1971) goes even further than Blackmun when, in the last line of her famous article, "A Defense of Abortion," she states: "A very early abortion is surely not the killing of a person." Ten years prior to Thomson's writing, H. J. McCloskey (1961) noted, "it would seem not to be the ordinary

Contemporary Debates in Bioethics, First Edition. Edited by Arthur L. Caplan and Robert Arp.

person's view that the fetus is a human being, for when a woman has a miscarriage, especially early in her pregnancy, her friends sympathize with her but neither she nor they mourn the death of a human person" (p. 110).

Notwithstanding the claims of Blackmun, Thomson, and McCloskey, it is precisely the definition of personhood—as well as *who* or *what* counts as a person—that often is at the center of the abortion debate. In her important article, "On the Moral and Legal Status of Abortion," Mary Ann Warren (1973) lays out the following as constitutive of personhood: (a) consciousness (in particular, the ability to feel pain), (b) reasoning, (c) self-motivated activity, (d) the capacity to communicate, and (e) self-awareness. A being that meets these criteria is a person, and, as a person, such a being has the fullest of moral rights and privileges—including the right to live and not be harmed. No one denies that a fertilized human egg is a member of the species, *Homo sapiens*; what is debated is whether a human being at certain developmental stages of its life could be considered a person according to the aforementioned criteria (there are other criteria given by thinkers, too). At first blush, we can see that there is an obvious developmental distinction between a human zygote, a human embryo, a human fetus, an infant, a toddler, a teenager, and a middle-aged, fully coherent individual; researchers in physical and psychological human development document and explain these differences quite thoroughly (Kail & Cavanaugh, 2010; Sadler, 2011; Newman & Newman, 2012). And, we would surely maintain that the middle-aged, fully coherent individual has moral rights and privileges in a society. Thus, given the criteria for personhood, human zygotes, embryos, fetuses, and even infants simply are not persons. Warren maintains, "a fetus, even a fully developed one, is considerably less person-like than is the average mature mammal, indeed the average fish" (p. 48; also see Warren, 1997). If zygotes, embryos, and fetuses are not persons, then they have no moral rights and privileges, and we need not think that we have done anything immoral when we abort them. Of course, there may be other reasons not to abort zygotes, embryos, and fetuses; again, however, their being persons is not a legitimate reason for not aborting them on Warren's view.

There are a number of problems with Warren's view of personhood that critics have noted, chief among them being:

1. The view seems to allow for the killing of infants, as well as individuals who are severely mentally disabled, and persons in a persistent vegetative state. By the criteria mentioned, such beings do not qualify as persons, so it seems that we can kill them for similar reasons that we kill zygotes, embryos, and fetuses. Such a result strikes many as logically suspect and morally incorrect (Benn, 1973; Marquis, 1989, 1997).
2. It is difficult to delineate clearly between persons and nonpersons at a certain point in the development of a human life. It may be clear to most people that a zygote is not a person, while a middle-aged neurosurgeon is; but is a normal three-year-old a person? How about a gifted two-year-old? Or, a one-and-a-half-year-old who has learned some sign language? We can imagine numerous cases where it would indeed be tragic to deny a being moral rights and privileges because we think such a being to be a nonperson, only to discover or figure out later that such a being was in fact a person (Marquis, 1997).
3. The criteria mentioned—consciousness, reasoning, self-motivated activity, the capacity to communicate, and self-awareness—may not be enough for someone to be considered a person. In other words, they may be necessary, but not sufficient, for personhood. What about being held fully responsible for your actions, for example? That would seem to be a significant criterion for someone to have in order to be considered as deserving of moral rights and privileges. And we seem to associate full moral responsibility with full personhood in a society (Locke, 1990).

And there are other problems with Warren's view—and similar personhood views—as well as numerous responses, rejoinders, repairs, and re-workings of the personhood view (Warren's and others; see English, 1973; Dennett, 1978; Parfit, 1984; Barresi, 1999; Glynn, 2000; Shoemaker, 2007, 2008).

Above, Judith Jarvis Thomson's "A Defense of Abortion" article was mentioned and her claim that a "very early abortion is surely not the killing of a person." But in this seminal article, Thomson actually defends abortion, even if one considers zygotes, embryos, and fetuses to be full-fledged persons. She uses a thought experiment and argument by analogy to make her case that goes something like this: Imagine waking up one morning with a famous violinist's circulatory system plugged into yours, and the violinist needs your kidneys for the next nine months in order to live and fully recover from an ailment. After the nine months, he will be able to live just fine without your assistance, but if you unplug him before the nine months are up, he will die. Thomson now asks a simple question, "Is it morally incumbent on you to accede to this situation? No doubt it would be very nice of you if you did, a great kindness. But do you have to accede to it?" (pp. 48–49). Her response is a resounding *no*, since it is your body and, ultimately, the violinist has no right to use it. She then goes on to argue by analogy that the fetus also does not have the right to use your body, and that a woman may justly abort the fetus.

Since the early 1970s, when the views of Warren and Thomson were articulated, various pro-life and pro-choice positions have emerged, complete with political activist groups associated with the positions, especially in the United States (Maxwell, 2002; Feldt, 2004). The conservative pro-life position usually is characterized by the belief that, from the moment a human egg is fertilized, a new person exists. This human being/person is innocent, and has the same right not to be killed as any other full-fledged person walking the streets, irrespective of the fact that this being is living inside a woman's body. From this perspective, abortion is akin to the murder of an innocent person, is immoral, and should not be performed under any circumstances except, possibly, if the woman's life is in danger due to the pregnancy or the fetus is the result of rape or incest.

On the other hand, the liberal pro-choice position usually is characterized by the belief that the being living inside the mother's womb is not a person—à la Warren and Thomson—and does not deserve legal and moral rights. Even if the fetus is considered a person, some believe the mother could abort it, under certain circumstances, because she still has the right to do with her body what she wants. From this perspective, abortion is not murder, because it is justified by the mother's personal bodily rights—à la Thomson and *Roe v. Wade*—or to avoid less preferable or bad consequences for the mother and future child.

The positions are laid out on a continuum in Figure P4.1 for simple reference, and we realize that not only are they rough-and-ready characterizations, but also there are other ways to portray the ideologies surrounding the abortion debate. On one end of the continuum is the most extreme, strongest ultra-conservative pro-life position whereby abortion is never permitted under any circumstances whatsoever, even if the mother's life is in danger. The Roman Catholic Church is famous for holding this position (John Paul II, 1995; CCC, 2004). On the other end of the continuum is the most extreme, strongest ultra-liberal pro-choice position, whereby it is legitimate for a woman to abort for any reason that she gives or none at all. Such an extreme position is underscored by the following from an official report issued by the United States Senate Judiciary Committee in 1982: "As a result of the Roe decision, a right to abortion was effectively established for the entire term of pregnancy for virtually any reason, whether for sake of personal finances, social convenience, or individual lifestyle ... Thus, the Committee observes that no significant legal barriers of any kind whatsoever exist in the United States for a woman to obtain an abortion for any reason during any stage of her pregnancy" (SJC, 1982, pp. 3–4).

Among several responses to objections and fine distinctions, Judith Jarvis Thomson deals with the typical claim that is made by the anti-abortionist that, "Given that a woman voluntarily engaged in sexual intercourse, we have to conclude that 'she made her bed, so now she must lie in it'—so to speak—and she is now morally obligated to have the baby." Thomson isolates the act of abortion from the act by which a woman has become pregnant, whether through rape, incest, or voluntary sexual intercourse. The decision to abort can be made wholly detached from—morally and justly—the manner in which a woman has become pregnant in the sense that the two (decision to abort vs. manner in which a woman has become pregnant) need not

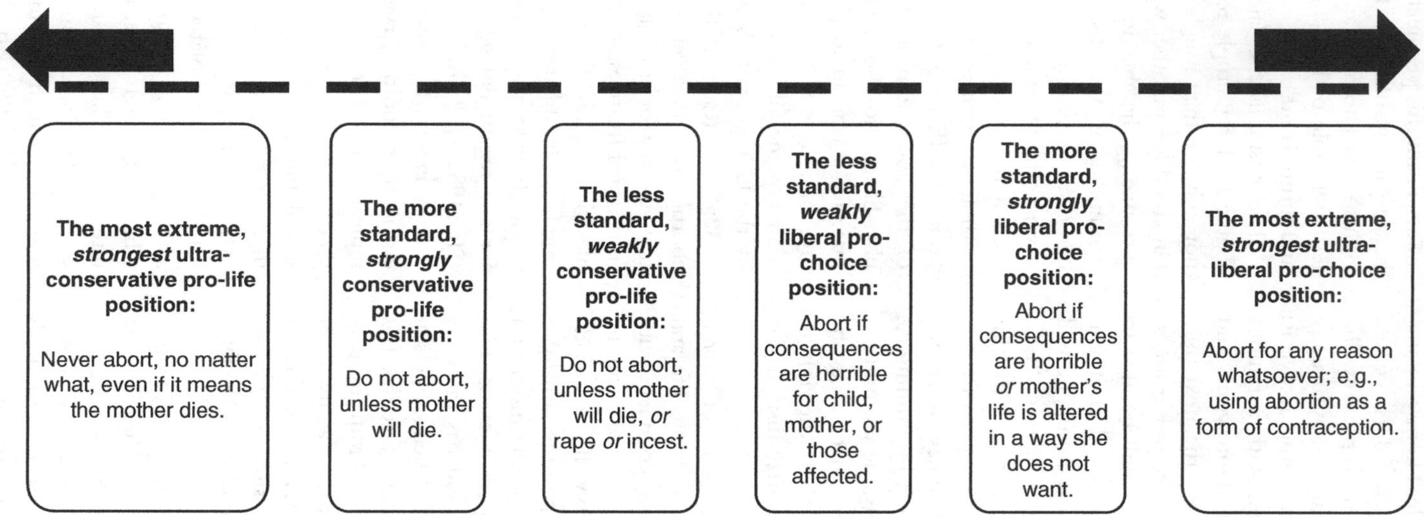

The most extreme, *strongest* ultra-conservative pro-life position:

Never abort, no matter what, even if it means the mother dies.

The more standard, *strongly* conservative pro-life position:

Do not abort, unless mother will die.

The less standard, *weakly* conservative pro-life position:

Do not abort, unless mother will die, *or* rape *or* incest.

The less standard, *weakly* liberal pro-choice position:

Abort if consequences are horrible for child, mother, or those affected.

The more standard, *strongly* liberal pro-choice position:

Abort if consequences are horrible *or* mother's life is altered in a way she does not want.

The most extreme, *strongest* ultra-liberal pro-choice position:

Abort for any reason whatsoever; e.g., using abortion as a form of contraception.

Figure P4.1 Continuum of positions on abortion

have anything to do with one another. The *consequence* of pregnancy is the same whether through rape, incest, or voluntary sexual intercourse, and the morality and justice of abortion should be kept separate from the morality and justice of rape, incest, or voluntary sexual intercourse.

It is a curious fact that many conservative anti-abortionists—specifically, those who hold what we call the *less standard, weakly conservative pro-life position* in Figure P4.1—think it is completely right and just for a woman to have an early-term abortion in the case of rape or incest when, again, whether one is impregnated through rape, incest, *or* the voluntary sex act, the same result of a pregnancy is the consequence. After all, abortion ends the human life, whether the life results from rape, incest, or the voluntary sex act. It would then seem that, to be logically consistent, anti-abortionists would be opposed to abortion even in the cases of rape and incest.

The arguments of the two authors in this section are among the most powerful for their respective positions. The liberal pro-choicer will find much with which to agree in Jeffrey Reiman's chapter, since he argues that the being living inside the mother's womb is not a person and does not have the same legal and moral right not to be killed as does a mother, mechanic, or monarch. But his reason why human zygotes, embryos, fetuses, and even infants do not deserve legal and moral rights has to do with the fact that such beings do not have what he calls "consciously-cared-about lives." They lack the ability to care about, or be concerned with, their own lives—their lives simply do not matter to them. His argument is put succinctly: "A fetus does not have a right not to be killed because losing its life cannot matter to it. It cannot matter to a fetus because it does not yet have a self—it is not yet a 'who'—to whom it could matter." Thinkers such as Ronald Dworkin (1993) and Bonnie Steinbock (1992) have made similar arguments about the right to life being based upon one's interest in continuing to live (cf. Tooley, 1972; Singer, 1979; Paske, 1998). Besides making his case for his argument, Reiman also points out that no matter if one is debating about abortion or anything else of moral substance: "people's moral beliefs may be influenced by emotions, affections, and fears, which may distort people's judgment so that they believe what is not rationally grounded." As rational beings, we are to resist these distortions and devise "independently reasonable theories" for why actions are right or wrong.

On the other hand, the conservative pro-lifer will agree that her/his position can be bolstered by the argument in Don Marquis' chapter. Marquis develops his now-famous *future of value view*: "We presume that a shorter life is a worse life than a longer life because the shorter life will, *ceteris paribus*, contain fewer goods than the longer life ... To deprive someone of *all* of the goods of her future life is to cause great harm to her ... Therefore, killing another human being is wrong because it deprives her of a future of value" (also see Marquis, 1989, 1997). Of course, Marquis is aware of special cases where killing another is not wrong—such as killing in self-defense, in wartime, or in justly administering the death penalty—but a standard abortion is wrong because the future of this potential person is obliterated. Whereas Reiman thinks that the *present state* of a human zygote, embryo, fetus, or even infant as a nonperson is what is decisive in making the decision to abort moral, Marquis thinks that the *future state* of a human zygote, embryo, fetus, or even infant as a person (Marquis calls it *future personhood*) is what is decisive in making the decision to abort immoral.

References

Bankole, A., Singh, S., & Hass, T. (1998). Reasons why women have induced abortions: Evidence from 27 countries. *International Family Planning Perspectives, 24*(3), 117–127, 152.

Barresi, J. (1999). On becoming a person. *Philosophical Psychology, 12*, 79–98.

Benn, S. (1973). Abortion, infanticide, and respect for persons. In J. Feinberg (Ed.), *The problem of abortion* (pp. 92–103). Belmont, CA: Wadsworth.

CCC (*Catechism of the Catholic Church*). (2004). Retrieved from: http://www.vatican.va/archive/ENG0015/__P7Z.HTM#-2C6

Dennett, D. (1978). *Brainstorms*. Cambridge, MA: MIT Press.

Dworkin, R. (1993). *Life's dominion: An argument about abortion, euthanasia and individual freedom*. New York: Alfred A. Knopf.

English, J. (1973). Abortion and the concept of a person. *Canadian Journal of Philosophy, 5*(2), 233–243.

Feldt, G. (2004). *The war on choice: The right-wing attack on women's rights and how to fight back*. New York: Bantam Books.

Finer, L., Frohwirth, L., Dauphinee, L., Singh, S., & Moore, A. (2005). Reasons US women have abortions: Quantitative and qualitative perspectives. *Perspectives on Sexual and Reproductive Health, 37*(3), 110–118.

GI (Guttmacher Institute). (2011). Facts on induced abortion in the United States. Retrieved from: http://www.guttmacher.org/pubs/fb_induced_abortion.html#2a

Glynn, S. (2000). *Identity, intersubjectivity and communicative action*. Athens: Paideia Project.

Henshaw, S., & Kost, K. (2008). Trends in the characteristics of women obtaining abortions, 1974 to 2004. *Alan Guttmacher Institute*. Retrieved from: http://www.guttmacher.org/pubs/2008/09/18/Report_Trends_Women_Obtaining_Abortions.pdf

Joffe, C. (1995). *Doctors of conscience: The struggle to provide abortion before and after Roe v. Wade*. Boston: Beacon Press.

Joffe, C. (2009). Abortion and medicine: A sociopolitical history. In M. Paul, E. Lichtenberg, L. Borgatta, D. Grimes, P. Stubblefield, & M. Creinin (Eds.), *Management of unintended and abnormal pregnancy* (pp. 1–9). Malden, MA: Wiley-Blackwell.

John Paul II. (1995). *Evangelium vitae: To the bishops, priests, deacons, men and women religious, lay faithful, and all people of good will on the value and inviolability of human life*. Retrieved from: http://www.vatican.va/holy_father/john_paul_ii/encyclicals/documents/hf_jp-ii_enc_25031995_evangelium-vitae_en.html

Johnston, W. R. (2011). Abortion and other statistics. Retrieved from: http://www.johnstonsarchive.net/policy/abortion/

Jones, R., & Koolstra, K. (2011). Abortion incidence and access to services in the United States, 2008. *Perspectives on Sexual and Reproductive Health, 43*(1), 41–50.

Kail, R., & Cavanaugh, J. (2010). *Human development: A lifespan view*. Belmont, CA: Wadsworth.

Locke, L. (1990). Personhood and moral responsibility. *Law and Philosophy, 9*(1), 39–66.

Marquis, D. (1989). Why abortion is immoral. *Journal of Philosophy, 86*(1), 183–202.

Marquis, D. (1997). An argument that abortion is wrong. In H. LaFollette (Ed.), *Ethics in practice* (pp. 91–102). London: Blackwell Publishers.

Maxwell, C. (2002). *Pro-life activists in America: Meaning, motivation, and direct action*. Cambridge: Cambridge University Press.

McCloskey, H. J. (1961). Practical implications of the state's right to promote the good. *Ethics, 71*(2), 104–113.

Newman, B., & Newman, R. (2012). *Development through life: A psychosocial approach*. Belmont, CA: Wadsworth.

Parfit, D. (1984). *Reasons and persons*. Oxford: Oxford University Press.

Paske, G. (1998). Abortion and the neo-natal right to life. In L. Pojman & F. Beckwith (Eds.), *The abortion controversy: 25 years after Roe v. Wade* (pp. 361–371). Belmont, CA: Wadsworth.

Paul, M., Lichtenberg, E., Borgatta, L., Grimes, D., & Stubblefield, P. (1999). *A clinician's guide to medical and surgical abortion*. Philadelphia: Churchill Livingstone.

Sadler, T. (2011). *Langman's medical embryology*. Hagerstown, MD: Lippincott, Williams & Wilkins.

Shoemaker, D. (2007). Personal identity and practical concerns. *Mind, 116*, 316–357.

Shoemaker, D. (2008). *Personal identity and ethics: A brief introduction*. Boulder, CO: Broadview Press.

Singer, P. (1979). *Practical ethics*. Cambridge: Cambridge University Press.

SJC (United States Senate Judiciary Committee). (1982). Report of the Committee on the Judiciary, United States Senate, on S.J. Res. 110, June 8, 1982. Retrieved from: http://thomas.loc.gov/cgi-bin/bdquery/z?d097:S.J.RES.110.

Steinbock, B. (1992), *Life before birth: The moral and legal status of embryos and fetuses*. Oxford: Oxford University Press.

Thomson, J. J. (1971). A defense of abortion. *Philosophy and Public Affairs, 1*, 47–66.

Tooley, M. (1972). Abortion and infanticide, *Philosophy and Public Affairs, 2*, 37–65.

Warren, M. A. (1973). On the moral and legal status of abortion. *The Monist, 57*, 43–61.

Warren, M. A. (1997). *Moral status: Obligations to persons and other living things*. Oxford: Oxford University Press.

Chapter Seven

The Deliberately Induced Abortion of a Human Pregnancy Is Ethically Justifiable

Jeffrey Reiman

To be an acceptable answer to the question of the morality of abortion, an answer must not simply match widely held moral beliefs, because we are fallible. It must be supported by a reasonable theory of what makes taking a human life wrong when it is wrong, and such a theory must account for the fact that the killing of one human being cannot be made up for by producing one or more other human beings. I contend that the only view that can satisfy these requirements is one that focuses on how humans care about their own lives, since humans care about their own lives asymmetrically—as not replaceable by others' lives. Killing a human offspring is only wrong once it starts to care about its life, which happens sometime during the first year of life. Thus, abortion is ethically permissible.

Introduction

Philosophers sometimes seem to like questions more than answers. But, philosophers like questions because they contain clues to their answers—just as keyholes tell us a lot about the keys that will open them. Consequently, I start my discussion with some reflections about the question of abortion: What does it ask? What can answer it? Later, I will use what we learn about the question of abortion to narrow its possible answers down to one. See Reiman (1999) for a fuller presentation of the arguments for this claim, and replies to objections not considered here.

The Moral Question of Abortion: Learning about the Key from the Keyhole

Those who think that abortion is ethically unjustifiable think that it is, morally speaking, the murder of a human being. I say "morally speaking" here because our question is about the moral status of abortion, not its legal status. Thus, *murder*, in the question, means the *gravely immoral killing* of a human being. The question of whether abortion is moral or immoral is separate from the legal question of whether it should be a crime, and should be taken up before the legal

Contemporary Debates in Bioethics, First Edition. Edited by Arthur L. Caplan and Robert Arp.

question. My focus, then, is strictly on the question whether killing a fetus is morally murder. I take it that, if abortion is not morally murder—if it is not gravely immoral killing—then a woman's right to control her body implies that abortion is ethically justifiable as long as it is authorized by the pregnant woman. And that will be a good reason for not treating it legally as a crime.

In asking whether killing a fetus is morally murder, I use the term *fetus* to refer to the offspring in a woman's uterus for the entire period of her pregnancy. In fact, scientists refer to this offspring by different terms as it develops in the womb: first it is a *zygote*, then a *blastocyst*, later still an *embryo*, only after about 60 days is it technically a *fetus* (Sadler, 2011). Nevertheless, for simplicity's sake, I will use the term *fetus* to apply to the offspring at any point from conception to birth. "Is killing a fetus morally murder?" should be understood as asking whether killing the offspring in a woman's uterus at any time during pregnancy is morally murder.

This question asks not what people *do* believe but what they *should* believe. It cannot be answered by surveying people's actual moral beliefs about abortion, anymore than it can be answered by putting it to a vote. We want an answer that we have good reason to believe is true; and we must recognize that what people actually believe may be false. This does not mean that people's beliefs play no role in answering our question. Since morality is about human judgments, moral beliefs are basic evidence for what is right that cannot be ignored. Moral philosophers often test their answers to moral questions by comparing them to widespread moral beliefs. This is appropriate because moral beliefs that are widely held have stood up against disagreement, and in the face of difficult experiences, for a considerable time. Nonetheless, widely held moral beliefs are not infallible. People may be mistaken. Even large numbers of people may be mistaken, as it seems they were for a long time about the moral implications of gender or racial differences.

The upshot of these considerations is that we tread a difficult course in seeking to answer the moral question of abortion. We must be guided by widely held beliefs, and yet we cannot simply accept them as true. We cannot answer our question just by finding the principle that is most compatible with people's actual beliefs. What is needed is a reasonable conception of what makes the taking of a fetus's life seriously morally wrong (if it is wrong). Such a conception will be part of a reasonable theory of what makes taking human life at any point wrong (when it is wrong). In other words, that our answer matches people's actual moral beliefs is important but not decisive. Our answer must stand on its own, by giving us a reasonable theory of what makes taking a human life wrong when it is wrong.

This is crucial in the abortion debate for several reasons. Most obvious is that people's moral beliefs about abortion clash. People's moral beliefs about the related issues of infanticide and euthanasia also clash, since there are many who think that there are conditions under which infanticide and euthanasia are morally permissible and others who think the opposite. Thus, some—even deeply held—moral beliefs about abortion (and euthanasia and infanticide) must be false.

Moreover, people's moral beliefs may be influenced by emotions, affections, and fears, which may distort people's judgment so that they believe what is not rationally grounded. This is a particularly strong risk regarding our attitudes towards infants and little children (or towards fetuses that look like little children), because of our evolutionary history. Compared to the offspring of other animals, human babies are born very early in their development and must, therefore, be tended to by their parents for a long time before they can get along on their own. That human babies continue to develop outside the womb has many evolutionary advantages, one of which is that it allows humans to develop larger brains than could fit through a woman's birth canal. It also surely means that humans have developed feelings of sympathy and affection for babies that motivate adults to provide the care that helpless little ones will need for many years. But these feelings may also get in the way of a rational assessment of little children's moral standing. Consequently, those who think that infanticide is terribly wrong may be overreacting to their natural affection for children, just as those who think that infanticide is acceptable may be overreacting to their desire to avoid the heavy responsibilities of childcare. Likewise, those who think that abortion is wrong because the fetus looks to them like a baby may be overreacting to their natural feelings about babies. In such cases, we must treat people's beliefs with some skepticism, a skepticism that can only be resolved by an independently reasonable theory of what makes taking a human life wrong when it is wrong—where "independently reasonable" means "based on plausible reasons independent of the theory's matching existing moral beliefs."

Thus, consideration of the moral question of abortion yields a guideline for identifying the question's answer: *Only an answer that can be supported by an independently reasonable theory of what makes taking a human life wrong when it is wrong (independently of the theory matching existing moral beliefs) can be a satisfactory answer to the moral question of abortion.* But there are other guidelines we can specify as well.

"Is killing a fetus morally murder?" is a question about the fetus's moral standing. Does it have moral standing like, say, that of normal human adults, such that killing it is gravely immoral? Here and elsewhere, I refer to the moral standing of "normal human adults" because both sides in the abortion debate agree that killing normal—innocent, nonthreatening, nonsuffering—human adults is gravely immoral. Or does it have moral standing like, say, that of sperm cells or mosquitoes, such that killing it is of little moral weight? These questions must be answered in terms of properties that the fetus has at the point at which killing it is considered. They cannot be answered simply by reference to properties that a fetus will have some time in its future. For this reason, philosophers have largely rejected arguments against abortion based on the fact that the fetus is potentially a human adult (Schwarz, 1990). This potentiality cannot mean that the fetus has the same rights as a human adult, because a human adult has those rights precisely because he is *actually* a human adult, not merely *potentially* one (cf. Feinberg, 1980). That an American infant is potentially president of the United States does not make that infant commander-in-chief of the US Armed Forces.

That the fetus's moral standing depends on its current properties will rule out other possible answers to our question. For example, some philosophers hold that what makes the ending of a human life wrong when it is wrong is that humans are rational beings, and it is morally wrong to kill a rational being (who is innocent and not posing a danger). Some of these philosophers will then add that, since the fetus has the genetic makeup that will lead to its developing a working brain, it is a rational being and therefore killing it is morally wrong (Beckwith, 2004; George & Tollefsen, 2008). But being rational requires that one already have a working brain. Rationality is not a current property of a fetus (surely not of a fetus prior to the development of a central nervous system at around the end of six months of gestation). A fetus is not now rational because it will develop a functioning brain, anymore than a fetus can now walk because it will one day develop legs.

Sometimes philosophers argue that the fetus is the *same entity* (albeit at a different point in time) as the adult it will become, and thus it must have the same essential properties, which include its basic rights. Then, the fetus has the same right to life as a normal human adult, and abortion is morally murder. But the idea that the fetus is the same entity as the eventual adult exaggerates the role of physical continuity in determining an entity's essential properties. An acorn is not an oak tree—a point noted by Judith Jarvis Thomson (1971), in her seminal essay, "A Defense of Abortion." Try giving your beloved rose seeds on Valentine's Day and tell her or him that they are the same as roses. You will quickly learn that things can be physically continuous without being the same thing.

It is not only anti-abortion writers who fail to see that an answer to the moral question about abortion depends on the properties of the fetus. Feminists who think that a woman's right to control her body decides the abortion issue in her favor are making the same error. A woman surely has the right to control her body. But, like other rights, that right is not unlimited. Its strength depends on what it comes up against. As lawyers say: "Your right to swing your fist ends where my nose begins." Though you have a right to swing your fist, that does not give you the right to use your fist to harm someone else who also has rights. By the same reasoning, a woman's right to control her body does not give her the right to kill another being that has similar rights over itself. The woman's right only prevails over the fetus if the fetus does not have the same rights over itself that the woman has over herself. And that will depend on the fetus's properties.

Thus, consideration of the moral question of abortion yields a second guideline for a satisfactory answer: *Only an answer based on properties that the fetus possesses at the point one is considering taking its life can be a satisfactory answer to the moral question of abortion.*

If this guideline is combined with the first, we get even more specific guidance. To see this, consider that some philosophers argue as follows: Human beings have rights not to be killed. A fetus is a human being. Therefore, it is morally wrong to kill a fetus (Kreeft, 2000). Abortion-rights defenders can respond by saying that there's a difference between being human in the *biological* sense, and being human in the *moral* sense. Being human in the biological sense means that one is the offspring of humans and is a member of the species *Homo sapiens*. In the moral sense, being human means that one is a member of the human moral community, "one of us," and thus entitled to the normal package of moral rights. The fetus is human in the biological sense. Does that entail that it is human in the moral sense?

Combining our two guidelines helps us answer this question. From the second guideline, the fetus's moral status must depend on its current properties. From the first guideline, the properties that are used to claim that the fetus is human in the moral sense, such that it has a right not to be killed, must provide reasonable grounds for granting the fetus that right. Biological species membership is not itself a reasonable ground for having the right not to be killed. Even if people do think that all members of *Homo sapiens* have that right, that they are *Homo sapiens* is not itself a good reason for it. To see why, consider that some philosophers have labeled basing rights on species membership *speciesism*, modeled on *racism*, and meaning an unjustified prejudice in favor of members of one's group (cf. Cohen, 1986; Ryder, 2005). If *Homo sapiens* have a right not to be killed, it must be because properties that members of the human species characteristically have—rationality, caring about their lives, capacity for love or creativity, or the like—provide reasonable grounds for that right, not merely because they belong to our group (cf. Warren, 1973; English, 1975; Parfit, 1984; Kamm, 1992; Merrill, 1998).

There is one more guideline. When we ask whether killing a fetus is morally murder, we want to know whether killing a fetus is wrong in the way it is wrong to murder a human adult. This wrongness has a very distinctive nature. For example, the wrongness of murdering a human adult is not canceled out or made up for in any significant degree if the murderer adds another human adult, or even several, to the human population (say, by the murderer producing and raising one or more children than he or she originally planned to have); whereas someone who, say, destroys your car can make up for that wrong significantly by giving you a new car or the money to buy one (or several). Or, consider that, while murder is gravely immoral, it is not gravely immoral to refrain from procreating—even though both murder and refraining from procreating mean that there will be one less human being in the human population.

These facts have the following surprising implication: Traits that make human life valuable—such as rationality, creativity, individuality, or the like—cannot themselves establish that killing a human being is morally murder. If the wrong of murder were that it destroys a being with one or more valuable traits, then we should expect that replacing the murdered one with another with those same valuable traits (another human), or more (several humans), would at very least significantly reduce the wrong of the murder—but it does not. Likewise, if the wrong of murder were that it removes a human being with valuable traits, then we should expect that refusing to procreate would also be significantly wrong because it also causes there to be fewer beings with those traits in existence—but we do not believe this about refusing to procreate. In short, the way we think murder is wrong implies that human beings are valued as *irreplaceable by beings of comparable value*. Or, as I shall say, the wrongness of murder implies that human life has *asymmetric value*.

Usually when we value something, we value it symmetrically. Our valuing it is about equally a reason for creating new ones *and* for not destroying existing ones. That is the symmetry in symmetric value. This is both a description of our conventional valuing practice, and a claim about the nature of valuing itself. Normally, when we value something, we think that thing is good, and that goodness applies to both existing ones and future ones. Such valuing applied to human life will imply that killing one human and replacing her with a new one yields no net loss in value, and that refraining from procreating deprives the world of as much value as does killing.

Asymmetric valuing is, of course, also quite common. We value friends and loved ones asymmetrically, and we value things that have personal (or sentimental) value that way too, a treasured possession from childhood, a gift from a lover, a diary, a work of art, and so on. The loss of such people or things could not be made up for by replacing them with others of equal value. But note that in such cases, we are valuing something that is in some way a special individual instance of its kind. When we value people we love asymmetrically, we are not valuing people generally, but valuing special ones; and when we value the ring given by a lover, we are not valuing rings generally, but valuing a special one. Such valuing cannot explain why murder is wrong, since the wrongness of murder must apply generally, not only to *special* individuals.

Moreover, we do value human beings symmetrically. Such valuing explains, for example, why it is good to keep the human race going. But it cannot explain the wrongness of murder. We need, then, to determine if there is anything about humans generally that justifies valuing them asymmetrically.

Thus, consideration of the moral question of abortion brings us to a third guideline for determining its answer: *Only an answer that accounts for the asymmetrical value of human life (implied by the special way in which we regard murder as wrong) can enable us to determine if killing a fetus is morally murder.*

Following our first guideline, we cannot satisfy this third guideline by simply asserting that people do in fact think that they and their fellows have asymmetric value. We need good reasons for believing that it is appropriate to treat humans as irreplaceable by beings of comparable value. And, by our second guideline, we have to find such reasons in properties that human beings actually have. Thus, we cannot account for the asymmetric value of human life simply by asserting that human life has *intrinsic worth,* or that human beings are *ends-in-themselves.* Such statements merely assert in different words that human life has asymmetric value. They do not show that it does; nor do they explain how it could. Rather we must proceed in the opposite direction: First, we must find one or more properties possessed by humans that provide a reasonable basis for asymmetrically valuing humans, and then *that* will enable us to explain how humans are ends-in-themselves or of intrinsic value.

A *utilitarian* ethic is one that aims at the maximization of some good, usually, happiness. A *deontological* ethic stresses duty or right conduct over the maximization of any good. A *virtue* ethic emphasizes the goodness of character over duty, right conduct, or the maximization of some good. Now, though I speak about how much value the world is deprived of by killing one human and replacing her with another, or by killing versus refusing to procreate, my argument is not limited to a utilitarian ethical framework or to one that thinks of value as quantifiable or maximizable. A deontologist may think that killing a human is worse than refusing to procreate because killing is a greater violation of duty, and a virtue-ethicist may think that killing is worse because it manifests a more evil character. The deontologist will have to explain why killing a human is a greater violation of duty than refusing to procreate, and the virtue-ethicist will have to explain why it manifests a worse character than refusing to procreate, when both acts result in there being one less human being. Both kinds of moral theorists will have to identify one or more properties that provide a reasonable basis for valuing human life asymmetrically.

We have established three guidelines that must be followed in answering the question whether killing a fetus is morally murder:

1. Only an answer that can be supported by an independently reasonable theory of what makes taking a human life wrong when it is wrong (independently of the theory matching existing moral beliefs) can be a satisfactory answer to the moral question of abortion.
2. Only an answer based on properties that the fetus possesses at the point one is considering taking its life can be a satisfactory answer to the moral question of abortion.
3. Only an answer that accounts for the asymmetrical value of human life (implied by the special way in which we regard murder as wrong) can enable us to determine if killing a fetus is morally murder.

We shall see that these guidelines dramatically reduce the possible candidates for answering the moral question of abortion. I shall argue that only one candidate is left standing, and thus it provides the answer we seek.

The Asymmetric Value of Human Life: Respecting Persons and Protecting Their Lives

Since imputing goodness to humans because of their distinctive properties is not asymmetric valuing, and since the reason that murder is wrong must apply generally and not merely to special individuals, I contend that only one thing can account for the way in which we think that murder of humans is wrong: *human beings' own subjective awareness of, and caring about, the continuation of their own lives*. Human beings care about their own particular lives asymmetrically. They do not think that losing their lives could be made up for by producing new people.

This is only part of the answer. Since it is we who are valuing human beings when we think it gravely immoral to kill them, we must be valuing consciously caring beings in a way that implies the asymmetric wrongness of killing them. This valuing cannot take the form of thinking that consciously-cared-about lives are good. Such valuing is symmetric; it implies that one consciously-cared-about life is about as good as any other, even a future one.

To arrive at the asymmetric valuing of human lives, then, we must value consciously-cared-about lives in a distinctive way. Instead of imputing goodness to consciously-cared-about lives, we must value *that* beings who consciously care about the continuation of their lives get what they care about. Valuing *that* caring beings get what they care about is asymmetric valuing because it applies only to beings who already care. Such valuing does not imply that it would be about as good to create new caring human beings as to preserve existing ones, because (in this way of valuing) we are not valuing caring beings as such (which would be symmetric valuing). We can value *that* beings who care about their lives continuing go on living without thinking that new living beings who care about their lives continuing should be brought into existence, much as we can value *that* starving beings get fed without thinking that new starving beings should be brought into existence.

Though this indirect valuing may seem odd at first, it is in fact quite common. *Respect* is just such indirect valuing: valuing that another get what he values. That is why we can respect people who make choices we would not make. Immanuel Kant (1785/1998) saw the indirect nature of the valuing in respect: "When I observe the duty of respect," he wrote, "I keep myself within my own bounds in order not to deprive another of any of the value which he as a human being is entitled to put upon himself."

Moreover, it is reasonable to respect human beings this way. It is reasonable because, once conscious caring has come on the scene, the ending of a being's life that is cared about causes a loss *to that being* that cannot be made good by replacing that being with another living being. The morality of the protection of human life makes sense as an agreement to protect every one of us against this unredeemable loss. Note that this reasonableness condition means that when, out of respect, we honor people's—even young children's—desire to stay alive, it is not only because they do so desire, but also because that desire is reasonable to honor.

There is another way in which this way of valuing human life is more familiar than it might seem at first: A being that consciously cares about the continuation of her life must be conscious *of herself*. She is not only conscious, but *self*-conscious. She is conscious of herself as the same self over time; otherwise she could not think of her life as continuing. A hallowed philosophical tradition defines personhood by this very awareness. John Locke (1689/1975, p. 335) defined a person as "a thinking intelligent being, that can consider itself as itself in different times and places." And Kant (1787/1963, p. 341) wrote, "That which is conscious of the numerical identity of itself at different times is in so far a person." The asymmetric valuing of human beings' lives is a form of what we know familiarly as *respect for persons*.

That killing is wrong if it kills a being who is conscious of and caring about the continuation of his life does not mean that killing a human being is wrong only when he knows that he is about to die—and thus not wrong when people are sleeping or unconscious (or, say, temporarily comatose). The point, rather, is that killing a being is wrong *when it is the killing of one for whom consciousness of self has begun, that is, a person*. To see why this is, consider the following.

When I awake after sleeping, my new waking experience seems to be happening to the same being that went to sleep a few hours before. For separate experiences that occur at different times to appear to happen to the same being requires an enduring point of view—one that is not equivalent to any one of the particular separate experiences—before which these experiences occur. This enduring point of view is the self. Philosophers differ on how it arises and of what it consists—Kant, for example, thought it was a necessary condition of our experiences fitting together as a coherent totality—but that it exists cannot be denied. The self's nature as an enduring point of view explains why personhood can be defined by awareness of one's identity (one's self-sameness) at different points in time. It is why our abiding traits remain ours (belong to our self) across periods of unconsciousness (Taylor, 1985; Unger, 1990; Schechtman, 1996). Einstein was a brilliant scientist even while asleep. The same applies to our abiding cares, such as the care about our continuing to live. It too belongs to one's self across periods of unconsciousness. Once a being has a self, its life happens before an inner audience—and that remains true even if the audience occasionally dozes off. Killing a person while asleep or unconscious is still a loss *to that person's self.*

And it is an asymmetric loss—a loss that cannot be made up for *to that self* by replacing that self's life with another self's life. Consequently, to value that beings vulnerable to this loss—*persons*—be protected against it implies that we believe that ending a person's life is far worse than not creating a new one. Thus, it implies neither that the wrong of murder can be made up for by adding new persons, nor that refusal to procreate is roughly as bad as murder. We value human life asymmetrically when we respect the persons whose lives they are.

The self begins at a point in time (when self-consciousness begins) and ends at a point in time (when self-consciousness ends for good). Killing a being who has not begun to be aware of its life, and to care about it continuing, is killing it before it has a self to whom its loss of life is an irreplaceable loss. For such a being, loss of its life is rather like its parents never having conceived it, a symmetric loss that cannot account for the wrong of murder.

Since the valuable traits of humans cannot account for asymmetric value, I contend that only our respect for people's subjective caring about their lives can account for the way in which we normally think murder is immoral. Since fetuses are not conscious that they are alive (and certainly not that their lives are continuing), they do not possess the property that is the object of asymmetric valuing. There is no ground for according them the special protection to which we think human life (at some point) is entitled. Consequently, abortion is not morally murder. Since women clearly have rights to control their bodies, it follows that the deliberately induced abortion of a human pregnancy is ethically justifiable as long as it is authorized by the pregnant woman.

Morality and Mattering: What Makes Killing Humans Wrong

A fetus does not have a right not to be killed because losing its life cannot matter to it. It cannot matter to a fetus because it does not yet have a self—it is not yet a "who"—to whom it could matter. This is also true of newborn infants. Awareness of themselves—and thus selfhood—does not happen to infants until at least well into their first year of existence. Thus, the argument made in the previous section does not imply that it is wrong to kill infants. Some people will respond to this by thinking that it proves that the approach taken here is wrong (Marquis, 2009; cf. Singer, 1993, pp. 175–217). That response is incorrect because of the first of the guidelines set out earlier. To reject the approach because it does not conclude that killing infants is gravely immoral is to take for granted the truth of one's moral belief that killing infants is morally murder. But we have already seen that there are good reasons for treating one's moral beliefs about infants with some skepticism.

Moreover, from the fact that the argument given in the previous section does not show that killing infants is wrong, it does not follow that there is nothing morally wrong with killing infants. What follows, rather, is that, if it is wrong to kill infants, it is wrong on grounds that are different from what makes killing human children and adults wrong. I think that there are grounds that make killing infants wrong, though not as gravely wrong as killing children and adults. These grounds condemn killing infants generally, though they leave room for infanticide of gravely defective newborns. To see what these grounds are, it will help to consider the conception of moral value that underlies the approach taken here.

The approach taken here bases moral value on *what* matters to beings, and on *how* what matters to them matters. So, for example, this view holds that it is wrong to inflict pain on animals, while it is not usually wrong to kill them painlessly. This is so because pain and avoiding it clearly matter to animals; but—with the possible exception of cetaceans and higher primates—animals have no consciousness of their futures and, thus, losing their futures cannot matter to them (cf. Boonin-Vail, 2003). This, we have seen, applies, not only to human fetuses, but also to newborn human infants.

However, even if infants' lives do not matter to them, human infants are universally objects of affection to human beings. And that means not only their parents and kin, but just about all normal human beings. This, as we saw earlier, is a product of our evolutionary history. We naturally respond warmly to human infants, to their cuteness and to their cries. Moreover, this affection is a good thing. It is part of the process by which human infants develop into psychologically healthy children and adults. Babies would not likely develop into well-balanced children and adults, if they were treated as disposable. Thus, what makes it wrong to kill infants is that they matter to virtually all normal human beings, and that it is good that they do.

But since this mattering is to others and not (yet) to themselves, it yields a weaker condemnation of killing newborn infants than of killing children or adults whose lives matter to themselves. This is because the loss of life to the one whose life it is, and who cares about it, is a more total loss than the loss of another's life is to one who cares about that other (Feitosa *et al.*, 2010). And this accounts for the permissibility of early infanticide of gravely defective newborns—an act that expresses care for infants by seeking to spare them suffering before their lives come to matter to them.

It might seem that we could apply the same argument to human fetuses. But that is false because, with the possible exception of the pregnant woman herself, no one can care about the particular fetus that is inside a woman. A person who thinks he does care about that particular one is really caring about his imaginative representation of a fetus, not the real one. Only the pregnant woman genuinely interacts with the fetus, and thus, only she has a chance of caring about the real one—and even then it is questionable how much of her care is directed to the real one, and how much to her mental image of it. Since the woman has a strong right to control her body, other people's imaginative caring about her fetus cannot possibly outweigh her right. Nonetheless, that people care about fetuses generally means on my view that fetuses should be treated with special care, even if they may be aborted.

It might seem that my argument implies that it is morally acceptable to kill older humans who, say, because of depression, do not want their lives to go on. This is not so because my view is part of a larger conception that grounds the morality of protection of life, and of rights generally, on how our lives matter to us, something which changes as we develop. Not only do newborn infants become little children with selves, and thus awareness of their lives and desire for it to go on; they continue to grow and mature. As they do, their lives start to matter to them in a new way. They come to see their lives no longer only as something they want to continue, but also as the arena of their living out their choices. As this way of caring about their lives develops, we shift from simply protecting children's lives to giving them increasing responsibility for making of their lives what they want. They are granted autonomy rights, even though these may be exercised only under parental supervision, or by the parents (or guardians) in the child's name.

This new way of the child's life mattering to it is still a form of caring about its future life, a desire that that life conform to its choices. Autonomy rights are a response to the child's new form of subjective caring about its life, just as the protection of its life was a response to the earlier form of simply desiring that its life go on. Normally the new form of caring joins and supplements the earlier form, but either could stand alone as a ground for protection of life. We respond to the new form by treating the child as owning its life, entitled to do with it what it wants—as far as is rational and morally acceptable. Accordingly, starting in childhood and developing from there, when people desire to end their life or lose the desire to go on due to depression or the like, we do not honor the desire or its lack because they are irrational. At the same time, treating people as owning their lives, we protect their lives for them, in trust, so to speak, until they can rationally decide what they want.

Thus, this view requires protecting the lives of those who irrationally do not want to go on living. But it also leaves room for a right of rational adults to choose euthanasia when they face pain-filled futures, or even to choose suicide when, upon sober reflection, they no longer want to go on living. What's crucial for my view is that all of this happens only once the self has already come on the scene, aware and caring about its life—and in response to that fact. Children whose selves fail to appear at all retain the moral status of newborn infants.

This account also explains our moral obligations regarding the lives of severely mentally defective adults. The vast majority of severely mentally defective adults still possess enough rationality to justify some autonomy rights, and nearly all possess the minimum self-awareness and caring about their lives that justifies protection of their lives. When people fall below this minimum, they revert to the moral status they had as newborn infants. There will be a strong rule against killing them because of how they matter to humans generally, though with exceptions that permit ending the lives of severely mentally defective people who are in terrible and unending pain.

Based on how life matters to the living being or to others, the approach to abortion taken here fits within a theory of how human life should be valued at all points from conception, through birth and maturation, to loss of capacities. Indeed, it goes even further. Though corpses cannot matter to themselves, they matter to virtually all normal people as "remains" of living people. Accordingly, we are obligated to take special care in treating and disposing of human corpses.

References

Beckwith, F. (2004). The explanatory power of the substance view of persons. *Christian Bioethics, 10*, 33–54.

Boonin-Vail, D. (2003). *A defense of abortion*. Cambridge: Cambridge University Press.

Cohen, C. (1986). The case for the use of animals in biomedical research. *The New England Journal of Medicine, 315*, 865–870.

English, J. (1975). Abortion and the concept of a person. *Canadian Journal of Philosophy, 5*, 233–243.

Feinberg, J. (1980). Abortion. In T. Regan (Ed.), *Matters of life and death: New introductory essays in moral philosophy* (pp. 256–293). New York: Random House.

Feitosa, S., Garrafa, V., Cornelli, G., Tardivo, C., & Carvalho, S. (2010). Bioethics, culture and infanticide in Brazilian indigenous communities: The Zuruahá case. *Cad Saude Publica, 26*, 853–865.

George, R., & Tollefsen, C. (2008). *Embryo: A defense of human life*. New York: Doubleday Broadway Publishing Group.

Kamm, F. M. (1992). Non-consequentialism, the person as an end-in-itself, and the significance of status. *Philosophy and Public Affairs, 21*, 354–389.

Kant, I. (1785/1998). *Groundwork of the metaphysics of morals* (M. Gregor, Trans.). (Section I: Transition from common rational to philosophic moral cognition). Cambridge: Cambridge University Press.

Kant, I. (1787/1963). *Critique of pure reason* (N. K. Smith, Trans.). London: Macmillan.

Kreeft, P. (2000). The apple argument against abortion. *Crisis, 18*, 25–29.

Locke, J. (1689/1975). *An essay concerning human understanding*. Oxford: Oxford University Press.

Marquis, D. (2009). Singer on abortion and infanticide. In J. Schaler (Ed.), *Peter Singer under fire: The moral iconoclast faces his critics* (pp. 133–152). Chicago: Open Court.

Merrill, S. B. (1998). *Defining personhood: Toward the ethics if quality in clinical care*. Amsterdam: Rodopi.

Parfit, D. (1984). *Reasons and persons*. Oxford: Oxford University Press.

Reiman, J. (1999). *Abortion and the ways we value human life*. Lanham, MD: Rowman & Littlefield.

Ryder, R. (2005). All beings that feel pain deserve human rights: Equality of the species is the logical conclusion of post-Darwin morality. *The Guardian*. Friday, August 5. Retrieved from: http://www.guardian.co.uk/uk/2005/aug/06/animalwelfare

Sadler, T. (2011). *Langman's medical embryology*. Hagerstown, MD: Lippincott, Williams & Wilkins.

Schechtman, M. (1996). *The constitution of selves*. Ithaca, NY: Cornell University Press.

Schwarz, S. (1990). *The moral question of abortion*. Chicago: Loyola University Press.

Singer, P. (1993). *Practical ethics*. Cambridge: Cambridge University Press.

Taylor, C. (1985). The concept of a person. In C. Taylor (Ed.), *Philosophical papers: Volume 1* (pp. 97–114). Cambridge: Cambridge University Press.

Thomson, J. J. (1971). A defense of abortion. *Philosophy and Public Affairs, 1*, 47–66.

Unger, P. (1990). *Identity, consciousness, and value*. Oxford: Oxford University Press.

Warren, M. A. (1973). On the moral and legal status of abortion. *The Monist, 57*, 43–61.

Chapter Eight

The Deliberately Induced Abortion of a Human Pregnancy Is Not Ethically Justifiable

Don Marquis

In this chapter, I describe several perspectives other than mine on the ethics of the abortion of a human pregnancy. I explain how each perspective seems initially plausible, but then go on to argue that each suffers from major difficulties. I then explain my own perspective on the abortion issue, which is called the *future of value view*. I argue that it shows that the deliberately induced abortion of a human pregnancy is not ethical.

The Reproductive Freedom Perspective

Most people who defend a woman's right to abortion appeal to the value of reproductive freedom (Thomson, 1971; English, 1973; Warren, 1973). There is much to be said for this perspective. The decision concerning whether to bring a child into the world is central to one's life plans. Unwanted children place a considerable burden on women, and are less likely to be loved and raised well. There seem to be many good reasons to respect a woman's right to reproductive freedom.

Some will object to the reproductive freedom perspective because they believe that life begins at conception. However, as Justice Harry Blackmun pointed out in *Roe v. Wade* (410 US 113, 1973) back in 1973, there is no consensus concerning when life begins. Further, many object to the reproductive freedom perspective based upon religious reasons of one kind or another. However, in a free society, even a majority may not limit important liberty rights of individual members of society when the limits on freedom are based on religion. As John Stuart Mill (1869/2011) argued in *On Liberty*, society is justified in restricting the liberty of one of its members only to prevent harm to another.

The reproductive freedom perspective, however, is open to an apparently devastating objection based upon Mill's harm principle noted above. Consider the product of conception—at least after the third week of pregnancy: it consists of cells that engage in metabolism; it grows; it is an integrated biological unit; therefore, it is certainly living. In addition, it certainly seems to be a very young biological organism that is a member of our species. Of what other species could it be a member? Therefore, human fetuses are living human beings, biological organisms who are members of the species *Homo sapiens*. This being the case, ending their lives is ruled out by Mill's harm principle, for to have an abortion greatly harms a human being by ending its life.

Contemporary Debates in Bioethics, First Edition. Edited by Arthur L. Caplan and Robert Arp.

The Innocent-Human-Life Perspective

Criticism of the reproductive freedom perspective opens the door to an opposed perspective on abortion ethics. According to this perspective, the right to life is a right of all human beings, or, at least of a right of all human beings who are innocent and have not waived their right to life. Therefore, all human fetuses have the right to life. The right to life trumps anyone's claimed freedom to end that life. Therefore, abortion is wrong (Noonan, 1970).

The innocent-human-life perspective is a powerful argument. It amounts to the syllogism:

1. All innocent human beings have the right to life.
2. All human fetuses are innocent human beings.
3. Therefore, all human fetuses have the right to life.

This syllogism is valid (*if* all of the premises are true, then the conclusion cannot be false). The first premise is a claim that all decent people would regard as too obvious to mention; think, for example, of what discussions of the evil of the Holocaust take for granted. The second premise is a true claim in biology. It follows that not only is the argument valid, but also it is *sound*—the conclusion must be true.

Note, also, that nothing in this argument rests on an appeal to religion: that all human beings have the right to life is a basic moral claim that virtually everyone takes for granted, whether religious or not. So, the claim that the pro-life view on abortion rests only on religion is clearly false.

In spite of its virtues, the innocent-human-life perspective is subject to two devastating criticisms set out most clearly by Peter Singer in his famous book, *Practical Ethics*, first published in 1979. Singer criticized the above syllogism in the only way it could be vulnerable to criticism: he attacked the first premise. He offered two objections to it.

First, Singer pointed out that when we condemn racism (as we should), we take for granted that any biological difference between Caucasians and non-Caucasians has, by itself, no moral significance whatsoever. And when we condemn sexism (as we should), we take for granted that any biological difference between males and females has, by itself, no moral significance. Therefore, Singer concluded that we should not take for granted that the biological property of being a member of our species has any moral significance whatsoever. In short, just as we believe that racism and sexism are unfounded, we should also believe that what Singer called "speciesism" is unfounded. Basing a moral right on a biological property—whether that biological property has to do with race, sex, or species—is unjustified.

Singer also pointed out that the claim that all human beings have the right to life is subject to what can be called the *over-commitment objection*. If all human beings have the right to life, then human beings who are rightly judged to be irreversibly unconscious have the right to life. There are good reasons for believing that some human beings who are irreversibly unconscious are functioning, integrated biological organisms of the species *Homo sapiens* and therefore are alive (Shewmon, 2001). Nevertheless, it is hard to believe that they really do have the right to life. If you, the reader, were irreversibly unconscious, would you really care if your life were ended? On the basis of these objections, Singer concluded that the first premise of the syllogism that represents the human life perspective ("All innocent human beings have the right to life") is arbitrary and, indeed, false. Singer's objections are compelling.

Warren's Personhood Perspective

Plainly what is needed is an account of the right to life that (1) explains why you and I have the right to life and (2) avoids the problems Singer raised. Mary Anne Warren (1973), in a famous paper titled, "On the Moral and Legal Status of Abortion," argued that the basis of this right is not our membership in a particular species, but the fact that we are *persons*. She understood being a person in terms of the traits of consciousness, reasoning, self-motivated activity, the capacity to communicate, and the presence of self concepts, noting, too, that her characterization of personhood was only rough and ready. She suggested that one could be a person if one possessed at least some of these traits, and that an individual who lacks them all is clearly not a person. Therefore, fetuses are not persons. They lack the right to life. So, abortion is morally permissible.

Warren's view has much to recommend it. For one thing, it attributes the right to life to all of those people who, by consensus, do have the right to life (if we waive problems regarding infanticide). For another, it explains why we would attribute the right to life to someone from another planet who happened not to possess human DNA, but who exhibited the manifestations of personhood, thereby avoiding the speciesism objection. In addition, it lacks the perverse consequence that we should treat the irreversibly unconscious as having the right to life, thereby avoiding the over-commitment objection. It explains why we say (without reflection) that all human beings have the right to life. It protects reproductive freedom, which we all agree is greatly to be valued.

Nevertheless, there are two major problems with Warren's personhood view. The first concerns her definition of personhood itself. If we take it quite literally, it is too narrow. Someone who is asleep is not conscious, is not reasoning, and is not exhibiting self-motivated activity. Nevertheless, such an individual is clearly a person and, moreover, is clearly a person in virtue of the capacity to exhibit those traits. Therefore, what is needed is an understanding of Warren's traits of personhood so that all of the traits are stated in terms of *capacities*. So far, so good, for Warren.

The trouble is that once we adjust Warren's views in this necessary way, we are confronted with the problem of how to understand the capacities in question. On the one hand, those who are fond of the innocent-human-life perspective will argue that these capacities should be understood in terms of the deep natural capacity for consciousness, reasoning, or self-motivation possessed by all human beings, even by fetuses at an early gestational age (Lee & George, 2008). On the other hand, those who wish to protect the value of reproductive freedom will argue that such capacities should be understood in terms of immediately exercisable capacities, capacities that one has because one has at least a minimally functioning brain. It is plainly unsatisfactory to treat the decision of who is a person and who is not as *only* a *decision*. To allow such a move is of a kind with allowing Nazis to make a decision concerning who is a person and who is not, and such an allowing is ruled out on grounds of common decency.

There is another problem with Warren's view. What is the connection between being a person and having the right to life? If what is wrong with the innocent-human-life perspective is that it requires making an inference from having a biological property to having a moral property, one wonders why one cannot criticize Warren's personhood perspective for requiring us to make an inference from a set of psychological properties to a moral property. If a defender of Warren's view should reply that it seems natural to connect those two properties, the defender of the innocent-human-life perspective can note that it seems natural to connect the biological property of being a member of our species with having the right to life. A major shortcoming of Warren's personhood account is that it fails to incorporate our values into our account of having the right to life or, alternatively, into the wrongness of killing (most) human beings.

The Pro-Attitude Perspective

Some of those who favor reproductive choice have a reply to the above criticisms. They argue that being a person is central to the correct account of the right to life because only persons have a self concept, that is, a concept of self as a continuing subject of experience. Only if one has a concept of self as a continuing subject of experience, can one desire to live. We have the strong desire to live. Our strong desire to live is the basis for our right to life. The reason the strong desire to live is the basis for the right to life is that everyone agrees that we have a presumptive obligation to respect the desires of others, especially to respect very strongly held desires. The desire to live is a strongly held desire because it is a desire that is a necessary condition of the fulfillment of our other desires. Accordingly, our strong desire to live is the basis for our belief that (most) human beings have the right to life (Tooley, 1972; Singer, 1979).

The pro-attitude perspective underwrites reproductive choice, of course. Fetuses do not desire to live, because they lack a concept of self as a continuing subject of experience. Therefore, they lack the property that is necessary for the right to life. It follows, then, that ending their lives is not wrong and abortion is morally permissible.

The virtue of this pro-attitude perspective is that it bases our view that killing post-natal human beings is wrong on the values we actually have. Warren's personhood perspective fails to do that. In addition, the pro-attitude perspective seems to have resources to get around the capacity problem that is a difficulty for her view. It is correct to attribute beliefs to individuals even if they are not, at present, thinking of their beliefs. Similarly, we believe that individuals can have the actual desire to live, even when they are not thinking of that desire or when they are asleep or unconscious. Ultimately, the basis of our view concerning people's desires or beliefs is our view that an individual possesses the right sort of brain state in virtue of which she holds a certain belief or has a certain desire. Plainly fetuses lack the requisite brain states. Therefore, the pro-attitude perspective does not suffer from either of the problems that afflict the Warren personhood perspective.

The pro-attitude perspective has another nice feature. It does not suffer from Singer's over-commitment problem mentioned above. People who are irreversibly comatose do not desire to live. Indeed, they lack the brain states in virtue of which they could possibly have any desires at all. Therefore, they lack the right to life. Therefore, the pro-attitude perspective, unlike the innocent-human-life perspective, does not underwrite the wrongness of killing them.

Pro-attitude perspectives are popular in the philosophical community. Singer (1979) and Tooley (1972) have argued that our right to life should be based on our desire to live. Harris (1999) has argued that our right to life should be based on the fact that we value our future lives. Steinbock (1992) and Dworkin (1993) have argued that our right to life should be based on our interest in continuing to live. Reiman (1999) has argued that our right to life is based on the fact that we care about continuing to live. Paske (1998) and Brown (2002) have argued that our right to life should be based upon our hopes for our future. No doubt there are even other variations. The differences between these perspectives should not be allowed to obscure their essential similarity: all of them refer to the pro-attitude you and I have toward our continued existence, and they all have the same virtues.

Unfortunately, they all suffer from a devastating problem. Consider someone with untreated bipolar disease who is greatly depressed and suicidal; or, someone who has been given a suicide pill by a mortal enemy and, after the pill takes effect, says sincerely she does not want to live; or, someone who has become convinced by his religious leader that all the members of their cult should commit suicide in order to obtain bliss in the afterlife. The pro-attitude view implies that it is not wrong to kill such folks. Therefore, any popular pro-attitude perspective is false.

Suppose a defender of the pro-attitude perspective tries to repair her view by arguing that the *rational* desire to continue to live is the basis for the right to life, and therefore, the above counterexamples are not counterexamples to the pro-attitude perspective as it is rightly understood. Such a repair is ineffective. If one lacks the desire to live, one lacks the *rational* desire to live. This move does not solve the problems posed by the counterexamples to pro-attitude perspectives.

The Future of Value View

Why are the counterexamples to the pro-attitude view really counterexamples? Are these counterexamples based on strong, but ultimately indefensible moral intuitions, or is there a reason why these counterexamples are persuasive? There is indeed a reason. Many people who are depressed can be treated with psychotherapy and/or psychotropic drugs and can go on to live lives they will value. We presume that, after the suicide pill wears off, the individual who took the pill will go on to live a life she will value. We presume that, after rescue and treatment, the deluded member of the religious cult can be deprogrammed and can go on to live a life he will value. This suggests that underlying the counterexamples is the belief that if an individual would have a future she will value if she does not die, it is wrong to kill her (Marquis, 1989).

This suggestion is borne out in other ways. Consider the class of people who do want to live. One could argue that it is wrong to kill them because if they are not killed, they will go on to live lives they will value. We believe that one's premature death from cancer, heart disease, or some other cause is a misfortune to her because that death deprives her of a future that she would value. Why is this? We presume that a shorter life is a worse life than a longer life because the shorter life will, ceteris paribus, contain fewer goods than the longer life. We believe that to cause someone's life to contain fewer goods than it would otherwise contain is to harm her. To deprive someone of *all* of the goods of her future life is to cause great harm to her. It causes her to suffer a great misfortune. It is wrong to cause others to suffer a misfortune. It is wrong to harm others, and it is certainly wrong to cause great harm to others. Therefore, killing another human being is wrong because it deprives her of a future of value. Reflection on the counterexamples to the pro-attitude perspective and reflection on our attitudes to death leads to a better account of the wrongness of killing.

The future of value view, like the innocent-human-life perspective, the pro-attitude perspective, or Warren's personhood perspective, is intended to provide us with a sufficient condition for the wrongness of killing, unless special circumstances obtain. Special circumstances include killing in self-defense, killing in time of war, and cases in which the death penalty may be the appropriate penalty for a crime. Discussion of these special circumstance cases takes for granted that ordinarily killing another human being is wrong, but there may be exceptions in cases involving the termination of other human life. However, these are all cases in which the killing needs careful justification. If these special circumstances do not obtain, then the future of value view, like the innocent-human-life perspective, and Warren's personhood perspective and the pro-attitude perspectives, is intended to provide us with a sufficient condition for the wrongness, indeed, the very serious wrongness, of killing.

Does the future of value view provide a necessary condition for the serious wrongness of killing? Consider those cases that cause difficulty for the innocent-human-life account: cases of human beings who have become irreversibly unconscious. Irreversibly unconscious humans lack futures of value; that is, they lack a future in which they would value their experiences. Therefore, the standard reason why killing a human being is wrong does not apply to them. However, it does not follow immediately that it is not wrong to kill anyone who is irreversibly unconscious. There may be another reason why such human beings should be kept alive. Perhaps a relative is willing to pay for the continuation of life supports. Perhaps the patient himself has made provisions to pay for his continued care. Usually, however, there is no such reason. Unless such a special situation obtains, ending the lives of people who are irreversibly unconscious is not wrong. In the absence of special situations, the future of value view of the wrongness of killing will function as a necessary condition for the wrongness of killing.

The future of value view of the wrongness of killing is, strictly speaking, too inclusive. Although it is easy to think only of cases of humans when considering the issue of wrongness of killing with special emphasis of the issue of abortion, the unqualified future of value view will imply that it is wrong to kill most mammals. Cows have future of value, as futures of value have been defined. Those who eat beef do not think that it is wrong to kill cows. Unless this difficulty is addressed, the future of value theory is subject to a serious objection.

It can be addressed in the following way. What is attractive about both Warren's personhood perspective and the pro-attitude perspective is that they take into account the moral importance of the lives of persons. In particular, Warren's perspective is attractive because it takes into account the common view that the lives of persons are far more morally important than the lives of those who are not. If the future of value view cannot provide us with insight into why Warren's perspective is wrong in this respect, we would have one reason for thinking that Warren's personhood perspective is superior to the future of value view.

We can put the difficulty another way. The reproductive freedom perspective and the pro-attitude perspective were criticized because they were too narrow. They made too much killing morally permissible. The innocent-human-life perspective was criticized because it was too broad. It made it wrong to end lives that it was clearly not wrong to end. Is the future of value view also too broad because it makes it wrong to end lives that most people think it is not wrong to end?

The P-Future of Value View

The future of value view can be qualified so that it deals with this objection. What are the arguments in favor of the future of value view? The arguments are based on analysis of why we believe that it is wrong to kill humans when it is wrong, and why we believe that it is permissible to end the lives of humans when it is permissible to end those lives. Those futures that we believe are so morally important that they are the basis of a strong moral prohibition of killing are the futures that can be characterized as the lives of persons. We believe that it is wrong to kill suicidal persons, or persons who have taken a suicide pill, or persons in the grip of a religious cult because they can have (after deprogramming) the kind of futures that persons have. We believe that death from cancer is a misfortune because it deprives someone of the kind of future that persons have. Thus, what is morally significant seems to be a future personal life. Call such a life a *p-future of value*. The p-future of value view does not imply that we must refrain from eating beef.

Accordingly, the objection that the future of value view makes too much killing wrong can be dealt with. Indeed, the p-future of value view recognizes the moral importance of the life of a person as much as does Warren's personhood perspective and the pro-attitude perspective. However, unlike those other perspectives, the future of value view recognizes *future* personhood. Therefore, it implies that abortion is not only wrong, but seriously wrong. It is wrong for the same reason that killing any post-natal human being is wrong. Birth is morally irrelevant.

A key concept in the p-future of value view is (of course) the notion of a p-future of value. What it is to have a p-future of value is (I suppose) intuitively obvious. However, there would be something wrong with the p-future of value view if one were unable to unpack the notion more precisely.

At an early age, we acquire a notion of a natural human life span. We recognize that our parents, grandparents, and great grandparents are located at later points in that life span. To end someone's life at some particular time is to deprive him of the years of a normal lifespan after that time. But what is that future of which he was deprived? It is not something that was actually part of his life if his life were ended prematurely. It is not necessarily something that he thought he had. Otherwise, the view would not imply that abortion is wrong, for a fetus is unable to have a concept of her future. An individual's future of value at a given age is one's *potential* at that age to live to a greater age and to have a future life that one would value. That potential is based on one's nature as a biological organism in much the same way as table salt's potential to dissolve if put in water (even if it is never put in water) is based on the chemical nature of NaCl (cf. McInerney, 1990).

There is nothing mysterious about this. Epidemiologists have data concerning one's median life expectancy at a given age and with respect to one's physical condition. One's median life expectancy refers to one's potential future life at a given age. One's future of value is just one's median future life expectancy on the assumption that one would value that future life.

This explication of the idea of a future of value shows how a common criticism of the future of value view is unsound. Norcross (1990) has argued that if fetuses have futures of value, then combinations of sperm and ova also have a future of value, for they can combine to form a zygote and then a fetus, and then a post-natal human being. However, not all combinations of sperm and ova could possibly have a future of value. Prior to fertilization there is no actual combination of a particular sperm and ovum, and, therefore, nothing to have the potential that is the basis for a future of value. There are only a multitude of possible combinations. Once a fetus exists, there is an actual entity with an actual potential to have a future of value. Misfortunes require actual victims.

The Superiority of the P-Future of Value View

Let us compare the p-future of value view to other accounts of the ethics of abortion. It is superior to the reproductive freedom perspective because it takes seriously the fact that fetuses are human beings and that, at least in the vast majority of cases, deliberately ending the life of another human being is wrong. It is superior to the innocent-human-life perspective because it is subject neither to the speciesism objection nor to the over-commitment objection. Unlike the innocent-human-life perspective, the p-future of value view does not make it wrong to end the lives of the irreversibly unconscious. Indeed, it does not rule out the moral permissibility of euthanasia and physician-assisted suicide. On the other hand, like Warren's personhood perspective and pro-attitude perspectives, it is open to the possibility that elsewhere in our universe there could be individuals with p-futures of value who lack human DNA.

The p-future of value view is superior to Warren's personhood perspective because it avoids the problem of being based on making an arbitrary decision about capacities and because it involves our values in a way that Warren's perspective does not. The p-future of value view is superior to any of the many pro-attitude perspectives because it deals correctly with cases in which, due to some mental aberration, a human does not desire to continue to live. Because there are other reasons why the p-future of value view is plausible, the p-future of value view is superior to alternative accounts of the wrongness of killing. The p-future of value view implies that abortion is seriously immoral. Therefore, abortion is seriously immoral.

The Ideal Desire Perspective

The p-future of value view justifies major restrictions on reproductive freedom. This is unfortunate. Boonin-Vail (2003) and Singer (2009) believe that an ideal desire perspective is superior to the future of value view. The ideal desire perspective is developed in the following way.

Pro-attitude perspectives concerning the wrongness of killing fail because they cannot account for the wrongness of killing an individual who lacks a pro-attitude toward her future life, where the absence of a pro-attitudes is, we are quite sure, irrational. So, instead of basing the account of the wrongness of killing on people's *actual* desires, the account of the wrongness of killing should be based on people's *ideal* desires. One's ideal desire to live is a desire an individual does have or would have if she were rational and fully informed. Therefore, those people referred to in the counterexamples to the actual desire perspective will all have an ideal desire to continue to live. It follows that an ideal desire perspective is not vulnerable to the counterexamples that afflict standard pro-attitude perspectives.

A close look at the ideal desire perspective reveals some problems, however. Recall that an actual desire version of a standard pro-attitude theory will justify abortion in terms of the following inference:

1. The basis for the right to life is one's strong desire to live.
2. Because fetuses lack a concept of self as a continuing subject of experience, fetuses cannot have a strong desire to live.
3. Therefore, fetuses lack the right to life.

The trouble with the actual desire version of a standard pro-attitude perspective is that point 1 is false. The ideal desire perspective patches up this inference in the following way:

1. The basis for the right to life is one's strong *ideal* desire to live.
2. Because fetuses lack a concept of self as a continuing subject of experience, fetuses lack a strong ideal desire to live.
3. Therefore, fetuses lack the right to life.

The basis for the idealization of the desire in this case involves full information and rationality about one's potential future. Clearly more is involved. One must also *have a future of value.* If you lack a future of value, all of the information in the world and perfect rational evaluation will not yield an ideal desire to live. The ideal desire perspective, when explicated in an obvious way, is *parasitic upon* the future of value view! The full information and the rational evaluation components are needed to get from having a future of value to a rational, informed desire to live. But if we present our account of the wrongness of killing in terms of one's future of value instead of one's *idealized* mental attitude, the full information components and the rational evaluation components drop out. This suggests that the mental attitude components of the ideal desire perspective are a part of the perspective only in order to generate conclusions concerning abortion that supports reproductive freedom. Accordingly, the preference for an ideal desire perspective rather than a future of value view can hardly *justify* reproductive freedom, on pain of circularity.

There is another problem. Versions of an ideal desire perspective that have been actually offered require having an actual desire at a time in order to have an ideal at that time. Boonin-Vail (2003, pp. 81–83) and Singer (2009, p. 156), for example, subscribe to this requirement. An ideal desire to live is an actual desire concerning one's future life that is corrected, when necessary, to account for imperfect information and imperfect rationality. Because no fetus has an actual desire to live or not live, no fetus has an ideal desire to live, and because no fetus has an ideal desire to live, no fetus has the right to life. One wonders, however, why a theory that involves *hypothetical* perfect information and *hypothetical* perfect reasoning requires as a component the *actual* capacity to desire. Suppose the *actual* capacity to desire component is omitted in favor of a *hypothetical* desire. Then, fetuses could have ideal desires to live just like the suicidal person. Unlike the original *actual* pro-attitude perspective, which was based on a fact about fetuses, the Boonin and Singer versions of the ideal desire theory are based only on a stipulation. An account of the wrongness of killing that is based on a stipulation is plainly unsatisfactory.

Thomson's Defense of Abortion Rights

The future of value view seems to provide us with an argument that abortion is wrong. After all, the loss a fetus would suffer by her life being ended is far greater than the loss a pregnant woman would suffer were she not permitted to procure an abortion. These considerations, plus the duty to minimize harm, imply that abortion is wrong.

Judy Thomson (1971) offered a famous thought experiment to show that the above argument is incorrect. Suppose that when you awaken one morning, you find that, while you were sleeping, you had been hooked up, bloodstream to bloodstream, to a famous violinist with a rare blood disease. As you are waking up, the president of the Society of Music Lovers explains that the violinist will die if you unhook yourself. The violinist has the right to life. Therefore, it is wrong to unhook yourself. Thomson suggests that most of us would regard the claim that we cannot unhook ourselves because the violinist's right to life outweighs our right to control our own body as outrageous. Her claim is certainly plausible. It is tempting to conclude that the famous violinist case is like pregnancy. Therefore, you have the right when pregnant to detach yourself from the fetus.

What is called the *responsibility objection* is a standard objection to Thomson's claim. According to this objection, in a pregnancy not due to rape the pregnant woman has acquired responsibility for there being another human being dependent on her.

Thomson (1971) argues that the responsibility objection does not succeed, however. She argues that just because you carelessly leave the windows to your house open and a burglar gets in, it is absurd to say that "she has given him a right to the use of her house—for she is partially responsible for his presence there, having voluntarily done what enabled him to get in" (p. 81). Will this do?

The responsibility objection is really two distinguishable claims: (1) A person who is pregnant has special, serious obligations to the dependent human being whose dependent existence is caused by her and whose continued existence is entirely dependent on her. (2) If (1) is true, then these obligations include the obligation to provide bodily life support for nine months.

Thomson's burglar analogy does not address (1) at all. No one thinks that you have any special, serious obligation to let the burglar stay. In the burglar case, we would hold the burglar entirely responsible for being in your house (note that you would not be charged with being an accessory to the crime). The fetus is not responsible to any extent for being in your body. Furthermore, the laws regarding property rights being what they are, the burglar has no right to be in your house at all, whether you left the windows open or not. To assume that the case of pregnancy is analogous is just to assume what needs to be shown.

There are two very good arguments for (1). Here is the first. All mammals have mothers. A fetus is a mammal. Therefore, a fetus has a mother. Only the pregnant woman qualifies to be the mother of the fetus within her. All mothers are parents. All parents (unless exceptional circumstances obtain) have serious, special duties of care to their children (think here of your reaction to deadbeat dads). Therefore, all pregnant women have serious, special duties of care to their children. Fetuses are children. Therefore, all pregnant women have serious, special duties of care to their fetuses. Therefore, (1) is true (cf. Pavlischek, 1993).

Here is the second. Suppose you are driving your car. You are negligent. You cause an accident in which another human being is harmed. Suppose this human being requires, as a consequence, expensive life-saving medical care for which he is unable to pay without going bankrupt. Do you have a moral obligation to pay his medical expenses, if you can? The answer is clearly *yes*. This suggests that we have special, serious obligations to another human for whose plight we are responsible when she would suffer a serious loss unless we aid her.

Either of these two arguments alone seems entirely sufficient to show that (1) is true. Nevertheless, a necessary condition of the truth of the anti-choice view is the truth of (2). Is (2) true? Well, (1) is rather empty if it is not.

Finally, however, independently of the merit of the responsibility objection, Thomson's defense of abortion fails. This can be seen by discussing a variant of the story of the famous violinist. Suppose that the violinist's blood disease afflicted everyone for nine months at some time in their lives, although medical science has been unable to determine yet just when. Suppose that one's bloodstream must be connected to another's for nine months in order to survive, but after such connection, one will be healthy again.

Now, suppose that we vote on whether the right to life in our society includes the right to bodily life support from another when one contracts this now universal blood disease. It would be in the prudential interests of all of us to vote that it does.

Note that the characteristics of this scenario are more like those of pregnancy than Thomson's violinist scenario. Few of us are famous violinists. All of us were dependent on bodily life support at one time in our lives. (It was very early.) These considerations show that the Thomson defense of abortion fails.

Conclusion

The future of value view is the best account of the wrongness of killing. Thomson's defense of abortion does not succeed. We may conclude that, unless a very special situation obtains, the deliberately induced abortion of a human pregnancy is not ethically justifiable. Such special situations may be pregnancy due to rape or pregnancy in which the life of the woman is threatened. I have neglected such special situations because their correct analysis is not simple. That analysis would detract from the major argument of this essay.

References

Boonin-Vail, D. (2003). *A defense of abortion.* Cambridge: Cambridge University Press.

Brown, M. (2002). A future like ours revisited. *Journal of Medical Ethics, 28,* 192–195.

Dworkin, R. (1993). *Life's dominion: An argument about abortion, euthanasia and individual freedom.* New York: Alfred A. Knopf.

English, J. (1973). Abortion and the concept of a person. *Canadian Journal of Philosophy, 5*(2), 233–243.

Harris, J. (1999). The concept of a person and the value of life. *Kennedy Institute of Ethics Journal, 2,* 293–308.

Lee, P., & George, R. (2008). *Body-self dualism in contemporary ethics and politics.* Cambridge: Cambridge University Press.

Marquis, D. (1989). Why abortion is immoral. *The Journal of Philosophy, 86,* 183–202.

McInerney, P. (1990). Does a fetus already have a future-like-ours? *The Journal of Philosophy, 87*(5), 264–268.

Mill, J. S. (1869/2011) *On liberty.* Whitefish, MT: Kessinger Publishing Company.

Noonan, J. (1970). An almost absolute value in history. In J. Noonan (Ed.), *The morality of abortion: Legal and historical perspectives* (pp. 51–59). Cambridge, MA: Harvard University Press.

Norcross, A. (1990). Killing, abortion, and contraception: A reply to Marquis. *The Journal of Philosophy, 87,* 268–277.

Paske, G. (1998). Abortion and the neo-natal right to life. In L. Pojman & F. Beckwith (Eds.), *The abortion controversy: 25 years after Roe v. Wade* (pp. 361–371). Belmont, CA: Wadsworth. 361–371.

Pavlischek, K. (1993). Abortion logic and paternal responsibilities: One more look at Judith Thomson's argument and a critique of David Boonin-Vail's defense of it. *Public Affairs Quarterly, 3,* 81–98.

Reiman, J. (1999). *Abortion and the ways we value human life.* Lanham, MD: Rowman and Littlefield.

Roe v. Wade (410 US 113). (1973). Retrieved from: http://scholar.google.com/scholar_case?case=12334123945835207673&q=Roe+v.+Wade+(410+US+113).&hl=en&as_sdt=2,26&as_vis=1

Shewmon, D. A. (2001). The brain and somatic integration: Insights into the standard biological rationale for equating 'brain death' with 'death.' *The Journal of Medicine and Philosophy, 26*(5), 457–478.

Singer, P. (1979). *Practical ethics.* Cambridge: Cambridge University Press.

Singer, P. (2009). Reply to Don Marquis. In J. Schaler (Ed.), *Peter Singer under fire: A moral iconoclast faces his critics* (pp. 153–162). Chicago: Open Court.

Steinbock, B. (1992), *Life before birth: The moral and legal status of embryos and fetuses.* Oxford: Oxford University Press.

Tooley, M. (1972). Abortion and infanticide. *Philosophy and Public Affairs, 2,* 37–65.

Thomson, J. J. (1971). A defense of abortion. *Philosophy and Public Affairs, 1,* 47–66.

Warren, M. A. (1973). On the moral and legal status of abortion. *The Monist, 57,* 43–61.

Reply to Marquis

Jeffrey Reiman

Don Marquis argues that murdering humans is wrong because it deprives them of a future personal life of value, and thus abortion is morally murder because it deprives a fetus of such a future life. In my chapter, I argued for three guidelines that determine the conditions of a satisfactory answer to the question whether abortion is morally murder: Such an answer: (1) must give us an independently reasonable account of the wrong of killing fetuses (if it is wrong)—that is, an account independent of its matching existing moral beliefs; (2) it must be based on properties the fetus possesses when we are considering killing it; and (3) it must account for the asymmetric value of life implied by the way that murder is wrong. "Having a future personal life of value" is a current property of fetuses. Thus, Marquis's view satisfies the second guideline, but it fails to satisfy the first and third: He does not provide an independently reasonable account of why killing fetuses is wrong, and he does not show that killing fetuses is wrong in the way that murder is wrong. Before I get to that, since Marquis makes much of the compatibility of his view with widely shared moral beliefs, I will start by showing how his view conflicts with three widely held moral beliefs, beliefs held even by many abortion opponents:

1. Marquis's view conflicts with the widely held moral belief that abortion gets worse the longer pregnancy goes on. For Marquis, killing a newly conceived zygote—a tiny cell not visible to the human eye, or after three weeks, a clump of cells barely visible to the human eye—is just as bad as killing a fetus a day before birth; indeed, just as bad as murdering an adult.
2. Marquis's view conflicts with the widely held moral belief that abortion is justified when pregnancy is the product of rape. Rape is not the fetus's fault, and thus rape cannot justify aborting the fetus if abortion is equivalent to murder. A rape by one being does not justify the murder of another. In his reply, Marquis says that, if the zygote is just "a bunch of cells, not an individual human being," then the morning-after pill would be okay for rape victims. But it is irrelevant whether the zygote is *human*; Marquis has recognized that that is an arbitrary appeal to a biological trait (also known as *speciesism*). What matters is whether the zygote is a *being* (of any sort whatever), which it is (it is a unified entity). So, what Marquis says here both allows early abortion, and denies that having a future of personal value suffices to give a being a right to life.
3. Marquis's view conflicts with the widely held belief that contraception is morally permissible (or if impermissible, not as immoral as abortion or murder). Since contraception deprives a sperm and an ovum of the possibility of joining together and forming a fetus, it deprives them each of a

Contemporary Debates in Bioethics, First Edition. Edited by Arthur L. Caplan and Robert Arp.

future that includes the same life of which abortion deprives the fetus. Marquis has replied to this objection by saying that nothing prior to conception has the property of having a future personal life of value. But that is false. Whenever it works, there was (at least) *one* actual sperm and *one* actual ovum that would otherwise have gotten together to form a fetus—otherwise pregnancy was not prevented. *That* sperm and *that* ovum (the particular ones that would have joined up in the absence of contraception) each had the property of having a future that included the same future of which abortion deprives a fetus. And they had the dispositional properties needed for this to be their potential future. Thus, on Marquis's view, contraception must be as immoral as abortion—indeed, as immoral as murder.

I turn now to what I think is the fatal flaw in Marquis's position: He has not shown that basing the wrong of killing fetuses on the fact that it deprives them of future personal lives of value is an *independently reasonable account of why killing fetuses is seriously morally wrong*. In his chapter, Marquis first suggests that "having a future life of value" is sufficient to make a being's life worth protecting. Realizing that this would make it wrong to kill cows and most other mammals, he revises this to "having a future *personal* life of value." The only justification we get for this change is that the new idea matches prevailing moral beliefs about which lives are wrong to end. We get no reason—independent of this match—for why having a "future personal life of value" entitles a being's life to protection, while having only a "future life of value" does not.

The "future personal life of value" account *seems* like an independently reasonable theory of why killing fetuses is immoral because *we* all regard the loss of our future lives as terrible losses. But *we* are already conscious and caring about those futures. What Marquis does not tell us is why loss of a future personal life of value is a terrible loss to a fetus that has never been aware of its future life. (Note the contrast with my view which explains that this would be a terrible loss to a person because a person knows and cares about his or her life continuing.) From the fetus' standpoint, losing its future personal life is no different from its not having been conceived. Why should the fetus be protected against a fate no different from not having been conceived, when such protection requires forcing a woman to carry that fetus for nine months against her will?

Aside from its matching some widely held moral beliefs, the only reason Marquis offers for why the fetus' ability to live out its future life should be protected is that the fetus has that future. *But that is a claim about what the fetus might lose; it is not a reason why the fetus should be protected against losing it.* In short, Marquis tells us that the fetus might be deprived of its future, but he tells us nothing about the fetus that justifies protecting it against this deprivation.

In fact, Marquis has not even justified his claim that the fetus can be deprived of its future. He assumes that the fetus can be deprived of its future simply because it has that future. But, not everything that *has* something can be *deprived* of it. Books *have* pages; but tearing out some pages does not *deprive the book* of anything (it may deprive the book's owner of something). Suppose that you plant roses in your garden. You put in seeds, and you water them. Seedlings pop up. But, then, a family emergency causes you to neglect to water them again. The seedlings wither and die. Your rose seeds have not been *deprived* of their rose futures. Those futures have simply failed to occur. By contrast, if you were murdered, you would certainly be deprived of your future. Some beings can be deprived of their futures, and others cannot. On this, abortion-rights advocates think that the fetus is more like the rose seed or the book than it is like you. Marquis must prove the reverse, but he does not try.

The difference between you and the roses is that you care about your future, and roses do not care about theirs. Thus, you have the basis for a moral claim on your future, and roses do not. This is what accounts for the fact that you can be deprived of your future, but roses cannot be deprived of theirs. Thus, in assuming that a fetus can be deprived of its future, in assuming that the fetus can be a victim in some morally significant sense, Marquis has treated the fetus as having the basis for a moral claim on its future, without telling us what that basis is. This amounts to assuming that the fetus is a moral being with moral rights, which is precisely what abortion-rights advocates deny and what Marquis must prove. Marquis has *assumed* from the beginning the conclusion that he must *prove*. His argument is circular. Thus, it fails the requirement of providing an independently reasonable theory of why killing the fetus is immoral.

But it also fails the requirement of showing that killing a fetus is wrong in the way that murder is wrong. Recall that the way that murder is wrong presupposes the asymmetric value of human life. If it is good that a fetus realize its future of value, what is wrong with aborting one fetus and replacing it with another that has a similar future? This leaves us with no net loss in value—so why is it wrong? To answer this, Marquis must show what it is about a fetus having a future of value that makes it wrong to kill that one *even though it could be replaced by another one with a comparable future*. But he does not try.

Marquis has not given us an independently reasonable argument for why abortion is gravely immoral, and he has not shown that abortion is wrong the way murder is wrong. The conclusion of my chapter stands: Abortion is ethically justifiable as long as it is authorized by the pregnant woman.

Reply to Reiman

Don Marquis

Jeff Reiman's criteria for the adequacy of an account of the morality of abortion are basically sound. According to Reiman:

1. Only an answer that can be supported by a reasonable theory of what makes taking a human life wrong (independently of the theory matching existing moral beliefs) when it is wrong can be a satisfactory answer to the moral question of abortion.
2. Only an answer based on properties that the fetus possesses at the point one is considering taking its life can be a satisfactory answer to the moral question of abortion.
3. Only an answer that accounts for the asymmetrical value of human life (implied by the special way in which we regard murder as wrong) can enable us to determine if killing a fetus is morally murder.

The parenthetical thought in criterion (1) is dubious. Obviously a theory of what makes taking human life wrong should match existing moral beliefs concerning whom it is wrong to kill when those moral beliefs are utterly uncontroversial. With this reservation, Reiman's criteria for the adequacy of an account of the wrongness of killing are entirely correct.

The p-future of value view I have put forward actually satisfies Reiman's three criteria. It matches moral beliefs we are not prepared to revise.

1. It is based on our judgments that: (a) premature death is almost always a great misfortune for an already-born human being, whatever the cause; (b) this misfortune is morally significant because it is the loss of a personal life; (c) birth is morally irrelevant since it is, after all, little more than a change in spatial location; and (d) to visit a great misfortune on another is wrong—although, of course, there are special exceptions.
2. The p-future of value view also is based on a property fetuses possess when they are fetuses: With rare exceptions, it is in the nature of a human fetus to possess, at the time she is a fetus, a *present* potential to have a future that will be valuable to her. You, reader, possess (at this very moment!) that potential. Therefore, what is wrong with killing fetuses is the same as what is wrong with killing you. This dispositional property is based on the nature of a human being, just as table salt's dispositional property of solubility is based on its nature. One may, of course, have a dispositional property at a time even though the disposition is not actualized until some future time or is never actualized at all. If you, reader, did not possess the present potential to have a future that would be valuable to you, that is, if you were irreversibly unconscious, then unless special considerations obtain, it would not be wrong to end your life. Think of the Terri Schiavo case.

Contemporary Debates in Bioethics, First Edition. Edited by Arthur L. Caplan and Robert Arp.

3. This dispositional property accounts for the asymmetrical value of human life. Nothing prior to conception has this dispositional property any more than the elements of a chemical compound when separated possess dispositional properties they will have when combined, or any more than the patio chairs I bought this spring could be sat on as long as they were in the box unassembled. Accordingly, the p-future of value view does not imply that either contraception or abstinence from sexual activity is wrong, even though not practicing contraception could result in more future valuable lives (cf. Singer, 1979, p. 142). This can be put in another way. Abortion victimizes a young human being. In the cases of contraception and abstinence, there is no victim. When there is no victim, there is no wrong. This can be put in still another way. Take *any* arbitrary human being; it is wrong to end her life unless very special circumstances obtain. Take any arbitrary sperm and ovum pair; it is not wrong to end the lives of any such pair.

Reiman says that the p-future of value view conflicts with three widely held moral beliefs. Whether, as he claims, the p-future of value view entails that "killing a newly conceived zygote, a tiny cell not visible to the human eye, is just as bad as killing a fetus a day before birth" is unclear. There are two issues here. First, does the p-future of value view entail what Reiman claims it entails? Some people believe that the entities that were our precursors during the first weeks after conception may be just a bunch of cells, not an individual human being with a future of value at all (van Inwagen, 1990, pp. 152–153; Olson, 1997, p. 93). Others do not (Lee & George, 2008, pp. 119–121). The issues here are difficult. Serious, careful discussion of them would make this reply unduly long. I believe the former view is correct, but I may be wrong. I have defended my view of this issue elsewhere (Marquis, 2007b).

Second, Reiman claims that, "many abortion opponents" believe that "abortion gets worse the longer the pregnancy goes on." I doubt that Benedict XVI—or anyone who accepts his view of these matters—would agree.

According to Reiman, the p-future of value view conflicts with the view that "abortion is justified when pregnancy is the product of rape." It is worth noting that "the responsibility objection" to Judy Thomson's defense of abortion does not apply to cases of rape. It is also worth noting that, if the early product of conception is "just a bunch of cells," then use of the morning-after pill after a rape (or on any other occasion) is morally unproblematic. There is clearly much more to be said about this matter, but this would also lengthen this response unduly.

I have made clear earlier in this response why Reiman's claim that the p-future of value view entails that contraception is wrong is incorrect.

Reiman believes that *only* his account of the wrongness of killing satisfies his three criteria. As I have made clear above, Reiman's claim is false. In addition, Reiman's account is subject to all of the difficulties of pro-attitude views I presented in my chapter.

The difficulty with Reiman's account can be presented starkly. Reiman says, "I contend that only one thing can account for the way in which we think that murder of humans is wrong: *human beings' own subjective awareness of, and caring about, the continuation of their own lives*" (Reiman's italics, p. X). When someone italicizes his thesis, one should take him seriously. This claim commits Reiman to:

1. It is wrong to end the life of a human only when that human cares about the continuation of her own life.
2. "No fetus cares about the continuation of her own life" is plainly true.

(1) and (2) entail:

3. It is not wrong to end the life of a human fetus.

This is the essence of Reiman's argument that abortion is morally permissible. Now consider the obviously true statement:

4. No person who is suicidal due to mental illness, or due to ingesting a suicide pill, or who wishes to commit suicide in obedience to his religious leader cares about the continuation of her own life.

(1) and (4) entail:

5. It is not wrong to end the life of someone who is suicidal due to mental illness, or due to ingesting a suicide pill, or who wishes to commit suicide in obedience to his religious leader.

(5) is false. Since (4) is plainly true, it follows that (1) is false. Therefore, Reiman's account of the moral permissibility of abortion is false. There is nothing exotic about this difficulty. It involves only simple logic and some indisputable truths.

Reiman seems to think he can avoid this difficulty with his view by talking about autonomy or rationality. Such talk is no more relevant to this issue than talk about whether the moon is made of green cheese. The argument I spelled out carefully above is a sound *deductive* argument. As with all sound deductive arguments, other considerations are totally irrelevant. There are other philosophical moves that surround this issue. Important discussions can be found in Tooley (1972), Boonin-Vail (2003), and Marquis (2007a). Peter Singer's defense of abortion is subject to the same difficulty as Reiman's (see Marquis, 2009; Singer, 2009).

Reiman's account of the wrongness of killing ordinary post-natal children is also unsatisfactory. (Set the case of infants aside.) Consider, for the moment, children who desire to live. The problem with Reiman's account is that, in general, the desires of children are not sufficient to anchor anything really morally important, such as the right to life. Children may desire—and desire strongly—all sorts of things that we do not regard as morally important. They may desire to play outside after it gets dark, even though it is past their bedtimes. They may desire not to be immunized because they are afraid of a needle. As these examples show, the desires of children are rather easily overridden. Why should the desire of a child to live (considered all by itself) be any different? In short, the easily overridden desires of children are not capable of doing the moral work that is needed for an account of the rarely, if ever, overridden serious wrongness of killing a child.

Reiman has responded to this by saying that we respect a child's desire to live because "it is a desire that it is reasonable to honor" (p. X). The trouble with this response is that we all believe that even if a child were brainwashed by some religious fanatic to desire not to live, we believe it would be wrong to kill the child anyway. This shows that the child's desire to live drops out of the picture in the account of the wrongness of killing children. It is redundant. It is *reasonable* to honor a child's desire to live, and it is *unreasonable* (in general) to respect a child's desire to die because that child has a future of value, and death would be a misfortune for her.

Here is another reason why the p-future of value view is reasonable. Think of yourself as a parent. We take for granted that our children should be raised with an eye to their futures. We think that children in general—and our own children in particular—should be raised with an eye to enabling them to be autonomous, flourishing adults, whatever their present desires. We believe that deliberately to refrain from promoting our children's potential in this regard is wrong. The p-future of value account of the wrongness of killing children is a trivial corollary of this common view. It explains why killing a child is one of the worst harms one can inflict on a child. By contrast, Reiman's care-based account does not fit well with a general account of our easily overridden duty to respect our children's desires.

Reiman believes that the p-future of value view is not supported by good reasons. In my chapter, I defended the p-future of value view on the grounds that it is a plausible theory of the wrongness of killing and that all other theories of the wrongness of killing are subject to fatal difficulties. Reiman has failed to offer a good reason to revise that judgment.

References

Boonin-Vail, D. (2003). *A defense of abortion.* Cambridge: Cambridge University Press.

Lee, P., & George, R. (2008). *Body-self dualism in contemporary ethics and politics.* Cambridge: Cambridge University Press.

Marquis, D. (2007a). Abortion revisited. In B. Steinbock (Ed.), *The Oxford handbook of bioethics* (pp. 395–415). Oxford: Oxford University Press.

Marquis, D. (2007b). The moral principle objection to human embryonic stem cell research. In L. Gruen, L. Grabel & P. Singer (Eds.), *Stem cell research: The ethical issues* (pp. 51–66). Malden, MA: Wiley-Blackwell.

Marquis, D. (2009). Singer on abortion and infanticide. In J. Schaler (Ed.), *Peter Singer under fire: A moral iconoclast faces his critics* (pp. 133–152). Chicago: Open Court.

Olson, E. (1997). *The human animal: Personal identity without psychology*. Oxford: Oxford University Press.

Singer, P. (1979). *Practical ethics*. Cambridge: Cambridge University Press.

Singer, P. (2009). Reply to Don Marquis. In J. Schaler (Ed.), *Peter Singer under fire: A moral iconoclast faces his critics* (pp. 153–162). Chicago: Open Court.

Tooley, M. (1972). Abortion and infanticide. *Philosophy and Public Affairs*, *2*, 37–65.

van Inwagen, P. (1990). *Material beings*. Ithaca, NY: Cornell University Press.

Part 5

Is It Ethical to Patent or Copyright Genes, Embryos, or Their Parts?

Introduction

According to the United States Patent and Trademark Office (USPTO), a *patent* can be defined as a type of intellectual property right—along with other types, such as *trademarks* and *copyrights*—that is granted (and enforced) by the legislative body of some society to an inventor so that the inventor may produce, utilize, and/or sell an invention for a period of time (usually 20 years). The invention itself is some object (device, machine, gadget), process (test, procedure), or methodology that must be wholly novel, but also non-obvious and useful. According to the USPTO: "Whoever invents or discovers any new and useful process, machine, manufacture, or composition of matter, or any new and useful improvement thereof, may obtain a patent therefor, subject to the conditions and requirements of this title." (USPTO, 2012). For example, in 1985, Joseph Enterprises, Inc. received a patent from the USPTO so that it could start selling the sound-activated electrical switch called The Clapper (US Patent # 5493618), which not only made its way into households all over the world so that one may "clap on" or "clap off" a lamp or stereo system, but also became the butt of many jokes over the years. An example of a patented process is Amazon.com's 1-Click technique (US Patent # 5960411), where a customer can use a credit card number and address that has been stored already in Amazon.com's database to purchase something in one click of the mouse.

A *gene patent* is a patent associated with a specific gene sequence, the chemical composition of that gene sequence, and/or the processes and procedures for obtaining or utilizing that gene sequence. At first blush, it may seem strange that it is possible to patent human-made devices like The Clapper, human-made processes like 1-Click, *as well as* genes like the breast-cancer-risk gene known as BRCA1—responsible for repairing the double-strand breaks in DNA—a clone of which was produced by Myriad Genetics and granted a US patent (US Patent # 5693473) in 1997. Nevertheless, according to the US Department of Energy's website devoted to the Human Genome Project, "In general, raw products of nature are not patentable. DNA products usually become patentable

Contemporary Debates in Bioethics, First Edition. Edited by Arthur L. Caplan and Robert Arp.

when they have been isolated, purified, or modified to produce a unique form not found in nature" (HGPI, 2012a). The reasoning here is straightforwardly that a gene in one's body is not patentable, given the fact that the gene is a natural entity residing in a natural environment; no one can lay claim to your body or any part therein. But genetic material that has been extracted from an organism by researchers is bioengineered in that it is manipulated, modified, and literally manufactured. Consider the fact that there are several ways to sequence DNA, and these methods usually entail not only fragmenting, isolating, and purifying it, but also "unwinding" it chemically, cloning it, and producing marked copies of it (Ossorio, 2002). The same reasoning holds, then, for proteins, human and animal parts, as well as embryos and their parts that have been bioengineered, for example, by cloning (USC, 2011).

Patenting genes and other biological objects, processes, and methodologies has been commonplace in the US since the US Supreme Court ruled that it is possible to patent a life form in *Diamond v. Chakrabarty* (447 US 303, 1980). That landmark case dealt with a genetic engineer named Ananda Chakrabarty, who sought to patent a bacterium he had developed that was capable of breaking down crude oil. In December 1980, some 6 months after the *Diamond v. Chakrabarty* decision, the USPTO granted Stanford University and the University of California at San Francisco three patents related to the recombinant DNA cloning procedure developed by Stanley N. Cohen (Stanford) and Herbert W. Boyer (UCSF) (Hughes, 2001). Using research in recombinant DNA pioneered by Paul Berg and his associates (Jackson et al., 1972; Yi, 2008), Cohen, Boyer, and their associates added a gene to a plasmid that elicits antibiotic resistance, and then inserted it into *Escherichia coli*, causing the bacteria to become zantibiotic-resistant (Cohen et al., 1973). These antibiotic-resistant bacteria are considered to be among the first genetically modified organisms (GMOs). Since then, GMOs have been used extensively not only in biomedical research and experimental medicine, but also in agriculture and the pharmaceutical industry (O'Connor, 1993; Parekha, 2004). In fact, you probably had some GMOs for breakfast since genetically modified foods such as corn, rice, soybeans, and canola are in the food supply in many parts of the world (Key et al., 2008; Hillstrom, 2012). It is estimated that as many as 5000 patents related to human genes, and 47,000 patents related to DNA or RNA generally, have been granted by the USPTO since 1980 (Cook-Deegan, 2008; THC, 2012).

Besides patents related to human genes, there are also patents for genetic tests, as well as for single nucleotide polymorphisms (DNA-sequence variations), proteins, nucleic acids, polypeptides, antibodies, hormones, and stem cells from the embryos of numerous animals (Caufield, 2003; EC, 2011). In 1988, Harvard researcher, Philip Leder, and his collaborators at DuPont Pharmaceuticals were granted a patent for the now-famous "Harvard Mouse" (US Patent # 4736866), understood to be the first US patent awarded for an animal (Anderson, 1988; OncoMouse™ is trademarked, too). In 2011, the biotechnology company, Advanced Cell Technologies, was awarded a patent from the USPTO for their single-blastomere technology (US Patent # 7893315), a method of harvesting stem cells from embryos without having to destroy them in the process (Klimanskaya et al., 2006, 2007). It is now commonplace to hear of, "patenting life" and its association with American biomedical research, especially recently with the passing of the Leahy-Smith America Invents Act, and the claim in Section 33(a) that, "Notwithstanding any other provision of law, no patent may issue on a claim directed to or encompassing a human organism" (LSA, 2011; USC, 2011). This law does not apply to human embryos and "methods for creating, modifying, or treating human organisms;" nor does it apply to: "cells, tissue, organs or other bodily components produced through human intervention, whether obtained from animals, human beings, or other sources; including but not limited to stem cells, stem cell derived tissues, stem cell lines, and viable synthetic organs" (LSA, 2011; USC, 2011).

Interestingly enough, while American researchers have been patenting life since 1980, such patents have been called into question, and subject to much legal scrutiny, by European researchers who abide by the rules laid out in the document produced by the European Patent Convention (EPC), which occurred in Munich in 1973 and established the European Patent Organisation.

The rules established in the EPC officially took effect in 1978, and they not only have gone through a few revisions since then (notably, one in 2000), but also have some 38 European countries that subscribe to them today. Article 53(c) of the EPC excludes "methods for treatment of the human or animal body by surgery or therapy and diagnostic methods practised on the human or animal body; this provision shall not apply to products, in particular substances or compositions, for use in any of these methods" (EPC, 1973/2012). It has been speculated by Chris Wadlow (2008) and others (Sterkcx, 2008; Kraβer, 2009) that one of the principal ideologies behind the EPC exclusion mentioned above has to do with the following:

> One of the distinguishing features of an organized profession is that its members are subject themselves to a higher code of practice and honour than mere tradesmen, exemplified in the case of medical practitioners by the so called Hippocratic oath . . . The proposition that medicine cannot simultaneously be a profession and an industry is consistent with the treatment of patentability of methods of diagnosis, surgery and therapy. (p. 378, n. 9)

The hesitation on the part of the EPC gives reason to carefully consider some of the ethical issues surrounding the patenting of genes and other biological objects, processes, and methodologies. Wadlow's point can be generalized to include any form of biomedical practice. There remains still an age-old debate about the extent to which the commercialization of biomedicine influences the biomedical disciplines and research ventures, possibly leading to problems associated with: a harmful product being manufactured because someone or some group is "out to make a quick buck;" for-profit insurance companies and hospitals refusing to serve nonpaying patients while at the same time taking what seems to be a substantial share of money from paying patients; altruistic, service-oriented virtues of care, compassion, and charity being replaced by egoistic, profit-oriented virtues of commoditization or even biopiracy, where outsiders use and take organisms and traditional knowledge from indigenous communities to make a profit without compensating those communities. There are many more problems, and the problems just mentioned are the subject of much debate (CQHE, 2007; Kirch & Vernon, 2009).

Narrowing the scope to genetic patents, an obvious effect has to do with the fact that anyone who would like to utilize the patented gene sequence—or composition of the sequence, and/or the processes and procedures for obtaining or utilizing that gene sequence—has to pay royalties to the owner of the patent. Usually, too, some person or company owning the patent on some gene sequence also patents the numerous single nucleotide polymorphisms and expressed sequence tags associated with that gene. So, the royalties paid out on numerous related patents may be quite costly; in which case, someone may be discouraged from pursuing scientific research utilizing the patents. And, one more discouraged researcher may mean one more possible cure or breakthrough never realized. Another concern closely connected to the one just mentioned has to do with a particular group—say, a biotechnology company—monopolizing the gene test market associated with a genetic patent they own—keeping out competitors who may have a more accurate test or more powerful cure to offer.

Monopolies are an economic and moral concern in any marketplace, but it is the very idea of patenting, producing, and pricing a natural entity is morally offensive to many. One argument against patenting human genes has to do with what is known as a *common heritage* objection. According to this objection, by virtue of its naturalness and universality in our species, the human genome is, and should be, collective property while a patent confers private ownership. If the genome belongs equally to all persons, then all should have equal access to the derived knowledge or beneficial uses of research on the genome, and it is unjust, therefore, to grant patents on the human genome (Eisenberg, 2002; Scola, 2011).

One response to this objection is that the patentable human genes and their products are those that are manipulated, modified, and manufactured through much effort, skill, and money, so, by virtue of this genetic engineering, they (the *specific* human genes and their products) are not common, natural, or universal. Add to this an underscore to the point that the group that bioengineered the human genes and their products invested a lot of effort, skill, and money in the project, and this gives further credence to private ownership, especially in an economic and political system like one finds in the United States (Ossorio, 2007; Scola, 2011); in which case, the response to *this* response might be something to the effect of, "Well, we shouldn't be meddling with Mother Nature in the first place." But, then the objection is really not against private ownership of the human genome; rather, it is an objection against the scientific endeavor in general vis-à-vis the sacredness of the human genome (Gustafson, 1994; Eisenberg & Schenker, 1997).

Many argue that, as representative of intellectual rights, patents are different from typical property rights concerning cars, boats, or homes; in which case, the criticisms just mentioned regarding private ownership, collective property, and monopolies are misdirected from the outset (Ossorio, 2002, 2007). A patent is distinct from a property right, it may be argued, not only because a patent has a set time period of exclusive ownership (usually 20 years)—whereas a property right extends ownership potentially indefinitely—but also that a patent exists as more of a device intended to ensure the common intellectual good of a society is served because researchers have an incentive to disclose their inventions to the intellectual community knowing that their inventions will be protected. And disclosed personal research is potentially helpful, common research.

This is the position of Lawrence Sung, whose chapter is the first one in this section. He notes that the "ugly truth is that intellectual property-rights policy is largely unconcerned with whether an author or inventor obtains a reward for his or her work or invention. The crux instead is whether the government grant of intellectual property rights is an efficient tool for driving national creativity and innovation … patent rights inherently foster innovation by demanding public disclosure of inventions in exchange for a temporary term of exclusivity." Sung reminds us of the fact that, without patents, not only would researchers be unwilling to disclose their inventions and instead rely on "trade secrets" and private pacts, but also researchers likely would be unknowingly duplicating work which may turn out to be futile or unnecessary. In the end, Sung's argument is straightforwardly utilitarian—namely, the end results benefit many people in terms of cures, breakthroughs, advancements, and the like—in that he argues not only for the existence of patents for genes and other life forms, but also for relaxed regulations of patent laws to help enable "the promise of medical advances that have yet to be seen."

In the second chapter in this section, David Koepsell is keenly aware of the utilitarian benefits associated with genetic patents. In fact, as he notes, "one of the most profitable uses to which human gene patents have been put is in diagnostic testing. Identifying a gene whose presence or mutation indicates the presence or propensity for a disease is extraordinarily helpful in medicine. Genetic screening now enables the early detection of genetic diseases, or the propensity to contract a disease. Knowing of this presence or propensity often increases both lifestyle and treatment options for patients." Koepsell calls our attention to the fact that, for the past 20 years, there have been numerous patents on genes and gene products applied for with, and granted by, the USPTO. This is primarily because of the work being done by researchers for the Human Genome Project, which officially began in 1990 and was completed in 2003—although, analysis of the human genome will continue for many more years to come (Venter et al., 2001; IHGSC, 2004; HGPI, 2012b).

However, despite his recognition of the utility of patents, Koepsell notes that, "science moves forward propelled largely by forces outside of profits, including the availability of public money for basic research, and scientists' desires for pursuing natural truths, as well as baser interests in their careers, fame, notoriety, etc." He also points to some research that seems to indicate that patents are "just an extra cost of doing business without any guarantee of reward," and that they hinder innovation, especially because of what are known as *patent thickets* which are, "an overlapping set of patent rights requiring that those seeking to commercialize new technology obtain licenses from multiple pantentees" (Carl Shapiro 2001, p. 119). Thus, utilitarian arguments for gene patents might not be as strong as people suppose.

The real moral rub for Koepsell, however, has to do with the fact that a patent on genetic processes means that, in theory, unless you pay royalties to the person or group that owns the patent, "you are prohibited from looking at portions of your own genetic code, even if you had access to the tools and the know-how to look for it." So, you cannot come to know something about your own genetic code without paying for it. And this violates a basic, deontological Kantian-inspired right to *free* ownership over—including, knowledge about—one's body. Koepsell supports one more Kantian-inspired argument against patenting genes and other life forms based in respecting the natural dignity of any life form. Life forms such as genes, Koepsell argues, can be considered as having a quasi-right to be free and "simply cannot be possessed or controlled to the exclusion of others." To this extent, Koepsell's argument is a species of the common heritage objection to patenting genes and other life forms mentioned above. Interestingly enough, Koepsell's argument also harkens back to the very roots of bioethics, which has certain affinities with what today is called environmental ethics.

Paying for biomedical products and services, as well as paying for research and development concerning biomedical products and services, is a fact of life. Tests, procedures, operations, studies, therapies, drugs, prosthetics, and the like not only cost money to administer and manufacture but also are commodities to be bought and sold, as well as insured and protected, in the marketplace. The concepts and arguments in this section prompt questions regarding the extent to which humans can manipulate, control, and own parts of the natural world. René Descartes (1596–1650)—the so-called Father of Modern philosophy who was also a mathematician (he is the inventor of analytic geometry and the Cartesian coordinate system) and strong advocate of the medical sciences—noted in Part Six of his *Discourse on Method of Rightly Conducting One's Reason and of Seeking Truth in the Sciences* (Descartes, 1637/1998) that we need to prolong our lives through advances in medicine so that we can become "masters and possessors of nature" (p. 35). Such is the dream of anyone involved in bioengineering.

References

Anderson, A. (1988). Oncomouse released. *Nature, 336*, 300.

Caufield, T. (2003). From human genes to stem cells: New challenges for patent law? *Trends in Biotechnology, 21*, 101–103.

CQHE (*Cambridge Quarterly of Healthcare Ethics*). (2007). *Cambridge Quarterly of Healthcare Ethics: Special Section on Commercialism in Medicine, vol. 16.*

Cohen, S., Chang, A., Boyer, H., & Helling, R. (1973). Construction of biologically functional bacterial plasmids in vitro. *Proceedings of the National Academy of Sciences: USA, 70*, 3240–3244.

Cook-Deegan, R. (2008). Gene patents. In M. Crowley (Ed.), *From birth to death and bench to clinic: The Hastings Center bioethics briefing book for journalists, policymakers, and campaigns* (pp. 69–72). Garrison, NY: The Hastings Center.

Descartes, R. (1637/1998). *Discourse of method and Meditations on first philosophy* (D. Cress, Trans.). Indianapolis, IN: Hackett Publishing Company.

Eisenberg, R. (2002). How can you patent genes? *American Journal of Bioethics, 2*, 3–11.

Eisenberg, V., & Schenker, J. (1997). Genetic engineering: Moral aspects and control of practice. *Journal of Assisted Reproduction and Genetics, 14*, 297–316.

EC (The European Commission). (Ed.). (2011). *A history of patenting life in the United States with comparative attention to Europe and Canada.* Saarbrücken: Dictus Publishing.

EPC (The European Patent Convention). (1973/2012). Exception to patentability. Retrieved from: http://www.epo.org/law-practice/legal-texts/html/epc/2010/e/ar53.html?popup=yes

Gustafson, J. (1994). A Christian perspective on genetic engineering. *Human Gene Therapy, 5*, 747–754.

Hillstrom, K. (2012). *Genetically modified foods.* Farmington Hills, MI: Lucent Books.

HGPI (Human Genome Project Information). (2012a). Genetics and patenting. Retrieved from: http://www.ornl.gov/sci/techresources/Human_Genome/elsi/patents.shtml.

HGPI (Human Genome Project Information). (2012b). Home page. Retrieved from: http://www.ornl.gov/sci/techresources/Human_Genome/elsi/patents.shtml.

Hughes, S. (2001). Making dollars out of DNA: The first major patent in biotechnology and the commercialization of molecular biology, 1974–1980. *Isis, 92*, 541–575.

IHGSC (International Human Genome Sequencing Consortium). (2004). Finishing the euchromatic sequence of the human genome. *Nature, 431*, 931–945.

Jackson, D., Symons, R., & Berg, R. (1972). Biochemical method for inserting new genetic information into DNA of simian virus 40: Circular SV40 DNA molecules containing lambda phage genes and the galactose operon of *Escherichia coli. Proceedings of the National Academy of Sciences: USA, 69*, 2904–2909.

Key, S., Ma, J., Drake, P. (2008). Genetically modified plants and human health. *Journal of the Royal Society of Medicine, 101*, 290–298.

Kirch, D., & Vernon, D. (2009). The ethical foundation of American medicine: In search of social justice. *Journal of the American Medical Association, 301*, 1482–1484.

Klimanskaya, I., Chung, Y., Becker, S., Lu, S-J., & Lanza, R. (2006). Human embryonic stem cell lines derived from single blastomeres. *Nature, 444*, 481–485.

Klimanskaya, I., Chung, Y., Becker, S., Lu, S-J., & Lanza, R. (2007). Derivation of human embryonic stem cells from single blastomeres. *Nature Protocols, 2*, 1963–1972.Nicholl, D. (2008). *An introduction to genetic engineering*. Cambridge: Cambridge University Press.

Kraβer, R. (2009). Purpose and limits of the exclusion from patentability of medical methods, especially diagnostic methods. In W. Prinz zu Waldeck und Pyrmont, M. Adelman, R. Brauneis, & J. Drexl (Eds.), *Patents and technological progress in a globalized world* (pp. 275–288). London: Springer.

LSA (Leahy-Smith America Invents Act). (2011). The Leahy-Smith America invents act. Retrieved from: http://www.uspto.gov/aia_implementation/bills-112hr1249enr.pdf

O'Connor, K. (1993). Patents for genetically modified animals. *Journal of Animal Science, 71*, 31–40.

Ossorio, P. (2002). Legal and ethical issues in biotechnology patenting. In J. Burley & J. Harris (Eds.), *A companion to genethics* (pp. 408–419). Oxford: Blackwell.

Ossorio, P. (2007). The human genome as common heritage: Common sense or legal nonsense? *The Journal of Law, Medicine & Ethics, 35*, 425–426.

Parekha, S. (Ed.). (2004). *The GMO handbook: genetically modified animals, microbes, and plants in biotechnology*. Totowa, NJ: Humana Press.

Scola, A. (2011). Uncommon genes, unpatentable subject matter, *Seattle University Law Review, 34*, 909–934.

Shapiro, C. (2001). Navigating the patent thicket: Cross licenses, patent pools, and standard setting. In A. Jaffe, J. Lerner & S. Stern (Eds.), *Innovation policy and the economy I* (pp. 119–150). Cambridge, MA: MIT Press.

Sterkcx, S. (2008). The European Patent Convention and the (non)patentability of human embryonic stem cells—the Warf Case. *Intellectual Property Quarterly, 8*, 478–495.

THC (The Hasting Center). (2012). Gene patents. Retrieved from: http://www.thehastings center.org/Publications/BriefingBook/Detail.aspx?id=2174

USC (United States Congress). (2011). Congressional record—extensions of remarks, June 23, 2011. Retrieved from: http://patentreform.info/Legislative%20History%20PDFs/Transcript%20of%20House%20Judiciary%20Comm's%20Markup%20of%20its%20bill/Smith%20extension%20remarks%206.23.11.pdf

USPTO (The United States Patent and Trademark Office). (2012). Patents. Retrieved from: http://www.uspto.gov/patents/index.jsp; also 35 USC. 101 Inventions patentable. Retrieved from: http://www.uspto.gov/web/offices/pac/mpep/documents/appxl_35_U_S_C_101.htm

Venter, J. C., Adams, M., Myers, E., Li, P., Mural, R., Sutton, G ... Zhu, X. (2001). The sequence of the human genome. *Science, 291*, 1304–1351.

Wadlow, C. (2008). Regulatory data protection under TRIPS Article 39(3) and Article 10bis of the Paris Convention: Is there a doctor in the house? *Intellectual Property Quarterly, 8*, 355–415.

Yi, D. (2008). Cancer, viruses, and mass migration: Paul Berg's venture into eukaryotic biology and the advent of recombinant DNA research and technology, 1967–1980. *Journal of the History of Biology, 41*, 589–636.

Chapter Nine

It Is Ethical to Patent or Copyright Genes, Embryos, or Their Parts

Lawrence M. Sung[1]

This chapter addresses the question: Is it ethical to patent or copyright genes, embryos, or their parts? Intellectual property rights (IPRs), such as patents and copyrights, are legislative attempts to embrace innovation and public access to knowledge, and, when necessary, to prioritize these societal goals. The procurement, exploitation, and enforcement of IPRs are explained in this chapter, particularly with attention to the misapprehension that IPRs govern science. In this regard, this chapter recognizes IPRs as mere catalysts for technology development, and offers that the ethics of obtaining IPRs to genes, embryos, or their parts depends entirely on the ethical nature of the underlying science.

Introduction

In the United States, the question "is it ethical to patent or copyright genes, embryos, or their parts" implicates the intellectual property rights established by the US Congress. The US Constitution authorizes the legislative enactment of laws "To promote the Progress of Science and useful Arts, by securing for limited Times to Authors and Inventors the exclusive Right to their respective Writings and Discoveries" (USC, 1787/2012). The copyright and patent laws are codified at Title 17 and Title 35 of the US Code.

With respect to copyrightable subject matter, the laws provide protection "in original works of authorship fixed in any tangible medium of expression, now known or later developed, from which they can be perceived, reproduced, or otherwise communicated, either directly or with the aid of a machine or device," but such protection may not "extend to any idea, procedure, process, system, method of operation, concept, principle, or discovery, regardless of the form in which it is described, explained, illustrated, or embodied in such work" (17, § 102). With respect to patentable subject matter, the laws provide that "[w]hoever invents or discovers any new and useful process, machine, manufacture, or composition of matter, or any new and useful improvement thereof, may obtain a patent therefor, subject to the conditions and requirements of this title" (35, § 101). The US judiciary has traditionally interpreted these statutes to apply universally with regard to the nature of the creative work or invention. Indeed, the subject-matter provisions for copyright and patent protection in the United States antedate the scientific elucidation of molecular genetics and the realization of modern biotechnology.

This chapter addresses the applicability and wisdom of according intellectual property rights in the form of US copyright and patent exclusivity to biologic subject matter generally, as well as genes, embryos, and

Contemporary Debates in Bioethics, First Edition. Edited by Arthur L. Caplan and Robert Arp.

their parts, specifically. As charged by the editors of this book, this chapter seeks to enhance the contemporary debate in bioethics by advocating why it is ethical to copyright and patent genes, embryos, and their parts. As with all good debates, reasonable minds may differ. Yet, the attention to certain perceptions, and perhaps misperceptions, about the interplay between law and science may offer some helpful guidance.

Intellectual Property Rights

Commentators often refer to copyrights and patents as intellectual property, which, by virtue of the name, implants the notion of these legal rights as real property like a home or a car. Intellectual property rights, however, arguably have little in common with real property. Although the subject matter of a copyright or patent may reflect aspects of personhood, the grant itself is a matter of government largesse, not natural entitlement. In this regard, a copyright or patent is only a means to an end, and as such, they constitute a societal good only to the extent the intended goals are achieved. The ugly truth is that intellectual property rights policy is largely unconcerned with whether an author or inventor obtains a reward for his or her work or invention. The crux instead is whether the government grant of intellectual property rights is an efficient tool for driving national creativity and innovation. And at the heart of this consideration is the public disclosure of the seeds of individual imagination to grow the fruits of societal knowledge.

Creativity and Innovation Policy

A public-policy rationale for the grant of intellectual property rights—particularly, copyrights and patents—is the incentive to create or invent and the incentive to invest in the creativity and innovation that exclusivity supports. Although there are distinct theoretical underpinnings for copyright and patent protection in the United States, the elements of each are sufficiently aligned for purposes of this discussion to treat these intellectual property rights in common. With patents, the operation of this concept may be observed at several stages along the development cycle of new technologies. For example, the basic research conducted at academic institutions may be funded in part by the transfer of this technology through the assignment or licensing of patent rights to the private sector. In turn, the industry may obtain further investment based on the patent rights to support efforts to develop and commercialize innovative products and processes. The cycle is complete as the financial rewards of enhanced commercial competitiveness through patent exclusivity are realized and available for reinvestment in other basic research.

This dynamic, however, is open to criticism focused on the third stage of the cycle described above, where the patent exclusivity may give rise to licensing practices and patent enforcement that hinder or block public access to innovations having cognizable benefits for public health, safety, and welfare. Indeed, the appreciation of intellectual property rights is perhaps further from universal acceptance today than ever before. Beyond continuing rallies against the notions of patent exclusivity as engines of innovation generally, the skepticism ignores the underlying premise that patent rights inherently foster innovation by demanding public disclosure of inventions in exchange for a temporary term of exclusivity. Perhaps unprecedented is the pervasive readiness to disavow this quid pro quo between the public and the inventor when the disclosed invention culminates in a product or process that achieves market demand.

Particularly with medical technology, compromising patent exclusivity in the face of the public wants and needs for novel medical prevention, diagnosis, and treatment seems a compelling case. But as with most operations of law, the specific events that present the easiest justifications to succumb to current social pressures at the expense of principles create the true test of established legal doctrines.

In any event, a commonly less recognized but perhaps more important public policy is the incentive to disclose that copyright and patent law seeks to embody. To the extent a government grant of temporary exclusivity is unavailable, authors and inventors may be less willing to disclose their works and inventions openly and instead rely upon controlled public access through restrictive covenants and trade secrecy. Aside from the consequential suboptimal dissemination, the reduced information transparency facilitates wasteful, duplicative efforts by other would-be authors and inventors. Accordingly, the societal benefits of intellectual property rights are worthy, but often ignored by the popular media, which finds their vilification irresistible in the face of human-interest stories.

Ethics and Morality

Some define ethics as a set of moral values, while others view ethics as merely a set of governing principles of conduct. The distinction is meaningful here because the former interpretation presupposes a guiding externality ex ante, whereas the latter may arise from experience. The copyright and patent statutes do not contain provisions that distinguish subject-matter eligibility on the grounds of ethics or morality. Rather, the debate over intellectual property rights is often framed generally as the tragedy of the anticommons, concerns over access to knowledge restrictions, and the propriety of the ownership of products of nature. Rarely have there been bona fide challenges to copyrightable and patentable subject matter discretely as unethical or immoral.[2] Indeed, the development and dissemination of controversial works and inventions, such as racially insensitive media, pornography, nuclear weaponry, birth control, gambling, and substance abuse, all of which society has at one time or another labeled as injurious to human life and/or the public order, typically are not blamed on the availability of intellectual property rights to such subject matter. To what extent should copyrights and patents be reformulated to aid only that creativity and innovation, which is deemed at that moment in history to be ethical or moral?

Myths and Legends

The societal impact of intellectual property rights may be the subject of misapprehension where a consideration focuses only on specific cases rather than the system as a whole. Whereas US copyrights are subject to registration, US patents are subject to substantive examination to determine patentability. To be sure, the US patent application process is costly and arduous, and many patent applications are rejected or abandoned. For example, the United States Patent and Trademark Office (USPTO) reported that 289,419 out of 553,549 patent applications—roughly 53%—were abandoned in 2010 (USPTO, 2011).

Beyond the qualification as statutory subject matter under 35 USC § 101, a successful patent applicant must present an invention that satisfies the remaining conditions for patentability (utility, novelty, and nonobviousness) under 35 USC §§ 101–103, and the patent application must satisfy the disclosure requirements under 35 USC § 112. These standards help ensure that the public receives a valuable benefit from the disclosure of an innovative technology in return for a grant of temporary exclusivity to the patent owner. One inherent problem with making sense of the patent law vis-à-vis biologic inventions in particular is the temporal distortion that occurs between the time patent claims are filed and the time the USPTO and/or federal courts pass on the patentability or invalidity of those claims. Particularly with biologic inventions, a decade or more can separate these two events, which can exacerbate misperceptions arising from historical accuracy and hindsight. The jurisprudential trend in US patent law is moving in favor of making it increasingly difficult for patent applicants to obtain claims having broad coverage.

To receive patent protection, the invention must be novel, i.e., not anticipated by the prior art under 35 USC § 102. An invention is anticipated if a single prior art reference expressly or inherently discloses each and every limitation of the claimed invention (Scripps, 1991). Thus, a prior art reference without express reference to a claim limitation may nonetheless anticipate by inherency.[3] Inherency is not necessarily coterminous with knowledge of those of ordinary skill in the art. Artisans of ordinary skill may not recognize the inherent characteristics or functioning of the prior art. In *Schering Corporation v. Geneva Pharmaceutical* (339 F.3d 1373, 1377, Fed. Cir. 2003), the contention that inherent anticipation requires recognition in the prior art was rejected.

The new realization alone does not render that necessary prior art patentable. In *Bristol-Myers Squibb Company v. Ben Venue Laboratories, Inc.* (246 F.3d 1368, 1376, Fed. Cir. 2001), it was explained that newly discovered results of known processes are not patentable because those results are inherent in the known processes, and in *Verdegaal Brothers, Inc. v. Union Oil Company of California* (814 F.2d 628, 633, Fed. Cir. 1987), it was held that the recognition of a new aspect of a known process is not a patentable invention of a novel process. This evolution of the doctrine of inherent anticipation may make it more difficult for applicants to obtain gene patents, particularly those claiming only certain fragments of a gene, which is otherwise disclosed in the prior art.

To receive patent protection, an invention must also be nonobvious at the time of the invention to one of ordinary skill in the relevant art under 35 USC § 103. In *KSR International Company v. Teleflex Inc.* (550 US 398, 2007), the Supreme Court rejected a rigid application of the Federal Circuit's approach known as the teaching, suggestion, or motivation (TSM) test, under which a patent claim is proved obvious only if some motivation or suggestion to combine the prior art teachings can be found in the prior art, the nature of the problem, or the knowledge of a person having ordinary skill in the art.

The Court opined that inventions in most, if not all, instances rely upon building blocks long since uncovered, and claimed discoveries almost of necessity will be combinations of what, in some sense, is already known. According to the Court, the obviousness analysis cannot be confined by an overemphasis on the importance of published articles and the explicit content of issued patents. The Court noted that granting patent protection to advances that would occur in the ordinary course without real innovation retards progress and may, in the case of patents combining previously known elements, deprive prior inventions of their value or utility. The Court admonished that when there is a design need or market pressure to solve a problem, and there are a finite number of identified, predictable solutions, a person of ordinary skill has good reason to pursue the known options within his or her technical grasp. If this leads to the anticipated success, it is likely the product is not of innovation but of ordinary skill and common sense. This relaxation of the obviousness standard may also make it more difficult for applicants to obtain gene patents, particularly those claiming a novel combination or other use of known genes and/or gene fragments.

In any event, the exclusivity of a copyright and patent is only as robust as the ability and willingness of the federal courts to enforce it. Despite common notions that a copyright and patent convey absolute control over the claimed subject matter by their private owners, the reality bears little resemblance. Copyrights are subject to compulsory license and fair use, and both copyrights and patents are subject to the discretion of a federal court to refuse to enjoin infringers against continued infringing activity. Moreover, in *eBay Inc. v. MercExchange, L.L.C.* (547 US 388, 2006), the US Supreme Court tightened the standards for granting injunctive relief in patent cases. Although US patent law does not expressly recognize compulsory licensing of patents, the denial of a permanent injunction in conjunction with the award of ongoing reasonable royalty damages is a compulsory license de facto.

The US government itself has a direct effect on US patent rights. For inventions supported in whole or in part with federal funds, any patent rights to such subject inventions retained by the government grant recipient or contractor are subject to a nonexclusive, nontransferable, irrevocable, paid-up license to practice or have practiced for or on behalf of the United States the subject invention throughout the world. In addition, the US government may (albeit it has never actually done so) exercise "march-in" rights to transfer licensed subject invention rights to others where the subject invention has not been sufficiently exploited by the existing licensee within a reasonable amount of time (35 USC § 203). The US government may also use (or authorize others to use on behalf of the US government) a copyrighted work or patented technology without permission anytime, with the sole recourse of the copyright or patent owner to sue the US government to recoup "reasonable and entire compensation" for such use (see 28 USC § 1498 (a), pertaining to patents, and § 1498 (b), pertaining to copyrights).

There are several other defenses against patent infringement that limit the reach of intellectual property rights. State governments and state institutions are exempt from patent infringement liability under the Eleventh Amendment immunity from private suit (USC, amendment XI). A statutory defense to US patent infringement liability exists under 35 USC § 271(e)(1), which acts as a safe harbor for activity reasonably related to the preparation and submission of an application for federal regulatory approval. Such activity may include experimentation and other data gathering. In this regard, § 271(e)(1) can be fairly characterized as an experimental or research use defense applicable only in the specific context of regulatory compliance.[4] Medical practitioners and related healthcare entities are also shielded from patent infringement liability under 35 USC § 287(c) with respect to the performance of a medical or surgical procedure on a body.

Accordingly, public concerns based on specific examples of incorrectly granted or overbroad patents arguably fail to appreciate the significant governmental resources allocated to achieve only reasonable grants of exclusivity to support continued innovation. Still, legislative efforts remain pending to further improve the US patent system (PRA, 2011). But at bottom, it is not as easy as one might think to obtain a patent, and even if granted, a patent does not convey the legal effect one might expect.

Genes, Embryos, and Their Parts

For the most part, the copyrightability of genes, embryos, and their parts has been generally dismissed on the grounds of lack of originality and/or authorship as well as intrinsic utilitarian function. The patentability of such subject matter, however, is the focus of greater contemporary debate. The controversy over the broad scope of patent eligibility generally has reinvigorated a discussion over the propriety of patenting biologic subject matter.

The terms *gene* or *embryo* patents are not part of a nomenclature with a customary or universally accepted meaning. For example, the term *gene patent* has been used generically to refer to patents as well as patent applications where all or just some of the claims pertain to subject matter ranging from a full-length DNA sequence that encodes a complete protein to a DNA sequence that has unknown biologic significance. Because the same term, *gene patent*, is often applied to very different things technically speaking, the legal governance of this technology is at sea without some measure of precision in the communication of what is being addressed.

Compounding the uncertainty that the science might carry is the vagary of our patent system that allows applicants to define their inventions in their own words, even where such definitions might otherwise contravene the customary meaning of such words to others skilled in the art. Accordingly, what one reads in a patent describing a "gene" may bear little resemblance to what a molecular geneticist would otherwise tell you a "gene" is as a matter of scientific truth. One can begin to appreciate the inherent difficulty in having confidence in a race where the starting line itself is debatable.

Although faced routinely with new technologies, our patent system has perhaps with no other class of inventions been so significantly challenged in dogma. In particular, a patent applicant must be able to teach the public about the invention by providing a reasonably clear answer to two fundamental questions: "What is it?" and "What does it do?" With regard to traditional gene patents, the response would include disclosure of the full-length DNA sequence that encodes a complete protein in conjunction with information about the protein and its potential beneficial uses. As a matter of scientific research, months, if not years, of characterization efforts might be entailed.

The Human Genome Project embodied breakthrough technology that made it possible for scientists to obtain vast numbers of genomic fragments by automated isolation and purification to facilitate chemical formula descriptions (high-throughput polynucleotide sequencing) without learning anything about their origin, fit, or function. The rub was that such an abstract process of invention hardly came with a complete answer to what the invention was, much less yielded any insight as to what the invention did. The dilemma of knowledge without wisdom came to the fore, and this change in the scientific paradigm relating to genomic discovery created significant problems for our patent system.

In the late 1990s, numerous patent applications were filed claiming thousands of genomic fragments with bare indications of what they were and even fainter disclosures of what they did. Moreover, these patent claims were of broad enough scope to capture as an infringer any user of a product derived from genomic material that included a patented DNA sequence. Such fears rekindled the public outcry over gene-patenting generally and its potential chilling effect on research and development. But the Patent

Gold Rush was on. Still, like most gold rushes, the dreams of riches from the ownership of genomic data alone began to fade almost as quickly as they arose. The USPTO established an instant moratorium on the examination of expressed sequence tag (EST) and single nucleotide polymorphism (SNP) claims (see USPTO Revised Utility Guidelines, 64 Fed. Reg. 71440, 71441, 1999).

The USPTO struggled with attempts to reconcile the applicability of traditional, generic principles of patent law to this emerging technology. The operative framework for meeting the utility requirements of 35 USC § 101 now includes the mandate for a patent applicant to articulate a specific, substantial, and credible utility. In the early 2000s, the USPTO refused to grant a patent to Monsanto's scientists Dane K. Fisher and Raghunath V. Lalgudi on the grounds that the ESTs they wanted to patent had no specific utility. After a court battle, the US Court of Appeals for the Federal Circuit ruled that a claimed invention must have a specific and substantial utility to satisfy 35 USC § 101; that an application must show that an invention is useful to the public as disclosed in its current form, not that it may prove useful at some future date after further research; and that an asserted use must show that that claimed invention has a significant and presently available benefit to the public where the asserted use must also show that a claimed invention can be used to provide a well-defined and particular benefit to the public (421 F.3d 1365, Fed. Cir. 2005).

In the words of the US Supreme Court about the utility requirement, "[A] patent is not a hunting license. It is not a reward for the search, but compensation for its successful conclusion" (*Brenner v. Manson*, 383 US 519, 536, 1966). Beyond § 101 utility, the standards for patenting inventions generally have become stricter in light of the evolving jurisprudence and will have a profound impact on the patenting of biologic inventions. Presently, the public spotlight is focused on § 101 statutory subject matter.

Patent Eligible Subject Matter

In *Diamond v. Chakrabarty* (447 US 303, 309, 1980), the US Supreme Court held that patent eligible subject matter included "anything under the sun made by man" when addressing the invention of a genetically engineered microorganism. This decision is widely credited as opening the age of modern biotechnology patenting. Now, more than 30 years later, the question of what should (and should not) be patentable, including genes, has reprised. In *Bilski v. Kappos*, the US Supreme Court held that the machine-or-transformation test is not the sole test for determining the patent eligibility of a process, but rather "a useful and important clue, an investigative tool, for determining whether some claimed inventions are processes under § 101" in concluding that a method of optimizing a fixed bill system for energy markets was an unpatentable abstract idea (561 US ___, 130 S. Ct. 3218, 2010). In the wake of *Bilski v. Kappos*, the appeal in *Association for Molecular Pathology v. US Patent & Trademark Office*, which is pending before the US Court of Appeals for the Federal Circuit, will consider the propriety of gene patents (No. 10-1406, Fed. Cir. 2011; reviewing 702 F. Supp. 2d 181, S.D.N.Y. 2010).[5]

On March 29, 2010, Judge Robert Sweet of the US District Court for the Southern District of New York, granted summary judgment invalidating seven US patents, which related to the BRCA1 and BRCA2 genes associated with breast cancer, that are owned or licensed to Myriad Genetics, Inc (Id. at 211–12, referring to US Patents No. 5,693,473, No. 5,709,999, No. 5,710,001, No. 5,747,282, No. 5,753,441, No. 5,837,492, and No. 6,033,857). Judge Sweet based his conclusions that the composition of matter patent claims were not directed to patentable subject matter on the fact that the claimed "isolated DNA" was not "markedly different" from the corresponding DNA found in nature. Judge Sweet focused on the expert testimony that genes are multifunctional with a dual nature as a chemical molecule as well as an information repository. In his view, the nucleotide sequence was the defining characteristic of both native and isolated DNA, and therefore, he concluded that the primary biological function of isolated DNA was the same as that of the corresponding native DNA. In so doing, he discounted Myriad's arguments that the differences between native and isolated DNA as chemical molecules should be the crux of the patentable subject-matter inquiry. Moreover, Judge Sweet abruptly dismissed concerns over the impact of his decision on the biotechnology industry as unfounded. In addition,

Judge Sweet embraced the Federal Circuit's recent patent eligibility precedents to invalidate the method claims of the Myriad patents.

Although the public reaction to the *Myriad* ruling has been mixed, the element of surprise seemed shared among all. For patient advocacy groups and medical practitioners, the decision lends credence to the notion that patent exclusivity for medical prevention, diagnosis, and treatment has been based on tenuous distinctions from the public domain and other "lawyer's tricks:"

> The claims-in-suit directed to "isolated DNA" containing human BRCA1/2 gene sequences reflect the USPTO's practice of granting patents on DNA sequences so long as those sequences are claimed in the form of "isolated DNA." This practice is premised on the view that DNA should be treated no differently from any other chemical compound, and that its purification from the body, using well-known techniques, renders it patentable by transforming it into something distinctly different in character. Many, however, including scientists in the fields of molecular biology and genomics, have considered this practice a "lawyer's trick" that circumvents the prohibitions on the direct patenting of the DNA in our bodies but which, in practice, reaches the same result. (Id. at 185)

For industry members and their patent attorneys, the decision represents an indefensible departure from decades of precedent as well as a significant undermining of established investment-backed expectations.

Now on appeal before the Federal Circuit, *Myriad* raises the question whether Judge Sweet was correct in his characterization of genomic fragments and synthetic polynucleotides as mere physical embodiments of the laws of nature that should be precluded from patentable subject matter. While many commentators expect the Federal Circuit to reverse the trial court on either substantive or procedural grounds, perhaps we are in store for further surprises. Precedent notwithstanding, only history will reveal whether Judge Sweet was simply the first to say the Emperor has no clothes.

Although DNA is naturally occurring as the biologic blueprint for living organisms, our patent system presently recognizes the subject matter as patentable where the claims set forth in a patent application properly distinguish the invention from the form of the genomic DNA found naturally. Because our patent system does not differentiate between the notions of invention and discovery, the elucidation of subject matter found in nature may nevertheless give rise to valid patent claims that relate to the natural product or process, at least under extant law.

A Path Forward?

The Federal Circuit has reminded us that "Congress never intended that the patent laws should displace the police powers of the States, meaning by that term those powers by which the health, good order, peace and general welfare of the community are promoted" (*Juicy Whip, Inc. v. Orange Bang, Inc.*, 185 F.3d 1364, 1368, Fed. Cir. 1999, quoting *Webber v. Virginia*, 103 US 344, 347–48, 1880). The US Congress has the power to exclude subject matter as it sees fit from copyright and patent exclusivity, including action based on a determination that it is somehow unethical to patent or copyright genes, embryos, or their parts. But the danger from such legislative action compels restraint.

The patent eligibility standard under 35 USC § 101 is the principal invitation of the patent laws to would-be innovators everywhere to bring forward the products of their inventive efforts. Using § 101 in a gatekeeping role projects a disenfranchising image of a system established, in the words of President Abraham Lincoln (1859), to add "the fuel of interest to the fire of genius." Without the continued openness of Section 101, this essential combustion that drives the engine of innovation may become a thing of the past. With public health priorities already taking center stage, we cannot afford to deny the promise of medical advances that have yet to be seen by restricting patent eligible subject matter, especially for biotechnology. Unlike the other conditions for patentability set forth under the patent statutes, namely novelty and nonobviousness, § 101 governs patent eligible subject matter and utility, neither of which requires a comparative assessment of the claimed invention against the prior art. Without such a measure, § 101 is ill suited to execute a gatekeeper function because it is relatively insensitive to the pace of innovation in a specific art.

Rather, § 101 looks more holistically to progress in the useful arts and best fulfills a role as a static prescription, which embraces existing technology and, more importantly, encourages the ingenuity of technology yet to come. Accordingly, attempting to refine § 101 to strike a normative balance today merely defers the debate until a new technology of concern arrives. But the true detriment of revising the patent eligibility standard now would be the incalculable lost opportunity from potential innovators discouraged from invention and public disclosure. In *Chakrabarty*, the US Supreme Court took the wise approach of interpreting § 101 as broadly inclusive in favor of allowing the other statutory conditions for patentability to more finely monitor what inventions may be patented vis-à-vis the prior art. Tinkering with § 101 in hopes of crafting a standard generally applicable to past, present, and future technologies, however well intentioned, may bring unforeseeable consequences, including the unfortunate chilling of future innovation.

Copyright or patent exclusivity to biologic subject matter does not confer "ownership" of life. Nor do these government grants conjure creativity and invention where none would have existed. What intellectual property rights do facilitate, however, is the placement of knowledge of such innovation in the public domain and the ability to use such technology freely following a temporary period of exclusivity. Even during the term of a patent, for example, technology transfer through assignments and licenses supports the public access to the patented technology, and such technology transfer is designed around efforts to help provide a roadmap to future innovation.

There are surely instances where copyrights or patent claims prevent a desirable event, at least for the moment for some. In certain cases, perhaps the intellectual property rights are accorded overly broad scope due to ambiguity or error in the grant or enforcement. However, the appropriate response would be the faithful application of existing standards, the reflective consideration of the continuing vitality of such standards, and change where change is warranted. What is imprudent is to allow rhetoric or less-than-fully-informed notions about the cost–benefit dynamic of intellectual property rights to cast unfair aspersions upon a vital component of the US economy that will only increase in dependency on innovation for global competitiveness. It is not only ethical to patent or copyright genes, embryos, or their parts, but socially desirable to do so.

Notes

1 I gratefully acknowledge the excellent research assistance of Pauline Pelletier, University of Maryland School of Law J.D. degree candidate, 2013. All statements in this text reflect the views of the author alone and should not be attributed to any other person or entity.

2 Justice Story's opinion in *Lowell v. Lewis*, 15 F. Cas. 1018 (C.C.D. Mass. 1817), is often cited as the common law origin for the proposition that inventions "injurious to the well-being, good policy, or sound morals of society" are unpatentable. As examples of such inventions, Justice Story listed "a new invention to poison people, or to promote debauchery, or to facilitate private assassination" (Id. at 1019). Although some courts have continued to recite Justice Story's formulation, see *Tol-o-matic, Inc. v. Proma Produkt-Und Marketing Gesellschaft m.b.H.*, 945 F.2d 1546, 1552–53, 20 USPQ 1332, 1338 (Fed. Cir. 1991); In re Nelson, 280 F.2d 172, 178–79, 126 USPQ 242, 249 (CCPA 1960), the principle that inventions are invalid if they are principally designed to serve immoral or illegal purposes has not been applied broadly in recent years. See *Juicy Whip, Inc. v. Orange Bang, Inc.*, 185 F.3d 1364, 1366–67 (Fed. Cir 1999) (disavowing as no longer good law other, earlier decisions that invalidated patents to gambling devices on the ground that they were immoral—*Brewer v. Lichtenstein*, 278 F. 512 (7th Cir. 1922); *Schultze v. Holtz*, 82 F. 448 (N.D. Cal. 1897); *National Automatic Device Co. v. Lloyd*, 40 F. 89 (N.D. Ill. 1889)).

3 See *Titanium Metals Corporation v. Banner*, 778 F.2d 775, 781–82 (Fed. Cir. 1985); In re Omeprazole Patent Litigation, 483 F.3d 1364, 1371 (Fed. Cir. 2007); *Abbott Laboratories v. Baxter Pharmaceutical Products, Inc.*, 471 F.3d 1363, 1368 (Fed. Cir. 2006); In re Crish, 393 F.3d 1253, 1258–59 (Fed. Cir. 2004) (holding asserted claims covering a gene's nucleotide sequence anticipated where the gene, though not its particular sequence, was already known to the art); In re Cruciferous Sprout Litigation, 301 F.3d 1343, 1349–50 (Fed. Cir. 2002) (ruling that an inventor's recognition of substances that render broccoli and cauliflower particularly healthy does not permit patent on identifying broccoli seeds or preparing broccoli as a food product).

4 See *Merck KGaA v. Integra Lifesciences I, Ltd.*, 545 US 193 (2005) (extending 35 USC § 271(e)(1) to all uses of patented inventions that are reasonably related to the development and submission of any information under the Federal Food, Drug, and Cosmetic Act (FDCA), including preclinical studies of patented compounds that are appropriate for submission to the FDA in the regulatory process; and clarifying that the statute did not exclude certain information from the exemption on the basis of the phase of research in which it was developed or the particular submission in which it could be included); see also *Integra Lifesciences I, Ltd. v. Merck KGaA*, 496 F.3d 1334 (Fed. Cir. 2007) (holding on remand that the criterion of whether the experimental investigation of a patented compound is reasonably related to the development of information for submission to the FDA is established at the time of the experiment, and does not depend on the success or failure of the experimentation or actual submission of the experimental results; stating that studies of compounds that are not ultimately proposed for clinical trials are within the § 271(e)(1) safe harbor, when there was a reasonable basis for identifying the compounds as working through a particular biological process to produce a particular physiological effect; and reasoning that the § 271(e)(1) safe harbor did not depend on a distinction between discovery and routine research, but on whether the threshold biological property and physiological effect had already been recognized as to the candidate drug; but see *Proveris Science Corporation v. Innovasystems, Inc.*, 536 F.3d 1256 (Fed. Cir. 2008) (clarifying that the § 271(e)(1) safe harbor does not immunize manufacture, marketing, or sales activity that is used in the development of FDA regulatory submissions, but is not subject to the FDA premarket approval process)).

5 On August 16, 2012, the US Court of Appeals for the Federal Circuit, in Association for Molecular Pathology v. US Patent & Trademark Office, 686 F.3d 1303 (Fed. Cir. 2012), reversed the district court's decision that Myriad's composition claims to isolated DNA molecules cover patent-ineligible products of nature under § 101. The Federal Circuit held that each of the claimed molecules represented a nonnaturally occurring composition of matter and, thus, constituted patent-eligible statutory subject matter. This decision awaits possible appeal to the US Supreme Court.

References

Lincoln, A. (1859). *Second lecture on discoveries and innovation.* In J. Nash & A. Blake (Eds.), *Discoveries and inventions: A lecture.* New York: Nabu Press.

PRA (Patent Reform Act). (2011). Patent Reform Act of 2011, 112th Congress, 1st Sess., S.23. Retrieved from: http://www.gpo.gov/fdsys/pkg/BILLS-112s23es/pdf/BILLS-112s23es.pdf

Scripps. (1991). *Scripps Clinic & Research Foundation v. Genentech, Inc.*, 927 F.2d 1565, 1576–77 (Fed. Cir. 1991). Retrieved from: http://openjurist.org/927/f2d/1565/scripps-clinic-research-foundation-v-genentech-inc-scripps-clinic-and-research-foundation

USC (The United States Constitution). (1787/2012). Article 1, § 8, clause 8. Retrieved from: http://www.house.gov/house/Constitution/Constitution.html

USPTO (The United States Patent and Trademark Office). (2011). Performance & accountability report FY 2010. Retrieved from: http://www.uspto.gov/about/stratplan/ar/2010/USPTOFY2010PAR.pdf

Chapter Ten

It Is Not Ethical to Patent or Copyright Genes, Embryos, or Their Parts

David Koepsell

In this chapter, I argue that according to two prominent ethical theories—namely a Mill-based utilitarianism and a Kantian-based deontology—it is unethical to grant patents over naturally occurring life forms and genes. After explaining the consequentialist/utilitarian theory behind the emergence of intellectual property law, and its intention to encourage innovation and dissemination of knowledge through state-granted monopolies, I argue that there is no evidence that patents over life forms, tissues, or genes fulfill the intentions of intellectual property law. In fact, patents may slow or otherwise hinder both the basic research and innovations that may result from the biosciences. Moreover, there are deontological reasons for prohibiting such patents. Patents over tissues, cells, genes, and other naturally occurring materials may violate our rights or duties to the scientific commons, that realm of the world that is discovered rather than invented. Finally, such patents may impede our equal dignity as humans, or the dignity of other living creatures, using both as instruments, or means to ends, rather than treating them as ends in themselves.

Introduction

Modern biotechnology is capable of great good. As scientists uncover the links between genes (which are the parts of DNA that direct the production of proteins) and phenotypes (how a life form looks, functions, etc.), the ability to create new medicine, treatments, and deeper understandings of both health and disease are improved. Particularly important in the field of human medicine has been the completion of the Human Genome Project (HGP), an international, largely publicly funded effort to map the contours of the human genome. Completed in 2003, the HGP was announced as uncovering the general map of mankind's "common heritage," the genetic code that all share, with only a very small amount of genetic distinction between any two human individuals (HGPI, 2012a, 2012b). DNA is actually a common heritage of all life, and the genes that compose us and comprise our functioning are shared among species as well. Nature has selected, over the billions of years of evolution on Earth, the genetic mechanisms of life. The most basic of these are shared widely, and each species has developed its own unique genetic traits; but the common heritage of all life as we know it is contained in our common DNA.

It was with during the course of the HGP that wide-scale patenting of DNA began (Varmus, 2010; *Science*, 2011). Patents are poorly understood by the general public, but their industrial value is enormous, and their applications widespread. Few people realize that DNA can be patented, or why. Most people are

Contemporary Debates in Bioethics, First Edition. Edited by Arthur L. Caplan and Robert Arp.

not aware that roughly 20% of the genes that compose all humans have some patent claim attached to them. Nor are they aware of what this means or involves. Slightly more people know that life forms themselves can be patented, but this too remains mysterious and detached from ordinary experience. What does it mean to say that an individual or entity holds a patent on a gene, protein, or life form? What then are the ethical implications of such patents?

Below I briefly examine the nature and history of intellectual property (IP), including patents and copyrights, as well as the arguments for and against IP in various technologies. Then, I review the history of the application of IP to life forms and now to genes. Finally, I outline the ethical implications and consequences of patenting DNA and life forms as this practice exists today, and where it might lead in the future.

Intellectual Property

Intellectual property is a rather recent invention in the law. Until about 200 years ago, there simply were no widely adopted laws or customs that guaranteed to those who made either aesthetic or utilitarian creations exclusive rights to the profits from them for a period of time. The very first patents and copyrights were originally granted by sovereigns (kings or queens) in European monarchies in the early to mid-1600s. Something called a *letter patent* was issued by a sovereign as an enticement for creative people to produce some innovative or lucrative art (including productive arts) so that they would either enter or stay within the kingdom. A letter patent was the grant by the sovereign of an exclusive right to practice that art within the domain of the sovereign for some specified time period (Blackstone, 1766; Bracha, 2004). Since their inception, intellectual property rights have been legal monopolies. The theory behind them has not changed since the first letter patent. The idea is that by granting an exclusive right to practice some art, or produce some product, innovation will be encouraged, and creators will be justly rewarded for their contribution to the nation's wealth. While in France, following the revolution, the dominant argument for creating monopolies for authors was based upon a *moral* right to the reproduction and profit from original expressions, the bulk of the nations that came to adopt IP did so on purely utilitarian grounds (Dutton, 1984).

Thomas Jefferson (1743–1826)—third president of the United States, as well as prolific author and inventor—was an early proponent for adopting the clause in the US Constitution that enabled Congress to pass laws creating IP rights in the United States (cf. Mossoff, 2006). The US has since become the model for the spread and creation of IP regimes elsewhere. But Jefferson was fully aware that the creation of IP was a practical issue, not determined by any *rights*, and to be measured only by the effects of IP laws on both creating incentives for the arts and productive sciences. The monopoly rights to be created by patents and copyrights were also to remain limited, as part of the goal of creating monopoly incentives for a time was to prevent secretiveness (an extra-legal way to enjoy some market advantage) and to move knowledge into the "public domain." The public domain is simply the set of knowledge that is freely available for all to use. Matters that are tied up in IP remain outside of the public domain, and remain the private domain of IP holders to do with as they will.

Creating legal institutions to promote investment of time and creativity into producing new, useful, and aesthetically appealing arts was deemed necessary partly because of the nature of their subjects. Once a new idea is expressed, either through the creation of some device, or by way of painting, novel, poem, etc., there is no natural way to exclude others from expressing the same idea. This is unlike other forms of property, like land or moveables (property that is not real estate, like a hammer, automobile, cow, etc.). Land and moveables are rivalrous, meaning that the possession of them is exclusive by nature. If you and I both want to exert control over rivalrous goods, we literally have to fight it out physically (or negotiate) until one of us possesses the thing to the exclusion of the other. The old saying that "possession is nine-tenths of the law" is true, and it is based upon the assumption that the current possessor of an object or piece of land is the proper possessor (and thus the owner) who is entitled to maintain his or her quiet, unimpeded possession against all other claims to ownership.

Ideas are not like land or moveables (cf. Gordon, 1992). They are neither rivalrous nor exclusive. When you and I both possess an idea, we deprive the other of nothing. Each can use the idea to his or her heart's content without injuring the originator or first expresser of the idea. Even when we each express the same idea, no matter who originated it, no one is deprived of anything. IP is nonrivalrous and nonexclusive by nature. This is why IP laws were deemed to be necessary. It was believed that without some limited monopoly right over an expression, creators would not invest the time or money necessary to create something innovative, valuable, and new. Thomas Jefferson, who led the effort to create a patent system in the US, recognized the practical arguments in favor of IP, as well as the *moral* need to limit IP, stating in one of his letters:

> It would be curious then, if an idea, the fugitive fermentation of an individual brain, could, of natural right, be claimed in exclusive and stable property. If nature has made any one thing less susceptible than all others of exclusive property, it is the action of the thinking power called an idea, which an individual may exclusively possess as long as he keeps it to himself; but the moment it is divulged, it forces itself into the possession of every one, and the receiver cannot dispossess himself of it. Its peculiar character, too, is that no one possesses the less, because every other possesses the whole of it. He who receives an idea from me, receives instruction himself without lessening mine; as he who lights his taper at mine, receives light without darkening me. That ideas should freely spread from one to another over the globe, for the moral and mutual instruction of man, and improvement of his condition, seems to have been peculiarly and benevolently designed by nature, when she made them, like fire, expansible over all space, without lessening their density in any point, and like the air in which we breathe, move, and have our physical being, incapable of confinement or exclusive appropriation. Inventions then cannot, in nature, be a subject of property. Society may give an exclusive right to the profits arising from them, as an encouragement to men to pursue ideas which may produce utility, but this may or may not be done, according to the will and convenience of the society, without claim or complaint from anybody. (Jefferson, T. 1813/1984)

Jefferson believed in the necessity of a limited period of protection, and headed the US Patent Office for a time after it was formed. But the operative word is *limited*, and over time, IP laws have extended the periods of protection for both authors and inventors significantly. Originally, patents were valid for 14 years, and so were copyrights. This meant that authors and inventors held the exclusive right to the production and dissemination of their works for 14 years, after which anyone might copy them and disseminate those copies. Currently, the patent term is 20 years, and authors enjoy a monopoly for their entire lifetime, *plus* an additional 70 years after they die (USPTO, 2012).

It is certainly debatable now whether the patent term, and certainly the copyright term, is sufficiently limited to balance the competing goals of IP regimes. Do new, useful, and enjoyable arts move quickly enough into the public domain? Are such long monopolies strictly necessary to promote the progress of the useful arts and sciences? IP law itself is subject to criticism, both based upon first principles (it is a limited restriction on otherwise free expression, after all) and from a pragmatic standpoint: Are the terms of protection sufficiently balanced against the demand for enriching the public domain?

Moreover, the expansion of IP into sciences and arts never contemplated in Jefferson's time raises further ethical and practical challenges. Specifically, within the past 50 years or so, patents have been extended to protecting inventive life forms, and now genes. What ethical concerns suggest that these sorts of things ought not to be patentable? There are both deontological (duty-based) and utilitarian (consequence-based) ethical arguments against the sorts of patents now routinely granted to both life forms and genes.

Before we examine those arguments, let us briefly review the history of *how* the present practice came into being. Perhaps this history will clarify the ethical arguments against the practice, by illuminating the nature of the slippery slope that led to the current aberration in the law.

Patenting "Life"

At one time, it was unthinkable that one could patent an animal. Section 101 of the US Patent Act of 1952 provides a list of patent-eligible things, including processes, machines, manufactures, and compositions of matter. Patent-eligible things fitting one or more of these categories can become patented if they are "new, nonobvious, and useful." One might well wonder how plants, animals, and genes came to be considered to be patent-eligible, then.

On April 10, 1790, George Washington signed the first Patent Act of the United States into law. For some 140 years, both the United States Patent and Trademark Office (USPTO) and inventors tacitly agreed that life was excluded as products not of invention but of nature. But in the 1930s, plants became explicitly recognized as patent-eligible subject matter under the Plant Patent Act (PPA) of 1930, which stated at 35 USC. § 161: "Whoever invents or discovers and asexually reproduces any distinct and new variety of plant, including cultivated sports, mutants, hybrids, and newly found seedlings, other than a tuber propagated plant or a plant found in an uncultivated state, may obtain a patent therefor, subject to the conditions and requirements of this title." This act was passed to satisfy the demands of plant breeders who created new, valued strains of plants. But it is important to note that the protection only extends under the PPA to all asexually reproduced derivatives of a uniquely created hybrid. It does not restrict independent production of the same or similar hybrid and sales of its asexually reproduced derivatives. Nonetheless, the PPA served as one of the cases that led us to where we are now. Even following the PPA, however, the courts refused to extend patents beyond mere plants to other living organisms, denying patent eligibility to a bacterium in the case *In re Arzberger*, 112 F.2d 834 (CCPA 1940).

The slope that carried us to patenting genes began in part with *Parke-Davis v. H.K. Mulford & Company* 189 Fed. 95 (1911). In *Parke-Davis*, Judge Learned Hand considered whether an isolated and purified form of adrenalin was patentable. The adrenalin, as patented in US Patent No. 753,177, was extracted from suprarenal glands as a salt, and then further purified as a base. The court concluded that because adrenaline had been isolated and purified from its original state, the utility of the isolated and purified substance deviated greatly from the substance in its natural form, suggesting that the novelty requirement was met. This is both because the purified substance does not simply occur in nature and because the extraordinary or unexpected results that are achieved when the substance is isolated or purified are indicative of patentable invention. Thus, a natural compound was considered patent-eligible based upon the *theory of isolation and purification*. We will come back to the impact of the "isolation and purification" theory of patenting life shortly.

Another critical case broke down the barrier to patenting nonplant life forms in 1980. In *Diamond v. Chakrabarthy*, 447 US 303 (1980), the Supreme Court overturned the Patent Office's rejection of a patent on a "new" bacterium, created by Chakrabarthy, which was developed to help consume hydrocarbons. The Supreme Court held that, while "laws of nature, physical phenomena, and abstract ideas are not patentable, respondent's claim is not to a hitherto unknown natural phenomenon, but to a nonnaturally occurring manufacture or composition of matter—a product of human ingenuity 'having a distinctive name, character [and] use.'" Finally, the doors were wide open to patent new life forms, presumably as compositions of matter. Given that the Patent Act itself did not explicitly prohibit the patenting of life forms, and given that Chakrabarthy had created a new, useful, and nonobvious composition of matter, the court reasoned there was no good reason not to extend patent-eligibility to the bacterium (Hughes, 2001; EC, 2011).

In the age of genetic modification, this reasoning has been used to patent all sorts of genetically engineered life forms, including the famous OncoMouse™ or "Harvard Mouse." Genetically engineered life forms do not occur in nature, they are arguably the product of human inventiveness, they are clearly compositions of matter, and they are frequently useful. The Harvard Mouse is a very useful model for conducting drug trials requiring a nonhuman model of cancer. The patent on the Harvard Mouse has earned Harvard University millions of dollars, and in turn, the availability of the Harvard Mouse to researchers has immeasurably aided the development of new cancer treatments. The Harvard Mouse was created through clever splicing of a known mutation into a mouse to create a mouse more susceptible to cancers. Rather than relying on pure natural chance, this engineered mouse serves a function that enhances the ability to do cancer research and meet human needs. It is the result of *changing* nature, and creating something new. But the reasoning that led to the Harvard Mouse also supported attempts to patent *unmodified* genes, and stands as perhaps the greatest dilemma in the realm of life-form patents (Anderson, 1988; Marshall, 2002; Murray, 2010).

During the course of the HGP, the first big wave of patents on genes began to be filed. Under the reasoning of the cases cited above, those patents became routinely approved, and now nearly one-fifth of the genes common to all humans have some patent claim against them. The reasoning behind granting these patents includes the notion that there is no general, legal prohibition to patenting life forms, the genes for which the patents were issued are all isolated and purified, and genes are all compositions of matter, and thus patent-eligible.

One of the most profitable uses to which human gene patents have been put is in diagnostic testing. Identifying a gene whose presence or mutation indicates the presence or propensity for a disease is extraordinarily helpful in medicine. Genetic screening now enables the early detection of genetic diseases or the propensity to contract a disease. Knowing of this presence or propensity often increases both lifestyle and treatment options for patients. Companies that have patented disease genes can ensure that their diagnostic tests have a monopoly of the market of testing for a particular disease or disorder.

While a number of people and organizations have challenged the practical and ethical implications of disease gene patents (including myself in my book *Who Owns You?* Wiley-Blackwell, 2009), it was not until recently that a court case challenged the legality of such patents. In the recent case, *AMP v. USPTO*, a number of plaintiffs, including an organization representing tens of thousands of physicians, have challenged Myriad's (a Utah-based corporation) patents on two mutations of the BRCA genes BRCA 1 and 2 whose presence indicates a significantly increased propensity for developing breast and ovarian cancer. The District court judge held in favor of the plaintiffs in early 2009, finding that the patents to the isolated (not even purified) genes were invalid patents on a naturally occurring product. This case will surely be challenged all the way to the Supreme Court and will define the legality of such patents, but we might well consider the history cited above from an ethical perspective. What moral considerations suggest that patents on life forms and genes ought not to be tolerated? Arguments can be made against such patents from several ethical perspectives.

Consequentialism

Intellectual property is an inherently utilitarian undertaking. According to basic utilitarian moral principles originating with Jeremy Bentham (1748–1832) and John Stuart Mill (1808–1873), acts that bring about the most benefit, good, or pleasure for the most people are the right ones to pursue, while acts that bring about the most harm or pain for the most people are the wrong ones to pursue (Mill, 1863/2001; Hooker, 2000). As described above, IP regimes were created because of a natural inability to prohibit others from expressing ideas, and a desire to create incentives to create new and useful things, and to move those ideas into the public domain after a period of time. Given that IP rights are not natural rights, but rather creations of the positive law meant to enhance utility, whenever they are in practice antithetical to utility, they ought to be revised or scrapped. In the case of gene and life-form patents, it is likely that these patents are undermining utility generally speaking.

While cases like the Harvard Mouse strongly suggest that happiness is increased because of patents, there are significant gaps in the argument. The argument assumes that advances like the Harvard Mouse would not be made without a patent incentive. There is simply no evidence for this point of view. In fact, most of the history of human science and technology took place without any IP incentive. Moreover, funding for the basic science behind advances like the Harvard Mouse comes from federal grants, and not from a profit incentive. Science moves forward propelled largely by forces outside of profits, including the availability of public money for basic research, and scientists' desires for pursuing natural truths, as well as baser interests in their careers, fame, notoriety, etc. So it is not possible to claim validly that medical advances of any kind are dependent upon the monopoly incentive of a patent.

Patents, moreover, do not ensure profits. Many great inventions consume terrific amounts of investment in research and development, and prove unprofitable anyway. Holding a monopoly never ensures that there is any market demand. Patents are, in many cases, just an extra cost of doing business without any guarantee of reward. There is, in fact, a growing body of evidence from the field of economics that shows that IP provides a *drag* on innovation given the nature and length of patent terms (Lemley, 2001; Gallini, 2002; Jaffe & Lerner, 2006; Holman, 2009; Huang & Murray, 2009; Torrance & Tomlinson, 2009; Williams, 2010). If patents are disincentivizing innovation in medicine, the overall effect on utility would presumably be greater than in other technological areas.

Patents also affect basic research. In basic science, which investigates natural truths, as well as in technology, which applies natural truths to some practical end, the existence and effect of so-called *patent thickets* are well known. Patent thickets emerge when patents in a particular scientific-technical area are granted "too far upstream." Consider natural laws as belonging to the upstream part of the spectrum, and particular practical applications of natural laws to a technology to lie downstream. If patents are granted too close to the natural laws themselves, then both the scientific investigation of those laws and their practical applications can suffer. In the life sciences, we can argue that unmodified genes and other natural phenomena are too far upstream, and that by granting monopolies to these phenomena, both the basic research into the natural laws involved and their creative applications by others through technologies are impeded. The effect on general utility is clear.

As a case in point, consider the effects of the Myriad patents on the BRCA 1 and 2 genes. These patents cover not merely the application of the particular, naturally occurring genetic mutation sequence to a particular test, but the *sequence itself*. Among the first claims specified in the patent are monopoly claims to the isolated sequences identified as causing a propensity for breast and ovarian cancer. The inventive step that is claimed to have made the patents valid was in identifying and isolating the sequence.

But nature itself isolates genetic sequences through natural processes. A gene is not just a random string of nucleic acids. Rather, it encodes, using known and well-understood processes, the *instructions* for the production of proteins in cells. Promoter codons (three-nucleic acid strings) and stop codons mark the beginnings and ends of genes in the 3 billion base pair string that is the human genome. Nature devised the beginnings and endings of the BRCA 1 and 2 genes, and when they function correctly, they produce proteins that inhibit cancers. When mutations to these genes occur then they cease to function as evolution devised them.

Now, scientists *discovered* the link between the presence of these mutations and an increased propensity to suffer breast and ovarian cancer. Granting patents to the sequences themselves arguably decreases general utility in a number of ways. Women (and men) who have a family history of such cancers can now only test for having the BRCA1 and 2 mutations by paying a single company for the right to see whether they possess that genetic mutation. Myriad charges about US$3000.00 for this test, making hundreds of millions of dollars per year, even while the actual cost of conducting such tests is roughly US$300.00 and falling every day (Ahmad, 2012).

Myriad has also sued clinical researchers who, using the publicly available knowledge of the genetic code of the BRCA1 and 2 mutations (published in the patent), dared to perform tests for their presence in their own labs as part of clinical studies. Myriad has the right to prevent such studies, as they own the exclusive right under the patent to the use of those sequences in testing for the presence of those sequences. But blocking clinical studies also arguably negatively affects general utility. While Myriad's vast profits measure in favor of an increased utility for Myriad, there is good evidence that overall utility, for researchers, patients, and the general public (who helped finance the discovery of the BRCA 1 and 2 genes through federal grants), is reduced disproportionately. Thus, on utilitarian grounds, Myriad's patents are actually immoral.

We should continue to allow patents on genes and life forms only if we know that, without them, general utility will decline. There is no evidence that it would, and there is an accumulating body of evidence that suggests that it would actually increase if we did away with such patents altogether. Without patents, there would still be basic research into both existing genomes and recombinant technologies by which the

Harvard Mouse was created. Basic research, if it might be profitable, would continue to be available to anyone, once published, for application through some technology. Without the fear of patent thickets, basic research might well flourish, and technical advances may well increase. Innovation and research proceed apace in other fields without the patent incentive.

An example is particle physics. Most basic science in particle physics moves forward with public financing, and without the potential or promise of monopolies through patents, much less commercially viable innovation except by way of rare spin-off technologies (Pickering, 1984; IM, 2003, appendix). Yet the public funds this research, advances are made routinely, and the pursuit of the science involves massive capital expenditures. It seems likely that medical research and technology would similarly move forward without patents, especially given the public's much more intimate connection with the fruits of medical research and biotechnology compared with particle physics. There seems to be little in the way of consequentialist support for maintaining the current practice of biotechnological patents, especially at the upstream end near the fruits of the basic research.

Deontological Arguments

Even setting aside utilitarian arguments, and even were we to assume that the balance of utility favored patenting life forms or genes somehow, there might yet be reasons to oppose the practice on other grounds. We might well argue that patenting life forms and genes violates some duty we owe, or violates the rights of others, utilizing Kantian-based deontological arguments. Immanuel Kant's (1724–1804) formulations of the categorical imperative have been used by numerous thinkers to argue (1) that one has a fundamental right over one's body and (2) that one has a duty to treat another with respect and never use another *merely* as a means to an end (Kant, 1785/1998; Korsgaard, 1996; Baron, 1999). Let us consider what rights or duties are implicated, and whether patenting life forms or genes ought to be prohibited under deontological ethics.

The potential stakeholders in debates about bio-patents include the public, individual donors of tissues, prospective patients, basic researchers, and those who take basic research and turn it into marketable products. Who among these stakeholders has a right to genes or life forms, and what rights are encumbered by patents?

Patents do not inhibit any possessory rights. Myriad's patents do not prevent your "use" of the genes in your body, in the sense that your body is perfectly, legally entitled to go about its business without paying Myriad a royalty. But patents do grant an *exclusionary* right to Myriad and other patent holders over both natural and engineered biotechnologies. What this means is that Myriad and other patent holders can exclude you from doing certain conscious things with your genetic material, or with the material of engineered life forms. You cannot reproduce the protected genetic sequences, or use them in new inventions, without paying a royalty to Myriad. That prohibition is significant in the field of genetic research, because in order to look for the presence of a genetic sequence in anything, you first must make multiple copies of the searched-for sequence. The process is called polymerase chain reaction (PCR), and it amplifies the presence of genetic material by making multiple copies of a sequence. PCR technically violates a patent if it involves reproduction of a patented gene, and so it is disallowed under a strict interpretation of the patent law. In essence, this means you are prohibited from looking at portions of your own genetic code, even if you had access to the tools and the know-how to look for it. Actually, Salzberg and Pertea (2010) developed a computational screen that "tests an individual's genome for mutations in the BRCA genes, despite the fact that both are currently protected by patents" (p. 1). Instead, you must pay a royalty to Myriad to look for the presence of genes in your own body. This is, in fact, exactly how Myriad has enforced its patents.

Arguably, this violates a right at least to know something vital about yourself. There is no greater, basic right than that of ownership or dominion over your own body, as numerous Kantians have argued (e.g., Korsgaard, 1996; Calder, 2006). Yet patent laws now prohibit your acquiring this knowledge except through license from some third party, which has claimed exclusive rights to portions of the DNA common to everyone. I have argued that there are simply parts of the world over which no control can ethically be exerted (Koepsell, 2009). I call these *commons by necessity*. While in economics we often hear the term *commons* used to describe portions of the world over which we *choose* not to allow ownership claims, I contend that there are still other parts of the world over which no ownership claims could logically be exerted. A state park is an example of a commons-by-choice, whereas I argue that DNA and other similar things simply cannot be possessed or controlled to the exclusion of others as a matter of logical or material necessity. We have a categorical duty to respect the commons by necessity.

Among other similar entities are things like radio waves, which cannot be enclosed in any meaningful fashion. One can broadcast on a certain frequency, and maintain a monopoly by force (like possessing a hammer) over that band of the spectrum for some limited circumference, but only until the next person comes along and broadcasts on the same frequency. Then, we have a classic tragedy of the commons in which we each, through force, attempt to maintain our monopolies. But because of the nature of radio waves, over which we can never exert a totally exclusive monopoly, we must instead reach some agreement. This, I contend, is a classic case of a commons-by-necessity, because radio waves are not naturally capable of being exclusively controlled by anyone.

DNA and nonsterile life forms are similar. DNA is a complex object, whose existence (once begun, whether by nature or by human design) is beyond the control of any individual. Natural, evolutionary forces define the ongoing shape of the domain, altering it according to natural laws, even in the case of engineered life forms, as long as they are nonsterile. Like radio waves, any attempt to exert exclusive control over a life form that is free to undergo the processes of evolution will fail. It simply cannot be enclosed.

Genomes, once freed, are nonexclusive and nonrivalrous goods. Unlike machines, manufactures, processes, or compositions of matter of other kinds, their continued existence and state of constant flux are not dependent upon humans. It may even be the case that engineered life forms enjoy a "right," just like nonengineered life forms, to reproduce freely, pursue their life-goals, and *evolve* without owing anything to their creators. It is certainly plausibly and arguably the case that nonengineered life forms share this right (Attfield, 2003; Keller, 2010), and attempts by anyone to exert some exclusive control over the information in their genes, or the expression of that information by any means, violates individual autonomy, privacy, and the right to self-determination.

There is yet another deontological, categorical duty implicated in attempts at owning genes and life forms: the duty to respect the equal dignity of others. The value of life is not instrumental; rather, it is absolute. No person can be used as a means to an end, and we are all under an ongoing duty to treat everyone with equal, inherent dignity. Allowing patents on life forms violates our categorical duty to treat others with inherent, equal dignity, and makes life and its constituent elements instrumental values, rather than categorical.

While this argument is typically extended only to persons, one could well argue that this is an arbitrary distinction, especially in light of the nature of genetic material. Genes know no bounds. Individual genes are often shared by numerous species. Genes that appear in fruit flies also appear in humans, and many other species. The nature of DNA in general, as a commons-by-necessity, means that not only does it evade any conscious attempt to contain it, but also there is no natural constraint on its extent. Respecting dignity extends not only to the community of human beings who share our common genetic heritage, but also to the community of creatures that share this heritage. It is our shared evolutionary history as various species that define the borders of each species. These borders themselves are ill defined. Treating any species, even if it is engineered, as instrumental for some other goal violates the fundamental right of dignity of each member of any species.

There is no converse duty owed to those who discover or express new things. Expressing some new idea does not carry with it some right to be compensated for that expression. No such right flows from expressions because they too are nonrivalrous and nonexclusive. Once expressed, any idea may be freely used without depriving the expresser of any right. Nor is any duty to compensate implied by another's expression even of a valuable expression. Some have argued there is a moral duty to compensate those who enrich us through their discoveries or inventions. If there is such a duty, it is difficult to see how such a duty could become ethically, legally imposed through IP law, although each person who benefits might well be *inclined* to pay those who benefit them in some way for their supererogatory acts. While Thomas Edison should certainly be compensated for each light bulb he sells, must everyone else be precluded from making competing light bulbs, or selling them for a profit? This is a general argument against the ethics of intellectual property itself, which forecloses the free expression of ideas of others, even in the case of innocent, independent discovery or invention. This argument becomes even more compelling in the case of life forms and genetic material in light of the clear nature of such things as commons-by-logical/material-necessity.

Conclusions

In sum, there are few arguments in favor of the existence of any duties or rights supporting IP claims against life forms or genetic material, and a number of arguments in favor of rights and duties that are explicitly impeded or violated by such claims. Moreover, the fundamental right of dignity is clearly implicated in IP claims, at least to human genetic material, and arguably to genetic material in general.

IP law ought not to be extended to the protection of claims against either genetic materials, engineered or naturally occurring, or life forms. IP claims made for genetic materials or life forms fail under both utilitarian and deontological arguments. There is no evidence that IP increases general utility at all, and especially in the field of biotech and medical research. Given the availability of state-funding for basic medical and biotech research, and the potential impediments to access, through patent thickets and monopolistic pricing, utilitarian arguments fail to support the continued use of IP in these domains. In fact, there is an increasing body of evidence being generated by economists, and also based upon the experiences of various sectors of the economy that thrive even in the absence of IP, that IP might well be a drag on innovation and development.

Further, deontological arguments do not support life form, genetic, or biotech patents. DNA and individual species are arguably commons-by-necessity, not prone to exclusive control. No rights are impeded if patents on these domains disappear, whereas clear rights are violated with their application. Finally, there is a strong argument that dignity requires that genetic material, life forms, and similar technologies remain free, unimpeded by the extension of a state-sanctioned monopoly, and available to all for mutual benefit, investigation, and use.

References

Ahmad, A. (2012). Myriad Genetics acquires patent on another breast cancer-linked gene. BioNews, January 23. Retrieved from: http://www.bionews.org.uk/page_118750.asp

Anderson, A. (1988). Oncomouse released. *Nature, 336*, 300.

Attfield, R. (2003). *Environmental ethics: An overview for the twenty-first century*. Cambridge: Polity Press.

Baron, M. (1999). *Kantian ethics almost without apology*. Ithaca, NY: Cornell University Press.

Blackstone, W. (1766). *Commentaries on the laws of England, 346*. Oxford: Clarendon Press.

Bracha, O. (2004). The commodification of patents 1600–1836: How patents became rights and why we should care. *Loyola of Los Angeles Law Review, 38*, 177–244.

Calder, G. (2006). Ownership rights and the body. *Cambridge Quarterly of Healthcare Ethics, 15*, 89–100.

Dutton, H. (1984). *The patent system and inventive activity during the Industrial Revolution, 1750–1852*. Manchester, UK: Manchester University Press.

EC (The European Commission). (Ed.). (2011). *A history of patenting life in the United States with comparative attention to Europe and Canada*. Saarbrücken: Dictus Publishing.

Gallini, N. (2002). The economics of patents: Lessons from recent US patent reform. *Journal of Economic Perspectives, 16*, 131–154.

Gordon, W. (1992). On owning information: Intellectual property and the restitutionary impulse. *Virginia Law Review, 78*, 149–215.

HGPI (Human Genome Project Information). (2012a). Genetics and patenting. Retrieved from: http://www.ornl.gov/sci/techresources/Human_Genome/elsi/patents.shtml

HGPI (Human Genome Project Information). (2012b). Home page. Retrieved from: http://www.ornl.gov/sci/techresources/Human_Genome/elsi/patents.shtml

Holman, C. (2009). Learning from litigation: What can lawsuits teach us about the role of human gene patents in research and innovation. *Kansas Journal of Law & Public Policy, 18*, 215–229.

Hooker, B. (2000). *Ideal code, real world: A rule-consequentialist theory of morality*. Oxford: Oxford University Press.

Huang, K., & Murray, F. (2009). Does patent strategy shape the long-run supply of public knowledge? Evidence from human genetics. *Academy of Management Journal, 52*, 1193–1221.

Hughes, S. (2001). Making dollars out of DNA: The first major patent in biotechnology and the commercialization of molecular biology, 1974–1980. *Isis, 92*, 541–575.

IM (Institute of Medicine). (2003). *Large-scale biomedical science: Exploring strategies for future research*. Washington, DC: National Academies Press.

Jaffe, A., & Lerner, J. (2006). *Innovation and its discontents: How our broken patent system is endangering innovation and progress, and what to do about it*. Princeton, NJ: Princeton University Press.

Jefferson, T. (1813/1984). Letter to Isaac McPherson, 13 August 1813. In M. Peterson (Ed.), *Thomas Jefferson: writings, autobiography, notes on the state of Virginia, public and private papers, addresses, letters*. New York: Library of America.

Kant, I. (1785/1998). *Groundwork of the metaphysics of morals* (M. Gregor, Trans.). (Section I: Transition from common rational to philosophic moral cognition). Cambridge: Cambridge University Press.

Keller, D. (Ed.). (2010). *Environmental ethics: The big questions*. Malden, MA: Wiley-Blackwell.

Koepsell, D. (2009). *Who owns you? The corporate gold rush to patent your genes*. Malden, MA: Wiley-Blackwell.

Korsgaard, C. (1996). *Creating the kingdom of ends*. Cambridge: Cambridge University Press.

Lemley, M. (2001). Rational ignorance at the patent office. *Northwestern University Law Review, 95*, 15–50.

Marshall, E. (2002). DuPont ups ante on use of Harvard's OncoMouse. *Science, 296*, 1212.

Mill, J. S. (1863/2001). *Utilitarianism*. Indianapolis, IN: Hackett Publishing Company.

Mossoff, A. (2006). Who cares what Thomas Jefferson thought about patents? Reevaluating the patent "privilege" in historical context. *Cornell Law Review, 92*, 953–1012.

Murray, F. (2010). The oncomouse that roared: Hybrid exchange strategies as a source of distinction at the boundary of overlapping institutions. *American Journal of Sociology, 116*, 341–388.

Pickering, A. (1984). *Constructing quarks: A sociological history of particle physics*. Chicago: University of Chicago Press.

Salzberg, S., & Pertea, M. (2010). Do-it-yourself genetic testing. *Genome Biology, 11*, 1–4.

Science. (2011). *Science: Special Series, Human Genome 10th Anniversary, 331*, Parts I–IV.

Torrance, A., & Tomlinson, B. (2009). Patents and the regress of useful arts. *Columbia Science and Technology Law Review, 10*, 130–168.

USPTO (The United States Patent and Trademark Office). (2012). Patents. Retrieved from: http://www.uspto.gov/patents/index.jsp; also 35 USC. 101 Inventions patentable. Retrieved from: http://www.uspto.gov/web/offices/pac/mpep/documents/appxl_35_U_S_C_101.htm

Varmus, H. (2010). Ten years on—the human genome and medicine. *The New England Journal of Medicine, 362*, 2028–2029.

Williams, H. (2010). Intellectual property rights and innovation: Evidence from the human genome. *National Bureau of Economic Research Working Paper Series*, Working Paper 16213. Retrieved from: http://www.nber.org/papers/w16213.pdf

Reply to Koepsell

Lawrence M. Sung

In asserting that it is unethical to patent or copyright genes, embryos, or their parts, Dr Koepsell ably challenges the notion that intellectual property protection is essential to innovation. He asserts that patent rights fail utilitarian and deontological justification, particularly with respect to medical technology, and, thus, concludes that intellectual property protection for such subject matter lacks societal benefit.

The ethics of legal governance are hardly ever binary, i.e., no absolute rights and no absolute wrongs. Rather, the law most often seeks to balance competing priorities, whether social, economic, or ethical—the lesser of two evils, if you will. The same is the case with the issue of patenting or copyrighting genes, embryos, or their parts.

Can patent rights frustrate certain behavior that may have its own moral imperative, such as low- or no-cost access to a particular medical treatment? Perhaps, but because they might, the legislature wisely limited the duration of patent exclusivity, and the executive and judiciary have remained mindful of cabining the scope of exclusivity to comport only with the precise subject matter that the inventor has brought to the public. Accordingly, the patent system promotes an incentive to innovate and to invest in innovation, as well as facilitates the public knowledge of cutting-edge technology, but precludes free riding on the inventor's efforts for a finite period. And while this balance of competing priorities may not be achieved optimally in every case, there are countless examples where technology would not have been made available to the public as quickly, if at all, had exclusivity been unavailable through intellectual property protection or other regulatory measure.

Can equivalent innovation and the public knowledge of such innovation occur without patent protection? Perhaps, but only if the inventive resources universally adhere to the pristine principles of robust collaboration, prompt publication of reliable data, and open access to research tools and materials. This effective dynamic has been demonstrated in certain scientific research initiatives, but always where the inventive resources are exclusively embodied in an identifiable and manageable number of entities, and often where governments commit the primary financial support and have the ability to regulate the behavior of the inventive entities. Where such externalities are missing or inadequate to accomplish the research and development mission to the shared success of the members, the cooperative disintegrates. Moreover, where foreseeable commercial exploitation exists, the allure of competitive advantage may manifest, arising from rogue member behavior and/or third-party market entry. Even well-conceived and managed, large-scale collaborations, such as the Human Genome Project or International HapMap Project, are not immune from such destabilizing influences.

Contemporary Debates in Bioethics, First Edition. Edited by Arthur L. Caplan and Robert Arp.

But alternatives aside, can we afford to disarm medical technology innovation by eliminating patent protection for genes, embryos, or their parts? If the development of novel diagnostics and therapeutics is enhanced by the patent system, even if only for a few conditions or diseases and even if only by weeks or months, would it be unethical to unwind the legal mechanism that supports the enterprise? An application of the precautionary principle also suggests that before any such action, the assurance that public harm would not result is warranted.

The potential injury to the public good that arguably occurs with the wholesale withdrawal of patent exclusivity to genes, embryos, or their parts may also include the unintended consequences of decreased funding availability for basic medical research generally. Where the goal of innovative diagnostics and therapeutics involving genes, embryos, or their parts remains vital, a reduction in private investment must be matched by an increase in government funding to maintain status quo. The relative inelasticity of public funding makes this problematic, which can lead to a loss of dedicated funding for research involving genes, embryos, or their parts, a dilution of funding for basic medical research generally, or both. Moreover, setting specific research priorities a priori is not an easy function for any government to administer. Allowing the market to identify the demand for certain medical products and services is optimal.

So, is there common ground? The patent law, like laws generally, is meant to be a dynamic system that reflects our shared moral and ethical values. The existing standards for obtaining a patent to genes, embryos, or their parts may be carefully tailored and/or rigorously applied to ensure that the public receives the true benefit of the invention disclosed as measured against the impact of the temporary grant of exclusivity awarded to the inventor. Moreover, the courts have the discretion to refine this balance further by withholding the grant of injunctive relief and/or limiting money damages where patent infringement is found. Indeed, the legislative agenda on patent reform has included the consideration of the apportionment of patent infringement damages to recognize the true value of the invention over the prior art, and this represents a movement away from broad patent enforcement.

At bottom, there is room within the existing US patent system to work to embrace the goal of bringing new medical technology involving genes, embryos, or their parts to the public as quickly as possible with intellectual property incentives that ultimately have minimal impact, even during the temporary terms of exclusivity, on patient access and future medical technology innovation. Striking the proper balance in this regard will require the cooperative participation of stakeholders and depend upon the continuing agreements and disagreements among reasonable minds, such as the lively and thought-provoking discourse the Contemporary Debates in Bioethics has afforded here.

Reply to Sung

David Koepsell

I appreciate Professor Sung's attempt to defend the legal system's current approach to patenting of life and genes. It is in every way what lawyers (including myself) do when making a defense case based upon precedent. The law certainly supports the current state of affairs. But sometimes, the law is wrong from an ethical or even logical perspective. Law and morality are often related because the law frequently reflects ethical or moral principles. Sometimes, however, it takes a little while for the law to catch up to morality.

History is replete with instances of legally allowed, but immoral, behaviors. In fact, at times the law has specifically *sanctioned* what we now generally agree to be institutionalized immorality, such as in the case of slavery, or the use of human subjects in science without proper protections, purpose, or consent. Especially in issues surrounding emerging technologies, the law may lag far behind moral or ethical expectations. This is the case, I contend, with the application of IP laws to genes, tissues, and life forms. While Sung makes the case well that the law permits the current state of affairs, he has not addressed the primary ethical arguments I suggest challenge the practice.

He appeals to utility primarily in making the case that IP is legally (and presumably ethically) applied to life forms, genes, etc. Against this argument remains the problem of a general lack of evidence. As I have argued already, the burden is on those who wish to promote a state-sponsored monopoly that curtails free speech and freedom of conscience (as copyright and patent do by prohibiting free re-expression of protected ideas, objects, and processes) to show that such restrictions are necessary, and that the good outweighs their evils. Most of the history of human progress proceeded without IP, and there is simply no evidence that the past few hundred years of progress would not have occurred without IP. Utilitarians who wish to suggest that IP on life forms, genes, and tissues is necessary to promote progress can point to no utilitarian calculus or historical evidence that promotes their case. They can cite correlation, but no causation. As I have mentioned, much of the basic scientific research that later becomes protected by IP is conducted with public funds to begin with. By taking that taxpayer money, and then diverting profits to private entities, the taxpayer is then forced to pay monopolistic rents to companies or institutions that benefitted in the first place from their tax dollars in order to reap any clinical reward.

Moreover, there are a number of studies that show that the utilitarian arguments for IP protection are ill founded, and not supported by the actual evidence starting with research by Machlup and Penrose (1950) and Machlup (1958) more than a half century ago. It seems that research and progress are, in many cases, hindered by state-created, artificial monopoly "rights"

Contemporary Debates in Bioethics, First Edition. Edited by Arthur L. Caplan and Robert Arp.

as researchers such as Wright (1999), Barnett (2000), Lemley (2001), Moser (2003), Bell (2006), and Torrance and Tomlinson (2009) have argued. Also, Turner (1998) is dubious about the efficacy of the patent system as a means of inducing invention, and would argue against having a patent system if this were its only justification. Merges and Nelson (1990) have noted that most economic models of patent scope and duration focus on the relation between breadth, duration, and incentives to innovate, without giving serious consideration to the social costs of greater duration and breadth in the form of retarded subsequent improvement. And Cotter (2002) claims that, "empirical studies fail to provide a firm answer to the question of how much of an incentive [to invent] is necessary or, more generally, how the benefits of patent protection compare to the costs" (p. 149).

It is taken as a matter of unchallenged faith by Sung and others who promote IP in general that IP is a necessary means to an end without which progress in the useful arts and sciences would not be motivated or proceed apace. But they have failed to meet their burden of proof, and where such elemental matters such as the genes, tissues, organs, and offspring are at stake, and monopolistic rights are sought over them, we ought to demand that the burden be met before allowing such control. IP rights grant the right to the holder to exclude others from their monopoly, which necessarily impedes the ability to publish the protected expressions and freely research about or make copies of protected objects or processes, and otherwise interferes with rights to free expression that we take for granted. Accordingly, such monopolies should be granted hesitatingly, if at all, and under a utilitarian framework only if the good clearly outweighs the bad. No such calculus has been supported by IP proponents, and it is their burden of proof.

Moreover, there may be more at stake than mere utility, and as I have argued there are various duties that are inviolable and that are nonetheless impeded by IP rights over organs, tissues, genes, and embryos. If, as I argue, there is no moral basis to grant exclusive control over objects belonging to the commons-by-necessity, or if, as others have argued, our dignity is impaired by the grant of IP rights, then no claim of utility can morally justify the grant of IP rights over genes, tissues, organs, or embryos.

Ultimately, the law should change. It cannot be relied upon as a measure of what is right, only what is permitted by states. As before, when laws changed slowly in reaction to cultural awakenings about various ongoing, inherent injustices, IP law must cease being applied to create monopolies for those who would tie up those things that belong not to any one person, but to humanity as a whole, or to nature's own designs. Whether by utilitarian or deontological analysis, IP proponents fail to argue convincingly otherwise.

References

Barnett, J. (2000). Cultivating the genetic commons: Imperfect patent protection and the network model of innovation, *San Diego Law Review*, *37*, 1008–1095.

Bell, T. (2006). Prediction markets for promoting the progress of science and the useful arts. *George Mason Law Review*, *14*, 37–92.

Cotter, T. (2002). Introduction to IP Symposium. *Florida Journal of International Law*, *14*, 147–152.

Lemley, M. (2001). Rational ignorance at the patent office. *Northwestern University Law Review*, *95*, 15–50.

Machlup, F. (1958). US Senate subcommittee on patents, trademarks & copyrights: An economic review of the patent system, 85th Cong., 2nd Session, Study No. 15. Retrieved from: http://www.archives.gov/legislative/guide/senate/chapter-13-judiciary-1947-1968.html

Machlup, F., & Penrose, E. (1950). The patent controversy in the nineteenth century. *Journal of Economic History*, *10*, 1–10.

Merges, R., & Nelson, R. (1990). On the complex economics of patent scope. *Columbia Law Review*, *90*, 839–870.

Moser, P. (2003). How do patent laws influence innovation? Evidence from nineteenth century world fairs. *National Bureau of Economic Research Working Paper Series*, Working Paper 9099. Retrieved from: http://www.nber.org/papers/w9909

Torrance, A., & Tomlinson, B. (2009). Patents and the regress of useful arts. *Columbia Science and Technology Law Review*, *10*, 130–168.

Turner, J. (1998). The nonmanufacturing patent owner: Toward a theory of efficient infringement. *California Law Review*, *86*, 179–210.

Wright, D. (1999). Optimal patent breadth and length with costly imitation. *International Journal of Industrial Organization*, *17*, 419–436.

Part 6
Should a Child Have the Right to Refuse Medical Treatment to Which the Child's Parents or Guardians Have Consented?

Introduction

"Do you realize you are going to die and your children are going to be motherless?" This was the question one of the anesthetists posed to Rachel Underhill during her emergency Caesarean section in a British hospital in 1999. Underhill was a Jehovah's Witness, and according to the doctrines of that faith, "blood must not be eaten or transfused, even in the case of a medical emergency" (Singelenberg, 1990; WTBTS, 1990, 2008; Carbonneau, 2003). British law is similar to American law in respecting a person who qualifies as within the so-called *age of majority*—the legal term associated with adulthood—and at 24 years of age, Underhill clearly was an adult who could assume control over her own actions, decision, and person. So, the hospital respected her wishes not to be transfused during the C-section, where her twin girls were delivered prematurely at 30 weeks of pregnancy. Underhill survived the procedure without transfusions, and she ate beetroot and received iron injections to restore her hemoglobin counts to normal levels. After a 6-week stay in a neonatal intensive care unit the twins survived, too (BBC, 2007; Underhill, 2012). There are other accounts of Jehovah's Witnesses who were not so lucky, however, dying as a result of not receiving blood transfusions (Hull et al., 2007; BBC, 2010; JW, 2012).

Many people agree that an adult's decision to do what they see fit ought to be respected, as long as the decision does not harm or potentially harm someone else, even if the decision actually harms the adult making the decision. The Kantian-based position whereby one's rationally informed act should be respected (Kant, 1785/1998; Baron, 1999), along with the Millian-based harm principle whereby a person's action should be prevented if it will harm another

Contemporary Debates in Bioethics, First Edition. Edited by Arthur L. Caplan and Robert Arp.

(Mill, 1859/2008; Wolff, 2006, pp. 104–124), both act as the justification for freely made, adult decisions, such as Underhill's. As a 24-year-old adult woman, Underhill was perfectly within her rights to deny a blood transfusion in this obviously serious situation, just as any adult with advanced cancer may decline the radiation and chemotherapy treatments recommended by the oncologist, or the schoolteacher decline to be treated by EMTs at an auto accident, or the professional football player may opt to check out of the hospital against the wishes of the ER doctors who would like to keep him overnight for observation because of the likely concussion he received in a game earlier that day.

Even *more* people—including many Jehovah's Witnesses (Gillon, 2000)—would agree that, despite one's right to freely exercise decisions, Underhill nevertheless made a poor decision to not receive blood transfusions precisely because of the potential harm to herself. On reflection, Underhill herself admits this and, since her C-section, has given permission to doctors so that her daughters may receive transfusions (BBC, 2007; Underhill, 2012). A C-section is an invasive, open surgery that requires cutting through the walls of the abdomen and uterus. On average, a woman can lose anywhere from 5 to 15% of her blood during the procedure, with the possibility always there of complications of one sort or another leading to much more blood loss (Larsson et al., 2010; Schorn, 2010).

What if Underhill did die as a result of not receiving a blood transfusion during her C-section? Or, what if her newly born twins required a blood transfusion as a result of some complication during the C-section? If it is the case that many people think that Underhill made a poor decision for herself, it is arguably the case that *many more* people think that she was being foolish and downright immoral for (1) potentially leaving her children without their mother (recall the anesthetist's question), as well as (2) signing her own children's potential death warrant by refusing a transfusion for herself and her children. It could be argued that Underhill violated the harm principle by setting up the conditions for her children to be put in harm's way. And—put colloquially—it is one thing for Underhill to put herself in harm's way; it is quite another to put her children in harm's way. An 11-year-old girl's death in Wisconsin due to diabetes acidosis, and a 15-month-old baby girl's death due to bacterial pneumonia (both in 2008; see Caplan, 2008; FDS, 2008) could have easily been avoided with common, everyday medical treatments. The parents in both of these cases turned to prayer and their faith instead of medicine.

So, moral discussions, debates, and debacles abound surrounding Underhill's case and those similar to it, prompting fundamental questions such as: Does a parent have the right to refuse treatment for his/her child on religious grounds, or any other grounds? But what if the tables were turned and it is a child (a minor who has not reached the age of majority) who is the one refusing medical treatment? One would be hard pressed to find someone who thinks that the 6-year-old has a right not to have his broken arm set and placed in a cast, or that the 13-year-old can refuse a spinal tap to determine if she has meningitis. But, what if some fairly precocious and strong-willed 16-year-old in the US needed a blood transfusion to save his life, but vehemently is opposed to the transfusion because he is a Jehovah's Witness? What if his parents—who are "disfellowshipped" and no longer subscribe to the tenets of the Jehovah's Witness faith—want to force him to receive the transfusion. Does a parent have the right to *enforce* treatment for his/her child on religious grounds, or any other grounds? Also, should minors have the right to refuse treatment, even when against the will of their parents or guardians?

The following cases include examples of parents respecting the choices of their children to refuse medical treatment, as opposed to forcing their children to do something they do not want to do outright. Because of the personal relationship that is fairly common between a parent and child, and the fact that a parent has a tremendous influence on the thoughts and beliefs of a child, cases where a child makes a significant medical decision for her/himself that is in direct opposition to the wishes of her/his parents are certainly few and far between. And, when it is claimed by a parent that, "I am respecting the thoughts and choices of my child with respect to X," we can almost always read into this claim that, "I am respecting the thought and choices of my child (*which are really just my thoughts and choices voiced through her/him*) with respect to X." Further, as any parent who has had the misfortune of going through this experience is keenly aware of, seeing your own child in pain or suffering with a life-threatening illness is horrible, and the parent usually not only would happily trade places with her/his child, but also may honor the wishes of the child, even if those wishes do not seem to be in the child's best interests in the long term.

Abraham Cherrix was 15 years old when he was diagnosed with Hodgkin's lymphoma. After one round of chemotherapy, he decided that he did not want to endure the nausea and other effects of the therapy anymore (Caplan, 2006; AJ, 2012). Embracing alternative medical approaches, his parents respected his decision and took Abraham to Tijuana, Mexico to undergo Hoxsey Therapy, which includes a paste of arsenic, sulfur, bloodroot, zinc, and other herbs for topical treatments of skin cancers such as melanoma, or a liquid made of potassium iodide, red clover, barberry, prickly ash bark, and other ingredients that one ingests for basically every other kind of cancer (MDA, 2012). Not only was the sale of this treatment outlawed by the US government in 1960 with straightforward references to it as "quackery" as well as numerous studies showing that it does not work (and, in many cases, actually *causing* more harm to the person treated; see Austin et al., 1994), but the US Food and Drug Administration, the National Cancer Institute of the National Institutes of Health, the American Cancer Society, the American Medical Association, and numerous other persons and groups all over the world have derided this therapy and seriously caution against it to treat any form of cancer (ACS, 2012; WHO, 2012). Ironically—and maybe even with a bit of poetic justice—the father and founder of this treatment, Harry Hoxsey, developed prostate cancer in 1967, and opted for standard treatment and surgery when his own method failed to work on himself (Ward, 1988; Young, 1992; Brinker, 1995; Caplan, 2007)!

As a result of the decision to stop Abraham's chemotherapy treatment, his parents were taken to court in 2006 by the Accomack County Department of Social Services in Virginia (*Virginia v. Cherrix*) and found guilty of medical neglect of a minor. The court ruled in that case that Abraham must continue his chemotherapy, but a circuit court reversed the decision on appeal. A compromise was eventually reached whereby Abraham could receive treatment from a board-certified oncologist who also utilizes alternative cancer treatments (Barisic, 2007). In 2008, after five treatments of concentrated doses of radiation and immunotherapy consisting of vitamin supplements, Abraham turned 18—the age of majority in the US—and showed no signs of the disease (Simpson, 2008). In essence, Abraham's oncologist followed standard medical procedures for this kind of cancer that, if treated in this standard way, has a high rate of success with some 90% or more people being cured.

A 13-year-old from Minnesota named Daniel Hauser made news in 2009 when he, too, refused to go through full treatment for his Hodgkin's lymphoma. Eschewing standard medical practices in general, Daniel's mother subscribes to the tenets and healing practices of the Nemenhah Native Americans—believing they are "100% effective" in treating cancer by "starving it, not feeding it" (Nesbitt, 2009; Landis, 2010)—and so she took Daniel and fled the state of Minnesota after only one round of chemotherapy, disregarding the appellate judge's order to have her son finish off the four-round treatment. Eventually she and Daniel returned to Minnesota and, after a custody hearing—complete with X-rays as evidence showing that one of Daniel's tumors had increased in size—Daniel was ordered by the judge to complete the chemotherapy treatment, which he did. In August of 2011, it was announced by a family spokesperson that Daniel's cancer was in remission (Carlyle, 2011).

A sadder case concerns a 16-year-old named Shannon Nixon who, with the consent and support of her parents, refused treatment for her diabetes and died in 1996. Instead of seeking medical attention, she and her parents opted to pray for her diabetes in their church in Altoona, Pennsylvania just before Shannon lapsed into a diabetic coma. Her parents were actually charged and convicted of involuntary manslaughter and endangering the welfare of a child and, after rejected appeals, began serving their sentence in 2001 (SCP, 2000). "Why didn't we seek medical treatment? The answer is we didn't feel it's right because of our religion," was the claim made by Shannon's older brother, Dennis Nixon, Jr, in a 2001 interview (Gibb, 2001). Ten years prior, in 1991, the Nixon's lost their 8-year-old son to an ear infection that doctors say could have easily been treated with antibiotics.

Most countries in the world set 18 as the age when they can be considered to be fully in the *age of majority*, namely, an adult who legally can assume control over their own actions, decisions, and person. At 18, one is no longer a *minor*, but a *major*, so to speak. Because of the fact that 18 can be a somewhat arbitrary number with obvious cases of teenagers under the age of 18 acting like 30-year-olds (and 30-year-olds acting like teenagers, unfortunately!), there are a number of court cases where the judge recognizes someone under the age of 18 to be a *mature minor*, which in effect grants her/him the rights and privileges of someone who is at the age of majority. So, while it is widely agreed by most legislative and judicial systems that parents are the ones who are ultimately responsible for the actions of their children, the well-being of their children, providing medical care for their children, and other similar kinds of obligations (see the US Supreme Court decision, *Parham v. J.R.* 442 US 584, 1979), there are US state legislatures that recognize mature minors as possessing certain privacy rights and abilities to consent to a few types of medical treatment without parental involvement. A significant ruling concerning mature minors occurred in 1992 in the West Virginia Supreme Court case, *Belcher v. CAMC* (422 SE2d 827), where the following factors were considered central in determining whether someone can qualify as a mature minor: age, ability, experience, education, training, degree of maturity, degree of judgment exhibited, past conduct, demeanor, and the capacity to appreciate the nature, risks, and consequences of a procedure.

Examples that would seem to encompass the spirit of the mature minor doctrine include the State of Pennsylvania allowing minors to be tested for STDs or pregnancy, or seek substance abuse treatment or psychotherapy, or even decide to have an abortion, without the knowledge or consent of their parents. Also, in Pennsylvania, an emancipated minor (one who is financially independent and responsible for her/his own medical care) is able to make certain medical decisions without parental consent (PAC, 2012).

William Winslade underscores the value of the mature minor doctrine in the first chapter of this section. However, cognizant of the fact that not every legal decision—such as the mature minor doctrine—is a moral one, and vice versa, Winslade offers moral reasons that justify the right of a minor to refuse medical treatment, even when against the will of a parent or guardian. His argument is based in the idea that a competent and rational person's autonomy and bodily integrity should be respected. Concerning certain medical decisions, then, minors are deserving of the same rights and privileges as any adult, and "their level of competence should be assessed in the context of the specific medical circumstance." He bolsters this argument with the practical observation that, "adolescents who actively participate in medical decisions affecting their bodies and their lives are more likely to form a better relationship with their physicians." And a better relationship with a physician oftentimes means more efficient diagnoses and treatments for the patient.

In the other chapter in this section, Catherine Brooks begins by wisely noting something that applies to this debate, as well as any legitimate, rational debate: "It is in taking care to understand the precise language to be employed that overly broad, generalizing propositions may be avoided, and unintended consequences may be limited. In paying attention to the words themselves, we may engage in a more nuanced discussion of the complexities of the issue presented in the title statement." And a nuanced discussion is precisely what she gives the reader.

After offering a history of important US court cases that have led to the idea that parents are the primary medical decision-makers for their children, Brooks goes on to clarify and qualify the concept of *consent* in relation to lawful adulthood (the age of majority). She notes, "autonomy is the hallmark of adulthood in our jurisprudence: the adult person is self-determining" and that minors in general are viewed as not being autonomous and self-determining. Whereas Winslade points to some evidence indicating that there are minors who can understand the consequences of their actions quite well, Brooks points out the fact that by the time someone reaches the age of 16, sensory-seeking, impulsive, and risk-preferring kinds of behavior are at their height. And, of course, such behaviors oftentimes can be associated with negative outcomes for these adolescents in terms of car crashes, unwanted pregnancies, and the like. In the end, although Brooks argues that to "impose on the child, without recourse to proofs of maturity, the right and corresponding responsibilities of medical decision-making places an unreasonable burden on the child," she offers her own nuanced position, maintaining that there are/can be cases where medical decision-making is a wholly reasonable burden that may be placed on the child who is mature enough to carry it.

References

ACS (American Cancer Society). (2012). Hoxsey herbal treatment. Retrieved from: http://www.cancer.org/Treatment/TreatmentsandSideEffects/ComplementaryandAlternativeMedicine/HerbsVitaminsandMinerals/hoxsey-herbal-treatment

AJ (Abraham's Journey). (2012). Website: Abraham's journey. Retrieved from: http://www.abrahamsjourney.com/

Austin, S., Dale, E., & Dekadt, S. (1994). Longterm followup of cancer patients using Contreras, Hoxsey and Gerson therapies. *Journal of Naturopathic Medicine, 5*, 74–76.

Barisic, S. (2007). Floyd teen who fought against chemotherapy is in remission: Starchild Cherrix's case spurred debate on the government's role in family medical decisions. *The Roanoke Times*, September 15.

Baron, M. (1999). *Kantian ethics almost without apology*. Ithaca, NY: Cornell University Press.

BBC (British Broadcasting Company). (2007). Refusing blood "source of regret." November 6. Retrieved from: http://news.bbc.co.uk/2/hi/uk_news/england/sussex/7080902.stm

BBC (British Broadcasting Company). (2010). Teenage Jehovah's Witness "died after refusing blood": A teenage Jehovah's Witness crushed by a car as it crashed into a West Midlands shop is thought to have died after refusing a blood transfusion. May 18. Retrieved from: http://news.bbc.co.uk/2/hi/uk_news/england/west_midlands/8690785.stm

Brinker, F. (1995). The Hoxsey treatment: Cancer quackery or effective physiological adjuvant. *Journal of Naturopathic Medicine, 6*, 9–23.

Caplan, A. (2006). Parents vs. judge: Who picks teen's cancer care? Cherrix's disease is curable with traditional medicine—not licorice root. *NBC News*, August 17. Retrieved from: http://www.msnbc.msn.com/id/14351658/ns/health-health_care/t/parents-vs-judge-who-picks-teens-cancer-care/#.UIG6grRn-04

Caplan, A. (2007). Challenging teenagers' right to refuse treatment. *Virtual Mentor, 9*, 56–61.

Caplan, A. (2008). Children's health can't be left to faith alone: When parents won't seek medical care, they must be punished by law. *NBC News*, March 31. Retrieved from: http://www.msnbc.msn.com/id/23885944/ns/health/t/childrens-health-cant-be-left-faith-alone/#.UIG5NLRn-04

Carbonneau, A. (2003). *Ethical issues and the religious and historical basis for the objection of Jehovah's Witnesses to blood transfusion therapy*. London: Edwin Mellen Press.

Carlyle, E. (2011). Anthony Hauser, father of boy who refused chemo, dies at 56. *Citypages*, August 31. Retrieved from: http://blogs.citypages.com/blotter/2011/08/anthony_hauser_son_refused_chemo_dies.php

FDS (Finding Dulcinea Staff). (2008). Parents face charges after children die from treatable conditions. *Finding Dulcinea: Librarian on the Internet*, April 29. Retrieved from: http://www.findingdulcinea.com/news/health/March-April-08/Parents-Face-Charges-After-Children-Die-from-Treatable-Conditions.html

Gibb, T. (2001). Prayerful parents in prison for death. *Pittsburgh Post Gazette*, June 1. Retrieved from: http://old.post-gazette.com/regionstate/20010601faith5.asp

Gillon, R. (2000). Refusal of potentially life-saving blood transfusions by Jehovah's Witnesses: Should doctors explain that not all JWs think it's religiously required? *Journal of Medical Ethics, 26*, 299–301.

Hull, L., Dolan, A., & Newling, D. (2007). Jehovah's Witness mother dies after refusing blood transfusion after giving birth to twins. *MailOnline*, November 5. Retrieved from: http://www.dailymail.co.uk/news/article-491791/Jehovahs-Witness-mother-dies-refusing-blood-transfusion-giving-birth-twins.html

JW (Jehovahs-Witness.net). (2012). 21-year old dies refusing medical aid. Retrieved from: http://www.jehovahs-witness.net/watchtower/medical/27725/1/21-YEAR-OLD-DIES-REFUSING-MEDICAL-AID

Kant, I. (1785/1998). *Groundwork of the metaphysics of morals* (M. Gregor, Trans.). (Section I: Transition from common rational to philosophic moral cognition). Cambridge: Cambridge University Press.

Landis, P. C. (2010). Nemenhah declaration of existence as an indigenous people. Retrieved from: http://www.nemenhah.org/images/pdf/NemenhahDeclaration

Larsson, C., Saltvedt, S., Wiklund, I., Pahlen, S., & Andolf, E. (2010). Estimation of blood loss after cesarean section and vaginal delivery has low validity with a tendency to exaggeration. *Acta Obstetricia et Gynecologica Scandinavica, 85*, 1448–1452.

MDA (MD Anderson Cancer Center). (2012). Constituents of the Hoxsey formula. Retrieved from: http://www.mdanderson.org/education-and-research/resources-for-professionals/clinical-tools-and-resources/cimer/therapies/herbal-plant-biologic-therapies/hoxsey-constituents.pdf

Mill, J. S. (1859/2008). *On liberty*. Oxford: Oxford University Press.

Nesbitt, (2009). Court to hear boy's testimony in private today. *The Jounral*, May 9. Retrieved from: http://www.nujournal.com/page/content.detail/id/506825.html

PAC (The Pennsylvania Code). (2012). 35 P.S. §10101, 35 P.S. §10103, 71 P.S. §1690.112, 50 P.S. §7201. Retrieved from: http://www.pacode.com/secure/data/055/chapter5320/chap5320toc.html, http://statecasefiles.justia.com/documents/pennsylvania/superior-court/a33035_08.pdf?1318293407, http://www.pacode.com/secure/data/055/chapter 3680/s3680.52.html

Schorn, M. (2010). Measurement of blood loss: Review of the literature. *Journal of Midwifery & Women's Health, 55*, 20–27.

SCP (Supreme Court of Pennsylvania). (2000). Commonwealth of Pennsylvania v. Nixon: Opinion. Retrieved from: Pennsyhttp://novalis.org/cases/Commonwealth%20of%20 Pennsylvania%20v.%20Nixon.html

Simpson, E. (2008). Cherrix turning 18, free of cancer signs and court oversight. *The Virginian-Pilot*, June 5.

Singelenberg, R. (1990). The blood transfusion taboo of Jehovah's Witnesses: Origin, development and function of a controversial doctrine. *Social Science Medicine, 31*, 515–523.

Underhill, R. (2012). Rachel's story. EXJW | Reunited website. Retrieved from: http://www.exjw-reunited.co.uk/Stories.htm

Ward, P. (1988). History of Hoxsey treatment. Prepared for the Office of Technology Assessment, US Congress, Washington, DC. Retrieved from: http://www.introductiontorife.com/refandres/files/papers_articles/History%20of%20Hoxsey%20Treatment.pdf

WHO (World Health Organization). (2012). Improving access to care in developing countries. Retrieved from: http://www.who.int/hiv/pub/prev_care/en/ImprovingaccessE.pdf

Wolff, J. (2006). *An introduction to political philosophy*. Oxford: Oxford University Press.

WTBTS (Watch Tower Bible and Tract Society). (1990). *How can blood save your life?* Brooklyn, NY: Watch Tower Bible and Tract Society.

WTBTS (Watch Tower Bible and Tract Society). (2008). *Keep yourselves in God's love*. Brooklyn, NY: Watch Tower Bible and Tract Society.

Young, (1992). *The medical messiahs: A social history of health quackery in twentieth-century America*. Princeton, NJ: Princeton University Press.

Chapter Eleven

The Child Should Have the Right to Refuse Medical Treatment to Which the Child's Parents or Guardians Have Consented

William J. Winslade

Black's Medical Dictionary (2009) defines adolescence as "that age which follows puberty and precedes the age of majority." This chapter defends the right of an adolescent sometimes to refuse medical treatment over the objection of their parents or physicians. The defense is based on moral considerations: respect for adolescents as persons, their capacity to rationally deliberate and make personal choices, and their physical integrity. Categorical legal incompetence is rejected in favor of individualized discussion and capacity assessments, and the circumstances, benefits, and burdens of the treatments.

Introduction

In American law, minors under the age of 18 are generally categorized as legally incompetent to make their own medical decisions. Parents are the authorized decision-makers unless an exception applies (such as emancipated or mature-minor rules, which are described below). The legal incompetence doctrine is based on the right and the duty of parents to act in what they consider to be the best interests of their children. *Black's Medical Dictionary* (BMD, 2009) defines adolescence as "that age which follows puberty and precedes the age of majority." In this chapter, I will argue that in some circumstances, some adolescents should have the right to refuse medical treatment over the objections of their parents and the recommendations of their physicians. These situations include some extremely burdensome and minimally beneficial treatments, futile treatments for dying children, or choices among more and less restrictive and intrusive treatments. I will argue that the legal incompetence policy is sometimes problematic, both morally and practically. It is morally suspect because it undermines respect for adolescents as persons and fails to acknowledge their rights to personal autonomy and bodily integrity. I will explain why these moral considerations should sometimes override the legal incompetence policy. As a practical matter, adolescents who actively participate in medical decisions affecting their bodies and their lives are more likely to form a better relationship with their physicians. This will enhance communication, trust, and compliance with treatment programs. Even competent adolescents, however, typically have dependence on their parents

Contemporary Debates in Bioethics, First Edition. Edited by Arthur L. Caplan and Robert Arp.

for emotional and economic support. Accordingly, parents usually do and should play a role in adolescents' medical decision-making. Incompetent adolescents, like incompetent adults, do not have a right to make their own medical-treatment decisions. Even in this situation, however, adolescents' preferences are relevant, even if not decisive. Respect for persons is manifested not only by respecting adolescents' choices, but also by the manner in which they are treated, even if their preferences are overridden.

To support my position, I will first discuss the ideas of competence and incompetence to refuse treatment as it applies to adults. Next, I will discuss adolescent development and why categorical age standards of legal competence are flawed. Adolescents should be evaluated for competency to refuse treatment on an individualized basis in the context of the specific treatment under consideration. I will then consider in detail why moral rather than legal reasons support adolescents' rights to refuse treatment. Although my position overlaps to some degree with the mature-minor legal doctrine, I contend that the moral reasons I offer provide a more convincing basis for permitting competent adolescents in some situations to refuse medical treatment. Next, I discuss the proper roles of parents and physicians, and occasionally judges, when an adolescent seeks to refuse recommended medical treatment. Finally, I will present illustrative cases where adolescents' right to refuse treatment should be respected.

Competence and Incompetence

In the law, adults are presumed to be competent to consent to or refuse medical treatment, unless they have been adjudicated to be incompetent. Competent persons in a medical context must (1) sufficiently comprehend relevant information about diagnosis, prognosis, and treatment, (2) be able to assess and deliberate about their treatment options, (3) rationally evaluate risks and benefits of recommended treatments, and (4) make a voluntary choice whether to consent or refuse the recommendations (Beauchamp & Childress, 1979/2009, p. 71; USDH, 2009; BMA, 2011). Comprehension, deliberation, rationality, and voluntariness need not be perfect, but must be adequate and appropriate for the circumstances. A competent person must at least have the capacity to meet these criteria. On occasion, of course, a competent person's abilities and capacities may be diminished by psychological, physical, or environmental factors. Even persons that have the capacity for rationality may sometimes make irrational choices.

In the bioethics literature about the concept of competence, some commentators argue that competence is a threshold concept that is not a matter of degree (Buchanan & Brock, 1990). You are either competent or not. Others argue that competence is a gradient concept that admits of degrees (Grisso & Appelbaum, 1998; also Jonas, 2007; Kim, 2010). I find the latter approach to be more useful. Even if competence is a threshold concept, then the criteria by which it is determined whether competence has been established are gradient concepts. The important point is that competency determinations are often subtle and nuanced for both adults and adolescents.

Legal decisions concerning competency are based on the testimony of patients and physicians, and, sometimes, mental-health professionals. Failure to meet the standards for any of the four criteria for competence may render adults incompetent to make their own medical decisions. In such situations, either a surrogate or a judge will decide on behalf of the incompetent person whether or not to accept a treatment recommendation.

There are two specific situations in the US, however, that are exceptions to the judicial standard. Persons who have been diagnosed by a psychiatrist with a serious mental illness as a result of which they are a danger to themselves or others can be involuntarily detained in a psychiatric facility, though not necessarily treated without informed consent or a judicial order of incompetence (Geller & Stanley, 2005). Also, resulting from the court decisions in *Barnett v. Bachrach* (34 A.2d 626, 1943) and *Canterbury v. Spence* (464 F.2d 772, D.C. Cir. 1972), in a hospital emergency room, clearly competent adults may refuse treatment, but if someone is sick or injured with a life-threatening emergency and clearly incompetent (say unconscious) or seems to be obviously incompetent (incoherent, delusional, etc.), emergency-room physicians can treat that person without consent, at least to stabilize her/him. Otherwise, adults presumed to be competent and not judicially determined to be incompetent have a legal right to refuse recommended medical treatment, even if it may be life-saving.

For example, assume that an adult with emphysema comes to the emergency room with breathing difficulties. He is told that he needs to be placed on a ventilator and may become permanently respirator-dependent. The man, who had previously experienced brief periods of respiratory support, is not willing to risk respirator dependence despite the risk of respiratory arrest or failure. The man is legally permitted to refuse the recommendation and leave the emergency room.

Sometimes it is asserted that even though judges must make a competency ruling, physicians can determine if a patient has decision-making capacity. For example, suppose the man with emphysema is accompanied by a family member. Physicians may believe the man lacks decision-making capacity, and the family member may be asked to intervene and serve as a surrogate decision-maker. Strictly speaking, physicians are not legally authorized to make competency determinations. The decision-making capacity terminology sometimes usurps a legal determination of competency or incompetency. Physicians are even sometimes accused of presuming just the opposite of the law: that all patients are incompetent and that informed consent is a mere formality, if not a useless gesture. It is also sometimes said that physicians treat patients as incompetent if they disagree with a treatment recommendation and competent if they agree. Although this oversimplification may be somewhat misleading, it is not totally mistaken. Adults (and adolescents) are often unfamiliar with medical information and find it difficult to assess it (especially if they feel or fear that they are sick). This makes it challenging to evaluate treatment options rationally and to make voluntary decisions; it is often easier for patients to acquiesce to the recommendation. Although the legal and ethical issues raised about the difference between legal competence and decision-making capacity cannot be fully explored here, legal competence is more of a threshold concept, whereas decision-making capacity is more of a gradient idea (Buchanan & Brock, 1990; Wilks, 1997; Wicclair, 1999; Checkland, 2001; Kim, 2010).

Legal Incompetence of Minors and the Categorical Age Criterion

The American legal system typically relies on categorical distinctions to facilitate judicial decision-making. Judges dislike vagueness and ambiguity, and prefer bright line categories. This is partly to counter the way in which the adversary system polarizes debate by creating doubt, challenging credibility of witnesses, disputing the weight of evidence, etc. It makes it challenging for judges and juries to render clear-cut verdicts. The presumed legal incompetence of minors is usually reasonable when applied to infants or very young children. They generally lack the cognitive and psychosocial capacity to make their own medical decisions. Even here, however, very young and gravely ill children with chronic or terminal illness may display a precocious maturity that surpasses that of their anguished parents. Dying children sometimes display acute awareness, appreciate their situation, and come to terms with it sooner and better than their parents. This is especially true when parents cling to false hopes of cure and insist on painful treatment when a child understandably prefers palliative care. In St. Jude Children's Hospital in Memphis, each young child is individually evaluated by an interdisciplinary team for their capacity to participate in or even make their own medical decisions, especially when further treatment is both futile and painful.

With regard to adolescents, the categorical legal incompetence of minors up to the age of 18 is more problematic. Adolescents differ in several respects from very young children. Adolescents are often developing their own identities, seeking increasing independence from their parents, and cultivating their relationships with peers. Adolescents are in transition. They are beginning to be more reflective and more aware of their future and the consequences of their actions. Admittedly, adolescents are also sometimes impulsive, reckless, and irrational; so are many adults. Research has shown that adolescents, especially between 15 and 18, have acquired learning and reasoning skills that enable them to understand, deliberate, reason, and make voluntary choices (Kuther, 2003; Albert & Steinberg, 2011; Sarkar, 2011). They are evolving toward adulthood.

Adolescents vary widely in their level of maturity as well as competence to make their own decisions in many areas of their lives. The categorical age criteria become suspect if not arbitrary. For example, in the US, adolescents are permitted to drive at 16, vote at 18, and drink at 21. Which is the age of maturity for medical decision-making? Minors are sometimes permitted to seek treatment for sexually transmitted diseases without parental permission to pursue public-health goals and to relieve adolescents from fear of repercussions from telling their parents. Similarly, adolescents who want an abortion may seek authorization from a judge to protect the adolescents' constitutional right to privacy and bodily integrity as well as to avoid negative parental reactions. Emancipated minors, such adolescents who are married or living independently and financially independent may also make their own medical decisions. Some states, such as Pennsylvania, permit minors to obtain mental-health treatment without parental consent (O'Connor, 2009). A key underlying factor in some of these exceptions to the legal incompetence of minors to make their own medical decisions is their right to integrity of both their bodies and their minds. I will say more about this moral consideration later.

In some states, the mature-minor rule provides an exception to the legal incompetence of minors to consent to or refuse medical treatment. The classic statement of the mature-minor rule was formulated in 1987 in *Cardwell v. Bechtol* (724 S.W.2d 739, 748), a Tennessee case in which a physician treated a 17-year-old girl for back pain without parental consent. Although the trial judge ruled that the physician committed malpractice, the jury did not find the physician liable for failing to obtain informed consent from the parents. The Tennessee Supreme Court formulated the classic statement of the mature-minor rule as follows:

> Whether a minor has the capacity to consent to medical treatment depends upon the age, ability, experience, education, training, and degree of maturity or judgment obtained by the minor; as well as upon the conduct and demeanor of the minor at the time of the incident involved. Moreover, the totality of the circumstances, the nature of the treatment, and its risks or probably consequences, and the minor's ability to appreciate the risks and consequences are to be considered.

In other cases, courts have recognized the mature-minor rule. In one case, a minor was in a car accident, after which he was diagnosed as permanently unconscious. The parents, based on a discussion with their 17-year-old son prior to the accident, agreed with the physicians to discontinue using a feeding tube. After much litigation, the Maine Supreme Court (In re Chad Eric Swan, 569 A.2d 1202, Me. 1990) upheld the decision to remove the feeding tube on the basis of the clearly expressed antecedent preferences of a normally mature high school senior. Other courts have permitted mature minors to discontinue treatment based on the debilitating side effects of treatment. For example, a 15-year-old who had undergone two liver transplants—one at age eight and another at age 14—did not want to continue taking immunosuppressant drugs because of its debilitating side effects. A Florida judge upheld the adolescent's right to refuse the drugs because he was a mature minor (TN, 1994). Some courts have also allowed older adolescents who, based on their beliefs as Jehovah's Witnesses, refused physicians' recommended blood transfusions (see Carbonneau, 2003). Although mature-minor cases of treatment refusal are rare, they call attention to the legal right of competent minors to make their own medical-treatment decisions.

In the context of consent to or refusal of medical treatment, whether or not adolescents agree or disagree with their parents or their physicians, I believe adolescents should be assessed individually to determine their level of competence to make their own personal medical decisions. They should be presumed to be neither competent nor incompetent. Instead, their level of competence should be assessed in the context of the specific medical circumstance. It is common to underestimate the capacities of adolescents. With empathic listening and appropriate inquiries, parents and physicians, sometimes with the assistance of other health professionals, can determine an adolescent's capacity to make their own healthcare decisions. Even if adolescents lack the capacity to participate fully in giving informed consent to or refusal of medical treatment, it is possible for them to express assent or dissent to treatment options. Their preferences may not always be decisive, but they should always be taken into consideration.

The Moral Rights of Adolescents to Consent to or Refuse Medical Treatment

The legal doctrine of the categorical incompetence of all minors, including adolescents, is a bright line favored by judges. For parents, it provides legal grounds for continuing parental authority over their adolescent children. Although I think parents do and should play a key role when adolescents are sick or injured, there are significant moral and practical reasons why the authority of parents, despite the prevailing legal policy, should be reconfigured. The first part of my argument for modifying parental authority in the context of medical decisions regarding adolescents rests upon three interconnected moral considerations: respect for persons, personal autonomy to make decisions, and personal control over one's body.

Respect for persons is an essential moral norm in the US, despite the fact that it is often violated. All persons, young and old, are vulnerable to exploitation, manipulation, and harm, especially when they are sick or injured. Our normal level of competence is threatened by anxiety, fear of disability or death, ignorance of medical technicalities, concern about unforeseen consequences, loss of income, etc. These psychological and existential concerns are distractions from our usual ability to meet the criteria for competence, namely, comprehension, deliberation, rationality, and voluntariness.

Incompetent adults are vulnerable in slightly different ways. They are more vulnerable to exploitation and manipulation because of their incompetence. Their families as well as health professionals acting with good intentions and with the idea that they are acting in the best interests of incompetent adults, especially the seriously disabled, may subject the chronically ill and the fragile elderly to aggressive interventions, when palliative care might be more appropriate.

Respect for competent persons as patients is manifested by robust informed consent practices and by recognizing that competent adults have a legal and a moral right to give or withhold consent. But respect for persons is not merely about informed consent or refusal of medical treatment. It is also manifested in the manner persons are treated. Competent adults want to be treated with empathy, with respect for their personal values, and with sensitivity to their personalities and preferences. Incompetent persons also deserve respect, but the manner in which they are treated often lacks empathy and sensitivity to their compromised capacities and overemphasizes their incompetence. This can occur when physicians talk directly to family members without giving adequate attention and due regard to the sensitivities of the incompetent person who may be demented but not wholly incompetent. All patients, competent or incompetent, should be treated with respect as persons. The manner in which incompetent patients are given individualized and personalized care is an essential feature of respect for persons.

My position is that adolescents, as persons in various stages of moral and psychological maturity, should also be treated with respect. Adolescents are particularly sensitive when their status as persons is diminished merely because of age. The injured or ill adolescent is after all the person whose mind and body are the direct target of treatment. In the context of consent to, or refusal of, treatment, adolescent persons should be presumed to be neither competent nor incompetent. They should be assessed individually in the context of treatment issues. Respect for adolescent persons in the first instance is to recognize that they are the patients, and it is their minds and bodies that are directly affected by treatment. Good adolescent physicians and, for that matter, good pediatricians of younger patients focus on their patients as persons first.

Parents and other family members are not the patient. I am reminded of an incident when my young daughter at age six visited her dentist. She complained—rightly—that the dentist talked to me rather than her. She said that the dentist should ask her permission to work on her teeth. "After all," she said, "it's my mouth." She understood why she needed dental work, what he was recommending, and why it was beneficial. She believed, with justification, that his failure to speak directly to her and seek her consent, failed to respect her competence, autonomy, and bodily integrity. She neither liked nor trusted the dentist.

It is common to underestimate the capacities of adolescents because of their sometimes-flippant attitudes or cautious passivity. They often have unarticulated feelings, sensitivities, and personal preferences regarding decisions about their minds and bodies. Even if an adolescent is not fully competent, it is important that they be treated as a primary participant in their own healthcare. Respect for adolescents as patients means remembering to address them and their health needs directly. Physicians and parents alike should give deference to adolescents to the degree they have the capacity to make their own healthcare decisions. This not only respects them as persons, but also acknowledges their evolving need for personal autonomy, especially over their minds and bodies. This is important not only because it is morally appropriate, but also because it enhances the effectiveness of physician–patient relationship and contributes to better outcomes.

Adolescents with an illness or injury may need time to reflect on their situation or come to terms with the recommended treatment. If adolescents make their own decision to endorse what their health professional and their parents recommend, they may be better able to cope with risk, pain, treatment programs, and even the outcomes. It is one thing to be forced to be treated and quite another to agree to it. Also, adolescents are more likely to be aware of their desire and need for respect and autonomy than young children or old demented adults.

Adolescents who feel that they are respected and that their interests and well-being are the primary focus of the physician–patient relationship are more likely to promote truthful discourse, trust, compliance with a treatment plan, and cooperation with their parents. In fact, even when adolescents are in agreement with their parents and a physician's recommendation, it is important for adolescents to feel that they are the primary participant. To the extent that adolescents are presumed to be incompetent or immature, especially when that is erroneous, that disrespects them both as patients and as persons (Ladd & Forman, 1995; Kuther, 2003).

Treatment-Refusal Situations

When should an adolescent's treatment refusal be accepted? Adolescents who have experienced lengthy, painful, and unsuccessful treatments for a terminal condition may be better able to judge when to refuse aggressive treatments and accept only palliative care. For example, a 14-year-old who knew she was dying from leukemia asked her pediatrician to admit her to the hospital for hospice care rather than continuing debilitating and futile chemotherapy. Her parents finally realized that their daughter was rational and realistic. The parents were in denial and harboring false hope of a cure. The adolescent's refusal to continue chemotherapy was endorsed and accepted by her physician who was also able to persuade the parents to respect their daughter's decision (Haga, 2011).

This case is representative of a class of cases encountered in children's hospitals that treat extremely ill and often dying children. Dying children may recognize that they are on a dying trajectory and that their bodies are overwhelmed by drugs and disease before their parents do. At some children's hospitals, a multidisciplinary team carefully assesses children on an individual basis to determine their degree and desire to participate in decision-making. For example, if an experimental treatment is being considered as a last resort to a seemingly intractable disease, even if parents consent to treatment, adolescent patients may be allowed to dissent. Physicians may come to agree with the adolescent that palliative, rather than aggressive and painful, treatments are medically appropriate. For example, pediatric oncologists have experimented with bone-marrow transplants for some cancers where chemotherapy is ineffective. The risk of graft versus host disease, a painful consequence of failed bone-marrow transplants, might cause an adolescent to refuse treatment.

It is the adolescent patient who benefits from, or endures the burdens of, medical treatment or refusal. Parents and physicians have every right to discuss the adolescent's medical needs and help them appreciate the treatment options, the possible consequences of treatment, or refusal. But the decisions of competent adolescents should not be usurped or ignored by parents or physicians. Even if parents have a legal right to override an adolescent's preferences, that power should not undermine respect for adolescents as persons, their personal autonomy, and their control over their minds and bodies. If adolescents, parents, and physicians mutually agree, and the adolescents participate in the decisions, they are more likely to comply willingly with the treatment plan or accept the consequences of refusal. Especially in situations where treatment is painful and causes suffering, it is essential to remember whose mind and body directly experiences pain and suffering. Pain and suffering can be endured or accepted if a person has made his or her own choice rather than having a decision made unnecessarily or even unwisely by others. Parents and physicians may have the duty and right to act in adolescents' best interests, but parents and physicians may not always be the best judge of best interests.

Another situation where an adolescent's right to refuse treatment should be taken seriously concerns mental healthcare. In US law, parents of adolescents are generally permitted to seek mental-health treatment for their children or even admit them to a psychiatric facility against their will. Suppose an adolescent is clinically depressed but not suicidal; nevertheless, the parents want to hospitalize their child. Some states, such as California (In Re Roger S., 141 Cal. Rptr. 298, 1977), give adolescents between the age of 14 and 18 a right to judicial hearing if they object to hospitalization. I would go further. A competent adolescent should have the right to refuse institutionalization in a psychiatric hospital unless they are dangerous to themselves or others. Even if mental-health treatment is necessary, adolescents should have a right to less restrictive alternatives that are available, such as outpatient care. Parents should not have the unilateral authority to make such significant mental-health treatment decisions.

What if parents of obese children decide that some form of weight loss surgery is in their child's best interests? And the parents have found a surgeon who agrees with the surgical treatment? Obesity may be a health problem, but it does not mean that obese adolescents are incompetent (Farmer, 2012). Competent adolescents should be permitted to refuse surgery in favor of a less invasive approach to weight loss. It is particularly important that adolescents not be coerced into enduring a treatment that imposes physical and psychological risks that they prefer not to take.

These examples are drawn from situations in which a court might invoke the mature mirror exception to the general legal rule that minors are presumed to be legally incompetent to consent to or refuse medical treatment. I have presented moral rather than legal reasons why adolescents as patients should be treated with respect and, if competent, the same as adults. Although similar to the mature-minor legal doctrine, my position rests also on the principle of respect for persons, personal autonomy, and control over access to persons' body and mind. I have argued that both informed consent to and refusal of treatment should be respected if adolescents are competent. I think, however, that there are relatively few situations in which a competent adolescent is likely to refuse effective treatment recommended by a physician.

I want to make it clear that I am not suggesting that parents and physicians should automatically accept a refusal of treatment from a competent adolescent. Parents and physicians should reason and negotiate with an adolescent who wants to refuse treatment. It is important for adolescents to participate fully in the discussions about treatment and to explore both their reasons and emotions related to the treatment. Sometimes refusal of treatment by adolescents (or adults) is premature, based on mistaken beliefs, or a result of miscommunication. But it is also important for parents and physicians, in the treatment refusal situations described above, to understand and appreciate the reasons that support an adolescent's refusal. Sometimes it is in the best interests of the adolescents whose minds, bodies, or lives are at risk to make their own decisions.

References

Albert, D., & Steinberg, L. (2011). Judgment and decision making in adolescence. *Journal of Research on Adolescence, 21*, 211–224.

Beauchamp, T., & Childress, J. (1979/2009). *Principles of biomedical ethics*. Oxford: Oxford University Press.

BMA (British Medical Association). (2011). *Assessment of mental capacity: A practical guide for doctors and lawyers*. London: BMA House.

BMD (*Black's Medical Dictionary*). (2009). *Black's medical dictionary*. London A&C Black.

Buchanan, A., & Brock, D. (1990). *Deciding for others: The ethics of surrogate decision making*. Cambridge: Cambridge University Press.

Carbonneau, A. (2003). *Ethical issues and the religious and historical basis for the objection of Jehovah's Witnesses to blood transfusion therapy*. London: Edwin Mellen Press.

Checkland, D. (2001). On risk and decisional capacity. *Journal of Medicine and Philosophy, 26*, 35–59.

Farmer, (2012). Obesity surgery in children—Too much, too soon! *Education.com*. Retrieved from: http://www.education.com/reference/article/obesity-surgery-children/

Geller, J., & Stanley, J. (2005). Outpatient commitment debate: Settling the doubts about the constitutionality of outpatient commitment. *New England Journal on Criminal and Civil Confinement, 31*, 127–138.

Grisso, T., & Appelbaum, P. (1998). *The assessment of decision-making capacity: A guide for physicians and other health professionals*. Oxford: Oxford University Press.

Haga, C. (2011). Grand Forks girl dies of cancer dies one week after public celebration of her life. *Grand Forks Herald*, January 25. Retrieved from: http://www.parkrapidsenterprise.com/event/article/id/26978/

Jonas, M. (2007). Competence to consent. In R. Ashcroft, A. Dawson, H. Draper, & J. MacMillan (Eds.), *Principles of healthcare ethics* (pp. 255–262). Chichester, UK: Wiley.

Kim, S. (2010). *Evaluation of capacity to consent to treatment and research*. Oxford: Oxford University Press.

Kuther, T. (2003). Medical decision-making and minors: Issues of consent and assent. *Adolescence, 38*, 343–358.

Ladd, R., & Forman, E. (1995). Adolescent decision-making: Giving weight to age-specific values. *Theoretical Medicine and Bioethics, 16*, 333–345.

O'Connor, C. (2009). What rights do minors have to refuse medical treatment? *The Journal of Lancaster General Hospital, 4*, 63–65.

Sarkar, S. (2011). In the twilight zone: Adolescent capacity in the criminal justice arena. *Advances in Psychiatric Treatment, 17*, 5–11.

TN (Transplant News). (1994). Florida Court allows teenager to stop taking immunosuppressive drugs. *Transplant News*, June 30. Retrieved from: http://www.highbeam.com/doc/1G1-44799374.html

USDH (United States Department of Health). (2009). *Reference guide to consent for examination or treatment*. Retrieved from: http://www.dh.gov.uk/en/Publicationsandstatistics/Publications/PublicationsPolicyAndGuidance/DH_103643

Wicclair, M. (1999). The continuing debate over risk-related standards of competence. *Bioethics, 13*, 149–153.

Wilks, I. (1997). The debate over risk-related standards of competence. *Bioethics, 11*, 413–426.

Chapter Twelve

The Child Should Not Have the Right to Refuse Medical Treatment to Which the Child's Parents or Guardians Have Consented[1]

Catherine M. Brooks

In this chapter, I argue that the child, specifically the adolescent young person, should not have a right to refuse medical treatment to which the adolescent patient's parent has consented, particularly in matters that do not involve fundamental, constitutionally protected rights of the young patient. In consultation with the child patient, physicians and parents are presumed to act in the patient's best interest with mature, adult judgment that has not yet been attained by the patient. Where there is proof of the child's maturity and proof of the unreasonableness of the parent's choice of medical treatment, the law already provides remedies to the youthful patient. To impose on the *child*, without recourse to proofs of maturity, the right and corresponding responsibilities of medical decision-making place an unreasonable burden on her/him. Also, expansion of rights is also an expensive and inefficient use of court resources for resolution of the inevitable disagreements between young patients and their parents. Instead, the use of patient counseling by medical professionals to provide important guidance to children and adolescents and their parents can help to guide young patients toward understanding the information and the complexities of available medical treatment and the reasons for their parents' treatment choices.

Introduction

The child, specifically the adolescent young person, should not have a right to refuse medical treatment to which the adolescent patient's parent has consented, particularly in matters that do not involve fundamental, constitutionally protected rights of the young patient. The law does recognize the right of adolescent patients to make medical decisions in an important but limited number of circumstances, where the patient has proved maturity sufficient for the decision or where other governmental or community goals are met by allowing the adolescent patient independent access to physical- and mental-health services. To illustrate present law, several historic US Supreme Court cases are reviewed, showing the law's recognition of the parent's right to raise his or her child without undue intrusion from others or from the state itself. Allowing the adolescent child a right to counter a parent's medical consent does not fit within this jurisprudence, and

Contemporary Debates in Bioethics, First Edition. Edited by Arthur L. Caplan and Robert Arp.

good reasons exist for not expanding the existing medical decision-making rights of young persons to veto their parents' treatment choices. Where there is proof of the child's maturity and proof of the unreasonableness of the parent's choice of medical treatment, the law already provides remedies to the youthful patient. The mature minor doctrine and the rubric of the "emancipated minor" already confer rights in the child to make medical decisions autonomously when the child is deemed mature by a judge. To create greater legal rights in the child to refuse the care consented to by his or her parent is to place the parent in an unreasonable position of ongoing responsibility where his or her guidance carries no weight. To impose on the child, without recourse to proofs of maturity, the right and corresponding responsibilities of medical decision-making places an unreasonable burden on the child. To enlarge this remedy beyond the existing limits is to ignore the preparatory role of childhood and adolescence for a person's adult responsibilities. Expansion of rights is also an expensive and inefficient use of court resources for resolution of the inevitable disagreements between young patients and their parents. Instead, the use of patient counseling by medical professionals to provide important guidance to children and adolescents and their parents can help to guide young patients toward understanding the information and the complexities of available medical treatment and the reasons for their parents' treatment choices. In consultation with the child patient, physicians and parents are presumed to act in the patient's best interest with mature, adult judgment that has not yet been attained by the patient. Respect for the dignity of the young person is better met by the counseling component of medical interactions than by imposing the responsibility concomitant with the right to veto his or her parents' decisions.

Speaking the Language of Rights in the Vernacular of the Law

To understand the issue debated in this chapter, one must appreciate the legal import of the words comprising the title statement. Respecting the careful use of language paves the path to the law's best responses to human problems, and in our society, a discussion of rights is a discussion cast in jurisprudence, the culture of law that frames and supports the way we abide with one another. To proceed here, one must be equipped for an analysis that, at its heart, is the careful study of the language used in the discourse of this debate. It is in taking care to understand the precise language to be employed that overly broad, generalizing propositions may be avoided and unintended consequences may be limited. In paying attention to the words themselves, we may engage in a more nuanced discussion of the complexities of the issue presented in the title statement.

The words that will occupy the central focus of this chapter are, therefore, the words of the title: rights, child, parent, refuse, and consent. In understanding the context in which they exist in the law, the reader may come to understand the title statement as a rational conclusion, as it should be understood that the position and argument here are not blunt instruments used to undermine the dignity of the child or adolescent in medical decision-making. Rather, this discussion accounts for the dignity of the youthful patient who is the subject of medical care and the decision-making required in that care. It behooves the reader to understand the title statement as a conclusion that seeks to find a balance among the competing forces present in medical decision-making. Nuance and complexity quickly surface here, as in any address of rights in law that seeks to arrive at a conclusion based in rationality and logic.

The discussion begins with a foundation designed to allow analysis of the problem presented: The first section will address how the law recognizes medical decision-making in the family, particularly in the context of third-party conflicts when parents and the state disagree and when the parents and their child's medical care provider disagree. Analysis of the roles of parents and the state in family decision-making, as subjects of federal constitutional decisions and state action, takes into account the reasoning of the United States Supreme Court in the legal conclusions it has drawn. The second section addresses the law's concerns with decision-making capacity, particularly of children and adolescents who necessarily have less than fully adult capacity. Knowledge gained from the professional study of psychological, social, and neurological development of children and adolescents, including studies of adolescents in legal decision-making roles in juvenile court, will be examined for its application to children and adolescents in medical decision-making. Further, as the incapacities of childhood and adolescence are accommodated in law in a number of contexts, knowing the legal issues in medical care consent is fundamental to understanding the legal questions inherent in medical decision-making by children and adolescents. The third section addresses medical decision-making for and by children and adolescents that takes into account parents' roles, the law's expectations of medical practitioners, and the need for children and adolescents to have time to practice decision-making without being required to bear the legal and personal burden of errors in judgment. A third conflict scenario, when parents and their child disagree about medical care, is reserved for discussion in this section. The conclusion offers an alternative perspective on parental roles in medical decision-making in childhood and adolescence.

A Foundation in Law: The Child and the Parent

In order to understand the law's perspective on whether to recognize and enforce a child's rejection of a parent's medical care decision made on the child's behalf, it is necessary to look first at the cases the Court regards as the foundation for the parent's right to make the decision in the first place. Throughout the past century, the United States Supreme Court developed a body of law recognizing the rights of parents to act on their children's behalf without undue interference from others, including federal, state, and local governments, and related and unrelated other persons. There are four critical Supreme Court opinions to understand, as they comprise the foundation of the parent–child relationship in American law and provide the basis for any discussion of rights of parents to make medical decisions for their children.

In *Meyer v. Nebraska* (1923), the Court addressed the nature of legal protection to be afforded parents in raising their children when it was asked whether a parent could obtain instruction for a child in a language other than English in the face of a state statute banning non-English education for children who had not yet completed the eighth grade. In *Meyer*, a schoolteacher had used a German-language bible, with the apparent knowledge and permission of the child's parents, to instruct a 10-year-old boy in reading, a violation of the state's ban on educating younger children in any language other than English, Latin, Greek, or Hebrew (at 401). The Court analyzed the interest of the state, the state's method of giving effect to that interest through its statutory ban on education in modern foreign languages, and the interests of the parents in having their children educated in a manner they selected. The Court concluded that parents have a constitutionally protected liberty interest in raising their children and that the state had improperly intruded on parents' right to raise their children as those parents saw fit. The Court also acknowledged the power of the state to intrude when warranted to further the important, legally sound interests of the state, for example, exercising its parens patriae power to protect a child from a parent's harm. In *Meyer*, the state's interest in creating compulsory education was to produce a literate citizenry, capable of intelligent and voluntary choice, vital to an elected, representative government. In limiting the languages with which a parent might choose to provide that education to a child, the state went beyond what it could justify as necessary to effect its interest in a literate citizenry and intruded into the sphere of parents' liberty interest in making choices about how to raise their children.

Two years later, in *Pierce v. Society of Sisters of the Holy Names of Jesus and Mary and Hill Military Academy* (1925), the Court was again asked about parents' rights to make decisions for their children without state intrusion. The question in *Pierce* was whether a state could limit a parent's right to make decisions about where the child's education took place. Oregon had enacted a law requiring that compliance with the state's compulsory education law could only be met by attendance at a state-created and state-funded public school. The Court did not disturb the compulsory education law, as it furthered the state's legitimate interest in creating a literate, competent citizenry, but it did rule that the place of education could not be so limited by the state as to deny parents the right to educate their children in privately supported institutions, provided those private schools met the requirements of the curriculum established by the state.

In 1944, the issue of parents disregarding a state law enacted to protect children from danger while at work was presented in a third case, *Prince v. Massachusetts* (1944). In *Prince*, a person standing in the place of a child's parent, in loco parentis, had allowed her young niece to distribute religious tracts one evening at a place on the street where the aunt could watch her. The canvas sack hanging from the niece's shoulder held the pamphlets she was distributing and bore a printed notice on its side that "The Watchtower" could be purchased for five cents. The state charged these words brought the girl's activity under the control of a law protecting newsboys from working on the street in the evening. The aunt, when prosecuted for the law violation, argued the child's activity was protected religious speech, falling under the rights of free exercise afforded by the first amendment to the US Constitution. The Supreme Court addressed the state's interest in the safety of the children within its borders, under parens patriae potentas, and found the state's interest took priority over the religious practice in which the aunt and her niece were engaged. Observing that "parents may be free to become martyrs themselves" (at 170), the Court held that parents could not make martyrs of their children "before they have reached the age of full and legal discretion when they can make that choice for themselves." (Id.) *Prince* has long since been held up as the legal precedent for denying parents the authority to impose religious and other practices on their child to the detriment of their child's health and well-being.

A fourth case, *Parham v. J.R. and J.L. et alia* (1979), gave the Court an opportunity to address directly the decision-making power of parents in seeking medical care for their children. In *Parham*, the plaintiffs were children in the State of Georgia who were committed to medical institutions for the treatment of mental illness and behavioral disorders, including J.L., committed by his parent, and another boy, J.R., committed by the state's Department of Family and Children Services, acting in loco parentis on behalf of its ward. The plaintiffs also included all children similarly situated as patients committed to mental-health institutions in Georgia. On behalf of this class of young plaintiffs, lawyers argued that the children who were at risk of losing their liberty by institutionalization for mental illness should be entitled to access to the legal procedures protecting adults from unwanted, unnecessary commitments. The Court was not persuaded of the need for legal procedure in addition to what already existed, namely, review of a parent's request that a child be committed to an institution for treatment of mental illness by the superintendent physician at the hospital to which the child would be committed, with subsequent reviews by that physician of the need for continued confinement.

In rejecting additional safeguards for the child patient, the Court found "the natural bonds of affection" (at 602, quoting Blackstone) that parents have for their children and the likelihood that parents act in their children's best interests in making decisions about their medical care were sufficient to protect a child from unnecessary institutionalization. Emphasizing the medical nature of the decision being made, the Court also relied on the professional consideration provided by the superintendent physician. What the Court did not address were the difficult cases of a child who was inadequately supported by a system of foster care and other placements, a state office where caseworkers might be overburdened by caseload responsibilities, and a physician whose information was less than comprehensive. What little is known about the two named plaintiffs, J.R. and J.L., provides enough information to know that neither child would have been particularly easy to care for at home or in stranger-care settings of foster homes and that recourse to institutionalization suited the needs of the adults involved. What is not known is whether the boys' indefinite commitments were necessary or merely convenient: J.R., removed from his home as an infant to protect him from neglect and moved through seven foster placements, was placed at Georgia's Central State Hospital indefinitely because the state had "nowhere else to place him."

Parham has come to stand for its legal conclusions that not only do parents have the right to raise their children as they see fit, free from undue state intrusion, but also that parents are presumed in law to act in their children's best interest in making medical-care decisions. The Court also did not address the quality of decision-making that should be standardized, beyond the professional opinion of the reviewing physician. Any concerns about the quality or quantity of information available to the reviewing physician on which to base the decision about a child's care were left to the physician.

Such deference is not to say, though, that parents are free of limitations in their medical decision-making about their children. Every state has statutory safeguards to protect children from harm and neglect by their parents or by those standing in a parent's place, including harms arising from parents withholding medical care for a child who needs medical intervention. Cases of medical neglect range from parents withholding standard medical care, because of their own religious beliefs, to instances where parents seek nonstandard interventions that are challenged or disavowed by a medical provider on behalf of the child patient.

Other limitations on parental medical decision-making arise from the nature of the medical issue the child presents. A number of states have statutes allowing medical decisions by minors for particular medical conditions or services without the knowledge or consent of their parents, including statutes allowing medical consent by minors for sexually transmitted diseases, reproductive contraception, and drug and alcohol treatment. The statutes allow medical providers to accept a minor's consent to treatment as if that consent were given by an adult. The minor's maturity for medical consent is presumed; no recourse to parents or persons acting in loco parentis is needed. The state's interest in promoting treatment in these limited areas is considered superior to its concerns about the sufficiency of the minor patient's consent.

Another limitation on parents' participation in medical decision-making for their child occurs when a minor seeks pre-natal care or a termination of her pregnancy. The Supreme Court has held that the adolescent (or near-adolescent) girl's right to control her reproduction, once she is pregnant, is superior to the right of her parents to make decisions for her about her pregnancy. Many states require the pregnant girl to give notice to or gain consent from a parent before exercising her right to terminate a pregnancy. Where such notice or consent requirements exist, the Court has held that the pregnant girl must have alternate means to exercise her right to reproductive control. Thus, the pregnant girl may circumvent the state's notice or consent requirements by seeking a confidential court ruling that she is sufficiently mature to choose to terminate her pregnancy without parental involvement. In these "bypass" judicial procedures, the pregnant girl must prove to a judge that she is mature enough to make decisions about her pregnancy without her parents' assistance. When she cannot make the case for her maturity, the judge may decide nonetheless that termination of the pregnancy is in her best interests after hearing evidence about her situation. Cases in which a pregnant girl, seeking an abortion, is subject to abuse by one or both of her parents provide clear illustrations of instances where a judge could find termination of the pregnancy to be in her best interests. (Evidence of child abuse or neglect coming to the court's attention will result in allegations of abuse or neglect being reported to the local state social-service agency.)

In sum, the law recognizes in parents the right to raise their child without intrusion from the state, absent an important reason of state purpose for that intrusion. Medical decision-making by the parent on behalf of a child is presumed to be in the child's best interest; that presumption, however, can be rebutted by contrary evidence. Under circumstances where the state's interest rests in removing obstacles to treatment, as in drug and alcohol rehabilitation or medical responses to sexually transmitted diseases, many states allow the minor patient to consent to treatment as if she or he were an adult. In the particular case of pregnancy, the pregnant girl makes decisions about her pregnancy as if she were an adult, except in those state jurisdictions where there is a statutory requirement that she provide notice to or seek consent from a parent; in states requiring parental involvement, there must be provision for an alternate, judicial procedure whereby the girl may prove her maturity sufficient to avoid parental involvement or that her circumstances warrant the abortion without parental involvement for good cause shown to the court. These case-by-case decisions about a girl's maturity serve as a counterpoint to the general rule that a person who has not achieved adulthood is not mature enough, in law, to make medical decisions on her or his own. Maturity, a quality of consent required for legally binding decisions, is considered below.

The Law, Psychology, and Neurology: Consent and Refusal to Consent, or Dissent

The law has a long history addressing the question of consent: when it is required, what makes it sufficient, what the consequences of its absence or its insufficiency are, and who bears the risk of its absence or insufficiency. In medical care, the requirement that a person consent to any treatment upon him- or herself follows the common law rule that a person has a right to be undisturbed in his or her physical self and that an unconsented touching may be grounds for recompense in law. Unconsented touching is commonly known as a battery, regardless of the degree or form of harm suffered. To qualify as a true consent, the consent must be knowingly given; it must be based on the fullest information available about the contact and its consequences. Further, the consent must be intelligently and voluntarily given.

In deciding the sufficiency of the consent given, courts examine the quality and thoroughness of the information provided to the patient by the medical provider about the contact—the medical treatment—and its known and knowable consequences. Courts also consider the ability of the patient to make a valid consent, to understand the information that has been given. The ability of the legally adult patient to make decisions on his or her own behalf is so well established that it is presumed in law; it does not need to be proved to allow the adult patient's decision-making—but its absence may be shown to suspend the adult patient's right to make decisions. Absent information suggesting an impaired ability to make rational judgments that the medical care provider could determine from the circumstances of the adult patient, the law allows the provider to rely on the autonomy of the adult patient to make decisions of self-determination. It is the accepted autonomy of the adult patient that frees the provider from the task of assessing the capacity of the adult patient who gives no sign of impairment to make the decision to give consent. Autonomy is the hallmark of adulthood in our jurisprudence: The adult person is self-determining.

Persons who have not yet reached adulthood are considered to be under a legal disability that disqualifies them from self-determining autonomy. That legal disability also affords them protection from inexperienced or otherwise faulty decision-making capacity, derived from their presumed inability to appreciate sufficiently and to consider with full adult intelligence the complete range of consequences of their decisions, thus making them unable to consent knowingly to those otherwise legally binding consequences.

Even adult patients, though, having received the fullest information available about medical treatment from the medical care provider, may be subject to influences that make consent less than voluntary. Those influences can be overt; for example, a patient may defer to the concern of a spouse who places emphasis on the financial implications of the procedure while the patient emphasizes the physical-health benefits to be gained. Or they may be subtle: A patient may know from experience that the person financially responsible for the cost of the medical procedure resists the expenditure of funds for healthcare and so defers to unspoken pressure, declining medical care. Pressures experienced by the patient detract from his or her ability to consent or refuse voluntarily. Where one is dependent upon someone else for payment of medical care costs, consent to or refusal of treatment from the patient may not be as voluntary as it appears. The law accepts the likelihood that adult decision-makers take nonmedical factors and the concerns of others into account in accepting or rejecting treatment and that the autonomy of adulthood includes the right to discern what weight to give such overt and subtle influences. However, the law protects the vulnerable adult who is unable to resist the imposition of improper influence of others on the patient.

When a medical-care provider or other involved person alleges that an adult is subjected to undue pressure in medical or other decision-making, the vulnerable adult's decisions will be assessed for their voluntariness. If a court finds that voluntariness is lacking, the improperly influenced decisions will be set aside; the person exerting undue influence will be removed from proximity to the vulnerable adult; and the vulnerable adult may also be provided with someone who will act in his or her interest to assist in making decisions. Of course, the problem of timely discovery of the improper influence is always present. Once discovered, the legal process can be expedited to address the issue of possible harm to the patient quickly. Matters involving children are often expedited in the courts, with priority given to them before other calendared cases. The question of maturity of the pregnant teen is one that is often heard almost immediately upon the filing of the case.

The law protects the patient from the unreasonable influence of the medical provider, by finding liability in that provider for unreasonable pressure on the patient to act in one way or another. The ethics of medical practice also underscore the need for the doctor to support the patient's decision-making free from manipulation by others outside the decision dyad of physician and patient, but within the sphere of the patient's daily life, influences amounting to manipulation may not be visible to the medical-care provider. Discerning those influences on a child or adolescent making a decision about his or her own medical care may be far more difficult. For the minor patient, there are additional considerations of dependence on near family members and the desire to meet their expectations, a not-unusual response of persons dependent upon those others who may be tempted to exert influence. With the minor patient, there is the additional consideration of payment for services when the decision-making minor is not the named holder of insurance coverage, cannot obtain insurance as a minor, and is left without a financial safety net for any decisions s/he would make in the absence of governmental social-security funds. For now, the discussion of dependence and the inability to pay for chosen medical services serves to underscore the issue of others' influence on the minor patient's decisions about medical care. As with other components of legal consent, social-science research has brought fresh understanding to the lesser ability of the child and adolescent to withstand the pressures from others who would influence decision-making.

Much has been learned in the last quarter century from social-science research, particularly in the areas of developmental psychology about the progress of the person, through childhood and adolescence, in acquiring the skill and understanding necessary for mature decision-making, required in law for valid consent. Under the auspices of the MacArthur Foundation, prominent social-science investigators and research psychologists engaged in extensive studies of the decision-making capacities of juveniles and young adults (11–24 years old). While the target of the research was an exploration of the competence of adolescents to participate in legal procedures adjudicating charges against them, the research and its conclusions are instructive in the debate here about medical decision-making. In medicine and law, the quality of a young person's participation is dependent upon an ability to interpret accurately the factual basis upon which decisions are to be made, to decide rationally after that information has been given by the professional provider—of either legal or medical services—what the preferred goals are, and finally to accept the consequences, known and unknown at the time of the decision, of the path decided upon by the client or patient, in consultation with the professional provider.

Discussion of minor patients' medical decision-making can benefit from the investigation into the decision-making of minor clients within the legal system, particularly in the juvenile courts. Extensive research into how minor clients participate in those legal processes serves to illustrate the issues in the present discussion. In law, the lawyer is responsible for choosing the strategies by which a client's goals are to be achieved, while the goals of the legal service are for the client to decide. The means by which the client decides upon the goals to pursue or to put aside is a counseling process in which the lawyer takes on the roles of teacher and translator. The success of the client counseling process is dependent upon both the lawyer's ability to communicate the information the client needs and the ability of the client to understand and act on—make decisions based on—the information offered by the lawyer. The client's ability to understand the lawyer is repeatedly assessed by the lawyer so the lawyer is assured the client grasps what is needed for rational decision-making. The issue of rational decisions is based not only on the client's appreciation of the facts provided by the lawyer, but also on the client's capacity to understand and act in a mature, intelligent way. The client will have to postpone gratification (e.g., a resolution of distressing uncertainty), comprehend his or her role in the outcome (e.g., the decision to accept or reject a plea agreement belongs to the client; it is not the defense lawyer's decision to make), tolerate the likelihood that not all outcomes can be identified in advance, and grasp the agency nature of the lawyer in the lawyer–client relationship. Each aspect of the legal decision-making process for the client has an analogue in the medical decision-making process for the patient. Both situations present issues of stress in which help is sought from a professional for the resolution of a problem. Both situations involve a language and processes outside the common experience of the layperson. Yet navigation of each requires the principal, client or patient, to bear personally the results of the decisions made and to accept those outcomes in advance, often without the benefit of prior experience. Understanding the extent to which a young person's linguistic and cognitive skills have developed and can be used in choosing among outcomes was significant in the recommendations that emerged from the research conducted under the auspices of the MacArthur Foundation.

The MacArthur Foundation research project involved investigation of the competence of young clients as participants in the decisions necessary to legal representation. Its findings are valuably instructive: Impulsive, sensation-seeking, risk preference behaviors all improve with increased age in adolescence; preference for risk peaks at ages 16–17 years and then decreases into early adulthood; impulsivity decreases from a high at 10–11 years through early adulthood; sensation-seeking decreases from 12 to 13 years through early adulthood as well. Conversely, the amount of time given to thought before taking action (deliberating for an outcome), directing one's thinking towards the future (evidence of understanding the longitudinal nature of outcomes), and the ability to delay gratification (experiencing the outcome) all improve with increasing age into early adulthood.

Neuroscience studies of the brain's development through childhood and adolescence (Giedd *et al.*, 1999) provide support for the MacArthur findings: The traits of the maturing person have counterparts in the maturing brain. The more emotionally based decisions of childhood and early adolescence, evidenced by MRI brain studies, give way to the more rationally based decisions of late adolescence and early adulthood, also evidenced in MRI brain studies. Increased communication circuitry between the hemispheres, a characteristic of the more mature brain, allows greater, faster access to more data stored in the brain that the "jury" processes of the brain can use in decision-making. (Id.) The logic of withholding the responsibilities of decision-making until the person reaches adulthood is highlighted by the knowledge offered by this research into the structural development of the human brain.

The Right to Decide: Consent and the Refusal of Consent

The law's treatment of decision-making in adolescence, well described by Scott and Grisso (2005), comprises a variety of approaches, two of which focus on the type of medical condition: For some medical decisions where a public-health interest of the state is involved, the minor is treated as fully adult, capable of consenting to treatment; for medical decisions involving pregnancy where the state has legislated a requirement of notice to or consent by a parent prior to their daughter terminating her pregnancy, the minor is treated as an adult upon proof of maturity. For all other medical decisions, there is no clear policy in law allowing minor patients to act on their own behalf by consenting to or refusing medical care. There are a number of instances where courts have addressed the question of whether a minor's consent to treatment—or refusal to consent—will be given legal effect, but no single line of responses points to the development of national policy. In one instance where a minor refused treatment to which a parent had consented, the question before the court was whether a minor could be forced to abort a pregnancy solely on the consent to treatment by her parents (*In re Smith*, 1972). The court, vindicating the girl's right to reproductive self-determination, allowed the girl's refusal to consent to control the outcome.

Absent the issue of pregnancy, there are few reported cases in which the minor patient is deemed in charge of his or her medical care. One of those cases involved a refusal to accept treatment by an adolescent close to adult age (*In re E.G.*, 1989). Her desire not to be treated in a way that violated her religious beliefs was resisted by the treating physician; the refusal, in her case, to accept blood products of another person, meant her death would be imminent or her ability to live independent of invasive medical support would be severely compromised. Because she was able to persuade the court of her maturity in making the decision to refuse blood products, and because she was close to the age of adulthood at the time of the court's decision, the minor patient was able to defeat her physician's petition to provide medical services against her will. (E.G. was an adult by the time the case reached the appellate court, but the case was heard nonetheless because of the importance the court placed on vindicating the young woman's refusal of treatment.) Because she was supported in her decision by her parent, the court was not required to rule against a parent in allowing the minor patient to choose death over medical care. The case illustrates the exception in law known as the mature-minor doctrine, discussed by Professor Walter Wadlington in his seminal article in 1973, in which the categorical, age-based consent rule gives way to the minor patient's desire to control his or her medical treatment when that minor patient can demonstrate to a judge the necessary maturity for medical decision-making and good cause for the parent to be overruled (Wadlington, 1973).

A second set of mature-minor cases exists under the rubric of the "emancipated minor." Emancipation ordinarily occurs at the age of majority, freeing a person from the constraints imposed by parents and freeing the parents from the duty to support their child. Other emancipating events in an adolescent's life may occur prior to majority age, with the permission of a parent, such as military-service enlistment and marriage. Also, an adolescent may petition the court for an order of emancipation when his or her parent does not consent to emancipation before majority age. Events emancipating an adolescent are deemed to be proof of the person's maturity, and medical decision-making that follows emancipation is legally binding, as if made by an adult. Thus, the emancipated minor is a person who, though below the age of adulthood, is deemed legally responsible for him- or herself in medical decision-making, payment for medical services, and all other aspects of life.

In every discussion of legal rights, including this one on medical decision-making, there is the premise of responsibility. To be autonomous and self-determining, one must be able to take responsibility for the outcomes—to oneself and others—created by one's acts of will. In not recognizing a minor's right to decide medical care, the law protects that minor patient from bearing liability for the consequences of those decisions—financially, physically, and psychologically. Inevitably, any decision can result in unintended, unwanted outcomes. The burden of choosing in the face of risking an unsatisfactory outcome is a necessary component of exercising consent in medicine. Ideally, the parent who makes medical choices on behalf of his or her child does so in light of life experiences, including the experience gained in caring for the child; the parent acts with the advice of the medical professional providing the care; and the parent is aware of and takes all possible precautions to prevent unwanted outcomes. The parent follows through with the child's care afterwards to maximize the desired outcomes and serves as an important component of the medical procedure, upon whom the medical provider depends as a channel for information flowing from and to the patient. When the parent is removed from the care of the minor patient—because the parent's choice of care has been vetoed by the child—a similarly informed and informative substitute is not available to provide what a parent gives the minor patient.

Conclusion: Respecting Childhood and Adolescence

The title of this debate, "The child should not have the right to refuse medical treatment to which the child's parent has consented," is a statement made in the reality of an imperfect world where inadequate information and resources co-exist with an evolving science of medicine and an incomplete understanding of the developing human cognitive, emotional, and rational capacities to comprehend the full vista of medical and personal outcomes. The creation of a right for children, with legal import, must be considered in the context of the law's recognition of existing rights and responsibilities within the family. In recognizing parents' rights to raise their children without undue intrusions, the law imposes responsibility on parents to provide for the health and well-being of their children. The parental duty of support, long recognized in American jurisprudence, requires the parent to provide and to pay the obligations incurred for the necessary medical care of the child. The common law "doctrine of necessaries" demands the parent to be responsible for payment to third parties who provide the necessities of life, including medical care, to a child. When parents fail to provide necessary medical care for their children, they are subject to civil and criminal neglect statutes. When they attempt to provide care, and their child refuses it, parents are required to overcome their children's resistance without causing harm to the child. And when parents seek to impose medical decisions that are not supported by the medical profession, those parents' choices are subject to being overruled by the court, upon application of the dissenting medical-care provider.

Parents may even be removed from their parenting role in their child's medical care because of their *own* wrongdoing in medical decision-making. In those instances, the state provides substitute care and remains liable for any inadequacies in that substitute care. Parents may be removed from the medical treatment of their child because their medical-care choices do not comport with the prevailing medical advice or practices in the community at that point in time. Again, in those instances, the state provides substitute care and remains liable to the child patient for inadequacies in that substitute care. However, when the parent is removed by the child patient's choice, not because of any wrongdoing or lapse by the parent, there is no provision in law for substitute care; nor does the law provide a parental legal duty to pay for the alternatives chosen by the child patient.

Most importantly, the law allows for childhood and adolescence to be a time of learning; it protects the child and adolescent from the full impact of their choices in most instances and provides the minor the time necessary to practice the skills, gain the experience, and allow the growth and development of the physical self—including the brain as it continues to develop through adolescence—in preparation for the requirements of adulthood. Medical decision-making is a learned skill, requiring the attributes of the mature person; it requires information, practice, and the qualities of full consent. Adolescence is the time during which one acquires those qualities, learns to apply what is learned, and gains experience in what not to do as well as what to do. Today, the law protects that time of preparation, but not unreasonably so. The law allows for the exercise of decision-making in limited spheres, where the balance is struck in favor of public health, reproductive rights, and proven maturity, as against the risk of error and the burden of unwanted, unintended outcomes, but outcomes often foreseeable to the adult decision-maker.

To create a legal right in the child to refuse the care consented to by his or her parent is to place the parent in an unreasonable position of ongoing responsibility where his or her guidance carries no weight. To impose on the child, without recourse to proofs of maturity, the right and corresponding responsibilities of medical decision-making is to place an unreasonable burden on the child. Where there is proof of a child's maturity and proof of the unreasonableness of the parent's choice of medical treatment, the law already provides remedy to the minor patient. To enlarge this remedy beyond these limits is to ignore the preparatory role of childhood and adolescence for a person's adult responsibilities.

Note

1 Professor Brooks is grateful to her research assistants, Ryan D. Portwood, class of 2011, and Lillian A. Rehrmann, class of 2012, for their able assistance in the preparation of this chapter, and to Elizabeth A. Brooks, Ph.D., for her careful reading and valuable comments.

References

Giedd, J. N., Blumenthal, J., Jeffries, N. O., Castellanos, F. X., Liu, H., Zijdenbos, A., …, & Rapoport, J. L. (1999). Brain development during childhood and adolescence: A longitudinal MRI study. *Nature Neuroscience, 2*, 861–862.

In re E. G. (1989). 133 Ill.2d 98, 139 Ill. Dec. 810, 549 N.E.2d 322 (Illinois Supreme Court).

In re Smith (1972). 16 Md.App. 209, 295 A.2d 238 (Maryland Court of Appeals).

Meyer v. Nebraska (1923). 262 US 390.

Parham v. J. R. & J. L. (1979). 442 US 584.

Pierce v. Society of Sisters of the Holy Names of Jesus and Mary and Hill Military Academy (1925). 268 US 510.

Prince v. Massachusetts (1944). 321 US 158.

Scott, E. S., & Grisso, T. (2005). Developmental incompetence, due process, and juvenile justice policy. *North Carolina Law Review, 83*, 793.

Wadlington, W. (1973). Minors and health care: The age of medical consent. *Osgoode Hall Law Journal, 11*, 115.

Reply to Brooks

William J. Winslade

Professor Catherine Brooks has carefully and cogently described many of the legal rights and duties of parents towards their children. She reviews States Supreme Court cases that restrict the state's power to intrude upon parents' rights to educate and raise their children in accordance with family and religious value.

But the state may intervene to protect the safety of children. It is important to note that these cases protect parents and families from state intrusions. None of these cases shed any light, however, on the rights of children. What if a child does not want to learn German or attend a parochial or private, rather than public, school? Should children have a right to participate in key decisions affecting their personal, educational, and social life? Of course, many parents do consider their children's preferences. But the law gives parents virtually exclusive authority to make these decisions. Perhaps it is time to reconsider the rights of children to challenge their parents' legal authority or at least to recognize that children have a right not only to voice their preferences, but to assent, if not consent, to such significant decisions. The law addresses only parents' rights on the presumption that they will act in the best interests of their children. I submit that parents, like physicians, should show respect for their children as persons by treating them in a respectful manner and giving due regard for the preferences of a competent child and the reasons that support them. But the law intervenes only when parents neglect, abuse, or compromise the safety of their children.

In the one Supreme Court case dealing with medical decisions for children, once again the parents and the health professionals make the decisions. While this is reasonable in the care of very young children, adolescents should have a right to challenge and seek judicial review of their parents and professionals decisions about psychiatric hospitalization as the California Supreme Court ruled in *Landeros v. Flood* (1976).

As Professor Brooks points out, adolescents do have some rights to make their own intensely personal decisions about their bodies with regard to sexually transmitted diseases, reproductive contraception, drug treatment, and pregnancy. What I have argued is that we should respect adolescents as persons by including them in all medical decisions that affect their own bodies. Adolescents, even many incompetent adolescents, can participate meaningfully in the medical decisions affecting their bodies. Even if, in most medical situations, parents and adolescent children agree about recommended medical care, the adolescent should be a participant in the consent process for both moral and practical reasons. The law presumes too much about the rights of parents and the wisdom of professionals, and overlooks the rights of adolescents to be treated with respect. The law also

Contemporary Debates in Bioethics, First Edition. Edited by Arthur L. Caplan and Robert Arp.

does not provide any guidance about the manner in which adolescents should be treated to maximize the benefits and to endure the burdens of treatment. I have argued that, as a practical manner, the more adolescents are participants in making medical decisions about their bodies, the more likely it is that adolescents will trust their physicians and accept their parents' decisions. Adolescents who are treated as mature participants are more likely to comply with a treatment program.

Professor Brooks rightly observes that the extent to which a young person has linguistic and cognitive skills significantly influences their ability to participate in legal decision-making in the juvenile courts. In addition, emotional maturity and capacity for rational choice are also key factors in assessing a person's ability to make their own decisions. Research about adolescents reveals that adolescents do have the capacity to consent to treatment in many contexts.

Research about adolescent brain development or personal maturity provides us with valuable general information. But it does not tell us about the cognitive or emotional maturity about any specific adolescent. My view is that each adolescent, like each adult, should be assessed for their level of development and competency in the context of the medical decisions regarding their bodies. Adolescents should not be presumed to be mature or immature-competent or incompetent. They should be evaluated in terms of their personal and specific capacities relevant to the particular medical issues affecting them.

The legal presumption that adolescents are incompetent to make their own medical decisions (in the absence of the specific exceptions mentioned by Professor Brooks and me) does a disservice not only to adolescents but also to the physician–patient relationship and the effectiveness of treatment. The law should not stipulate in advance how the adolescent–parent–physician relationship should be structured or implemented. My alternative proposal shifts attention away from general presumptions toward specific assessments. As I have already argued, this approach is morally preferable and practically desirable, and enhances, rather than undermines, parent–child relationships. Adolescents respected and treated as persons are more likely to act not only in their own but also in their parents' best interests.

Reply to Winslade

Catherine M. Brooks

In his fine piece, "The Right of An Adolescent to Refuse Medical Treatment," Doctor William Winslade begins with the premise that the proper focus of our discourse is on adolescence. We are in agreement that a discussion of medical decisions and creating medical decision-making rights in children before they have reached adolescence is not fruitful. Such a discussion, if based on the capacity to make decisions, would not progress far, given the young child's limited experience in the world, the limitations of the young brain to comprehend fully the consequences of allowing or disallowing a medical procedure or medication, and the limitations of the very young person to engage in voluntary decision-making and to be responsible for their decisions.

We both would suggest that young patients play important roles in their medical care, and acknowledgment of those roles by the young patient's medical caregivers and parents can lead to better delivery of care. Examples abound in the pediatric practice of doctors, nurse practitioners, nurses, and other medical professionals who, in gaining compliance from a child patient, are able to deliver care with less trauma, fear, and psychological stress for the child patient. Further, role-modeling ways to gain the child's compliance, rather than relying on the ordinary promises of rewards thought to be valued by the child, is an important teaching component that the medical professional provides for the parents and other caregivers of the child patient. Explaining a procedure in language the child can understand in advance of treatment, teaching the child about his or her role in the procedure in ways that acknowledge the dignity of the child patient and convey respect for the child's interest in accuracy, and providing an opportunity for the child to report afterwards on the experience of the procedure or prescribed medication to the medical provider are all valuable components of the relationship a medical professional has with the child patient. These interactions also give the child opportunities to realize and experience his or her own investment in the medical care outcomes and serve to teach the child about becoming a competent participant in his or her own medical care.

It is in his discussion of involving the adolescent in medical care—as a patient with dignity to be acknowledged and so respected—that Doctor Winslade excels in his argument. That involvement, however, is used to support a challenge to the way the law reserves full decision-making rights in the adult patient, which is cast as a deprivation of the adolescent's right to determine his or her medical care.

A second premise that is familiar to the law upon which Dr Winslade supports his argument is the use of the gradient approach to legal competency, as is the threshold approach (Winslade, p. 3); the former presents a staircase of increasing responsibility and a consequent increased recognition of rights while the

Contemporary Debates in Bioethics, First Edition. Edited by Arthur L. Caplan and Robert Arp.

latter can be described as a doorway to rights and responsibilities that the maturing person passes through at a particular age or event. In certain areas of medical care, the law's use of the gradient approach (e.g., the mature minor) is deemed necessary because of the stakes involved in a recognized fundamental right (e.g., reproductive care) or the proximity of the patient to adulthood where another fundamental right could be exercised (e.g., free exercise of religion). The gradient approach, when it requires individualized judicial approval of medical decision-making by adolescents, unfortunately, is a costly and inefficient use of the courts. It is, though, a reasonable component of a physician's counseling of an adolescent patient and his or her parents.

In his instructive discussion of adult rights in medical decision-making, Dr Winslade leads us to the heart of the issue at hand: Legal rights presuppose responsibilities from which the law protects that class of persons who may not yet be fully mature from the tasks of adulthood. Where the sufficiently mature adolescent patient is making a medical decision involving a right considered fundamental and therefore constitutionally protected, the courts are available to that patient whose parents or legal guardian are obstructing that minor patient's wishes. That such cases are not predominant in the courts may speak to the success of physicians counseling both patients and parents. Dr Winslade provides an excellent example of this more proper focus of decision-making counseling in his recounting the efforts undertaken at St. Jude Children's Hospital in Memphis, Tennessee.

The law's preference for the threshold approach is not limited to use at the bright line of majority age. Several events also serve as thresholds; beyond marrying and entering military service, which are emancipating events, for example, certain needs to seek diagnosis and treatment also create rights in the young person. Parental disagreement or even disapproval has led a number of states to extend limited consent rights to adolescents for drug and alcohol treatment as well as for diagnosis of and treatment for sexually transmitted diseases. These and other states also often extend consent rights to adolescents seeking treatment for mental-health issues.

The proposal, however, that "... adolescents should be assessed individually to determine their level of competence to make their own personal medical decisions" (Winslade, p. 8) is an impossibly expensive proposition for the legal system. While it is not clear from the language of the proposal that the courts should be the first forum for such an assessment, the assignment of the right and the plausible forecast of a parent's or a treating professional's disagreement when the right is exercised will involve the courts, at least as the last forum in the process of resolving the disputes that will arise.

Under the current legal system, an adolescent may ask for legal recognition of his or her maturity as sufficient to supplant parental involvement in a particular decision when a fundamental right is at stake in medical decision-making. Doctor Winslade's proposal would expand this practice to one in which the adolescent "... should be presumed to be neither competent nor incompetent. Instead, their level of competence should be assessed in the content of the specific medical context."

There is nothing in the law that prevents the medical professional from doing such assessments. In fact, the best practices endorsed by the authors of the MacArthur Foundation study of adolescent decision-making competence include such individualized assessments of juvenile court defendants. The MacArthur Foundation study recommends that the assessment results be used to guide the juvenile's lawyer in the lawyer–client relationship. In the medical sphere, a comparable use of the assessment should be a welcomed addition to pediatric practice.

The next step of creating a legally cognizable right to make one's own decisions, while a young person is still dependent upon his or her parents' care, not only places a costly demand on judicial and other legal resources to respond to disagreements between children and their parents but also creates an area of legal contention between parents and their children that is better resolved within the sphere of the teaching and counseling functions of the medical profession. A moving example of this perspective is offered by Dr Winslade in the story he tells, in the last section of his chapter, of the 14-year-old leukemia patient who asked for hospice care rather than chemotherapy. The physician, Dr Winslade relates, was instrumental in helping her parents come to accept her request. What would have been gained in this instance by resort to the courts when the dispute about treatment could be resolved with counseling from the child's physician? Had the parents continued to resist their daughter's wish to cease treatment despite the physician's counseling, the court would have been available to the young patient through her physician who believed the parents' treatment plan was unjustified. The doctor would have sought a judicial finding of medical neglect of the child, caused by the parents' insistence on fruitless, detrimental treatment of the child; the court would then have evaluated the doctor's assessment of the case—with reference to a court-appointed medical expert—and would have made a determination of whether the parents' were failing to act in their child's best interest. If the court so determines, a guardian is appointed by the court for the purpose of medical decision-making for the minor patient until the issue of medical treatment is no longer present or the minor patient is deemed sufficiently mature to make her own decisions or is emancipated.

Continued emphasis on the medical professional's relationship with the adolescent patient, and all pediatric patients, with its teaching and counseling components, is the right and worthy focus for developing a culture of respectful treatment of the minor patient's role in medical decision-making. Resolution of disputes that may arise between the parent and patient in the context of medical counseling—without resorting to the legal system—may prevent or at least de-escalate family suffering and a young patient's and parents' distress with one another. The medical professionals' involvement may prevent the parents and the young patient from becoming hard set into positions that have unwanted consequences wider and more profound than a discussion of children's rights might encompass. Keeping the decision about treatment in the context of medicine may allow the young patient and his or her parents to accept the hard truths they may face in the supportive and respectful presence of the medical professionals who are intimately involved in the family's process.

In sum, decisions about the treatment of young persons should be made in the environment of caring and well-informed medical professionals who are empathic and skilled at communicating with young patients. Legal protection for the young patient whose doctor and parents are aligned against his or her wishes is already available; the patient can access the courts through the state's protective services office and, once in court, must demonstrate the undesirability or ineffectiveness of the proposed treatment, compared to the alternative desired by the patient. The patient must demonstrate that his or her alternative is feasible, affordable, and effective to the standard used by the law to measure reasonable medical care in that community. For the young patient who wishes to continue treatment that the parents have decided to stop upon the physician's advice, the process would be essentially the same. He or she would need access to the courts and would have to prove that the decision to stop treatment was medically unreasonable, amounting to medical neglect; again, access would be gained through a telephone call to the local state social-services office.

According rights to adolescents in all instances of medical decision-making is likely to lead patients to the courts for resolution of cases where physician counseling and open communication among the doctor and patient and patient's parents would have been better used. Emphasizing the vindication of rights over the practice of good medical care-giving and counseling may not lead to better results for adolescent patients; it will surely, however, lead to delays in care-giving and increases in family stresses at a time when action based on competent, caring medical advice is needed.

Part 7
Is Physician-Assisted Suicide Ever Ethical?

Introduction

According to the Hippocratic Oath (ca. late 5th century, BCE)—an oath that virtually every medical student around the world takes—all doctors are supposed to ἐπὶ δηλήσει δὲ καὶ ἀδικίῃ εἴρξειν, that is, "refrain from doing harm." They are also to Δεν θα δώσω καμία θανάσιμη ιατρική σε οποιαδήποτε εάν ρωτιέται, ούτε προτείνω σε οποιαδήποτε τέτοιαδήποτε συμβουλή, that is, "give no deadly medicine to any one if asked, nor suggest any such counsel" (North, 2002). In fact, the American Medical Association's (AMA) Code of Medical Ethics (AMA, 2004) notes that the Oath "has remained in Western civilization as an expression of ideal conduct for the physician." Probably given that the Oath also asks doctors to "swear by the gods" and perform (or not perform) other antiquated and culture-specific things, it has been adjusted and modernized through the centuries (Orr et al., 1997; Rocca, 2008). Today, most medical schools in the US utilize some version of the Oath, and graduating med students are offered the option to swear by it (though, at many schools they need not do so). Still, it is likely the case that reciting the Oath is regarded by most med students as a kind of pro-forma ritual associated with upholding the tradition of the practice of medicine (Markel, 2004; Miles, 2004; Davis, 2011).

In 2008 at a University of Florida talk, Dr Jack Kevorkian noted that the Oath "wasn't discussed in medical school, and our class (University of Michigan, 1952) never took the oath. It isn't a medical oath; you pledge allegiance to all the gods and goddess, the pagan gods and goddesses of Greeks—what sense is that today?" He made the further point that the Oath was a "byproduct" of a sect of Pythagoreans that happened to be one of the only groups at that time (ca. late 5th century, BCE) opposed to a doctor helping a terminally ill patient end her/his life (Borghese, 2008). Kevorkian, like many other doctors and thinkers nowadays, had no use for the Oath, in direct opposition to those who continually appeal to it as the primary reason why physician-assisted suicide is immoral. Dr Hilary Evans (1997) is not alone in maintaining: "I personally oppose physician-assisted suicide on the ethical principles embodied in the Hippocratic Oath—'give no deadly medicine to any one if asked, nor suggest any such counsel'" (Kass, 1989; Hartmann

Contemporary Debates in Bioethics, First Edition. Edited by Arthur L. Caplan and Robert Arp.

& Meyerson, 1998). And US Congresspersons such as Asa Hutchinson have in the past appealed to the Oath as a basis for outlawing physician-assisted suicide (CR, 1999, pp. 270–273).

Obviously doctors are to refrain from doing harm, as they are devoted mainly to healing. But it is a matter of much debate as to whether the physician-assisted suicide of terminally ill patients either violates the no-harm principle part of the Oath (since death may be a welcomed relief) *or* should be sanctioned despite the "give no deadly medicine to any one if asked, nor suggest any such counsel" part of the Oath. Again, given that it is obviously antiquated and culture-specific in many respects, it seems wholly reasonable to many that the Oath should be interpreted as a guideline at best and modified as necessary according to an individual patient's need. Using the Oath as its basis, in 1957 the AMA outlined guidelines in its own Principles of Medical Ethics, which has been updated a number of times since then. The first of the nine principles reads: "A physician shall be dedicated to providing competent medical care, with compassion and respect for human dignity and rights" (AMA, 2001).

A name that has become virtually synonymous with physician-assisted suicide is Dr Jack Kevorkian, who died on June 3, 2011 at the age of 83. Kevorkian was a medical doctor with a specialty in pathology who is said to have assisted over 130 people with their own suicides using machines he designed and constructed like the Thanatron (named after the Greek god that personifies death, *Thanatos*). This was a device that allowed one to push a button that released deadly potassium chloride into one's body intravenously. He also built the Mercitron, a device that employed a gas mask that could be filled with carbon monoxide (Kevorkian, 1988; Roscoe et al., 2000; Dowbiggin, 2003; Nicol & Wylie, 2005; Schoifet, 2011). He was also referred to as "Dr Death," despite the fact that he repeatedly denied this moniker by claiming as he did in 2008: "My aim was not to cause death, that's crazy. My aim was to end suffering" (Borghese, 2008).

When Dr Kevorkian assisted in the suicide of Janet Adkins in 1990 with the Thanatron (his first assisted suicide), many utilized the "refrain from doing harm" and "give no deadly medicine to any one if asked" dictums from the Hippocratic Oath to condemn Kevorkian's actions. Kevorkian took things much further when he himself administered a lethal injection to Thomas Youk on September 17, 1998, and taped this homicide for later broadcast on national television. This act saddled him with a second-degree murder conviction and over 8 years of prison time (Johnson, 1999). Still, it has been argued that Kevorkian's lethal injection was a sympathetic action, along the lines of the Scottish doctor, John Gregory's, claim—made in the beginning of the nineteenth century—that a doctor, like any other human being, needs to have a "sensibility of heart which makes us feel for the distresses of our fellow creatures, and which, of consequence, incites in us the most powerful manner to relieve them" (Gregory, 1817, p. 22).

Due in part to the consciousness-raising actions of Kevorkian, in 1994 Oregon became the first US state—as well as one of the first places in the world—to permit physician-assisted suicide through the Oregon Death with Dignity Act (ORS 127.800-995). Washington followed suit with the Washington Death with Dignity Act (RCW 70.245) in 2008. In *Baxter v. Montana* (DA 09-0051, MT 449, 2009) on New Year's Eve in 2009, the Montana Supreme Court ruled that, "we find nothing in Montana Supreme Court precedent or Montana statutes indicating that physician aid in dying is against public policy," a ruling that effectively permits physician-assisted suicide in The Treasure State (Goldberg, 2011). Countries such as Canada, France, and Germany (there are others) have laws against assisted suicide of any form, while at present Belgium, Luxembourg, the Netherlands, and Switzerland permit physician-assisted suicide with various caveats (Humphry, 2011).

It is somewhat fascinating to note, however, that respecting a patient's request for a certain amount of pain-relieving drug (such as morphine), or allowing a patient to administer the pain-relieving drug to her/himself (at the push of a button, for example), *knowing* that the dosage will likely kill the patient not only appears to be a common practice all over the world (Quill et al., 1997; Fohr, 1998; Matzo & Schwarz, 2001; Schwarz, 2003), but also skirts the problem of the illegality and/or immorality of directly committing suicide or directly assisting in a suicide. Instead, one is either trying directly to stop the pain, or directly assisting one in trying to stop the pain by ingesting so much of the drug, with the unintended consequence, indirect result, or so-called *double effect* being that the person dies (Marquis, 1991; Garcia, 1995; Quill et al., 1997; Cavanaugh, 2006; Foster et al., 2011). A clear example of the sanctioning of this double effect can be found in the Australian Medical Association's Code of Ethics, where it is said of the dying patient that the physician should always: "Respect the right of a severely and terminally ill patient to receive treatment for pain and suffering, even when such therapy may shorten a patient's life" (AuMA, 2006, 1.4,c).

Interestingly enough, one of the strongest—if not, *the* strongest—arguments in favor of physician-assisted suicide can be grounded in the Hippocratic Oath's call for physicians to "refrain from doing harm." Many argue that the moral imperative to refrain from doing harm entails the moral imperatives "prevent harm" and "alleviate harm" as well (Snyder & Caplan, 2001). Stated simply and colloquially, you should not do harmful things; but you also should try to prevent harmful things from happening before they happen, as well as try to lessen, weaken, alleviate, diminish, mitigate, or remove harmful things that are in fact happening right now or have happened. In explicating the principle of beneficence, William Frankena (1973) argued that "One ought not to inflict evil or harm" includes "One ought to prevent evil or harm" and "One ought to remove evil or harm," and Tom Beauchamp and James Childress ratify this—with modifications—in their influential book, *Principles of Biomedical Ethics* (Beauchamp & Childress, 1979/2009, pp. 114–115).

The intuition is seen clearly when a dog owner has the veterinarian euthanize her beloved Fido, who is suffering from inoperable cancerous tumors all over his body, and lays around the house glassy eyed and listless when he is not urinating and defecating on himself, or hacking violently as a result of the great amount of pain medication in his system. Of course, Fido's owner wants to refrain from doing any harm to Fido by not kicking him, not starving him, not locking him outside on a freezing night, etc. And, of course, if she could have known about the first cancerous tumor next to his lung, she would have had it removed immediately, and Fido would have had a round of doggie chemo so as to try and prevent the cancer from spreading. But, by virtue of the fact that Fido's owner has made the decision to have Fido euthanized, rather than suffer the way he apparently is suffering for a few more days, weeks, or even months, Fido's owner thinks it is best to alleviate the harm being done to him in terms of his suffering. Apparently, in this case the (obvious) nonsuffering associated with Fido's death is the better alternative to the continued suffering associated with Fido's cancer, as this dog expert maintains: "the one thing you are able to do for your dog is alleviate undue pain and suffering. Arguably, no other decision you make about your dog will be as difficult as the one to euthanize, but in so many cases, it is the only humane option" (Dogtime, 2012).

The same "humane" intuition regarding ending Fido's life rather than letting him suffer can be applied to ending a human's life, too. Think of the now-cliché scene from some story in a book or movie where John Doe is incapacitated, in a lot of pain, and obviously going to die as a result of a stabbing, a gunshot, an explosion, being burned, or some other misfortunate experience, and he asks his friend, Jane Doe, to kill him. And then, somewhat reluctantly, Jane takes pity on an incapacitated John and ends his life as quickly and painlessly as possible, usually with another better-placed stabbing or gunshot to the heart or head. There are many who would argue that honoring John's wish to end his suffering is the right thing for Jane to do (Costello, 2005).

The first author in this section, John Lachs, shares the above intuition, noting, "we do not permit our animal companions to suffer: we ease them out of life with sorrow, painlessly. By contrast, we seem to take no pity on human beings, forcing them to live to the end, no matter how miserable they are. Visitors from another planet would find this a baffling and indefensible cruelty." He argues that a human life of value is one of "conscious and intelligent enjoyment," and if that enjoyment is no longer there—and especially if it is replaced with misery—then not only should suicide be an option, but *assisted* suicide should be an option for someone who is incapable of committing suicide. Lachs espouses a Mill-based utilitarian calculus as a sensible way to make such a difficult decision: if someone is miserable and wants to die, the people around that person are negatively affected by that person's misery, it is costing time and money to keep this person alive in misery, etc., then a suicide ends the misery and adds to the "net sum of good in the world."

Especially since Jeremy Bentham (1748–1832) and John Stuart Mill (1806–1873), utilitarians argue that an action is morally good insofar as its consequences promote the most "net sum of" good, beneficence, positivity, or pleasure for the most persons affected by the decision (Mill, 1859/2001; Pettit, 1993; Scarre, 1996). This view has been termed *utilitarian* because of the apparent usefulness to be found in generating such a huge amount of satisfaction for the group of persons (Driver, 2012). Part and parcel to utilitarianism has always been the idea that the "end" of bringing about good, beneficial, positive, or pleasurable consequences/results for the majority "justifies the means" or manner in bringing about those consequences/results, even if those means (a) violate some moral principle, or (b) create *minimal* evil, detrimental, negative, or painful consequences/results for the minority affected by the decision. So, if you need to tell a bald-faced lie (which is a violation of the moral principle, "One ought not lie") to the Nazis who have come to your door looking for the non-Aryan family you have hiding in your basement, then you are morally justified in doing so on utilitarian grounds. Also, you are morally justified in torturing the terrorist (creating *minimal* evil, detrimental, negative, or painful consequences/results, all things considered) to find out where he hid the bomb that will soon blow up the city, based upon utilitarian principles. Further, if we could rewind 20th-century history knowing that this history would play itself out exactly as it in fact did, there are strong utilitarian arguments in favor of executing Adolf Hitler, Josef Stalin, and Mao Tse-tung before they gained their megalomaniacal, murderous, and monstrous political momentums, which led to untold atrocities.

Lachs supports suicide and physician-assisted suicide based upon the utilitarian idea of the end justifying the means. In short, the *end* of stopping the suffering and gaining relief in death is a great good, beneficence, positivity, or pleasure for someone that *justifies the means* of utilizing suicide (or physician-assisted suicide) to achieve that great good. The second author in this section, Patrick Lee, essentially is diametrically opposed to this corollary of utilitarianism and argues that the end *should never* justify the means. The intrinsic value, worth, and dignity associated with human life are sacred and ought to be preserved at all costs—no matter what—such that even horrendous pain and suffering experienced by someone cannot justify suicide. In fact, Lee notes that those who claim that there can be death with dignity actually *undermine* their human dignity in the act of suicide: "to choose death to avoid indignities ... is to act against what has basic, intrinsic dignity for the sake of an ulterior end. But the end does not justify the means. Moreover, the very act of killing a person with the supposed justification that the one killed has lost her dignity, or is about to lose her dignity, denies the *intrinsic personal* dignity of the one killed." And further, Lee argues, death itself can be seen as the real loss of dignity—the "supreme indignity"—so we should be preserving our lives at all costs.

A point of debate between Lachs and Lee is one that has been going on since the dawn of utilitarianism, and it has to do with whether it is possible objectively and legitimately to assign weight and value to the pros and the cons associated with not only the *present state* of goods/pleasures and evils/pains surrounding events, but also the *future, expected* good/pleasurable or evil/painful consequences surrounding events. How do we measure psychological states like pleasure and pain, for example, which are by their very nature subjective phenomena? And, even though Bentham (1789/1988) himself claimed that it is not "expected" that a cost–benefit analysis "should be strictly pursued previously to every moral judgment" (p. 31), we still ask the question: how can we reliably forecast beneficial or detrimental consequences, when there are no crystal balls? And there are a whole host of other concerns regarding present and future consequences (Scheffler, 1982, 1988; Sosa, 1993; Sverdlik, 2011, ch. 3).

With respect to the present state of good/evils surrounding the decision to commit suicide, Lee maintains that "there is no objective standard by which one can measure the goodness as such of the pains and sufferings, on the one side, against life, continuing personal relationships, and so on, on the other side," while Lachs clearly thinks it is possible to perform such a measurement, especially if we approach each case with much care, concern, caution, and contemplation. With respect to the future, expected good/evils surrounding the decision to commit suicide, Lachs is comfortable with the good of pain relief found in death, while Lee is obviously uncomfortable with such a drastic solution. Despite his skepticism concerning utilitarianism and the legitimacy of weighing future pros and cons in moral decision-making, in the final lines of his reply to Lachs, it seems as if Lee utilizes a utilitarian argument *against* the utilitarian argument for suicide or physician-assisted suicide:

> But most problematic of all: the social acceptance of suicide as an apt solution to continuing pain, suffering, and loss of independence, when one is severely debilitated, would be a strong social affirmation that the lives of many of the weakest and most vulnerable among us are not intrinsically worthwhile. And so society would send the message to the elderly and the disabled, that when they become dependent and feel like burdens on their families, their life may very well lack inherent value. That itself will be a pressure—and not a very subtle one—on the elderly, and even on many disabled, to opt for death rather than life.

References

AMA (American Medical Association). (2001). Principles of medical ethics: Retrieved from: http://www.ama-assn.org/ama/pub/physician-resources/medical-ethics/code-medical-ethics/principles-medical-ethics.page?

AMA (American Medical Association). (2004). Code of medical ethics: Current opinions with annotations of the Council on Ethical and Judicial Affairs. Retrieved from: http://www.ama-assn.org/go/ceja

AuMA (Austrlian Medical Association). (2006). AMA code of ethics. Retrieved from: http://ama.com.au/codeofethics

Beauchamp, T., & Childress, J. (1979/2009). *Principles of biomedical ethics*. Oxford: Oxford University Press.

Bentham, J. (1789/1988). *An introduction to the principles of morals and legislation*. Amherst, NY: Prometheus Books.

Borghese, M. (2008). Jack Kevorkian speaks out against Catholic doctors, religion and Oregon's suicide law. *All Headline News*, January 17. Retrieved from: http://www.freerepublic.com/focus/f-news/1955767/posts

Cavanaugh, T. (2006). *Double-effect reasoning: Doing good and avoiding evil*. Oxford: Oxford University Press.

Costello, D. (2005). Assisted suicide at center stage once again. *Los Angeles Times*, March 7. Retrieved from: http://articles.latimes.com/2005/mar/07/health/he-assist7

CR (Congressional Record). (1999). Congressional Record V. 145, Pt. 19, October 26, 1999 to November 3, 1999. Retrieved from: http://bookstore.gpo.gov/actions/GetPublication.do?stocknumber=052-000-01151-5

Davis, M. (2011). Professional codes. In R. Chadwick, H. ten Have, & E. Meslin (Eds.), *The SAGE handbook of health care ethics* (pp. 63–72). Thousand Oaks, CA: SAGE Publications.

Dogtime. (2012). When to say good-bye to your dog. Retrieved from: http://dogtime.com/when-to-say-good-bye.html

Dowbiggin, I. (2003). *A merciful end: The euthanasia movement in modern America*. Oxford: Oxford University Press.

Driver, J. (2012). *Consequentialism*. London: Routledge.

Evans, H. (1997). Pitfalls of physician-assisted suicide. *Physician's News Digest*, September. Retrieved from: http://www.physiciansnews.com/commentary/997wp.html

Fohr, S. (1998). The double effect of pain medication. *Journal of Palliative Medicine, 1*, 315–328.

Foster, C., Herring, J., Melham, K., & Hope, T. (2011). The double effect effect. *Cambridge Quarterly of Healthcare Ethics, 20*, 56–72.

Frankena, W. (1973). *Ethics*. Englewood Cliffs, NJ: Prentice-Hall.

Garcia J. (1995). Double effect. In W. Reich (Ed.), *Encyclopedia of bioethics* (pp. 636–641). New York: Simon & Schuster.

Goldberg, S. (2011). *Death with dignity: Legalized physician-assisted death in the United States, 2011*. New York: Stuart Goldberg Publishing.

Gregory, J. (1817). *Lectures on the duties and qualifications of a physician*. Philadelphia: M. Carey & Son.

Hartmann, L., & Meyerson, A. (1998). A debate on physician-assisted suicide. *Psychiatric Services, 49*, 1468–1474.

Humphry, D. (2011). Assisted suicide laws around the world. www.assistedsuicide.org/suicide_laws.html

Johnson, D. (1999). Kevorkian sentenced to 10 to 25 years in prison. *The New York Times*. April 14. Retrieved from: http://www.nytimes.com/1999/04/14/us/kevorkian-sentenced-to-10-to-25-years-in-prison.html?ref= thomasyouk

Kass, L. (1989). Neither for love nor money: Why doctors must not kill. *National Affairs, 94*, 25–46.

Kevorkian, J. (1988). The last fearsome taboo: Medical aspects of planned death. *Medicine and Law*, 7(1), 1–14.

Marquis, D. (1991). Four versions of double effect. *The Journal of Medicine & Philosophy, 16*, 515–544.

North, M. (2002). Translation of the Hippocratic Oath. History of Medicine Division, National Institutes of Health. Retrieved from: http://www.nlm.nih.gov/hmd/greek/greek_oath.html

Markel, H. (2004). Becoming a physician: "I swear by Apollo"—on taking the Hippocratic oath. *The New England journal of Medicine, 350*, 2026–2029.

Matzo, L., & Schwarz, J. (2001). In their own words: Oncology nurses respond to patient requests for assisted suicide and euthanasia. *Applied Nursing Research, 14*, 64–71.

Miles, S. (2004). *The Hippocratic Oath and the ethics of medicine*. Oxford: Oxford University Press.

Mill, J.S. (1859/2001). *Utilitarianism*. Indianapolis, IN: Hackett Publishing Company.

Nicol, N., & Wylie, H. (2005). *Between the dying and the dead: Dr Jack Kevorkian's life and the battle to legalize euthanasia*. Madison, WI: University of Wisconsin Press.

Orr, R., Pang, N., Pellegrino, E., & Siegler, M. (1997). Use of the Hippocratic Oath: A review of twentieth-century practice and a content analysis of oaths administered in medical schools in the US and Canada in 1993. *The Journal of Clinical Ethics, 8*, 377–388.

Pettit, P. (Ed.). (1993). *Consequentialism*. Aldershot: Dartmouth.

Quill, T., Dresser, R., & Brock, D. (1997). The rule of double effect—A critique of its role in end-of-life decision-making. *The New England Journal of Medicine, 337*, 1768–1771.

Quill, T., Lo, B., & Brock, D. (1997). Palliative options of last resort: A comparison of voluntarily stopping eating and drinking, terminal sedation, physician-assisted suicide, and voluntary active euthanasia. *Journal of the American Medical Association, 278*, 2099–2104.

Rocca, J. (2008). Inventing an ethical tradition: A brief history of the Hippocratic Oath. *Legal Ethics, 11*, 23–40.

Roscoe, L., Dragovic, L, & Cohen, D. (2000). Dr Jack Kevorkian and cases of euthanasia in Oakland County, Michigan, 1990–1998. *The New England Journal of Medicine, 343*, 1735–1736.

Scarre, G. (1996). *Utilitarianism*. London: Routledge.

Scheffler, S. (1982). *The rejection of consequentialism*. Oxford: Clarendon Press.

Scheffler, S. (Ed.). (1988). *Consequentialism and its critics*. Oxford: Oxford University Press.

Schoifet, M. (2011). *Bloomberg*. June 3. Retrieved from: http://www.bloomberg.com/news/2011-06-03/jack-kevorkian-assisted-suicide-advocate-dies-at-83.html

Schwarz, J. (2003). Understanding and responding to patient requests for assistance in dying. *Journal of Nursing Scholarship, 35*, 377–383.

Snyder, L., & Caplan, A. L. (2001). *Assisted suicide: Finding common ground*. Bloomington: Indiana University Press.

Sosa, D. (1993). Consequences of consequentialism. *Mind, 102*, 101–122.

Sverdlik, S. (2011). *Motives and rightness*. Oxford: Oxford University Press.

Chapter Thirteen

Physician-Assisted Suicide Is Ethical

John Lachs

In this chapter, after noting that the typical bioethics case study is too detached from real-world experience, I argue that, if their misery is placing an undue burden on their existence, rational adults may legitimately ask for assistance in ending their lives. If conscious and intelligent enjoyment of life is absent for people—especially individuals suffering near the end of life—and they see their existence as no longer of value, then suicide or assisted suicide (in the event that a person is unable to commit suicide) is a legitimate and morally justified option. I refute some of the standard objections against physician-assisted suicide and offer provisos for the practical application of physician-assisted suicide in our society.

Introduction

A persistent weakness of bioethics discussions is their abstraction. A nameless individual or someone designated by a capitalized letter, without personal background and value commitments, is supposed to have drifted into the emergency room and presents us with a thorny moral problem. The age and gender of the individual are indicated, and his/her condition is described in a neat paragraph. That is all we know of the "case," and that is supposed to be enough to come to a medically defensible and morally conscientious decision (cf. Yin, 2009).

Physicians in emergency rooms may encounter such cases, but this way of presenting moral problems is ill adapted to getting sound answers. The current condition and future prospects of people cannot be detached from their histories. Treatment appropriate to them is not independent of their beliefs and values. Such abstract principles as "First, do no harm" and "Respect autonomy" lack meaning without an understanding of what, for the person involved, constitutes harm and counts as self-determination (Arras, 1993; Walker et al., 1995).

Magda

I will try to correct such vacuous abstractions by describing in considerable detail the ways and needs of a person seeking relief from existence. Her name was Magda, and she lived a long and rich life. She outlived a series of her physicians, all youngsters by comparison with her. She was massively healthy throughout life. Two broken hips in her 90s did not slow her down, and at 101 she cooked and needed no help to take care of herself.

Her husband died before she turned 70. As she aged, her closest companions also went to the grave. Undaunted, she made new friends and reached out to

Contemporary Debates in Bioethics, First Edition. Edited by Arthur L. Caplan and Robert Arp.

people she had known as a child. Over decades, she saw these buried as well. Eventually, only two or three friends remained, and they lived so far away that she could keep only in telephone contact with them.

Although Magda had no life-threatening illness, her organs began to fail. Macular degeneration robbed her of her sight, and she lost much of her hearing. She learned to walk with a cane, then with a walker, and finally gave up walking altogether, except for a step or two when someone would lift, steady, and support her. Her mind remained clear, which made things more difficult because she saw and understood how her life was closing down.

A vibrant woman who loved life and enjoyed its activities, Magda resisted the closing hour. She employed every mechanical aid available to support her organs. But she had always been fiercely independent and did not find it easy to have to rely on others for help with a growing number of activities. Her tendency was to offer help rather than to seek it, and her inabilities took a heavy toll on her self-image. She said that she was angry because she could no longer even attempt what she used to do without effort.

Magda understood how, as we age, the horizon narrows, and the activities of life become impossible to sustain. But she thought it was an indignity that she could not take care of her own private functions and could communicate with others only with great difficulty. At 103, she suffered compression fractures and found that moving caused excruciating pain. Going to bed became torturous, so she learned to live and sleep in a recliner. She had to wear diapers and rely on her son to clean her.

A mild case of pulmonary hypertension did not hold hope of terminating her life quickly. Living longer seemed to her utterly pointless: the pain, the indignity, and the growing communicative isolation overshadowed her native optimism and the joy she had always taken in being alive. She decided that she had had enough, and she was ready to die. She had foreseen this possibility in her younger years and stockpiled sleeping pills so that when the time came she could commit suicide. But the pills disappeared in the chaos of her apartment, and she was, in any case, unable to leave her chair to get them. She decided not to eat or drink, but there was enough love of life left in her to make this a regimen she could not sustain.

This leads us to the moral problem. Is it acceptable to provide her with aid in dying? Here is a more pointed way of putting it: Is it not outrageously wrong to let her shriek in pain and live disgusted with her condition for months and possibly years?

It may be worth mentioning that this was the story of my mother.

The Value of Human Life

In the name of what value past, present, or future could one deny Magda help with finishing her life? Clearly, no past value is at stake: her days of delight and generosity were over and would never return. The past has an integrity all its own, opening itself to grateful memory without ever changing. There is reason to be thankful for lives of kindness and sharing, but what was achieved in the past neither calls for, nor justifies, maintaining an existence after it turns barren.

Magda's life near its end has no present value. If we added up the positive aspects of her pained existence in the recliner and deducted her anguish, embarrassment, sorrow, and frustration, the sum would come in as a high negative number. Further deducting her sense that she is a burden on everyone and that her will is violated if she cannot die, we get an overwhelming indication that nothing in her present justifies continued life.

There are occasions when the hope of future good makes it appropriate to grit our teeth and fight through painful times. Cancer patients have reason to subject themselves to surgery, radiation, and chemotherapy. Husbands and wives divorcing suffer through dark days in anticipation of a better life. Soldiers endure the pains of basic training and young doctors the sleepless exhaustion of internship, expecting something better at the end of such torture. Nothing like this relates even vaguely to Magda. She had no future; all she could anticipate was release whenever it would come "naturally," that is, without the help of any human being.

She made it clear to me and to others that receiving no help in dying amounted, in her view, to abandonment. "Don't let me live like this," she pleaded, "No human being should be made to endure such a fate." I cannot think that in this assessment, she was wrong. With pity in our hearts, we do not permit our animal companions to suffer: we ease them out of life with sorrow, painlessly. By contrast, we seem to take no pity on human beings, forcing them to live to the end, no matter how miserable they are. Visitors from another planet would find this a baffling and indefensible cruelty.

Animal life is cheap, but human life is sacred, some might be tempted to say. Just exactly what is it that makes for this difference? The usual answer is that animals are valuable only as instruments, adding to our comfort and enjoyment, but humans represent an intrinsic and perhaps infinite value (Kant, 1785/1998; Haezrahi, 1961/1962; Pullman, 1996, 2002; CCC, 1994; Baron, 1999; Schaeffer, 2005, p. 69). As ends in themselves, possibly the only ones this side of God and the angels, humans deserve respect: we are not to shorten their lives or interfere with their fortunes. This is a hugely improbable position, a theory we may embrace in words but never honor in practice.

If we are to do nothing to extend human life, we have no business going to the doctor, taking medicines, driving cautiously, and even eating. And if we must not shorten our existence, hundreds of activities, including smoking, eating beef, overwork, and worry, become morally unacceptable. The human race has pronounced judgment on this theory long ago by happily taking control of human life, extending and shortening it according to what seems sensible and good at any given time. If slow and long-term self-destruction escapes moral censure, the immediate termination of life in suicide cannot be morally condemned.

This argument aside, however, we can ask what confers intrinsic value on human life. The idea that humans claim extraordinary status for humanity is immediately suspect (Singer, 1979, Ch. 10; Dunayer, 2004). Does it not sound like special pleading or species-ist foolishness? Cats maintain that humans are there to serve them and lions affirm their superiority by killing and eating everything in sight. If we could converse with chimpanzees and porpoises, would they not instruct us to view our existence as of no special concern because they are merely instrumental to their good? Those who do not spend time observing animals make the mistake of thinking that they lack value systems and intelligence.

The supposed intrinsic value of humans must be due either to some relationship or to a special feature of their lives. The prime candidate for the relation is the Deity who is supposed to have created us and placed us in a privileged position above the beasts (CCC, 1994; Schaeffer, 2005, p. 69; Soulen & Woodhead, 2006; USCCB, 2011). Without reference to something identifiably special in our experience, this relationship remains a theological supposition in need of evidence. That leaves the claim that there is something unique in human experience, something whose extinction would represent a momentous loss. The uniqueness of any feature of human experience is questionable, but let us make the best case for the view and say that the characteristic we are looking for is the conscious and intelligent enjoyment of life.

One can readily see that such enjoyment is of great value. In fact, it may be the only genuine good in the world (Mill, 1863/2001; Singer, 1979). But if this is what constitutes the intrinsic value of human beings, what becomes of that value when conscious and intelligent enjoyment is no longer possible? This was Magda's problem: her days of delight were over, and she could no longer perform the activities that make life worthwhile. She faced only suffering, and if the source of the intrinsic value of human existence consists of intelligent joy, then toward the end, her life was without value.

Confusing Essence with Existence

Opponents of suicide may here respond that intrinsic value can never be lost. That which is valuable in and of itself relies on nothing beyond itself for its value. For this reason, it is immune to changes in its surroundings: since nothing external gave it value, nothing external can take it away (Sulmasy, 2002).

Unfortunately, this argument is flawed. It confuses essence with existence, the characteristic of an object or experience with its presence. Certain experiences are valuable in and of themselves, and it may well be impossible to separate them from their value. But that does not mean that such events must happen or always do. Being special on account of a unique brand of intelligent enjoyment does not guarantee that that enjoyment will always be available to humans. So long as it is at hand, it may well be wrong to hasten death. But in Magda's case and in many others, the enjoyment is unavailable, eliminating the special status of humans and the obligations that go with it.

Opponents of suicide can attempt to reformulate their view by insisting that what makes humans special, and imposes restrictions on hastening their death, is not a set of events or experiences but the very constitution of human nature. Followers of Kant (1785/1996, 1785/1998) maintain that our uniqueness is due to our rationality or to the spontaneity of the human mind. It is notoriously difficult to give a precise account of what it means to possess reason, especially if this single factor is to be responsible for separating humans from all other animals.

The fact is that many species of animals show themselves capable of reasoning (Watanabe & Huber, 2006; Pearce, 2008). Their behavior reveals that they seem to understand what counts as evidence and can move unhesitatingly from premises to conclusions. In the sphere of morality, Kant believes that reason enables us to decide on our actions totally independently of desires and external pressure. But if such performances serve as conditions of being human, the large majority of our fellows belong to a different species. We cannot be sure that anyone in the human race has ever reached a level of purity of intention to satisfy Kant. Moreover, how can we maintain that reason is the hallmark of the human in the teeth of all the irrationality that surrounds us? Thinking of reason as a faculty present in all of us, if only potentially, amounts to embracing an unwarranted opinion.

Social and Political Reasons

Obviously, arguments on the basis of the quality of life and the constitution of human nature do not prevail against suicide. But many people who object to the practice do so for social or political reasons. On the social side, they think that permitting it sets a dangerous example: they fear mass suicides and the possibility that, not understanding what they do, children will join adults in terminating their lives. Politically, they maintain that the state has a legitimate interest in the protection of human life. They imagine that without legislation banning the practice, older people, the sick, the disabled, and the poor will likely be forced to end their days (Moreland & Geisler, 1990; Siegler, 1996).

The fear of mass suicides is altogether groundless. We do not have to outlaw starvation to get people to eat; living is sufficiently joyous and the alternative sufficiently frightening to motivate people to hang on with all their might. The way to reduce child suicides is by parental love and caring, and not by laws of whose existence the young are in any case unaware. Unavoidably, some young, jilted romantics will kill themselves under any regime, but here, too, the best hope of reducing their number is social vigilance and the investment of time to help them over their despair, rather than legislation and threats of punishment.

From the standpoint of justice and the protection of human life, there is nothing to fear from morally accepting and legally permitting suicide. In 1994, Oregon passed the Oregon Death with Dignity Act (ORS 127.800-995). The Oregon experience of legalization yielded significantly fewer suicides than had been anticipated (OHD, 1999; Werth & Wineberg, 2004). It is possible, of course, that heartless people will exert pressure on the old, the sick, and the less fortunate to remove themselves before their time, but this can occur whether suicide is legal or not. If there is evidence of it, laws can be introduced to control the unfeeling, and in any case, adequate safeguards can be developed against abuse when suicide is aided by physicians.

The state's interest in protecting life raises a troubling issue concerning the range of its power. Sometimes, this is expressed by the question of who owns our persons or our lives. The metaphor of ownership can be misleading, but it is useful because it points to social arrangements of which slavery was an integral part. The great historical development of banning slavery established the untouchable independence of human individuals. If no other person can own us, no group of people—such as the state—can either.

That God, having created us, has lost or ceded ownership control was clear as early as the Garden of Eden. He can order us about, but whether we obey him is a question for us to decide. The idea that we are somehow God's "children" and therefore lack the right to make decisions about our lives confers no credit on religion. One would want to make the commitment to a faith and its God as a responsible adult, with an understanding of the prospects and the costs. Acting like a child in such matters of the gravest import does not give moral credit to individuals and can hardly be acceptable to God.

The myth of a social contract carries a vital message concerning the relationship of citizens to their states. It reminds us that nations are derivative organizations built on the consent and cooperation of individual human beings. The state can impose a variety of demands and limitations on its citizens, though only ones that promote the common good. For example, a system of taxation, setting limits to one's control of one's earnings, is justified so long as the money extracted is used for projects that cannot be undertaken by individuals and that benefit everyone.

The state can and should protect individuals from others who may want to harm them. It exceeds its legitimate power, however, if it sets out to protect sensible people from themselves, interfering in the way they choose to run or end their lives. Specifically, keeping a person such as Magda going beyond the time she reasonably decides to be done with life is an abomination: there is no value in the name of which government officials can insist that she continue to suffer. The existence of people in excruciating pain, hardly capable of moving and without the prospect of improvement, contributes nothing to the common good. Striving to make suicide unavailable to them reminds one of hell where devils torture sinners instead of letting them expire in peace.

Since neither God nor the state owns us, we must learn to be our own masters. This is appropriate in many of the activities that make life interesting and precious, but especially when it comes to decisions concerning the quality and quantity of existence. People who choose to live as drunkards or as deans must be allowed to make their own decisions and bear the consequences. It is especially important for end-of-life choices to be left in the hands of directly affected individuals. Telling others what they should do is for the most part wrong, but making others carry on the burden of a horrible life when they want to be set free is nothing short of wanton cruelty.

Kant and Mill

The followers of Kant and Mill appear to agree in describing freedom as self-determination. The agreement, however, is only verbal because the selves they have in mind differ sharply. For Kant (1785/1996), the self that is to determine itself is what we might call the "higher" or rational element in us. This means that free actions are supposed to be devised solely by reference to duty or other stern moral values, without taking into account the influence of others or what we may desire. A free action is, in this way, inevitably also a moral action, and an immoral act is at once unfree.

Mill (1863/2001, 1863/2008), by contrast, views freedom as the ability to do what we desire. The self that determines our actions is the everyday agent we know, motivated by needs and wants, and seeking its happiness in a changeable, treacherous world. Here, freedom means the absence of external constraint, that is, the ability of people to frame purposes and to carry them out. Free or autonomous actions are, therefore, not necessarily moral: as Adam and Eve in the Garden of Eden, we can succumb to temptation and choose the wrong alternative.

The point of the contrast is not that Kant recommends the righteous path, and Mill is satisfied with the willful search for happiness. Both of them embrace moral standards, but Kant thinks happiness has nothing to do with them. He finds it difficult to identify with the everyday ambitions of ordinary people, restricting morality to the realm of austere duty. Mill, on the other hand, understands the yearning for untrammeled movement that frames the moral life; he attaches high value to being able to do what we want. Morality, for him, is constituted by desires freely formed and actions freely performed or restrained, enabling us to grow into responsible adults.

Kant and Mill represent the two great strands of accounting for moral action. Deontology, growing out of Kant, measures moral performance by its adherence to duty; teleology, perfected by Mill, insists on assessing the consequences of what we do. Oddly, Kant and Mill agree that suicide is impermissible, but neither has an argument that adequately supports that conclusion. Kant (1785/1996) thinks that suicide constitutes disrespect for human life: when we commit it, we use ourselves as a means to relieving us of some undesirable condition:

> To annihilate the subject of morality in one's person is to root out the existence of morality itself from the world as far as one can, even though morality is an end in itself. Consequently, disposing of oneself as a mere means to some discretionary end is debasing humanity in one's person. (6:423, p. 177)

Mill (1863/2008) believes that suicide and selling oneself into slavery do not fall within the range of our freedom because they are irreversible: choosing to destroy oneself is to put a permanent end to one's freedom to choose:

> He therefore defeats, in his own case, the very purpose which is the justification of allowing him to dispose of himself. He is no longer free; but is thenceforth in a position which has no longer the presumption in its favor, that would be afforded by his voluntarily remaining in it. The principle of freedom cannot require that he should be free not to be free. It is not freedom, to be allowed to alienate his freedom. (pp. 198–199)

Kant's argument is unconvincing because we use ourselves (and others), unobjectionably, as means in the course of ordinary life. I use myself to acquire the skill of playing the piano when I make myself practice, and I use the pilot to get me to my destination when I take a trip on an airplane. What makes such actions morally acceptable is that when I undertake them, I do not use humans as means *only*, but respect their freedom by asking for their consent. But that is precisely what happens in suicide. Designed to relieve a horrible situation, it does so with the sufferer's consent. Further, we can reasonably ask if it does not show greater respect for human life to terminate suffering rather than to let someone like Magda struggle for months with despondency and pain.

Mills' argument against suicide is equally weak. The irreversibility of the choice of self-destruction is shared by every decision. When I marry, I change my life permanently; choices that were once open disappear. In deciding to settle in one part of the country, I surrender a host of possibilities, and in choosing a profession I disable myself to practice many others. Admittedly, these choices close off many activities but not all, whereas killing oneself is, presumably, an end to everything. But this distinction is irrelevant in Magda's case. She was able to do very little and nothing that satisfied, so the loss of all is a net gain because it ends the suffering.

Another way to look at this is to examine duties and consequences more systematically. In taking my life, do I violate a duty? The language of obligation is not well adapted to capture the relation of individuals to themselves. We commit ourselves to values, formulate plans, undertake projects, and engage in activities as a result of what we want and what we think is good. We do not believe that we owe it to ourselves to do these things or that we are duty-bound to perform them. We do have obligations to others: parents, for example, have a duty to stay alive so they may take care of their underage children. But no such obligation existed in Magda's case. Her husband and her close friends had died long ago, her son had grown old, and her grandchildren were busy with their lives. No duty held her attached to existence.

Utilitarian or teleological calculation of the consequences of Magda's committing suicide yields a similar result. She had little on the positive side of the ledger. A few distant friends had the pleasure of occasional conversations with her, and her son and daughter-in-law took delight in bringing her food she particularly liked. For the most part, she ate only a few morsels. Her days were indistinguishable from her nights: her pain medication left her without knowledge of who or where she was, and when she awoke to a moment of lucidity, all she could call for was an end to it. Sadly, much as she would be missed, her suicide would have reduced the misery and thereby added to the net sum of good in the world.

The Morality of Suicide and Physician-Assisted Suicide

The first stage in arguing that physician-assisted suicide is morally permissible consists in showing that committing suicide is not always wrong. If we can find even one case in which the intentional termination of life by a human being is clearly justified, the abstract claim that it is always wrong is roundly defeated. The logic of the argument is that a single counter-example destroys a general theory. Magda's case is just such an example: no good could emerge from forcing her to continue to suffer. This establishes the legitimacy of suicide at least in some cases.

The next task is to show that it is morally acceptable for doctors to aid people when they wish legitimately to terminate their existence. The modern world values life and makes it difficult for people to end it. People who want to kill themselves by jumping from high places find it difficult to identify a suitable venue. The windows of skyscrapers do not open, and high fences protect the walkways on bridges. Slitting one's arteries is a bloody and distasteful affair. Most people do not have guns or are untutored in their use. In any case, one might miss, as did the German generals when they tried to commit suicide after their unsuccessful attempt on Hitler's life. That leaves pills, with which everyone today is thoroughly familiar. They hold the hope of a smooth and rapid transfer, the painless end to pain and misery.

Unfortunately, however, people do not know the power of pills: they tend to be ignorant of which ones end life and which put them in the hospital. In any case, ordinary people have no access to powerful drugs without the intervention of doctors, and physicians are notoriously reluctant to make drugs suitable for suicide available to their patients. The question of why doctors should assist in suicides is easy to answer: the medical profession has monopoly power over drugs (Light, 2010). Since society conferred this vast and lucrative power on physicians, they are under an obligation to help individuals who have a legitimate reason to hasten their death.

The standard objection to this consists of reminding us that doctors are supposed to return us to health rather than aid our demise. "As physicians, we're not supposed to be in that role," many would claim, as Dr Andy Harris did when he commented on a case dealing with a Baltimore doctor who was acquitted of physician-assisted suicide in 2011 (May, 2011). But what if health is never to be restored? There was simply no hope of improvement in Magda's situation; at her age, any intervention was like trying to stop the tides. Would it not be appropriate for her physician to offer help when she cried out to die? This question opens a distinction between two conceptions of the proper function of physicians, one narrow and one much broader.

The narrow notion is characterized by the claim that physicians should treat diseases so that their patients may recover. This tends to be the view of medical specialists, who arrive on the scene to practice their marvelous art and depart as soon as the problem gets resolved. One might think of them as hired guns employed by the sheriff to help restore order in town. They have little interest in their patients as people, asking little about the values and personal history of the individuals they treat. Such information is not necessary for the cure and may in fact interfere with it: doctors are supposed to solve problems by means of pills or surgery and, when all goes well, return patients to their normal lives.

The broader conception of the task of medicine was in complete possession of the field 150 years ago when many physicians lived in small communities and cared for their patients from birth to death. Doctors in those days took an interest not only in the physical status, but also in the psychological condition and social relationships of their patients. In the belief that personal health is inseparable from the flourishing of society, some went so far as to demonstrate vital concern for the well-being of the families and communities of their patients. Family practice physicians come closest to this conception today, though financial pressures make it difficult even for them to spend much time with their patients.

Not surprisingly, doctors who subscribe to the dominant narrow conception of their duties have difficulty understanding how they could be called on to aid a patient's suicide. Their role is to treat the disease and, when there is nothing further they can do, to declare the case one of medical futility, making room for hospice care and palliative measures. The idea that patients have life histories, purposes, desires, values, and fervently held beliefs appears irrelevant; the possibility that they might not want to waste away waiting for death is given no consideration. The result is that just when we need good doctors the most, they become unavailable.

Even if the broad conception of physician duties is no longer viable, we must insist that doctors help us through every stage of life. They need to provide empathy no less than specialist knowledge and learn to view their contributions to our lives as informed suggestions and kindly advice. Most important, they must be there for their patients at the great crises of life, helping in the difficult task of making decisions concerning the dark days. This does not mean that they have to stand ready with pill or syringe to honor every wish of the depressed. But, unless they have personal or religious objections to suicide, they must be on hand to provide, when appropriate, the means to a peaceful and dignified departure.

The original version of the Hippocratic Oath forbids physicians to make deadly drugs available to their patients (North, 2002). It is essential, however, to remember that in the days of Hippocrates people did not live very long. Many died in the prime of life, and virtually no one reached old age in a debilitated condition. Magda would have expired long before she reached her 103rd birthday and hence would not have needed physician help to terminate her life. Enlisting doctors in the quest for a peaceful and dignified death is a need and an activity unique to the contemporary world. It grew out of the success of medicine in keeping people alive and the political decision to control drugs and vest their distribution in the medical profession. The vast and continuing increase in the number of the very old will likely intensify the pressure on physicians until our laws come to reflect the moral acceptability of terminating life.

Does this mean that suicide is morally permissible at any age and under all conditions? Not at all. Here it may be useful to distinguish between what we are free to do and what is good to undertake. A generous reading of human freedom leaves it open for adults to finish the book of life at any time they desire. If they are young and healthy, their doing so is a lamentable error. But they are at liberty to do what is sad and wrong, as Adam and Eve were when they disobeyed God's command. The source of the liberty is the fact that no one has a right to force life on people when they want to die.

Friends and neighbors incur responsibilities when people they know decide to exit life. They must speak with them, stressing the beauty and goodness of life, along with the irreversibility of death. They have to ask them to reconsider or at least to wait until they see more clearly. If they can truthfully say it, they might even indicate how much they mean to their friends and how intensely they will be missed. But just as God did not use His power to stop Adam and Eve, the freedom of individuals blocks us from employing force to prevent their suicide. We cannot be expected to stand idly by while people kill themselves, yet morally we can stop them only by persuasion.

This means that exercising freedom is by no means the same as following moral rules. The freedom to commit suicide gives us more operational leeway than moral principles allow: we have the right to terminate our lives even if it is wrong to do so. But healthy young adults who propose to kill themselves cannot demand aid from others. Helping someone commit an immoral act is itself immoral, so there can be no obligation to provide gun or pills. The situation is altogether different with suicide that is justifiable. As in trying to do what is right or at least permissible, so here also, one can legitimately enlist the aid of friends and physicians. Such a right to ask, if exercised, imposes an obligation on those in a position to help.

Naturally, the duty is dissolved if the request violates the physician's moral commitments. But it is binding if aid is just bothersome or inconvenient. The demand is valid even if meeting it is dangerous or may lead to severe repercussions. This is why Dr Kevorkian must be seen as a pioneer who was willing to risk criminal censure to affirm in his actions the responsibility of the medical profession for help with suicide. Many found his manner of providing deadly drugs to terminal patients disquieting or even grisly, but he used a parked van only because honest ways of committing suicide are banned in hospitals. The objection to his efforts that the people he aided in dying were not his patients is fatuous; he stepped in only because the attending physicians did not shoulder their responsibility.

Being Careful, Cautious, and Conscientious

How can we tell whether a proposed suicide that requires physician assistance is morally acceptable? There are no easy answers to such questions. In the moral life, everything is a matter of judgment, with no recipe for making them. A careful examination of the facts, conscientious reflection on the values involved, and a savvy understanding of needs and alternatives will still not guaranty the correct result. But it may be helpful to remember Magda's case and use it as a measure by which other problem situations may be evaluated. Her predicament establishes a standard that other potential cases of physician-assisted suicide must approximate.

First, there must be adequate reasons for terminating life, and they have to be both objective and subjective in nature. On the subjective side, nihilistic mood and temporary despondency do not amount to a justification. We have to begin with objective facts: the patient must be near the end of life and in significant pain or discomfort. The phrase "near the end of life" is vague and requires case-by-case interpretation. No one knew how close Magda was to the end of her life, but it was clear that past her 103rd year, with pulmonary hypertension, she could not live very long. A precise number of days or weeks that would govern universally is impossible to postulate, but we know that, in most cases, a life expectancy of a year or more would be too long.

As important as the amount of time left is the quality of it. People who are likely to be able to operate to the end and then slip away peacefully are not candidates for physician assistance in killing themselves. Sick persons who are not in excruciating pain but experience their debility as a crushing burden, on the other hand, may well be justified in seeking help to get permanent relief. In any case, if people have significant obligations they can discharge only by living on, they forfeit the right to look for help with dying. How significant these duties need to be is another question to which there is no general answer. Having promised someone to go to lunch next month is obviously not weighty enough; earning money to feed one's children who would otherwise go hungry clearly is.

Provisos

A few common sense provisos need to be added at this point. Even if it is morally acceptable for people to seek expert help in hastening death and for doctors to provide it, patients do not have the right to approach *any* physician with their request. There must be an established doctor–patient relationship between the parties that makes the call for help legitimate. Furthermore, it is wise for society to establish a variety of safeguards to make abuse of the practice of physician-assisted suicide difficult and improbable. The state may require application to a board, examination of the patient by at least one physician uninvolved in the case, and a waiting period. Regular reassessment of the practice may suggest additional safeguards and procedures (see, for example, OHA, 2012).

It took multiple calls to Magda's physician to get him to order hospice on the scene. When representatives of this worthy organization arrived, they brought a powerful morphine solution. They assured her caregivers that any dosage necessary to still her pain and any frequency of applying the drug were acceptable. This was essentially, in my view, an invitation to suicide, assisted in this case not by a physician but by benevolent hospice nurses. Hiding behind the double-effect of morphine, they offered pain relief at the price of depressed lung function and accelerated death. Our current laws make it impossible to help needy people die peacefully without this subterfuge.

References

Arras, J. (1993). Principles and particularity: The roles of cases in bioethics. *Indiana Law Journal, 69*, 983–1014.

Baron, M. (1999). *Kantian ethics almost without apology*. Ithaca, NY: Cornell University Press.

CCC (Catechism of the Catholic Church). (1994). Part three: Life in Christ, section two, chapter two, article six. Retrieved from: http://www.vatican.va/archive/ccc_css/archive/catechism/p3s2c2a6.htm

Dunayer, J. (2004). *Speciesism*. Herndon, VA: Lanetern Books.

Haezrahi, P. (1961/1962). The concept of man as end-in-himself. *Kant-Studien, 53*, 209–224.

Kant, I. (1785/1996). *The metaphysics of morals* (M. Gregor, Trans.). Cambridge: Cambridge University Press.

Kant, I. (1785/1998). *Groundwork of the metaphysics of morals* (M. Gregor, Trans.). (Section I: Transition from common rational to philosophic moral cognition). Cambridge: Cambridge University Press.

Light, D. (2010). Health care professions, markets and countervailing powers. In C. Bird, P. Conrad, A. Fremont, & S. Timmermans (Eds.), *Handbook of medical sociology* (pp. 270–289). Nashville, TN: Vanderbilt University Press.

May, A. (2011). Baltimore doctor accused of helping people commit suicide is acquitted. *CBS Baltimore*, May 22. Retrieved from: http://baltimore.cbslocal.com/2011/05/22/acquitted-baltimore-doctor-helped-people-commit-suicide/

Mill, J. S. (1863/2001). *Utilitarianism*. Indianapolis, IN: Hackett Publishing Company.

Mill, J. S. (1863/2008). *On liberty*. Oxford: Oxford University Press.

Moreland, J., & Geisler, N. (1990). *The life and death debate*. Westport, CT: Greenwood Press.

North, M. (2002). Translation of the Hippocratic Oath. History of Medicine Division, National Institutes of Health. Retrieved from: http://www.nlm.nih.gov/hmd/greek/greek_oath.html

OHA (Oregon Health Authority). (2012). About the Death with Dignity Act. Retrieved from: http://public.health.oregon.gov/ProviderPartnerResources/Evaluation Research/DeathwithDignityAct/Pages/faqs.aspx

OHD (Oregon Health Division). (1999). Oregon's Death with Dignity Act: The first year's experience. Retrieved from: http://public.health.oregon.gov/ProviderPartner Resources/EvaluationResearch/DeathwithDignityAct/Documents/year1.pdf

Pearce, J. (2008). *Animal learning and cognition: An introduction*. New York: Psychology Press.

Pullman, D. (1996). Dying with dignity and the death of dignity. *Health Law Journal*, *4*, 197–219.

Pullman, D. (2002). Human dignity and the ethics and aesthetics of pain and suffering. *Theoretical Medicine and Bioethics*, *23*, 75–94.

Schaeffer, F. (2005). *A Christian manifesto*. Wheaton, IL: Crossway Books.

Siegler, M. (1996). Is there a role for physician-assisted suicide in cancer? No. In V. DeVita, S. Hellman, & S. Rosenberg (Eds.), *Important advances in oncology* (pp. 281–291). Philadelphia: Lippincott-Raven Publishers.

Singer, P. (1979). *Practical ethics*. Cambridge: Cambridge University Press.

Soulen, R., & Woodhead, L. (Eds.). (2006). *God and human dignity*. Grand Rapids, MI: Wm. B. Eerdmans Publishing.

Sulmasy, D. (2002). Death, dignity, and the theory of value. *Ethical Perspectives*, *9*, 103–118.

USCCB (United States Council of Catholic Bishops). (2011). To live each day with dignity: A statement on physician-assisted suicide. Retrieved from: http://www.priestsforlife.org/magisterium/bishops/bishops-statement-physician-assisted-suicide.pdf

Walker, L., Pitts, R., Hennig, K., & Matsuba, M. (1995). Reasoning about morality and real-life moral problems. In M. Killen & D. Hart (Eds.), *Morality in everyday life: Developmental perspectives* (pp. 371–408). Cambridge: Cambridge University Press.

Watanabe, S., & Huber, L. (2006). Animal logics: Decisions in the absence of human language. *Animal Cognition*, *9*, 235–245.

Werth, J., & Wineberg, H. (2004). A critical analysis of criticisms of the Oregon Death with Dignity Act. *Death Studies*, *29*, 1–27.

Yin, R. (2009). *Case study research: Design and methods*. Thousand Oaks, CA: Sage Publications.

Chapter Fourteen

Physician-Assisted Suicide Is Not Ethical

Patrick Lee

I argue that physician-assisted suicide is morally wrong because one ought not deliberately assist someone to do what is objectively morally wrong. Though not morally required to adopt excessively burdensome means to sustain our lives, we are morally required to have respect for all human lives, our own included. Every human life, including the life of someone in extreme pain and suffering, is intrinsically worthwhile. Life is not merely instrumentally valuable, nor does one's life cease to have intrinsic value with pain and suffering. Loved ones and healthcare professionals should act to mitigate pain and suffering, not destroy persons as a means of removing pain and suffering.

Introduction

Physician-assisted suicide is one of various types of end-of-life decisions debated in bioethics and legal circles. It is obviously closely related to euthanasia, and its various types (voluntary, nonvoluntary, etc.), and to suicide itself. The question here is about the *morality* of the choice of a physician to assist suicide, not directly about the *legal* issue. Although the moral and legal issues are closely related, they are quite distinct and involve different considerations. Thus, the question here is not about what the state should or should not allow, or about what is Constitutional or not; those questions regard social policies, actions of the political community as a whole. The question we address is: setting aside the legal issue, if you or I were a physician, would it ever be morally right for us to choose to assist someone to commit suicide?

Of course, whether a choice to help someone do something is morally right depends, at least partly, on whether that something is morally right. For that reason, in what follows I will focus almost solely on the choice to commit suicide. Would it ever be morally right for me to commit suicide? If the choice to commit suicide is morally wrong then one's deliberately helping someone else to do that is morally wrong also. Compare: if adultery is morally wrong, then deliberately helping someone to commit adultery is morally wrong. By *deliberately*, I mean: to intend that the act be done, not just to do something else which facilitates someone else's act as a side effect. Thus, I set aside here questions about "material cooperation" (assistance that is not intended but a side effect of what one does). The question here is about *formal cooperation*, that is, whether it is right for a physician to choose to help someone commit suicide where the physician intends that this person succeed (Keenan & Kopfensteiner, 1995). I will argue that none of us should commit suicide and that, thus, no one should formally assist someone else to commit

Contemporary Debates in Bioethics, First Edition. Edited by Arthur L. Caplan and Robert Arp.

suicide. From this, it follows, a fortiori, that physicians should not formally assist people to commit suicide. I will address what I think is objectively morally right or wrong: someone who makes a choice that is objectively wrong is not at fault for a morally bad choice if she thought what she was doing was right and was not at fault for this mistaken judgment—often referred to as an inculpably erroneous conscience.

Why Intentionally Killing Innocent People (Including Oneself) Is Morally Wrong

In ethical discussions, the following type of hypothetical scenario has often been described. Suppose, at a modern hospital with an advanced emergency department, intensive care unit, and a transplant team that happens to be on call, a fairly young homeless man, Charlie, is admitted to the emergency department. Charlie has fallen and undergone a severe but recoverable brain injury. The social workers at the hospital discover that Charlie has recently become severely depressed, and has begun drinking heavily. One of the medical personnel—no one quite remembers who—hits upon a bright idea. If Charlie is admitted, recovers, and returns to the streets, he will most likely continue his downward spiral. Also, sadly, Charlie has no family or friends who will miss him. On the other hand, Charlie's organs are still in very good shape. He has two good kidneys, a healthy heart, a good liver, lungs, and so on. If Charlie were disaggregated, then his organs could be used to save six people who have bright futures. The downside, of course, is that this will involve killing Charlie. But—one of the team argues—although this action will involve killing one person with (probably) a very dim future, it will save *six* people with bright futures—a better outcome. Would this be morally justified?

Almost everyone agrees that this would *not* be morally right, despite the fact that real-life cases similar to this one have been documented in history (AP, 1992; Roach, 2004). It seems that there are some choices (such as intentionally disaggregating a living human person) that cannot be morally justified by a good end (saving six people).

Of course, this story will not by itself convince every consequentialist (someone who holds that the standard for what is morally right is what will produce the best consequences, or the least bad consequences, in the long run, in other words, that the end *does* justify the means; see, for example, Mill, 1861/1998, p. 81; Hooker, 2000; Driver, 2012). A consequentialist might argue that killing Charlie would set a bad precedent, or lead to a slippery slope—and so it would not lead to a better outcome. Or a consequentialist might bite the bullet and say that in some cases killing Charlie would be morally right. Nevertheless, I submit that killing Charlie would be wrong. The question is: what is it about killing Charlie that makes it wrong? I suggest that what makes it wrong is that it is a choice contrary to the intrinsic good of an innocent human person. I use the word *innocent* here simply to set aside the questions about capital punishment and just war. Henceforth, I will usually assume that restriction. Intentionally killing a human person seems to involve treating his or her life as if it were merely an instrumental good rather than—what it actually is—worthwhile in itself. Killing Charlie treats his life as if it were merely instrumentally valuable, or as if his life could be outweighed by certain other goods. But Charlie's life is intrinsically worthwhile, and the attempt to measure his life against the benefits that could be obtained by killing him is suspect (Kant, 1785/1998; Dworkin, 1993; PCJP, 2005, 11,III,c; O'Neill, 2008).

Morality concerns the difference between good choices and bad choices, and how we should shape our lives by our choices. Both morally good choices and morally bad ones involve pursuing some benefit (or avoiding some harm) for ourselves and for others we care about. Some benefits are only instrumentally good, for example, medicine and money. But not every benefit can be merely instrumentally good; some objects or conditions must be good in themselves, intrinsically worthwhile.

Which objects or conditions are basic goods is not a matter of further choice. We do not select what condition will be actually good in itself for us and other persons. Rather, what is good in itself for us and other human persons is what genuinely fulfills us, what realizes the basic potentialities we have as human persons. Thus, human life, health, understanding, excellence in work or play, friendship, for example, are aspects of genuine human fulfillment and are basic goods. These goods are worth pursuing, promoting, and protecting, not as mere means to some other condition, but as worthwhile in themselves.

To choose in a way that implicitly denies the intrinsic goodness or worthiness of an instance of a basic good—such as life, health, knowledge of truth, friendship, and so on—is to act unreasonably, that is, immorally. Such a choice diminishes one's respect, or caring, for some aspect of the intrinsic good of persons.

Human life itself is a basic human good. For, the basic goods are real fulfillments of us as human persons, and our being alive is the same as our continuing to exist. Human life is not something we have; rather, one's life is identical with one's concrete reality, that is, identical with oneself. So, a choice to kill a human being is a choice contrary to a basic good of a person. This is true both of killing ourselves and of deliberately assisting others to kill themselves.

Intentional Killing vs. Accepting Death as a Side Effect

This does not mean, however, that we must always take all measures possible to preserve someone's life, our own included. It can be morally right to forgo life-sustaining treatment, foreseeing that this will result in dying more quickly than one otherwise would. Hence, there is a crucial distinction between intentionally killing, on the one hand, and choosing to forgo treatment, foreseeing (but not intending) the death or hastening of death, that will occur as a side effect, on the other hand. For example, someone with cancer may forgo the offer of chemotherapy on the grounds that in this particular case, it may prolong life only for a short time, would be quite expensive, and would block spending time with one's family. Such a choice is quite distinct from intentional killing—say, choosing to kill oneself by means of swallowing lethal pills. A choice to forgo excessively burdensome treatment does not involve a failure of respect for the intrinsic good of life. Rather, it is a choice not to use certain means of prolonging life in order to avoid the burdens of that treatment.

We cannot pursue all instances of basic goods all of the time. When choosing to pursue one instance of a good, other instances of goods are not realized or not promoted. Choosing one good while not pursuing another is not the same as choosing against a basic good, and does not necessarily involve a lack of appreciation or openness to those goods not realized. The same may be true if the side effect of carrying out one's choice is the damaging or destruction of an instance of a basic good. We do have some responsibility for causing bad side effects (since we could have chosen the option that did not cause them). Yet, since our will is not directed precisely against the instances of basic goods thus harmed, the moral norms governing causing bad side effects are not the same as the moral norms regarding intentionally destroying, damaging, or impeding an instance of a basic good. Intentionally killing human persons is always morally wrong, but causing death as a side effect is sometimes (not always) morally right. The former type of choice is incompatible with an openness and respect for the basic intrinsic good of human life.

Sometimes not doing something can be chosen as a means of bringing about some end. So, it is possible to choose an omission as a way of bringing about someone's death. For example, if a husband wanted to be rid of his wife, he might withhold needed insulin from her so that she would die. In that case he would intend her death just as much as if he had deliberately dropped arsenic in her orange juice. Similarly, if the point of withholding treatment is to get it over quickly, then death is intended, even though the means chosen is an omission. Critics of traditional morality on killing and accepting death as a side effect sometimes say there is no difference between the two, and point to cases like the husband withholding insulin from his wife as illustration (Rachels, 1975; Tooley, 1999). But the important moral difference is not between whether one physically does something that results in death or not, but whether one wills to bring about death either as an end or as a means—and this may be by an omission or a commission.

Why is the distinction between intentional killing and accepting death as a side effect important? In a given case, the difference in outcome between intending to destroy or damage a basic good on the one hand, and accepting the destruction or damage to a basic good as a side effect of what one does (or as a side effect of one's not doing something), on the other hand, may seem nonexistent. For example, the difference between killing a patient and not resuscitating a patient (because he requested a Do Not Resuscitate order) may seem slight or unimportant, since in both cases the patient dies. Still, the moral difference is immense (Aquinas, 1265/1989; Glynn, 1999; Cavanaugh, 2006). By our choices not only do we bring about one type of external outcome rather than another, but in the act of choosing we dispose our will (the capacity for choosing, intending, loving, and hating, intelligible goods and bads) in a certain direction. By our choices, we constitute a certain type of self (Anscombe, 1958; Hursthouse, 1999). Thus, if I commit to learning and choose in accord with that commitment, and respect the good of truth in my choices, I constitute a self that is open to and appreciative of that good, and the same with other basic goods. By contrast, if I choose to kill, then I direct my will *against* an instance of the basic good of life; in that choice, I *diminish* my love of and respect for the intrinsic good of human life.

The Denial That Life Is in Itself Valuable

To defend suicide and assisted suicide, one might, first, argue that human life is not in itself valuable, that it is only instrumentally good; or, second, one might hold that although life is valuable in itself, it can in some circumstances cease to be valuable; or third, one might hold that life is valuable in itself and always remains valuable, but that its value is outweighed by pain and other burdens so that killing becomes permissible (Graber, 1981; Singer, 1994; Hardwig, 1997; Szasz, 2002). I reply to the first alternative in this section, to the others in subsequent sections.

I have argued that human life is itself valuable or worthwhile, and so a choice to kill an innocent person is always morally wrong. However, someone contemplating a life filled with suffering and despair may view her continued living as something bad, in that it continues the pain and suffering. In other words, on this view, human life is only instrumentally good—a means toward realizing good experiences, achievements, and so on, but when it no longer makes those possible, it ceases to be valuable. There is no point—it might be argued—in prolonging life when it is no longer worthwhile.

In reply, this view implicitly identifies the self—the person who would be benefited by death—with something other than the human organism that is killed. The idea that one's life—sometimes in these contexts referred to as "mere biological life"—can be a severe imposition on one's well-being implicitly supposes that the subject of well-being is something other than the human, bodily entity (George, 2012). Bodily life is treated as merely an interesting tool or instrument—good just insofar as, and for as long as, it enables *us* to have and enjoy various experiences. But the body is not—on this view—part of the person or the self.

This view cannot be sustained. We are not just consciousnesses or spirits that inhabit or use bodies; we are living bodily entities (Nussbaum & Rorty, 1992; Leftow, 2001). Now, those who wish to deny that we are physical organisms think of *themselves*, what each of them refers to as *I*, as the subject of self-conscious acts, or of conceptual thought and willing. But we can show that this agent—the one who has self-awareness and conceptual thought—is identical with the subject of physical, bodily actions, and so is a living, bodily being (an organism).

Sensation is a bodily action, an action performed by the organism as a whole (and not just its brain). The act of seeing, for example, is an act that an animal performs with its eyeballs and optic nerve, just as the act of walking is an act that he performs with its legs. But it is clear in the case of human individuals that it must be the same entity, the same single subject of actions, that performs the act of sensing and that performs the act of understanding. When I know, for example, that *This is a book*, it is by my understanding, or a self-conscious intellectual act, that I apprehend what is meant by *book*, apprehending what it is (at least in a general way). But the subject of that proposition, what I refer to by the word *This*, is apprehended by sensation or perception. Clearly, it must be the same thing—the same I—which apprehends the predicate of a judgment and the subject of that same judgment. So, it is the same substantial entity, the same agent, who understands and who senses or perceives. Hence, the entity that is referred to by the word *I* (namely, the subject of conscious, intellectual acts) is identical with the physical organism which is the subject of bodily actions such as sensing or perceiving.

So, it is mistaken to say that human life is valuable only as a means toward bringing about other conditions that are valuable in themselves. As I briefly indicated before, the basic reasons for action are the various forms of personal perfection or fulfillment for ourselves, and others like us. That is, what makes a condition or activity intrinsically valuable, worth pursuing for its own sake, is that it is *fulfilling*. But it makes no sense to hold that the fulfillment of an entity is intrinsically valuable and yet that the entity itself is not. The entity itself cannot be viewed as a mere instrumental good, or as a mere condition for the fulfillment or perfection of that entity. Thus, my genuine good includes my *being*—and so my life—as well as my *full*-being or fulfillment.

Moreover, while it is true that an intrinsic *part* of myself can be viewed as in some way instrumentally valuable (my bodily parts are called *organs*, from the Greek word for instrument, όργανο), it is impossible actually to view my whole self as merely instrumental to another good. One must value, at least implicitly, one's own being as in itself good. So, to view one's whole biological life as merely instrumentally valuable is indeed, though perhaps only implicitly, to identify oneself with something other than that living bodily entity, which is false.

Can Innocent Human Life Lose Its Value?

Next, one might grant that one's life is intrinsically valuable, but insist that it can *lose* that value, either because one waives one's right to life, one is exercising one's autonomy by suicide, or one's life has lost its dignity.

Autonomy

One might argue that one's life can cease to be valuable because one waives her right to life. On this view, while human life is in itself valuable, it is not unconditionally valuable—it ceases to be worthwhile if the owner of this life waives her right to life, or no longer values it.

One way of expressing this objection is to argue that what makes intentional killing wrong is, not that it is a choice contrary to an intrinsic good of a person, but that it violates someone's rights, and that in suicide and assisted suicide, the person being killed waives her right not to be killed. What makes killing usually wrong (on this view) is that it violates someone's *autonomy*. But suicide is the exercise of one's autonomy (if done by someone with decision-making capacity), and assisting someone to commit suicide promotes that autonomy.

But let us return to our hypothetical scenario. Suppose Charlie—the homeless candidate for transplant of vital organs—woke up, learned of the idea (of distributing his organs to save six others), and demanded that we go ahead with our plan. Would that make killing him for his organs morally okay (either on his part or ours)? It does not seem so. To thwart someone's will is not the only way of harming a person or of failing to respect that person. Although an act may not violate a person's autonomy (that is, may not restrict or go against that person's will), it may still be contrary to the intrinsic good of that person and morally wrong for that reason.

To this, one might rejoin that in Charlie's case, the reason why his consent would not justify his being killed is that he would be consenting to being used for the sake of others. His conception of what he wants for his own life, however, or what is in his own interests, *would* morally justify killing him (see Fishkin, 1982; Murphy, 1993). However, this does not seem right either. If Charlie embraced a bizarre religion and wanted with all his heart to be sacrificed to the gods, neither his act nor ours would thereby be morally justified. Again, a choice to waste my talents is morally wrong, and not only because it deprives the community of gifts I could have contributed. It is wrong because I have failed to respect my own welfare; I have made less of myself than I should have—without violating my autonomy. Hence, the fact that a choice to commit suicide may be both an exercise of one's autonomy and in accord with one's own self-interpreted interests does not morally justify that choice. Nor would assisting someone to commit suicide be morally justified on those grounds.

Appropriate Death

Another way of construing death as in some cases actually good is to argue that death is the boundary of life, related to one's life somewhat the way a picture frame is related to a picture. And so, just as a picture frame may add to or detract from the picture, so dying in this way or that may add to or detract from one's self-created life as a whole, and so death carried out in this manner would be a good thing.

However, while life is like art in many ways, there are important dissimilarities that make this argument unsound. We do constitute our characters by our choices—and so there is an important analogy; but the goodness or badness of the biological and intellectual dimensions of ourselves is not wholly constituted by our designing or shaping them. Human life (including health) and knowledge of truth are in themselves good *prior to* their being pursued by choice, and their structures are not directly subject to free or artistic design. Most importantly, death itself is simply not an artistic product. There may be various desirable *effects* of the death: for example, its timing may be more or less apt for various reasons. But death itself is the destruction of one's life. One's own death itself is not an act that one performs: although one can choose to kill, and one can do something that causes one's death, one's actual death is something that, whether one wishes it or not, occurs to a human being rather than an action one performs. This is because it is a *ceasing to be*, not the actualization of any potentiality one possesses. Therefore, death as such is the privation of the life of a living being, and so death itself is in no way a good. There could be aesthetic *effects* of one's dying or there could be a certain appropriateness about when one dies, but these are in reality distinct from the death itself. That being so, the object of choice in a suicide adopted as a means toward shaping one's "life as a whole" in an appropriate manner (though how it does so is obscure, to say the least) remains the destruction of one's life. This is a bad means chosen to bring about a (possibly) good end and so is morally wrong.

Dignity

Still another way of arguing that human life can lose its intrinsic value is by appeal to the concept of *dignity*. It might be argued that there are various conditions that make continuing to live a severe *in*dignity, and therefore in choosing to kill, one is not choosing to destroy what retains intrinsic value. Granted, one might contend, one ought not to kill any person whose life retains dignity or intrinsic worth. Still, to live in a persistent vegetative state, or as severely demented, or as completely dependent on others and burdensome to them—to continue to have biological life but without *meaningful life*—is a fate worse than death. A different way of expressing this argument is to say that there are two types of death: death *with* dignity and death *without* dignity, and the former is to be preferred to the latter, and thus it can be morally right to choose it (Graber, 1981).

To reply to this argument, we must clarify the different things that may be referred to by the word *dignity* (see the papers in Dillon, 1995). There are different types of dignity, but in each case the word refers to a property or properties—different ones in different circumstances—that cause one to *excel* and thus merit respect from others. First, there is the dignity of a person or personal dignity. The dignity of a person is that whereby a person excels other beings, especially other animals, and merits respect or consideration from other persons. In my judgment, what distinguishes us from other animals, what makes us persons rather than things, is our radical capacity for (that is, the basic nature which orients us toward) shaping our own lives, our ability to chooses deliberately. This basic, natural capacity is possessed by every human being, even those who cannot immediately exercise it. Dignity in this sense derives from the kind of substantial entity one is, a human being—and this is dignity in the most important sense. Because it is based on the kind of being one is, one cannot lose this dignity as long as one exists. Someone in a so-called persistent vegetative state has a nature orienting her toward shaping her own life, though circumstances block the actualization of that nature.

A second type of dignity is dignity *in action or choice*. Thus, one can distinguish between *having* dignity and *acting with* dignity. Acting with dignity is an action or choice that manifests an underlying dignity; the action itself also is dignified, in the sense that it excels other types of action and being acted upon. Of course, one speaks of dignified action usually in the moral sense of excellence. Thus, one can make choices and live one's life in a dignified manner in relation to severe suffering and indignities (of other types).

Third, there is a type of dignity that varies in degrees, which is the *manifestation* or *actualization* of those capacities that distinguish us from other animals. Thus, slipping on a banana peel (being reduced for a moment to a passive object) and losing one's independence and privacy (especially as regards our baser functions) are events that detract from our dignity in this sense. However, while this dignity seems to be harmed by various situations, it never seems to be completely removed. Moreover, this dignity, which varies in degrees, is distinct from the more basic dignity that derives from the kind of substantial entity one is.

In addition to the different types of real dignity, one must distinguish one's sense of dignity. Something may harm one's *sense of* dignity without removing one's real dignity. Everyone who becomes dependent on others *feels* a certain loss of dignity. Yet their dignity, in any of the first three senses distinguished above, may not have been diminished at all. Often one's sense of dignity can be at variance with one's real dignity (in all of the first three senses). Those who are sick and who bear their suffering in a courageous or holy manner often inspire others, even though they themselves may feel a loss of dignity.

So, in truth, every human being has a basic real dignity based simply on being a person—that whereby she excels other animals and has in her what makes her deserving of respect and consideration from all other persons. This is one of the crucial truths at stake in the debate about suicide and euthanasia.

Some conditions harm our dignity in the third sense discussed earlier (the manifestation of our more basic dignity)—conditions such as being dependent on others, loss of privacy, and preoccupation with pain. These conditions are certainly bad. None of us desires to be in these conditions, and we should work to remove or alleviate such conditions in sick and elderly people as much as possible. But that does not mean that it would be right to kill someone (or oneself) to prevent those indignities. First, the life of a person is itself distinct from the suffering and other burdens that may mistakenly seem to detract from that person's dignity. Death itself is bad, the destruction of an intrinsic good. So, to choose death to avoid indignities (in the sense of loss of independence, which is the *manifestation* of an underlying dignity) is to act against what has basic, intrinsic dignity for the sake of an ulterior end. But the end does not justify the means. Moreover, the very act of killing a person with the supposed justification that the one killed has lost her dignity, or is about to lose her dignity, denies the *intrinsic personal* dignity of the one killed. It also is worth remembering here that there is a distinction between death and the process of dying. The process of dying may in many ways assault our dignity, in the sense of its manifestation, but it is not a loss of one's basic dignity as a person, and it need not involve a loss of dignity in action. It must be conceded that death itself, since it is one's ceasing to be or destruction, is a loss of dignity. But that point argues *against* hastening death, not for it.

No one wants to die without dignity. But we do not really want to die now *with* dignity either. Death itself is never a dignity—it is, in a way, the supreme indignity. We may bear suffering and death well, and whether we do so depends, in part, on whether we continue to treat ourselves as well as others as persons with intrinsic dignity; that is, persons who have dignity simply because they are persons.

Can the Intrinsic Value of Life Be Outweighed by Other Considerations?

Someone might concede that human life is intrinsically valuable, and that it remains valuable to the end, but insist nevertheless that its value can be outweighed or overridden. Almost all admit that there are times when forgoing life-sustaining treatment is morally permissible, and of course death, or the hastening of death, results. But, it might be argued, isn't the decision to forgo treatment in those situations based on the judgment that relief of pain, or avoidance of all the difficulties being experienced, is a greater good for the patient, and the loss of life a lesser evil? But if that is a morally sufficient reason for forgoing treatment, why would it not also be a morally sufficient reason for choosing to hasten death? In other words, it seems that one who holds that it can be morally permissible to forgo life-sustaining treatment, is admitting that sometimes the harm of death is outweighed by the good of relief of pain and avoidance of other burdens.

However, this argument assumes that the only standard for rationally and morally preferring one option with bad results over another with different bad results is that one option offers a greater net benefit than the other. But this assumption cannot be sustained. The basis on which one reasonably determines that it is morally permissible to forgo life-sustaining treatment does not involve measuring the consequences of treating versus those of not treating, and finding that not treating will result in a greater amount of good.

Suppose I have badly damaged my knee and the orthopedists propose surgery. To decide whether to have surgery or not, I must of course consider the pros (eventual complete knee repair and greater ability to run, play sports, etc.) and the cons (cost of several thousand dollars, and time lost from my physically demanding job). Suppose I decide I ought to forgo the knee surgery, and suppose that is a reasonable judgment. Is that because I have measured the benefits and burdens of surgery against the benefits and burdens of forgoing surgery, and concluded that the latter has a net greater good or lesser evil? Clearly not. The burdens and benefits in the different options here cannot be measured against one another; they are of different types and so cannot be placed on a common scale to weigh them against each other. One cannot objectively measure—prior to moral norms, which is what this objection says we must do—the costs of missing work for a short but significant time, against decreased athletic ability over a longer time. One cannot say that one option (forgoing surgery) contains all the good that the other one does (surgery), plus more. But one would have to do that in order to make the judgment that the results in one option *outweigh*—in terms of sheer goodness or badness—the results in the other option. Instead, the moral judgment that I ought to forgo surgery is based on my discerning a greater moral responsibility involved in one option (in this case, to my family to remain employed in the near future) than in the other option.

Now, the same point is true when the treatment is life-sustaining and an effect of forgoing treatment is loss of life. No more here than in the knee surgery case can one measure the consequences in the options against one another just in terms of the amount of good or bad produced. Of course, one can compare the options in relation to a moral standard, such as the moral demand for fairness, or the golden rule. But the assumption of the objection is that one can measure the benefits and burdens of the option directly against each other, to arrive at a premise—this option produces greater net good than the other—that, when joined with the general ethical norm that one should benefit persons, will yield a moral conclusion (Griffin, 1986; Chang, 1997). Rather, moral norms measure choices, not outcomes. So, there are other moral norms, such as that I should be motivated by concern for genuine goods, not mere fear, or that I should not be motivated merely by a greater emotional attachment to some persons rather than others, instead of a concern for genuine goods, including specific types of relationships—that can distinguish when one should forgo treatment and when one should not. Hence, moral judgments that one may (or should) forgo life-sustaining treatment do not presuppose that the value of a human life has been overridden or outweighed by other considerations.

The judgment that the value of a human life is outweighed by the avoidance of suffering and other goods brought about by the act of killing is unfounded. Indeed, it is hard to see how one could say that killing Charlie to obtain his organs is morally wrong, if one held that view. If one chooses to kill in order to end suffering, one sees (at least initially) that continuing to live instantiates a basic human good, but that escaping pain and other burdens also would instantiate a basic good. To act *against* the first reason (as opposed to simply not acting on it), one must judge that the second reason (escaping pain) is preferable to it. But one can make such a judgment only on the supposition that the good offered by the second alternative (escape from pain) is of a higher order than the good offered by the first alternative (a human life). But it could be of a higher order only if human life were not a basic and intrinsic good. Thus, the choice to kill a human person as a means toward escaping pain and other burdens involves the attitude that human life is not a basic and intrinsic good. A choice to kill a human life is incompatible with a love for that life. Such a choice involves the judgment or attitude that some lives are not worth living, that this life—which is in truth identical to the human person himself or herself—is not an instance of a basic and irreducible good. Suicide, then, is an objectively morally wrong choice, and so, formally assisting suicide is also objectively morally wrong.

References

Anscombe, G. E. M. (1958). Modern moral philosophy. *Philosophy, 33*, 1–19.

AP (Associated Press). (1992). Colombian says he killed 50 to supply school with bodies. *Los Angeles Times*, March 6. Retrieved from: http://articles.latimes.com/1992-03-06/news /mn-3345_1_medical-school

Aquinas, T. (1265/1989). *Summa Theologiae*, IIa–IIae Q. 64, art. 7. (T. McDermott, Trans.). Notre Dame, IN: Christian Classics.

Cavanaugh, T. (2006). *Double-effect reasoning: Doing good and avoiding evil.* Oxford: Oxford University Press.

Chang, R. (1997). *Incommensurability, incomparability, and practical reason.* Cambridge, MA: Harvard University Press.

Dillon, R. (Ed.). (1995). *Dignity, character, and self-respect.* New York: Routledge.

Driver, J. (2012). *Consequentialism.* London: Routledge.

Dworkin, R. (1993). *Life's dominion: An argument about abortion, euthanasia, and individual freedom.* New York: Vintage Books.

Fishkin, J. (1982). *The limits of obligation.* New Haven, CT: Yale University Press.

George, R. (2012). Terminal logic: Everyone is a person—no one is "mere biological life." *Touchstone: A Journal of Mere Christianity.* Retrieved from: http://www.touchstone mag.com/archives/article.php?id=19-02-032-f.

Glynn, K. (1999). "Double effect": Getting the argument right—physician-assisted suicide. *Commonweal, 126*, 36–39.

Graber, G. (1981). The rationality of suicide. In S. Wallace & A. Eser (Eds.), *Suicide and euthanasia: The rights of personhood* (pp. 51–65). Knoxville: University of Tennessee Press.

Griffin, J. (1986). *Well-being.* Oxford: Clarendon Press.

Hardwig, J. (1997). Is there a duty to die? *Hastings Center Report, 27*, 34–42.

Hooker, B. (2000). *Ideal code, real world: A rule-consequentialist theory of morality.* Oxford: Oxford University Press.

Hursthouse, R. (1999). *On virtue ethics.* Oxford: Oxford University Press.

Kant, I. (1785/1998). *Groundwork of the metaphysics of morals* (M. Gregor, Trans.). (Section I: Transition from common rational to philosophic moral cognition). Cambridge: Cambridge University Press.

Keenan, J., & Kopfensteiner, T. (1995). The principle of cooperation. *Health Progress, 76*(3), 23–27.

Leftow, B. (2001). Souls dipped in dust: Aquinas on soul and body. In K. Corcoran (Ed.), *Body, soul and survival: Essays on the metaphysics of human persons* (pp. 120–138). Ithaca, N.Y.: Cornell University Press.

Mill, J. S. (1861). *Utilitarianism* (R. Crisp, Ed.). Oxford: Oxford University Press, 1998.

Murphy, L. (1993). The demands of beneficence. *Philosophy and Public Affairs, 22*, 267–292.

Nussbaum, M., & Rorty, E. (Ed.). (1992). *Essays on Aristotle's De Anima.* Oxford: Oxford University Press.

O'Neill, O. (2008). Kant and utilitarianism contrasted. In J. Arthur & S. Scalet (Eds.), *Morality and moral controversies: Readings in moral, social and political philosophy* (pp. 78–83). Upper Saddle River, NJ: Prentice-Hall.

PCJP (Pontifical Council for Justice and Peace). (2005). *Compendium of the social doctrine of the Church.* Washington, DC: United States Conference of Catholic Bishops.

Rachels, J. (1975). Active and passive euthanasia. *New England Journal of Medicine, 292*, 78–80.

Roach, M. (2004). *Stiff: The curious lives of human cadavers.* New York. W. W. Norton.

Singer, P. (1994). *Rethinking life and death.* New York: St. Martin's Press.

Szasz, T. (2002). *Fatal freedom: The ethics and politics of suicide.* Syracuse, NY: Syracuse University Press.

Tooley, M. (1999). An irrelevant consideration: Killing versus letting die. In B. Steinbock & A. Norcross (Eds.), *Killing and letting die* (pp. 103–111). New York: Fordham University Press.

Reply to Lee

John Lachs

Professor Lee's essay against physician-assisted suicide is an eloquent statement of a traditional position. He thinks that suicide is always wrong, and intentionally aiding someone who performs such a culpable act is itself morally unacceptable.

Unfortunately, Professor Lee's argument suffers from at least six major flaws. The weaknesses take the form of questionable assumptions, unexplicated claims, and inadequate arguments. I will deal with them in turn.

Objective Values

Professor Lee thinks that values are objective, that is, that they are independently existing realities. This means that good things are good prior and without reference to being pursued. Facts and values are on a par: both are open to investigation and discovery, and when we grasp what is good, we are inclined to devote ourselves to its service. We can be just as mistaken about right choice as about the location of the nearest Wal-Mart. Morality consists of finding the true precepts of moral action and choosing according to them.

If any of this were true, the moral life would be marvelously easy. In reality, however, it is overwhelmingly difficult to make conscientious moral judgments. The good is not like the seashore, ready to be visited and loved; different people pursue different activities and, with equal fervor, judge them to be good. How do we tell who is right? Professor Lee offers us no tools for choosing among competing accounts of what is right or good. When there is so much disagreement, what reason do we have for supposing that any of them is objectively true?

Human Nature

Professor Lee supposes that there is a single, uniform human nature. He expresses this by saying that there are "basic goods" and fulfilling activities valued by everyone. Unfortunately, however, the basic goods he mentions are far from being universal. Health, knowledge of truth, friendship, and excellence at play, along with many other activities, are valued at best generally and for the most part, though clearly not by everyone.

Declaring that certain characteristics are universal, even if we do not display them, is of no avail. We lack a basis for attributing latent or potential tendencies to people who show no traces of them. Human nature is so diverse that the prevailing values and most sacred features of one individual or society may well be anathema to others. Consequently, any attempt to build an edifice of values on the basis of "the intrinsic good" of human beings in order to house an unconditional commitment to life is doomed to failure.

Contemporary Debates in Bioethics, First Edition. Edited by Arthur L. Caplan and Robert Arp.

Shaping Lives

The theory of dignity advanced by Professor Lee is built on the difference between animals and humans. Dignity is supposed to be the just demand we make to be respected on account of our excellence. The others we excel are not human beings, or else some of us would have more dignity than others. Instead, any human excels any animal because we have "a radical capacity for shaping our own lives," and other living things do not. This radical capacity for choice characterizes each of us and is not lost even in a persistent vegetative state. Suicide, according to Professor Lee, runs afoul of this human dignity.

Anyone who thinks animals lack the capacity to shape their lives has never lived with a cat. Careful observation of animal behavior makes it abundantly clear that they can choose, decide, plan, and calculate. They do not discuss these feats the way humans tend to do, and their limited ability to conceptualize the future renders their foresight unimpressive. But there is not a shred of evidence to support the idea that there is a sharp line between animals and humans. Further, the notion that individuals in a persistent vegetative state retain the ability to make decisions is a fiction. Since such unfortunate people do not excel anyone and do not direct their lives, they lack what Professor Lee calls basic dignity. The collapse of the argument from dignity knocks out a main pillar of the case against suicide.

Life as a Basic Good

Professor Lee announces, without a supporting argument, that life is a basic good. A basic good, presumably, is something the attainment of which satisfies us. But whether life does indeed satisfy us is a factual question, and it is well known that under some circumstances it does not. Since it would be devastating for his position, Professor Lee attempts to sidestep this consideration by saying that one's life is identical with one's intrinsically valuable self, and it cannot therefore be used as a means to relieving one's suffering.

This argument strikes me as somewhat murky. But whatever intrinsic merit it may possess, it misrepresents what happens in suicide. People who decide to kill themselves do not view their existence as a means to anything beyond. Instead, they recognize that their lives serve as the condition of their misery, and they want to end their suffering. The confusion is between the ideas of means and condition. If something is a means to something else, it contributes to bringing it about. A condition, by contrast, only makes events possible, without causing them.

Being a woman, for example, does not conduce to pregnancy, so it is not a means to it. But it makes impregnation possible, and so it is a condition without which pregnancy cannot occur. Similarly, being alive is a neutral state that opens the door to both joy and misery. There is nothing morally wrong with eliminating a condition that leads to constant suffering. It is morally permissible to pull the tooth that perpetually hurts.

Benefits and Burdens

In order to justify suicide, one has to assess the benefits and burdens of terminating life and measure them against the consequences of continued existence. Professor Lee maintains that such comparisons are impossible. Strange as this sounds, he thinks that the amount of good produced by one of the alternatives is incommensurable with that generated by the other. The reason, he says, is that the comparison requires measuring both options against a moral standard, and such standards gauge choices, not outcomes.

This is a remarkable argument. It declares impossible what we do many times each day. Most of our moral choices are determined by assessment of the reasonably expectable consequences of our actions. At least one half of moral philosophy is summarily dropped from consideration if we insist that pain, happiness, love, trust, caring, heartache, and despondency—consequences all—do not matter. If Professor Lee insists that we measure against a moral standard, why are good and bad consequences inadequate? Why do only right and wrong choices matter?

Losing Features

Professor Lee's world is crowded with beings that can never lose their characteristic features. Life can never lose its value, what is right can never quit being so, and, because we are substantial beings, we can never lose our dignity. Such a world is vastly reassuring: it provides moral compass and the cozy feeling that we already know everything important about the moral life. Since what is of intrinsic value can never change, painful and thorny moral problems dissolve into easily applied casuistry.

This is not the world inhabited by conscientious contemporaries. Unfortunately, because corrosive change is at the heart of everything, we cannot find any "substantial" beings. Species emerge from pre-existing forms, and their supposedly rigid essences melt into one another. Humans find new perfections to pursue; the luxuriant variety of our fellows makes it difficult to categorize or to condemn them. Moral values are themselves in process, confounding those who rely on ancient remedies for novel ills.

The earth is moving under our feet, and the sky is too cloudy to steer by distant stars. What was once right is now questionable; what was once good no longer satisfies. No being is assured of continued life, and no characteristic of it remains the same for long. Terrible moral problems beset us, creating confusion, testing the conscience, and offering only painful choices. What have never even been conceived in prior centuries now face us as urgent problems, and we have no one to turn to for help but ourselves.

The aging of our population and the rapidly growing power of medicine to keep people alive force us to confront the problem of physician-assisted suicide. Some people are simply done with life: they have had enough and want help with finishing it off. Under the right circumstances, their cry for help is justified, and we cannot morally deny them aid. There is reason to believe that our laws will soon have to follow the lead of our morality.

Reply to Lachs

Patrick Lee

Professor Lachs's essay presents a powerful emotional appeal in behalf of physician-assisted suicide (PAS), an argument for his position, and replies to some others. In my judgment, the emotional appeal is the strongest part. So, I will comment on both the emotional appeal and the arguments.

Lachs complains about the "abstractness" of many bioethical discussions. But the question is not whether a moral statement is abstract—every reasoned argument contains abstract statements—but whether any *relevant factors* have been omitted. Even Lachs's long story about Magda is abstract: many features of the situation—such as Magda's height, weight, hair color, place of residence—are omitted. But, plainly, that is because they are irrelevant to the ethical question. Where Lachs and I disagree is on which factors are relevant to the ethical question and which are not. Thus, it would be a mistake to hold that my position is abstract, while Lachs's position is concrete. Lachs later states that no physician should be compelled to participate in PAS if this violates his conscience; evidently, trying to make someone violate his conscience is a feature sufficient to make a choice to do that morally wrong. I agree, but I also hold that the fact that a choice includes the intention to destroy an innocent human life is sufficient to make such a choice morally wrong.

Perhaps the complaint about abstraction means that an intellectual approach should give way to emotion—which does respond to the concrete. But, while emotions are not to be ignored, they must be evaluated by intelligent assessment of how one's choices are related to the genuine human goods at stake in that choice. What we react to with emotional repugnance is, precisely, the suffering itself of someone who is dying, and in severe pain, gradually losing their vigor and faculties, becoming dependent on others, and perhaps feeling despair. I share that emotional repugnance, and I believe that we *should* have such an emotional response. But it is a different thing altogether to assert that, given that emotion, the best way to act—the best way of helping someone in that condition—is to help her kill herself. The problem with Lachs's appeal to emotion—as with many other appeals to emotion—is that the conclusion it is meant to support confuses what the appropriate emotion is actually directed to: we rightly abhor the pain and suffering, but not the person himself or herself in that condition. It is right to try to remove the pain and suffering; it is *not* right intentionally to destroy the person, as a means of removing that pain and suffering.

A related confusion grounds the absurd accusation that those who refuse to assist someone's suicide are forcing them to endure pain and suffering. This accusation rests on Lachs's repeated failure to distinguish between *intentionally* doing something bad (such as intentionally making someone suffer), on the one

Contemporary Debates in Bioethics, First Edition. Edited by Arthur L. Caplan and Robert Arp.

hand, and choosing not to do something, which results in something bad as a *side effect* (not assisting a killing, with the side effect that a person suffers more than if a killing had been assisted).

The argument Lachs advances to support PAS is that, first, life is not an intrinsic basic good, and only enjoyable experiences are intrinsically good; second, for people in situations like Magda's, the bad experiences far outweigh the good ones, and so, third, one can infer that for such persons, continuing to live is pointless.

On this view, life itself is merely an instrumental good: one's life is worthwhile only if one's future experience contains a net positive. But the idea that one can apply a utilitarian calculus and measure the good and bad effects brought about by an action depends on identifying what is intrinsically worthwhile only with experience. Even in his paradigm case, Lachs seems to have ignored important items on the positive side of the "ledger": the continuing relationship of Magda to others, including her son (Professor Lachs himself), for example. If what is worthwhile is not just experiences, but what is genuinely fulfilling for persons—including life itself—then it is impossible to perform the utilitarian calculation Lachs assumes is possible: there is no objective standard by which one can measure the goodness as such of the pains and sufferings, on the one side, against life, continuing personal relationships, and so on, on the other side.

Lachs attempts to rebut various rationales for the idea that life can be intrinsically valuable. In my judgment, these replies are weak. From the fact that human beings are often quite irrational, it simply does not follow that rationality—that is, having a rational *nature*, that is, a dynamic constitution orienting them to the stage where they can shape their own lives by their deliberate choices—is not a fundamental and distinguishing human feature. Lachs's assertion—with no argument—that "many species of animals show themselves capable of reasoning," is unconvincing. How many other animals manifest any pondering over whether they are doing the right thing or not? How many devise different manners of living together (as opposed to species-invariant modes of cooperation), different types of art, of architecture, and of mating rituals? Such activities manifest the possession of genuine reasoning—conceptual thought, based on apprehending the nature of a thing and what necessarily follows upon it, as opposed to perceptual thought and instinct. What is more, such activities *follow upon* the possession of reason, so that, if another species really did have such a basic capacity, then individuals of that species would at some point manifest those activities.

The ground for having intrinsic moral worth (or being a subject of rights) is being an individual with a rational nature. Moral worth is the reciprocal of a moral responsibility to respect or care for someone. Mere desires or urges—which we have in common with other animals—do not ground moral responsibilities. But the practical *understanding* that an activity or condition would be fulfilling for me and others like me does ground a moral responsibility. Such practical understanding is found in all, and only, rational beings. So, what is fulfilling for any rational being is a good worthy of pursuit, and every rational being has moral worth. And those who possess moral worth are the individuals with the basic capacity (nature) for such practical understanding—they have moral worth during those times of their lives they are not able immediately to exercise their capacity for rationality, such as when they are asleep, in a coma, very young, or senile. The person themself is intrinsically valuable, not just the "conscious and intelligent enjoyments" they have. And so their lives—which are identical to them—remain worthy of respect even when—and perhaps especially when—they are experiencing severe pain and suffering.

I briefly turn now to the legal issue. Since the original question posed was whether assisted suicide is *ethical*, not whether it should be legal, my first essay did not address that issue. Professor Lachs's essay moves back and forth between both questions. I agree with Lachs that the political community should confine itself to preventing public harms. But there are, in my judgment, several ways in which legalization of PAS is gravely unjust to all of those who are dying or disabled (and so, as unjust, is a public harm). Professor Lachs assures us that there will be effective safeguards to insure that mercy killings will be voluntary. But if death is considered to be in many cases a benefit, then how could it be withheld from those who lack decision-making capacity (including those with varying degrees of dementia and impaired infants)? Moreover, since most doctors are not trained to notice signs of clinical depression, the practice likely will lead to many who are incapacitated for rational choices opting for suicide; whereas, if they are treated for their depression—experience shows—most withdraw their request for death. Thus, in my judgment—and that of many others—a policy of making PAS available for the terminally ill who are enduring unbearable suffering will by its own logic and practice lead to nonvoluntary euthanasia (including on infants) undertreatment (due to less incentive to pursue alternatives to PAS) and less availability of hospice and palliative care.

But most problematic of all: the social acceptance of suicide as an apt solution to continuing pain, suffering, and loss of independence, when one is severely debilitated, would be a strong social affirmation that the lives of many of the weakest and most vulnerable among us, are not intrinsically worthwhile. And so society would send the message to the elderly and the disabled, that when they become dependent and feel like burdens on their families, their life may very well lack inherent value. That itself will be a pressure—and not a very subtle one—on the elderly, and even on many disabled, to opt for death rather than life.

Part 8

Should Stem-Cell Research Utilizing Embryonic Tissue Be Conducted?

Introduction

While looking at thin pieces of cork bark through his compound microscope in 1665, English naturalist, Robert Hooke (1635–1703), noticed what he would later refer to as "small rooms" butting up against one another in a pattern that reminded him of an aerial view of monks' chambers at an abbey. In his work related to his microscopic observations, *Micrographia* (Hooke, 1665), Hooke would dub these small rooms *cells*, after the Latin word for small room, *cellula*. Thus began the work that would lead to the *cell theory*—first articulated by the combined efforts of researchers doing work in microscopy such as Antonie Philips van Leeuwenhoek (1632–1723), Johann Jacob Paul Moldenhawer (1766–1827), and Ludolph Christian Treviranus (1779–1864), then Theodor Schwann (1810–1882), Matthias Jakob Schleiden (1804–1881), and Rudolf Virchow (1821–1902)—which still holds true today:

1. All living things are composed of cells.
2. The cell is the basic unit of structure and function in a living thing.
3. Cells contain hereditary information.
4. All cells derive from pre-existing cells.
5. All cells are similar in chemical composition in organisms of a similar species (Mazzarello, 1999; Alberts et al., 2009).

"It is the cells which create and maintain in us, during the span of our lives, our will to live and survive, to search and experiment, and to struggle." So maintained the Belgian biologist, Albert Claude, in his Nobel Lecture on December 12, 1974 (Lindsten, 1992, p. 145). The creative capacity of a cell that Claude colorfully and metaphorically spoke about is most clearly made manifest—quite literally—in a stem cell. Found in all multicellular organisms, a stem cell is a type of cell that has the ability (a) to renew itself through numerous cycles of cell division (both symmetric and asymmetric) and (b) to differentiate into numerous cell types. A primary function of stem cells (along with progenitor cells) is to repair tissues in organisms that have been damaged; thus, in line with Claude's claim above, stem cells truly help "maintain" us.

Contemporary Debates in Bioethics, First Edition. Edited by Arthur L. Caplan and Robert Arp.

According to the historical research of Ramalho-Santos and Willenbring (2007), it was Ernst Haeckel (1834–1919) who likely first used the term *Stammzelle* with the dual purpose of describing (1) the unicellular organism that predated multicellular organisms in evolutionary history, as well as (2) the fertilized egg from which all the other cells of an organism derive. In 1896, Edmund Beecher Wilson (1856–1939) was the first, however, to use the term to refer to an undifferentiated cell that becomes differentiated during development (Maienschein, 2003, p. 253). Aware of Haeckel's research, Theodor Boveri (1862–1915) and Valentin Häcker (1864–1927) described cells that give rise to the germline as stem cells, while Artur Pappenheim (1870–1916), Alexander Maximow (1874–1928), and Ernst Neumann (1834–1918) used the term for the cells from which an organism's blood system emerges.

Today, it is understood that there are two broad types of stem cells in mammals. *Embryonic stem cells* are derived from the inner cell mass of the blastocyst (an early-stage embryo composed of about 100 cells, or so) and are *totipotent*, meaning that they have the ability to differentiate into any one of the cells (more than 200 types) in a mammal's body. *Somatic (or adult) stem cells* are found all over the body in various tissues and are pluripotent or *multipotent*, meaning that they have the ability to differentiate into a number of closely related cells. There are also multipotent stem cells that are derived from amniotic fluid called *amniotic stem cells*, as well as artificially created *induced pluripotent stem cells* produced by gene insertions that have similar properties to that of embryonic stem cells. Finally, there are stem cells that are *unipotent*, meaning that they can only differentiate along one lineage; skin stem cells and many neural stem cells are unipotent (Lanza, 2009; Stein et al., 2011).

Given the pluripotent properties of stem cells, one can imagine the numerous ways in which they can be controlled and manipulated by researchers to yield any number of medical benefits. According to the US National Institutes of Health: "Stem cells, directed to differentiate into specific cell types, offer the possibility of a renewable source of replacement cells and tissues to treat diseases including Alzheimer's diseases, spinal cord injury, stroke, burns, heart disease, diabetes, osteoarthritis, and rheumatoid arthritis" (NIH, 2012). Besides medical benefits, stems cells can be used in testing the effectiveness and safety of drugs (SCRN, 2010), as well as in improving our understanding of life's basic processes.

One may argue on a variety of different religious and secular grounds that any kind of human manipulation of nature or natural processes whatsoever is immoral. If one holds this view, then the production and/or engineering of any kind of stem cell is wrong, and such actions should not be performed. Most researchers in the mainstream scientific world, as well as most religious leaders in the world, have no moral problem with producing and engineering *human* somatic stem cells, amniotic stem cells, and induced pluripotent stem cells. Likewise, most have no moral problem with producing and engineering *nonhuman* somatic stem cells, amniotic stem cells, induced pluripotent stem cells, *and* embryonic stem cells (Annas et al., 1999).

Martin Evans and Matthew Kaufman (1981) at Cambridge and Gail Martin (1981) at the University of California-San Francisco independently produced the first mouse embryonic stem cells in 1981. This research then led to the harvesting of stem cells in all kinds of organisms, including the human embryonic stem cell lines first produced by James Thomson and his group (Thomson et al., 1998) in 1998. Thomson and Nobel Laureate, Shinya Yamanaka, are credited with deriving the first induced pluripotent stem cells (Yu et al., 2007).

However, there are many who find the production and engineering of human embryonic stem cells to be immoral, the primary reason being that the standard procedure for harvesting stem cells results in the destruction of the embryo. There are also straightforward engineering problems associated with, as well as unintended consequences resulting from, harvesting stem cells that still need to be addressed, significant ones being the fact that the harvested stem cells often form tumors (Leeb et al., 2009; also the research in Skotheim et al., 2002), or may cause cancer (Mayshar et al., 2010). The procedure that has been standardly used to harvest embryonic stem cells is known as *somatic cell nuclear transfer* (SCNT). In SCNT, the nucleus of a somatic cell is transferred into a host egg cell that has had its nucleus removed (enucleated). The host egg cell with its new somatic-cell nucleus is then stimulated by electric shock or chemical influence and begins to divide, producing a blastocyst, which is an early-stage embryo composed of about 100 cells, or so. Between 5 and 7 days, stem cells are harvested from the inner cell mass of this blastocyst, and in the process, the blastocyst (embryo) is destroyed (Sutovsky, 2006).

In 2011, the biotechnology company, Advanced Cell Technologies, was awarded a patent from the United States Patent and Trademark Office for their single-blastomere technology (US Patent # 7893315), a method of harvesting stem cells from embryos without having to destroy them in the process that was pioneered by Robert Lanza and his colleagues (Lang, 2011). Given this technology—coupled with the fact that induced pluripotent stem cells are produced from adult stem cells having similar properties to that of embryonic stem cells—it would seem that the ethics of human embryonic stem-cell research might be side stepped altogether. Researchers could use human induced pluripotent stem cells for most of their work, and then for the work requiring human embryonic stem cells to yield the most effective results, single-blastomere technology could be utilized without destroying the embryos. Single-blastomere technology, however, is a controversial technique, since there is some research indicating that it is not possible for an embryo to grow normally following the harvesting of the stem cells (Bertolini et al., 2007).

There is also another method for harvesting pluripotent stem cells without destroying human embryos that has been proposed—but not yet utilized—by Stanford physician, William Hurlburt (2005), called *altered nuclear transfer* (ANT). In ANT, the "somatic cell nucleus or the enucleated egg contents (cytoplasm) or both are first altered before the somatic cell nucleus is transferred into the egg. The alterations cause the somatic cell DNA to function in such a way that no embryo is generated, but pluripotent stem cells (PSCs) are produced" (Hurlburt, 2012). Researchers have pointed out, however, that this proposal "raises the serious question of whether it is possible to know with confidence that this procedure generates a nonembryo, rather than merely an embryo with a deficiency" (Melton et al., 2004; Condic, 2008).

Despite the attempts of researchers to obviate the destruction of human embryos in stem-cell harvesting techniques, there are numerous people who agree with Fr. Tad Pacholczyk (2006) of the National Catholic Bioethics Center that, "in a gesture that reduces young humans to commodities or manipulable products ... embryonic humans should not be generated in laboratory glassware where they can be prodded, invaded, and violated." The official Catholic Church position is that human life begins at the moment of conception, and that this life is as dignified, valued, and deserving of protection as any other human life, no matter what stage of human development (zygote, embryo, fetus, infant, child, young adult, adult, elderly adult). Given this inherent value, a human embryo should never be harmed, even for the general good of medical and scientific improvements, or to save a woman's life (John Paul II, 2001; DHC, 2004; NCBC, 2009; O'Brien, 2011). One could argue for the same conclusion on secular grounds pertaining to inherent value, too (Kant, 1775–1789/1963, 1785/1998, 1797/1996; Dworkin, 1993; Lachmann, 2001; Novak, 2001; cf. Manninen, 2008).

An opposing camp of thinkers agrees with Friedrich's (2000) claim that "the early human embryo is too rudimentary in structure and development to have moral status or interests in its own right" (p. 681). Since the early 1970s with the worldwide emergence of the abortion debate, many thinkers have equated moral status and having interests with *personhood*, so it is precisely the definition of personhood—as well as *who* or *what* counts as a person—that often is at the center of the abortion *and* stem-cell debates. In her important article, "On the Moral and Legal Status of Abortion," Mary Ann Warren (1973) lays out the following as constitutive of personhood, which many would agree with some 40 years later:

1. consciousness (in particular, the ability to feel pain);
2. reasoning;
3. self-motivated activity;
4. the capacity to communicate; and
5. self-awareness, including a self-concept.

A being that meets these criteria is a person, and, as a person, such a being has the fullest of moral rights and privileges—including the right to live and not be harmed—in a society willing to grant such rights and privileges (such as in a constitutional monarchy like the UK, or in a constitutional republic like the US).

No one denies that a fertilized human egg is a human being and member of the species, *Homo sapiens*; what is debated is whether a human being at certain developmental stages of its life could be considered a person according to the aforementioned criteria (there are other criteria given by thinkers, too; see English, 1973; Dennett, 1978; Parfit, 1984; Barresi, 1999; Glynn, 2000; Shoemaker, 2008). At first blush, we can see that there is an obvious developmental distinction between a human zygote, a human embryo, a human fetus, an infant, a toddler, a teenager, and a middle-aged, fully coherent individual; researchers in physical and psychological human development document and explain these differences quite thoroughly (Kail & Cavanaugh, 2010; Sadler, 2011; Newman & Newman, 2012). And, we would surely maintain that the middle-aged, fully coherent individual has moral rights and privileges in a society. Thus, given the criteria for personhood just mentioned, human zygotes, embryos, fetuses, and even infants simply are not persons. Warren maintains, "a fetus, even a fully developed one, is considerably less person-like than is the average mature mammal, indeed the average fish" (p. 48; also see Warren, 1997). If embryos are not persons, then they have no moral rights and privileges, or interests in their own right (using Friedrich's words), and we need not think that we have done anything immoral when we harvest stem cells from them and discard them. Of course, there may be other reasons not to harvest stem cells from human embryos and discard them; again, however, their being persons is not a legitimate reason for not discarding them on Warren's view. And there are numerous doctors, scientists, philosophers, and others who think the same way (Green, 2001; Shannon, 2001; Lebacqz, 2003; Sandel, 2004; cf. Shoemaker, 2008).

In the first chapter of this section, Jane Maienschein is in full agreement with thinkers such as Friedrich and Warren that an embryo is not a person, noting that, "the only reason to pretend that this early blastocyst stage falls under the same description as later developmental stages is to support the a priori belief that 'embryos are persons' ... 'life' that begins then is biological cell division and only that." She offers the following argument to bolster her position: "For those who insist that fertilization and cell division makes a 'person,' then presumably a lineage of cells derived from a fertilized egg and developing in culture should be a person also. So, those cell lines that already exist because of past research should be considered persons, too, and that claim is either useless or absurd."

One interesting point she puts forward in her chapter is that people fallaciously draw the conclusion about what *is* the case regarding the nature of an embryo from a premise having to do with what *ought to be* the case regarding our use of persons in scientific research. Instead of committing an is/ought fallacy, then, one can be tempted to commit an *ought/is* fallacy. The is/ought fallacy occurs when we jump to the conclusion about what ought to be the case from a premise (or premises) about what is the case without offering any legitimate reasons for this (il)logical move. For example, the Catholic position that sexual relations of any kind ought to be performed only in the form of sexual intercourse with the intent to procreate *because* it is the case that sexual intercourse leads to procreation is often cited as a clear example of committing the is/ought fallacy. Counterargument examples that emphasize the fallacious nature of this is/ought way of thinking can be seen in the following:

1. Just because *it is the case that* children engage in self-centered behavior on a regular basis (premise) does not mean that they *ought to/should* engage in self-centered behavior on a regular basis (conclusion).
2. Just because *it is the case that* I want five pieces of cake for dessert (premise), does not mean that I *ought to/should* have five pieces of cake for dessert (conclusion).
3. Just because *it is the case that* students do not want to take a final exam (premise) does not mean that they *ought not/should not* take the final exam (conclusion).
4. Just because *it is the case that* sexual intercourse leads to procreation (premise), does not mean that it *ought to/should* lead to procreation (conclusion).
5. Just because *it is the case that* science can do it (premise), does not mean that science *ought to/should* do it (conclusion).

With respect to stem-cell research utilizing embryonic tissue, then, Maienschein thinks that an ought/is (rather than an is/ought) fallacy is committed, since many of the people who oppose this research think in the following way:

Premise: We ought/should not use persons in scientific research when persons are psychologically and/or physically harmed in this research.

Conclusion: Therefore, it is the case that human embryonic stem cells are persons.

The result is that such people "are attempting to draw *is* conclusions about the nature of embryos from their personal opinions. This is not good science, nor is it good ethics."

Even if a human embryo is not a person, the second author in this section, Bertha Alvarez Manninen, thinks that such a being is nonetheless sacred, and she is not alone in this thinking (Plau, 1996; DHC, 2004; RfP, 2008; Brodd, 2009; O'Brien, 2011). "Vulnerable human life, indeed *all* human life," she maintains, "deserves equal respect in all stages of development." Given this sacredness and respect, a human embryo should not be utilized in research experiments even if we know much good will come of it. Although researchers use human embryos "for a benevolent reason—to help persons debilitated by diabetes, Alzheimer's disease, Parkinson's disease, and spinal cord injury, among other ailments—it remains impermissible to instrumentalize human beings in this way, especially defenseless human beings and even in very early and rudimentary stages of development." To ground her position, Manninen appeals to Immanuel Kant's (1785/1998) second formulation of the categorical imperative: "act in such a way that you treat humanity, whether in your own person or in the person of another, always at the same time as an end and never simply as a means." She also couples Kant's idea with Don Marquis' (1989, 1997) *future of value* argument where the destruction of a human embryo in abortion or stem-cell research is considered wrong because it deprives one of a future life.

Despite their difference of opinion concerning the moral status of a human embryo, Manninen and Maienschein agree that research should be performed on human embryos that have already been produced through IVF, but which are considered "extras" that will be discarded anyway. While Manninen argues that we should not engineer human embryos for the specific purpose of performing research on them, she is in full accord with Maienschein regarding extra embryos that the "onus is on those who oppose their use to argue how incinerating embryos or flushing them down a drain does a better service to humanity than allowing the deaths of these embryos to positively contribute to the world."

References

Alberts, B., Bray, D., Hopkin, K., Johnson, A., Lewis, J., Raff, M ... Walter, P. (2009). *Essential cell biology*. New York: Garland Science.

Annas, G., Caplan, A., & Elias, S. (1999). Stem cell politics, ethics and medical progress. *Nature Medicine, 5*, 1339–1341.

Barresi, J. (1999). On becoming a person. *Philosophical Psychology, 12*, 79–98.

Bertolini, M., Bertolini, L., Gerger, R., Batchelder, C., & Anderson, G. (2007). Developmental problems during pregnancy after *in vitro* embryo manipulations. *Revista Brasileira De Reproduo Animal, 31*, 391–405.

Brodd, J. (2009). *World religions: A voyage of discovery*. New York: St. Mary's Press.

Condic, M. (2008). Alternative sources of pluripotent stem cells: Altered nuclear transfer. *Cell Proliferation, 41*, 7–19.

Dennett, D. (1978). *Brainstorms*. Cambridge, MA: MIT Press.

DHC (Document of the Holy See on Human Cloning). (2004). Retrieved from: http://www.vatican.va/roman_curia/secretariat_state/2004/documents/rc_seg-st_20040927_cloning_en.html

Dworkin, R. (1993). *Life's dominion: An argument about abortion, euthanasia and individual freedom*. New York: Alfred A. Knopf.

English, J. (1973). Abortion and the concept of a person. *Canadian Journal of Philosophy, 5*(2), 233–243.

Evans, M., & Kaufman, M. (1981). Establishment in culture of pluripotent cells from mouse embryos. *Nature, 292*, 154–156.

Friedrich, M. (2000). Debating pros and cons of stem cell research. *Journal of the American Medical Association, 284*, 681–682.

Glynn, S. (2000). *Identity, intersubjectivity and communicative action*. Athens: Paideia Project.

Green, R. (2001). *The human embryo research debates: Bioethics in the vortex of controversy*. Oxford: Oxford University Press.

Hooke, R. (1665). *Micrographia: or, some physiological descriptions of minute bodies made by magnifying glasses*. London: J. Martyn and J. Allestry.

Hurlburt, W. (2005). Altered nuclear transfer: A way forward for embryonic stem cell research. *Stem Cell Reviews and Reports*, *1*, 293–300.

Hurlburt, W. (2012). Altered nulclear transfer: How does ANT work? Retrieved from: http://alterednucleartransfer.com/

John Paul II. (2001). Pope's address to President Bush at Castel Gandolfo, Italy, July 23, 2001. Retrieved from: http://www.americancatholic.org/news/stemcell/pope_to_bush.asp

Kail, R., & Cavanaugh, J. (2010). *Human development: A life-span view*. Belmont, CA: Wadsworth.

Kant, I. (1775–1789/1963). *Lectures on ethics* (L. Infield, Trans.). Indianapolis, IN: Hackett Publishing.

Kant, I. (1785/1998). *Groundwork of the metaphysics of morals* (M. Gregor, Trans.). (Section I: Transition from common rational to philosophic moral cognition). Cambridge: Cambridge University Press.

Kant, I. (1797/1996). *Practical philosophy* (M. Gregor, Trans.). Cambridge: Cambridge University Press.

Lachmann, P. (2001). Stem cell research—why is it regarded as a threat? An investigation of the economic and ethical arguments made against research with human embryonic stem cells. *European Molecular Biology Organization (EMBO) Reports*, *2*(3), 165–168.

Lang, M. (2011). ACT awarded patent for stem cell generation technique. *Mass High Tech*, February 25. Retrieved from: http://www.masshightech.com/stories/2011/02/21/daily53-ACT-awarded-patent-for-stem-cell-generation-technique.html

Lanza, R. (Ed.). (2009). *Essentials of stem cell biology*. London: Elsevier.

Lebacqz, K. (2003). Stem cell ethics: Lessons from context. In N. Snow (Ed.), *Stem cell research: New frontiers in science and ethics* (pp. 85–99). Notre Dame, IN: University of Notre Dame Press.

Leeb, C., Jurga, M., McGuckin, C., Moriggl, R., & Kenner, L. (2009). Promising new sources for pluripotent stem cells. *Stem Cell Reviews and Reports*, *6*, 15–26.

Lindsten, J. (Ed.). (1992). *Nobel lectures, including presentation speeches and laureates' biographies, 1971–1980*. London: World Scientific Publishing Company.

Maienschein, J. (2003). *Whose view of life? Embryos, cloning, and stem cells*. Cambridge, MA: Harvard University Press.

Manninen, B. (2008). Are human embryos Kantian persons? Kantian considerations in favor of embryonic stem cell research. *Philosophy, Ethics, and Humanities in Medicine*, *3*(4). Retrieved from: http://www.peh-med.com/content/3/1/4

Marquis, D. (1989). Why abortion is immoral. *Journal of Philosophy*, *86*, 183–202.

Marquis, D. (1997). An argument that abortion is wrong. In H. LaFollette (Ed.), *Ethics in practice* (pp. 91–102). London: Blackwell Publishers.

Martin, G. (1981). Isolation of a pluripotent cell line from early mouse embryos cultured in medium conditioned by teratocarcinoma stem cells. *Proceedings of the National Academy of Science USA*, *78*, 7634–7638.

Mayshar, Y., Uri, B-D., Lavon, N., Biancotti, J-C., Yakir, B., Clark, A … Benvenisty, N. (2010). Identification and classification of chromosomal aberrations in human induced pluripotent stem cells. *Cell Stem Cell*, *7*, 521–531.

Mazzarello, P. (1999). A unifying concept: The history of cell theory. *Nature Cell Biology*, *1*, E13–E15.

Melton, D., Daley, G., & Jennings, C. (2004). Altered nuclear transfer in stem-cell research—a flawed proposal. *The New England Journal of Medicine*, *351*, 2791–2792.

NCBC (National Catholic Bioethics Center). (2009). *A Catholic guide to ethical clinical research*. Philadelphia: National Catholic Bioethics Center.

Newman, B., & Newman, R. (2012). *Development through life: A psychosocial approach*. Belmont, CA: Wadsworth.

NIH (National Institutes of Health). (2012). Stem cell information: What are the potential uses of human stem cells and the obstacles that must be overcome before these potential uses will be realized? Retrieved from: http://stemcells.nih.gov/info/basics/basics6.asp

Novak, M. (2001). The stem cell side: Be alert to the beginnings of evil. In M. Ruse & C. Pynes (Eds.), *The stem cell controversy: Debating the issues* (pp. 111–116). Amherst, NY: Prometheus Books.

O'Brien, N. (2011). Science, religion not in conflict, US bishops say in stem-cell document. *AmericanCatholic.Org*. Retrieved from: http://www.americancatholic.org/News/StemCell/stemcelldocument.asp

Pacholczyk, T. (2006). Guilt-free pluripotent stem cells? National Catholic Bioethics Center. Retrieved from: http://www.ncbcenter.org/Page.aspx?pid=287

Parfit, D. (1984). *Reasons and persons*. Oxford: Oxford University Press.

Plau, D. (1996). *Global communication: Is there a place for human dignity?* Geneva: World Council of Churches.

Ramalho-Santos, M., & Willenbring, H. (2007). On the origin of the term "stem cell." *Cell Stem Cell*, *1*, 35–38.

RfP (Religions for Peace). (2008). Common themes from religious background papers. Retrieved from: http://www.google.com/url?sa=t&rct=j&q=sacred%20dignity%20respect%20human%20life%20religious%20traditions%20around%20the%20world&source=web&cd=2&ved=0CCoQFjAB&url=http%3A%2F%2Freligionsforpeace.

org%2Ffile%2Finitiatives%2Flegal-empowerment%2Fexecutive-summary.doc&ei= qCCYT_W_KoXy2gWg7oysBw&usg=AFQjCNFV8XUonsJt08r1S7JwQnMkJ2Jtqg&sig2=o6CcHuL-2r8ejpGuOlyioQ

Sadler, T. (2011). *Langman's medical embryology*. Hagerstown, MD: Lippincott, Williams & Wilkins.

Sandel, M. (2004). Embryo ethics—The moral logic of stem-cell research. *The New England Journal of Medicine, 351*, 207–209.

SCRN (Stem Cell Research News). (2010). Stem cell research proves useful for pharmaceutical industry. *Stemcellresearchnews.net*. Retrieved from: http://stemcellresearchnews.net/News/StemCellResearchProvesUsefulforPharmaceuticalIndustry.aspx

Shannon, T. (2001). Human embryonic stem cell therapy. *Theological Studies, 62*, 811–824.

Shoemaker, D. (2008). *Personal identity and ethics: A brief introduction*. Boulder, CO: Broadview Press.

Skotheim, R., Monni, O., Mousses, S., Fosså, S., Kallioniemi, O., Lothe, R., & Kallioniemi, A. (2002). New insights into testicular germ cell tumorigenesis from gene expression profiling. *Cancer Research, 62*, 2359–2364.

Stein, G., Borowski, M., Luong, M., Shi, M-J., Smith, K., & Vazquez, P. (Eds.). (2011). *Human stem cell technology and biology: A research guide and laboratory manual*. Malden, MA: Wiley-Blackwell.

Sutovsky, P. (Ed.). (2006). *Somatic cell nuclear transfer*. New York: Springer Science.

Thomson, J., Itskovitz-Eldor, J., Shapiro, S., Waknitz, M., Swiergiel, J., Marshall, V., & Jones, J. (1998). Embryonic stem cell lines derived from human blastocysts. *Science, 282*, 1145–1147.

Warren, M. A. (1973). On the moral and legal status of abortion. *The Monist, 57*, 43–61.

Warren, M. A. (1997). *Moral status: Obligations to persons and other living things*. Oxford: Oxford University Press.

Yu, J., Vodyanik, M., Smuga-Otto, K., Antosiewicz-Bourget, J., Frane, J., Tian, S ... Thomson, J. (2007). Induced pluripotent stem cell lines derived from human somatic cells. *Science, 318*, 1917–1920.

Chapter Fifteen

Stem-Cell Research Utilizing Embryonic Tissue Should Be Conducted

Jane Maienschein

Moral claims against human-embryonic stem-cell research are based in a priori claims that include and often start from mistaken assumptions about the natural world. They amount, in effect, to deriving an *is* from an *ought*. The result is bad moral arguments, and also bad policy. This chapter looks at what stem cells are, what stem-cell research is, what embryonic stem cells are, why researchers want to do embryonic-stem-cell research, what leads opponents to their poorly informed moral positions, and then why such research should be at least allowed and even why it should be actually conducted.

Introduction

Centuries of moral philosophers, starting most notably with David Hume (1711–1776) in his work, *A Treatise of Human Nature* (Hume, 1739–1740/1975), have worried about the relationship between what is the case and what we think ought to be the case. The question has been whether it is possible to derive an *ought* from an *is*, and the answer has typically been *no*. Or at the least, it is accepted that what exists in the world is not sufficient to tell us about what is morally good (Falk, 1976). Attempting to do so has been labeled the *naturalistic fallacy* (initially by philosopher G. E Moore). And rejection of this fallacy has led generations of moral theorists to assume that scientific knowledge of the empirical world will not allow us to derive moral claims. A mistake in reasoning occurs also when one reasons from claims regarding what ought to be the case to claims regarding what is the case.

I argue that in fact there are cases of moral decision-making in which misunderstanding of the actual natural world leads to moral errors of this latter sort. This is the case with human-embryonic stem-cell research. Here, most of the moral claims against engaging in this research are based in strong a priori moral claims that include and perhaps begin from mistaken assumptions about the natural world. Starting with claims linked to bad science (or pseudo-science or nonscientific claims about nature), the result is bad arguments and, to the extent that these moral arguments influence political decisions, bad policies. This has surely happened with human-embryonic stem-cell research.

Let us look at what stem cells are, what stem-cell research is, what embryonic stem cells are, why

Contemporary Debates in Bioethics, First Edition. Edited by Arthur L. Caplan and Robert Arp.

researchers want to do embryonic stem-cell research in particular, what opponents seem to be thinking that leads them to their poorly informed moral positions, and then at arguments for why such research should be at least allowed and even why it should be actually conducted.

What Are Stem Cells?

The term *stem cell* goes back to the late nineteenth century embryological work of researchers when it was used to refer to those cells that are not yet differentiated into the diverse types of cells that come later (Maienschein, 2003). Stem cells have the capacity to self-replicate and also to give rise to cells that do become differentiated. Some stem cells are called *unipotent*, which means that they can become just one kind of differentiated cell; for example a neural stem cell can become only a nerve cell. At least this is the case under anything like normal conditions; we do not know about all the possible experimental conditions that might allow different results. *Multipotent* stem cells are just like they sound, so that they have the capacity to self-replicate like all stem cells do and also can become differentiated as at least two different kinds of cells. This is true of hematopoietic stem cells, for example. These are found in the bone marrow and have the capacity to self-replicate and also to become any of several different kinds of cells in the body. *Pluripotent* stem cells have the capacity to self-replicate and can become differentiated as any kind of cell. Embryonic stem cells are pluripotent, and researchers are now able to induce pluripotency in adult somatic stem cells, too. As far as we know, nearly all stem cells that we can actually find in the body are these kinds of stem cells: uni, multi, or pluripotent stem cells (see the NIH website or any number of textbooks on stem-cell research for definitions and distinctions).

The nature of uni- and multipotent stem cells had already been well established in humans since the 1950s when researchers discovered that hematopoietic stem cells in the bone marrow could produce blood cells after the marrow was transplanted from a donor to a patient. Early cases, in France through the research of Jean Dausset (1958) and then elsewhere, showed that bone-marrow transplants could help leukemia patients or patients who had been exposed to excessive radiation or for a few other conditions. This led to the study of what it was that allowed those particular cells to become blood cells, and it raised questions about how much transplantation of other cells might be possible and to what effect.

As often with human experimentation, unless there is a desperate immediate medical need, we do research in other animals before experimenting with humans. Researchers therefore learned a lot about mice, and how and why the bone marrow has special capacities that other tissues and cells do not have. They also learned much about cell culture from cancer cells, including the famous HeLa cells that proved easy to reproduce and very powerful for a wide variety of research questions. Hannah Landecker (2007) has written an important study of such cells and their history, and Rebecca Skloot (2010) provides a wonderful story about the original donor, Henrietta Lacks.

Then, starting in the 1950s biologist Leroy Stevens was at the Jackson Laboratories in Maine studying early developmental stages in mouse cells (Lewis, 2000). He discovered a particular strain of mouse—number 129—that developed differently from normal. Inside the testes in many individuals within this lineage, there emerged a mess of hair, teeth, and other cells that obviously should not normally arise in testes. Stevens (1970a, 1970b) set out to understand why this strain behaved this way, and in 1970 he reported that what he named "pluripotent stem cells" from the blastocyst stage did not differentiate as they normally would in mice from strain 129. Instead, they settled in the testes and gave rise to these out-of-place types of cells.

What Are Embryonic Stem Cells?

Other researchers realized the importance of Stevens's work. By 1981, two groups—Martin J. Evans and Martin H. Kaufman (1981) in Cambridge and Gail Martin (1981) at the University of California San Francisco—had succeeded in isolating and culturing pluripotent cells directly from early embryos. Finally, in 1998, James Thomson and John Gearhart (Thomson et al., 1998) demonstrated the same ability to culture pluripotent stem cell lines in humans. This step is important because these pluripotent stem cells come from embryos, and unlike the uni- or multipotent cells found in the bone marrow, for example, these embryonic pluripotent cells are not yet differentiated at all. They are not totipotent, meaning that they do not have the ability to become the whole body with all its different types. Rather, they have "plural" rather than "total" potential and are therefore pluripotent.

Pluripotent stem cells may also exist in the developing or adult body, but not in large numbers and not in a way that can be isolated and studied. At this time, the only known significant source of many pluripotent stem cells is in the embryo. Experimental approaches have produced induced pluripotent stem cells (or iPS, which involves intervening by adding specific genes that can cause some adult cells to redifferentiate into cells that have some but not all of the capabilities of embryonic stem cells). The full capacities of these iPS cells remain unknown, and the cells do not seem to act *exactly* as embryonic pluripotent stem cells do (see recent discussions in response to 2012 Nobel Prize award to Shinya Yamanaka for stem-cell research).

Where do these stem cells come from? What happens in normal development is that the egg cell is fertilized by a sperm cell, and in those cases where the fertilization is successful (which is a relatively small percentage in humans) the cells begin to divide. The fertilized egg, which is one cell, divides into two, then into four, then into eight cells. These eight cells are actually all totipotent, and if they are separated from each other, they can often develop independently. We know this because of studies in mice as well as the fact that humans can give rise to multiple identical twins, triplets, up to octuplets. Since the cells up to the eight-cell stage in humans are totipotent, each can give rise to a whole new organism. Normally, however, the dividing cells will be held together to make up one individual.

After the eight-cell stage, the cells begin to divide at different rates and to divide many times. The cluster of cells goes through a stage called a *morula*, which looks like a blackberry with cells sticking out all around. Then, at typically day 3–5 and no later than day 14 after fertilization in humans, the blastocyst is formed. At this stage, there is a single layer of cells around the perimeter, and these will give rise to the placenta later if development progresses (which it often does not). Inside most of the space is a large cavity, yet there is also a cluster of cells that make up what is called the *inner cell mass*. These cells are completely undifferentiated but have lost their totipotency. They are now pluripotent stem cells. And they are called embryonic stem cells because they come from the embryo.

Normally, then, these embryonic pluripotent stem cells are neatly packed away inside the blastocyst, protected by the surrounding layer of cells that will eventually make contact with the woman's uterine wall. This blastocyst will in cases of normal development become implanted in the woman's uterus, and the two will begin to grow together. The blastocyst must be implanted or frozen by no later than 14 days (and often earlier), or it will stop cell division and die. Only a relatively small percentage of blastocysts actually become implanted and develop normally and fully to full term birth; there are many obstacles along the way.

At implantation, the embryo begins to exchange nutrients and eventually waste products with the woman host. Judging from what we know about mouse blastocysts, cells very quickly lose their pluripotency and their ability to self-replicate. They are no longer embryonic stem cells and instead become differentiated cells with increasingly determined roles.

Embryonic Stem-Cell Research

Because stem cells are self-replicating, they can be cultured in glass dishes to produce more and more of themselves. The number of cell division, or cell cycles, may be limited biologically, though that is not clearly established. At any rate, the cells can divide many times and provide a sustainable research material.

Because stem cells are not yet differentiated, a great many researchers working hard in numerous labs have figured out many of the conditions that will cause those cells to become particular differentiated cell types in the body. Because the cells are shaped by what they eat, it is possible to culture them with different food, that is to use a different culture medium, and they will differentiate in different ways. Culturing with a certain medium will lead to differentiation as, say, heart muscle cells, nerve cells, pancreatic islet cells, or any other cell type.

This means that researchers can largely control the kinds of cells that they can produce in culture. They can then study the factors involved in different cases: which genes are expressed in producing a heart muscle instead of a nerve, for example? Which environmental and genetic factors lead each nerve cell to differentiate in particular specialized ways? Researchers have learned a tremendous amount about the factors involved in many steps of development as a result of embryonic stem-cell research.

This has led to the hope that we can build on the scientific knowledge about developmental biology to understand what differentiates a stem cell in a particular way, and with that knowledge also understand what differentiates other cells. From the beginning, researchers and the public have eagerly hoped to produce particular kinds of cells with defined clinical applications. The bigger challenge is to understand what causes cells, once differentiated, to stay differentiated. Clinical successes will depend on being able to cultivate, say, a heart muscle cell in culture and then have it stay a heart muscle cell when transplanted to a patient's heart. This is very challenging, and every responsible party agrees that we should not try the experiment clinically until we understand the underlying science much better (see nih.gov for the latest on clinical trials and results).

Much of the work until recently has taken place in mouse cells, which are very instructive because they are parallel to human cells in many ways. But if we are going to confirm the knowledge about development in humans and then apply it in clinical treatments, which so many patients hope happens soon enough for them, researchers must also study human-embryonic stem cells. Fortunately, federal funding in the US and elsewhere, along with state support and philanthropic and industrial funding, has allowed research to progress. And progress it has, leading to increased knowledge and even the first applications in the US for approval to carry out a clinical trial.

The California biotech company, Geron, received approval for the first clinical trial using human-embryonic stem cells in early 2009. This approval came from the US Federal Drug Administration (FDA), which has come to have jurisdiction over medical procedures since the passage of the Pure Food and Drug Act in 1906. For various reasons, Geron did not proceed immediately but pulled back from the trial. In August 2010, they were again awarded approval to proceed and report that they are doing so; but in 2011, due to financial problems, they dropped their entire program devoted to human-embryonic stem-cell research (Frantz, 2012). Other trials have begun or are being planned, and the US National Institutes of Health (NIH, nih.gov) and FDA (fda.gov) websites both provide updates on research and requests for clinical trials, respectively.

One challenge for clinical trials comes from outside science, because of the unstable political and economic environment in the United States. This makes investors nervous, for example, and it makes young researchers nervous about entering a field that is periodically under attack. That concern was very clear after the Federal District Court ruling on August 23, 2010 in Washington, DC, when Judge Royce Lamberth ruled that federal funding cannot be allowed to support human-embryonic stem-cell research on the grounds that it violates the intentions of the Dickey–Wicker Amendment (LC, 1995–1996; CR, 2010; Lamberth, 2010). The ruling had the effect of putting an immediate stop to federal funding of human-embryonic stem-cell research and was considered "shocking" by most researchers and congressional supporters, who vowed to work to gain explicit legislative support for the research. However, on July 27, 2011, due to a lift of Lamberth's injunction by the DC Court of Appeals on April 29, 2011, Lamberth actually reversed his ruling and dismissed the case entirely.

The problem in the US is that Congress has not yet passed clear legislation regulating or endorsing stem-cell research. Instead, we have legislative regulation of human-subjects research (HHS, 2009). And we have the Dickey–Wicker Amendment that was passed to restrict federal funding for embryo research, plus a series of presidential executive orders. Beyond that, we are left with a patchwork of state decisions, judicial decisions that some consider "legislating from the bench," and presidential orders (Matthews & Rowland, 2011).

President Bill Clinton issued an order that human-embryonic stem-cell research could be carried out, with federal funding through the NIH. President George W. Bush ordered that it could continue with federal funding on only those lines of cells that had already existed before he began his address on August 9, 2001. Then, President Barack Obama's executive order in 2009 allowed federal funding of the research once the NIH had adopted ethical and procedural guidelines, and the National Institutes of Health (NIH, 2012) began granting funds for the work. Judge Lamberth's ruling in the Federal District court on August 23, 2010 (Lamberth, 2010) provided a temporary injunction against federal funding and created confusion. For example, it immediately called into question the status of NIH grants already awarded and those in the final processes of being approved. It made it seem once again that the safest funding in the US is private funding, which unfortunately closes the results behind proprietary doors and limits the number and nature of labs able to pursue the research. This limitation obviously concerns researchers and those hoping for clinical treatments. The climate of confusion created by the series of appeals and proposals and temporary decisions, alongside unrealized promises for clarifying legislation, has kept researchers nervous and uncertain (Hurlbut, 2010).

The strong reaction to the District Court ruling reinforces the fact that the research community considers this research with human-embryonic stem cells to offer extremely rich possibilities both for advancing scientific knowledge of development and also for developing practical clinical applications. Researchers know that there is a long road ahead before we are likely to have many clinical results, and in fact the results are unlikely to be exactly what we would predict now. Yet uncertainty about the exact nature of expected results does not undercut the fact that gaining the scientific knowledge will surely lead to some valuable clinical applications.

Mistakes of Opponents

It is worth looking more closely at the case that led to the ruling by Judge Royce Lamberth, a self-avowed conservative from Texas who was appointed to the court by President Ronald Reagan. Lamberth based his interpretation in part on his mistaken views about the nature of the research, in part on his interpretation of the congressional intent of the Dickey–Wicker Amendment, and in part on his acceptance of two of the plaintiffs' arguments that they are harmed by federal funding of embryonic stem-cell research.

Since this case depends on some fundamental errors in moral reasoning, including assuming that *is* implies *ought*, as well as *ought* implies *is*, it warrants a closer look. We see an illuminating set of errors related to this case and from this judge who is known to be anti-abortion and sympathetic to conservative interpretations of the nature of life.

The legal case started in 2010 with *Sherley vs. Sebelius* (SvS, 2010) and involved a biologist named James Sherley, who had recently been denied tenure at MIT and moved to the Boston Biomedical Research Institute, and a researcher in Seattle named Theresa Deisher, who founded her company, AVM Biotechnology, "in response to growing concerns about the need for safe, effective, affordable and ethical medicines and therapeutic treatments" (http://www.avmbio tech.com/home.html). Sherley and Deisher were joined by Nightlight Christian Adoptions, plaintiff embryos (Shayne and Tina Nelson, William and Patricia Flynn), and the Christian Medical Association in their suit seeking to halt federal funding on embryonic stem cells.

In identifying the plaintiffs, the suit states that:

> Plaintiff Embryos include all individual human embryos that are or will be "created using in vitro fertilization (IVF) for reproductive purposes and [are] no longer needed for these purposes." 74 Fed. Reg at 32,171. The Embryos are persons that qualify for representation under Fed R. Civ. P. 17 (c). NIH's violation of the Federal Funding Ban will place the lives of these Embryos under a recurring risk of destruction. (SvS, 2010, sec. 9)

The case claims that the NIH was violating both the laws of various states that prohibit embryo research and the clear intent of the congressionally legislated Dickey–Wicker amendment that prohibits "research in which a human embryo or embryos are destroyed, discarded, or knowingly subjected to risk or injury or death greater then that allowed for research on fetuses *in utero* ..." (LC, 1995–1996, 45 C.F.R. 46.204(b); also Green, 2001).

In fact, the NIH, the National Research Council of the National Academy of Sciences, and other committees had determined that the NIH should fund only human-embryonic stem-cell research on cell lines that have already been developed in laboratories and that had been caused to exist without any use of federal funds and following specific ethical guidelines. No federal funds would be used to "destroy" embryos, but only those embryos that had already been discarded or donated according to established ethical guidelines could be used. The NIH guidelines following the Obama executive order, then, made clear that there is no reason not to study the lines that have come to exist with private donations and private funding.

This is a subtle, but very accurate and important, distinction between the process of generating stem-cell lines and the process of doing research with them, since it is a well-established fact that thousands of embryos are discarded every year, and since once the stem cell lines exist, they are like any other cell lines that are widely used for cancer and other biomedical-research purposes. The fact that those who have caused the embryos to exist can now donate them for research purposes rather than throwing them away has actually been regarded as a very positive ethical step by many (Hall, 2001).

Yet Sherley and Deisher are self-described social conservatives who are anti-abortion, and they have explained that what they consider "ethical" necessarily rejects any embryo research, including research on those embryos that the owners wish to donate explicitly for such research. They claimed in their suit that funding the research on cell lines will contribute to the destruction of embryos that researchers need and that presumably would not haven been destroyed otherwise, and the research therefore violates the Dickey–Wicker Amendment.

The case was rejected by the District Court initially, but on appeal, it was ruled that Sherley and Deisher did have legal standing to bring such a suit, which placed Judge Lamberth in the position to make a decision. On this point related to violation of the Dickey–Wicker Amendment, Lamberth made two mistakes in reasoning.

First, he made assumptions about how the science works, as if doing stem-cell research involves actually generating new cell lines in every case. This is a failure to understand the nature of stem-cell and cell-culture research. Related to that, he concluded that the process of destroying embryos to generate cell lines and then doing research on those cell lines is all one line of research, rather than separable parts of a larger complex process. To do research on the stem cell lines is necessarily to destroy embryos, he asserted, and there is no such thing as a "piece of research" out of a whole process (Lamberth, 2010; Cohen & Adashi, 2011).

This interpretation has many implications that legal scholars will undoubtedly continue to explore, but it reflects a serious failure to understand stem-cell science. Cell lines are generated, and since the cells can self-replicate, the lines are shared and used over and over by many different labs for many different research questions. There are, in fact, many different "pieces" of research. And the first step in many cases starts with salvaging the cells from blastocyst's cluster of cells that would otherwise be discarded. Lamberth's failure to accept the scientists' explanations of how they do their work and his assumption that stem-cell research always requires destroying embryos that would not be otherwise destroyed are mistaken. Erroneous assumptions also led him to conclude that the research violates Dickey–Wicker, since he mistakenly believed that doing research on the cell lines is the same research as generating the cell lines.

A third factor in Lamberth's ruling relates to the fact that both of the plaintiffs who were ruled by the appeals court to have legal standing in the case work on those uni- or multipotent stem cells found later in the body (called adult stem cells). They were allowed to bring suit against the NIH and Health and Human Services that support embryonic stem-cell research on the grounds that allowing federal funding for what they regarded as illicit embryonic stem-cell research would harm their own chances of obtaining funding for their adult stem-cell research. This is obviously a highly problematic claim for many reasons.

Their extensive claims that adult stem-cell research and even iPS research are scientifically and clinically "better" than embryonic stem-cell research are completely unfounded. Furthermore, though federal funding is limited, there is no evidence that funding was directly shifted from the kinds of work they do to embryonic stem-cell research or that they were harmed by any slight reduction in access to funds even if they could prove that such reduction occurred.

This part of Judge Lamberth's ruling raises many troubling questions. Does any researcher have a right to file suit against the NIH or other government funding agency because funding has shifted to a new initiative in a way that might have reduced funding for an older way of doing research? Or does that right hold only if the researcher claims (as they two did) that their way is "better science"? And if so, how will that be adjudicated? Surely we will not decide which is the best science through the judicial system! Nonetheless, this case went forward with precisely this kind of claim at its core and with Judge Lamberth's (2010) ruling that possible loss of funding would "threaten the very livelihood of plaintiffs Sherley and Deisher. Accordingly, the irreparable harm that plaintiffs would suffer absent an injunction outweighs the harms to interested parties" (sec. C). His conclusion is astonishing, given the facts of how federal funding processes actually work.

Judge Lamberth has ruled that Sherley and Deisher's case was likely to succeed and therefore could proceed. Fortunately, for the sake of scientific research, the US Circuit Court of Appeals disagreed with Judge Lamberth and held that the case was likely to fail. This sent the case back to Lamberth for reconsideration. On July 27, 2011, he made clear that he was not happy about the higher court decision, but he felt bound by it to accept that:

> This Court, following the D.C. Circuit's reasoning and conclusions, must find that defendants reasonably interpreted the Dickey–Wicker Amendment to permit funding for human embryonic stem cell research because such research is not "research in which a human embryo or embryos are destroyed."

This ruling settles the case related to interpretation and application of Dickey–Wicker, but it does not address other claims in the lawsuit. Some of these are likely to resurface in other arguments and other lawsuits.

For example, these researchers started with the assumption that others hold, namely that, "It is unethical to do research on persons, and embryos are persons." This statement amounts to the claim that "we believe for metaphysical reasons that have nothing to do with science or the research involved that embryos are persons." That is, they are seeking to impose their own personal ethical beliefs on others, and they are doing this by pretending that they have scientific reasons for doing so. The inclusion in their original case of the claim that "Potential donors are not told that many scientists believe that human embryos are human life or that many States hold that human life begins at conception," and then quoting Arkansas's reference to "the life of every unborn child," is legally clever but scientifically false.

Very few scientists would agree that life begins at conception in anything like the imputed sense that an individual's *personhood* begins then (Friedrich, 2000). Nor would they agree that the bunch of cells (which for humans is technically defined as an *embryo* up to the eight-week stage and then a *fetus* until it is born) is the same as an "unborn child"—a category, actually, that scientifically does not exist (Sadler, 2011). In *Roe v. Wade* (410 US 113), for example, Mr Justice Harry Blackmun rightly claimed that, "the unborn have never been recognized in the law as persons in the whole sense." The plaintiffs in *Sherley et al. vs. Sebelius* are playing a legal game, of course, but they are engaged in faulty reasoning that we should reject. They are starting from an *ought* and imputing claims about what *is*, which, as we have noted, is a fallacious move in reasoning.

Importantly, other legal decisions have explicitly rejected this claim that imputes a moral or legal status to a cluster of biological cells. For example, in Arizona's case of *Jeters v. Mayo* (1 CA-CV 04-0048, 2005), Judge Kessler ruled and was upheld on appeal that "3 day old embryos are not persons." Even President George W. Bush in his speech of August 9, 2001, while expressing his concern about embryonic-stem-cell research, understood the biological distinction between the early embryo and later stages of development. Bush explicitly accepted that there is a different status for "pre-implantation embryos" (which he also called "pre-embryos"), in which there has been no significant gene expression, no differentiation, and just multiplication of one cell into a cluster of cells.

This is not the place for an in-depth discussion of what counts as a person, or how we define personhood (start with Shoemaker, 2007, 2008), but the important point here is that developmental biologists agree that the early stages, when there is just a bunch of stem cells in the inner cell mass of the blastocyst, are biologically completely different from later developmental stages (Kail & Cavanaugh, 2010). Blastocysts and their stem cells cannot live independently without being implanted into a uterus, and most do not continue to live at all because they stop dividing or do not implant, or their owners choose not to try to implant them. Apparently, the only reason to pretend that this early blastocyst stage falls under the same description as later developmental stages is to support the a priori belief that "embryos are persons." That is, advocates of this view want to take moral *ought* beliefs and attempt to impose them on others. They are attempting to draw *is* conclusions about the nature of embryos from their personal opinions. This is not good science; nor is it good ethics.

These advocates—such as the Catholic Church (CCC, 2004; NCBC, 2009)—buy into an anti-abortion philosophy that assumes that life begins at fertilization, which they label "conception." In a simple sense, it is true that in normal development, the early steps on the road to development of an individual human organism start with egg and sperm, and fertilization. But, again, the "life" that begins then is biological cell division and only that. For those who insist that fertilization and cell division make a "person," then presumably a lineage of cells derived from a fertilized egg and developing in culture should be a person also. So, those cell lines that already exist because of past research should be considered persons, too, and that claim is either useless or absurd. They are not the same kinds of things as later-stage embryos or fetuses (as humans are called after eight weeks of development) that have differentiated significantly, eventually have developing sensory systems, and later acquire the ability to live independently.

Some of those such as the Nightlife Christian Adoptions group (nightlight.org) do argue that all embryos are persons and that therefore we should preserve all embryos so that they can be adopted. Such advocates may actually believe that there will be enough parents to adopt all the available embryos, but careful studies show that this is just not possible. This wish is not even close to realistic. There are thousands more embryos than would-be adoptive parents (see the research, for example, in Skene, 2009). They claim now that would-be adoption parents wait for embryos that they cannot get, but that is surely in part because of background checks and such regulations, and also because the owners of the embryos do not wish to have their embryos adopted. The numbers just do not add up.

The only possibility to follow through on their logic is government regulation, which will have to be the federal government to control interstate commerce. The government would have to either prohibit anyone from generating "extra" embryos or force the owners to give up any extras for adoption, and then force would-be parents to adopt them. Surely these embryo-rights advocates do not really want to demand federal government intervention in private lives in all these ways. Yet their assumptions about what "ought to be" and therefore the faulty conclusions about what an embryo "is" lead to such impossible conclusions.

We Should Allow Stem-Cell Research

Some of the owners of extra embryos want to donate their embryos for research (see the research, for example, in Islam et al., 2005). They are going to discard their embryos otherwise, do not want to allow adoption, understand what is involved, and also see the cluster of undifferentiated cells as a potentially rich resource for scientific knowledge. They accept the current NIH guidelines that were established by the Obama executive order. They want to support research in a way that accepts the guidelines not to use any federal funding to "destroy" the embryos, and in ways that make the resulting cells available for research, to gain knowledge, and perhaps eventually to bring clinical results. And they want federal funding to be available for the research so as to yield the highest possible public use and public good. This should be allowed.

In addition, some go further and insist that such research should be not just allowed but also actually conducted. These are two different claims, of course. The first involves assessing harms, while the second involves assessing the balance of harms and benefits. The first is an ethical and policy matter, the second a pragmatic decision. For the US, I argue here—and have argued elsewhere (Maienschein, 2003; Maienschein & Robert, 2010)—that at this time and given what we know now, we should both allow and conduct human-embryonic stem-cell research.

First, in the US, we accept that behaviors including carrying out research should be allowed if it does not involve significant harm to others. Doing scientific research is parallel to a speech act in this respect, with protections for such acts. We start, then, with the assumption that research is allowed. Then would come the burden for opponents to demonstrate that research does involve harm to others. Building nuclear or biological weapons or explosives in one's basement is not protected, for example. Carrying out research that involves torturing human subjects or violates animal-care guidelines: such research is prohibited. We develop a set of regulatory and legal guidelines to determine the extent and nature of limitations based on understanding of harms.

In the case of embryonic-stem-cell research, the majority of American citizens in repeated polls favor allowing the research and feel that there is no significant harm involved (Gardner, 2010). A minority do argue that embryos are harmed, but given the scientific facts that the pre-implantation of earliest developmental stages involves just a bunch of undifferentiated cells, it is difficult to see how these cells can be harmed, the way one harms a person on the street, for example. The usual sort of argument that the minority do not want to live in a society that would do research on embryos sits alongside other claims that a minority do not want to live in a society that eats meat or wears leather or lets doctors turn off a respirator when the patient has indicated a wish that that happen and when the family or guardians agree. Legally and ethically, as a society, we have decided that these are either not harms or not significant harms. The same should be true with embryo research.

Yes, there is the Dickey–Wicker Amendment to the Health and Human Services Funding bills. And, yes, that Amendment says (to expand on the earlier point) that federal funding will not be used for "(1) the creation of a human embryo or embryos for research purposes; or (2) research in which a human embryo or embryos are destroyed, discarded, or knowingly subjected to risk of injury or death greater than that allowed for research on fetuses *in utero*" (LC, 1995–1996). Yet, contra Judge Lamberth, the NIH, National Academy of Sciences, and many other scientific groups hold that embryonic stem-cell research on stem-cell lines generated without federal funding do not violate this legal restriction. Furthermore, the assumed harm to embryos comes in a budget amendment and is not based on any assessment or demonstration of actual harms.

Therefore, in the absence of demonstrated harms, human-embryonic stem-cell research should be allowed. And it should be allowed with federal funding, though there is no entitlement for any particular line of scientific research that it should receive federal funding. That is instead a pragmatic decision, and that is the second point.

Second, human-embryonic stem-cell research should be not only allowed but also actually conducted. Here, we have to show that there are actual benefits as well as no significant harms. That is, deciding what research should be conducted is a pragmatic matter, involving cost–benefit analyses. In this case, there is very significant actual benefit, as can be seen from the research provided by the NIH on their site devoted to stem-cell research (stemcells.nih.gov). Also see the European research (eurostemcell.org) and Chinese research (stemcellschina.com). We have learned a tremendous amount already from having carried out the research. In fact, much of what we know about adult stem-cell development and all the work on induced pluripotent cells builds on the knowledge gained from embryonic stem-cell research. This research should definitely be continued. Insofar as federal and other funding helps generate new knowledge, it is a good investment.

The clinical benefits remain unknown and potential. While groups such as Advanced Cell Technology (ACT, 2010, 2011; Schwartz et al., 2012) are undertaking the first FDA-approved clinical trials with embryonic stem cells, many informal experiments have begun and other carefully designed clinical trials are under preparation. In fact, it is not likely that clinical benefits will come quickly nor easily, and probably not even as originally envisioned. That does not, however, undercut the cost–benefit analysis results that weigh in favor of carrying out the research. And it does not mean that only this kind of research should be done. Instead, the best results are likely to come from comparative studies, drawing on knowledge generated from embryonic stem-cell research, iPS research, and continuing research on all other stem-cell lines.

Therefore, human-embryonic stem-cell research, carried out with cells from human embryos as well as other cell lines should be allowed and should be carried out.

References

ACT (Advanced Cell Technologies). (2010). Advanced Cell Technology receives FDA clearance for the first clinical trial using embryonic stem cells to treat macular degeneration. Retrieved from: http://www.advancedcell.com/news-and-media/press-releases/advanced-cell-technology-receives-fda-clearance-for-the-first-clinical-trial-using-embryonic-stem-cel/index.asp

ACT (Advanced Cell Technologies). (2011). ACT secures patent to generate embryonic stem cells without embryo destruction. Retrieved from: http://www.advancedcell.com/news-and-media/press-releases/act-secures-patent-to-generate-embryonic-stem-cells-without-embryo-destruction/index.asp

CCC (*Catechism of the Catholic Church*). (2004). Retrieved from: http://www.vatican.va/archive/ENG0015/__P7Z.HTM#-2C6.

Cohen, G., & Adashi, E. (2011). Human embryonic stem-cell research under siege—battle won but not the war. *The New England Journal of Medicine*, *364*, 48.

CR (Congressional Record of the United States Government). (2010). 45 CFR 46. Retrieved from: http://thomas.loc.gov/

HHS (Health and Human Services). (2009). Basic HHS policy for protection of human research subjects. Retrieved from: http://www.hhs.gov/ohrp/humansubjects/guidance/45cfr46.html

Dausset, J. (1958). Iso-leuko-antibodies. *Vox Sanguinis*, *3*, 40–41.

Evans. M, & Kaufman, M. (1981). Establishment in culture of pluripotent cells from mouse embryos. *Nature*, *292*, 154–156.

Falk, W. (1976). Hume on is and ought. *Canadian Journal of Philosophy*, *6*, 359–378.

Frantz, S. (2012). Embryonic stem cell pioneer Geron exits field, cuts losses. *Nature Biotechnology*, *30*, 12–13.

Friedrich, M. (2000). Debating pros and cons of stem cell research. *Journal of the American Medical Association*, *284*, 681–682.

Gardner, A. (2010). Most Americans back embryonic stem cell research: Wide range of support, including Republicans, Catholics and born-again Christians, Harris Interactive /HealthDay poll finds. *HealthNews*, October 7. Retrieved from: http://health.usnews.com/health-news/managing-your-healthcare/research/articles/2010/10/07/most-americans-back-embryonic-stem-cell-research-poll

Green, R. (2001). *The human embryo research debates: Bioethics in the vortex of controversy*. Oxford: Oxford University Press.

Hall, C. (2001). The forgotten embryo: Fertility clinics must store or destroy the surplus that is part of the process. *San Francisco Chronicle*, August 20. Retrieved from: http://www.sfgate.com/cgi-bin/article.cgi?file=/chronicle/archive/2001/08/20/MN 58092.DTL

HHS (Health and Human Services). (2009). Basic HHS policy for protection of human research subjects. Retrieved from: http://www.hhs.gov/ohrp/humansubjects/guidance/45cfr46.html

Hume, D. (1739–1740/1975). *A treatise of human nature* (Ed. P.H. Nidditch). Oxford: Clarendon Press.

Hurlbut, B. (2010). *Experiments in democracy: The science, politics and ethics of human embryo research in the United States 1978–2007*. Ph.D. dissertation, History of Science, Harvard University.

Islam, S., Rusli, B., Ab Rani, B., & Hanapi, B. (2005). Spare embryos and human embryonic stem cell research: Ethics of different public policies in the Western world. *International Medical Journal Malaysia*, *4*, 1–27.

Kail, R., & Cavanaugh, J. (2010). *Human development: A life-span view*. Belmont, CA: Wadsworth.

Lamberth, R. (2010). Memorandum opinion regarding Civ. No. 1:09-cv-1575 (RCL). Retrieved from: http://www.courthousenews.com/2010/08/24/embryo.pdf

Landecker, H. (2007). *Culturing life: How cells became technologies*. Cambridge, MA: Harvard University Press.

LC (The Library of Congress). (1995–1996). Bill summary & status, 104th Congress (1995–1996) H.R. 2880, all Congressional actions with amendments. Specifically, Pub. L. No. 104–99, § 128, 110 Stat. 26, 34 (1996). Retrieved from: http://thomas.loc.gov/cgi-bin/bdquery/z?d104:HR02880:@@@S

Lewis, R. (2000). A stem cell legacy: Leroy Stevens. *The Scientist*, *14*, 19.

Maienschein, J. (2003). *Whose view of life? Embryos, cloning, and stem cells*. Cambridge, MA: Harvard University Press.

Maienschein, J., & Robert, J. (2010). What is a healthy embryo and how do we know? In J. Nisker (Ed.), *The "healthy" embryo: Social, biomedical, legal and philosophical perspectives* (pp. 1–15). Cambridge: Cambridge University Press.

Martin, G. (1981). Isolation of a pluripotent cell line from early mouse embryos cultured in medium conditioned by teratocarcinoma stem cells. *Proceedings of the National Academy of Science USA, 78*, 7634–7638.

Matthews, K., & Rowland, M. (2011). Stem cell policy in the Obama age: UK and US perspectives. *Regenerative Medicine, 6*, 125–132.

NIH (National Institutes of Health). (2012). Retrieved from: http://stemcells.nih.gov/info/scireport/chapter5.asp

NCBC (National Catholic Bioethics Center). (2009). *A Catholic guide to ethical clinical research*. Philadelphia: National Catholic Bioethics Center.

Sadler, T. (2011). *Langman's medical embryology*. Hagerstown, MD: Lippincott, Williams & Wilkins.

Schwartz, S., Hubschman, J-P., Heilwell, G., Franco-Cardenas, V., Pan, C., Ostrick, R … Lanza, R. (2012). Embryonic stem cell trials for macular degeneration: A preliminary report. *The Lancet, 379*, 713–720.

Skloot, R. (2010). *The immortal life of Henrietta Lacks*. New York: The Crown Publishing Group.

SvS (*Sherley v. Sebelius*). (2010). 610 F.3d 69 (D.C. Cir. 2010) Civ. No. 1:09-cv-1575 (RCL). Retrieved from: http://www.cadc.uscourts.gov/internet/opinions.nsf/DF210F382F98EBAC852578810051B18C/$file/10-5287-1305585.pdf

Shoemaker, D. (2007). Personal identity and practical concerns. *Mind, 116*, 316–357.

Shoemaker, D. (2008). *Personal identity and ethics: A brief introduction*. Boulder, CO: Broadview Press.

Skene, L. (2009). Should women be paid for donating their eggs for human embryo research? *Monash Bioethics Review, 28*, 1–15.

Stevens, L. (1970a). The development of transplantable teratocarcinomas from intratesticular grafts of pre- and postimplantation mouse embryos. *Developmental Biology, 21*, 364–382.

Stevens, L. (1970b). Experimental production of testicular teratomas in mice of strains 129, A/He, and their F1 hybrids. *Journal of the National Cancer Institute, 44*, 923–929.

SvS (*Sherley v. Sebelius*). (2010). 610 F.3d 69 (D.C. Cir. 2010) Civ. No. 1:09-cv-1575 (RCL). Retrieved from: http://www.cadc.uscourts.gov/internet/opinions.nsf/DF210F382F98EBAC852578810051B18C/$file/10-5287-1305585.pdf

Thomson, J., Itskovitz-Eldor, J., Shapiro, S., Waknitz, M., Swiergiel, J., Marshall, V., & Jones, J. (1998). Embryonic stem cell lines derived from human blastocysts. *Science, 282*, 1145–1147.

Chapter Sixteen

Stem-Cell Research Utilizing Embryonic Tissue Should Not Be Conducted

Bertha Alvarez Manninen

This chapter functions as a survey of a few of the strongest arguments proffered by philosophers and ethicists against the moral permissibility of destroying embryos for stem-cell research. First, I explore the question concerning whether embryos ought to count as moral persons, concluding that any attempts to denote the commencement of personhood at any other biological threshold other than fertilization are subject to severe difficulties. Second, I will discuss two moral principles that are often appealed to in order to defend embryonic stem-cell research—*the nothing-is-lost principle* and *the principle of waste avoidance*—and illustrate why such defenses also fail. I end by calling attention to the increasing malleability of adult stem cells, and encourage researchers to continue to explore ways in which adult stem cells can come to resemble embryonic stem cells in terms of their potency without having to resort to destroying nascent human life.

Introduction

In the interest of full disclosure, I actually support the use of surplus in vitro fertilization (IVF) embryos for stem-cell research, and I have published articles to that effect (Manninen, 2007, 2008). However, I also believe that there are strong arguments against the use of embryos for stem-cell research, especially since adult stem cells are proving increasingly versatile (Zhou et al., 2009; Bhowmik & Yong, 2011; Seki et al., 2012). As a philosopher, I believe it is important to examine and understand the range of arguments when it comes to controversial issues. As John Stuart Mill (1806–1873) famously wrote in *On Liberty* (Mill, 1859/2008): "He who knows only his own side of the case knows little of that." With this in mind, this chapter will attempt to outline a strong argument against the moral permissibility of human-embryonic stem-cell research (hESCR).[1]

Respect for the Individual

Embryonic stem cells are derived from fertilized human eggs at the blastocyst stage of development, approximately 5 days after fertilization. The blastocyst comprises about 50–100 cells. The outer layer of the blastocyst, the trophoblast, contains the cells that will

Contemporary Debates in Bioethics, First Edition. Edited by Arthur L. Caplan and Robert Arp.

give rise to the embryonic and fetal auxiliary tissue, while the inner layer of the blastocyst, the embryoblast, contains the cells that will form the fetus. Stem cells are extracted from the embryoblast, a procedure that results in its destruction. The stem cells themselves are not totipotent, i.e., they cannot give rise to a whole human organism. They are, however, pluripotent, i.e., they can give rise to any cell-type of the body; indeed this capacity is the source of their desirability. It is not, then, that the stem cells themselves have the potential to create a distinct embryo or fetus; rather it is that the entity that is destroyed in order to obtain the stem cells, the human blastocyst, is a complete and genetically distinct human organism that, if implanted in the womb, had the potential to grow into a fetus, infant, child, and adult (Lanza, 2009; Stein et al., 2011). According to detractors of hESCR, this is sufficient for rendering the harvesting of embryonic stem cells morally impermissible.

A comic strip panel by John Cox and Allen Forkum from 1995 (coxandforkum.com) shows an illustration of President George W. Bush sticking his head outside of a tree house, with the label "Culture of Life Club" crudely drawn under the door. He is holding a beaker in one hand; below on the ground sits a child in a wheel chair with "Stem-cell research" written on the back of the chair. The caption for Bush reads, "Sorry, Billy ... some life stages are more sacred than others," while a sign that reads, "Embryos Welcome!" adorns the ground in front of the tree house. This, in short, is how advocates of hESCR regard those who oppose it: that the life of an embryo is worth more to them than the lives of the diseased.

This is a straw man of the anti-hESCR position. According to those who oppose the research, it is not that embryos possess *more* moral worth than sick individuals; it is that *all* human beings, at all stages of their lives, whether healthy, sick, vulnerable, or strong, have *equal* moral status and moral worth. Consequently, society ought not to endorse sacrificing the life and dignity of one group of human beings in order to aid or save the life of others. In other words, those who oppose hESCR shun a consequentialist approach to the issue; as noble as the desire to cure disease is, and as much as we should try to pursue this end as much as possible, this goal should not be attained via the destruction of human life, even at a rudimentary stage of development.

Such a moral imperative is not a new one, and indeed, when it has been violated in the past, society typically recoils in horror. Consider, for example, the Tuskegee syphilis experiment (1932–1972), which studied the effects of syphilis on impoverished African-American men, who were lured into the experiment by the promise of free medical exams and free meals. The men were never told they were infected with the disease, and they were never treated for it, even after the discovery of penicillin in the 1940s as an effective treatment. All the subjects were allowed to degenerate from a disease that could have been treated, and, in hindsight, such behavior is quite rightly held to be repulsive. No matter the wealth of knowledge obtained by such an experiment, it was (and remains) unethical to exploit the poverty, ignorance, and vulnerability of these men in order to conduct the research. As a result of the Tuskegee experiments, new rules regarding the use of human subjects in scientific research were devised, including requiring informed consent and full disclosure, all of which is currently overseen by the Department of Health and Human Services (Reverby, 2009).

In 1978, Robert McFall suffered from aplastic anemia, and consequently required a bone-marrow transplant to survive. After a long search, it was determined that his cousin, David Shimp, possessed matching bone marrow, yet Shimp refused to undergo the extraction procedure. McFall sued Shimp in the hopes that the Pennsylvania District Courts would compel his cousin to submit to further testing and ultimately the extraction itself. As the Court stated (MvS, 1978), the main ethical issue at stake was whether "in order to save the life of one of its members by the only means available, may society infringe upon one's absolute right to his 'bodily security'?" The judges answered this question in the negative:

> Our society, contrary to many others, has as its first principle, the respect for the individual, and that society and government exist to protect the individual from being invaded and hurt by another ... For our law to compel the defendant to submit to an intrusion of his body would change the very concept and principle upon which our society is founded. To do so would defeat the sanctity of the individual, and would impose a rule which would know no limits, and one could not imagine where the line would be drawn. (MvS, par. 3)

What we should not derive from this decision is that the judges felt no sympathy for McFall, or regarded his life as less sacrosanct than Shimp's. Rather, the appropriate conclusion is that the judges held that the rights of one human being (in this case the right to bodily autonomy) cannot be compromised, even to help another human being survive an affliction with a serious ailment (McFall died two weeks after the ruling).

Consider the blood shortages that pervade hospitals and clinics. Certainly, this can be solved if the workers in blood mobile trucks or vans grabbed random people from the street, strapped them down to a bed, and forcibly extracted their blood. The organ-shortage crisis would be significantly curtailed if all nonvital organs were forcibly extracted from random hospital patients, or if vital organs were removed after death regardless of the patient's wishes while still alive. In our society, however, we do not endorse such practices because, in the end, we respect the "sanctity of the individual," and we, therefore, do not support sacrificing some human beings in order to save others. According to detractors of hESCR, those who support the research wish to violate this deeply held moral imperative in regards to human embryos, who are some of the most vulnerable members of the human species, and whose vulnerability is being exploited in the interest of medical research. Although they wish to do so for a benevolent reason—to help persons debilitated by diabetes, Alzheimer's disease, Parkinson's disease, and spinal cord injury, among other ailments—it remains impermissible to instrumentalize human beings in this way, especially defenseless human beings and even in very early and rudimentary stages of development. Therefore, the basic tenet held by those who oppose hESCR is that, while we should no doubt work tirelessly to find cures for these devastating illnesses, we should not do so at the price of destroying the lives of human beings in one of their most vulnerable stages of development.

Are Embryos Persons?

The immediate response those who support the research can offer is that, unlike the victims of the Tuskegee studies and David Shimp, embryos are not persons; they are not moral subjects, nor rights-bearers (Tooley, 1972, 1985; Warren, 1973; Singer, 1979) and so disaggregating them by extracting stem cells is not analogous to a forcible bone-marrow extraction, nor to deceiving and refusing to cure unwitting human beings of syphilis. In response, detractors of hESCR will have to admit that destroying embryos causes them no pain or suffering, since they lack the capacity for sentience. Moreover, it is also true that extracting stem cells from blastocysts cannot be regarded as a compulsion (in contrast to forcibly extracting Shimp's bone marrow), since blastocysts are incapable of forming desires. Nevertheless, it may be retorted, we would think it morally wrong to, say, painlessly euthanize an infant for research purposes, even though the infant has no conscious desire to continue living.

The pertinent question that must be addressed, the one that most divides supporters from detractors of hESCR, is not whether embryos are human *life*, but whether they are human (normative) *persons*, that is, beings with moral status and moral rights. Certainly human embryos are human life: they are members of the species *Homo sapiens*, and they are biologically alive. Unlike other cells in the body, embryos, if implanted into a uterus, may commence a continuous growth that may end with the birth of a human infant. Embryos are distinct human organisms that possess a complete genetic code; already the future child's sex, phenotype, and even aspects of its personality are determined by the genetic information in the embryo.

Individuals who oppose hESCR maintain that there is no nonarbitrary line that can be drawn between fertilization and birth so as to clearly demarcate when an embryo crosses the line from a dispensable entity, to an entity with moral rights and value. Therefore, they argue, an embryo ought to be considered a person with moral status when it first comes into existence: at fertilization (JPII, 1995; Lee & George, 2008). Moreover, as will be illustrated below, any proposed time for attributing personhood to the embryo other than fertilization is fraught with difficulties.

Arbitrary Lines

First, let us consider what can be called *the argument from appearance*: since human embryos do not look like human persons, this means that they are not. Many individuals are taken in by how early in gestation a human fetus begins to resemble an infant. For example, although Judith Jarvis Thomson (1971) does not consider embryos or early fetuses persons, she does maintain that, "it comes as a surprise when one first learns how early in its life it begins to acquire human characteristics. By the tenth week, for example, it already has a face, arms and legs, fingers and toes; it has internal organs, and brain activity is detectable" (pp. 47–48). A human blastocyst may not yet possess fingers, toes, arms, or a face, but it decidedly *does* have human characteristics; it looks exactly what a human life is suppose to look like at that particular point in development. Moreover, appearance is not the determining factor of whether a human being has moral rights. Too often in United States history, from the treatment of Native Americans, to African slaves, and the Japanese during World War II, the fact that a human being does not look "like us" has resulted in inhumane and deplorable treatment. We should, therefore, avoid denying human embryos moral rights on these, or similar, grounds.

Second, there is the argument that embryos should be considered legally alive, and therefore legal persons, only after the onset of brain activity. Currently, human beings are considered legally dead, following the 1981 Uniform Determination of Death Act (UDDA), at the permanent cessation of any detectable brain activity (NCCUSL, 1981). Therefore, for the sake of parallelism, human life should be regarded as commencing at the beginning of any detectable brain activity, at about 6–8 weeks of gestation. Philosopher Baruch Brody (1975) supports this view, arguing that, as a result of the commencement of brain activity, "the fetus becomes a human being about the end of the sixth week after its development." Because there is no detectable brain activity prior to this, the fetus "is surely not a human being at the moment of conception" (pp. 109, 112).

This sounds initially plausible, but an understanding of why the UDDA is the current definition of death illustrates why such a criterion is inapplicable to embryos. Before the advent of life-sustaining technology, humans were considered legally dead at the permanent cessation of cardio-pulmonary functions. This was the point of organismic death. However, with the development and widespread use of technologies such as respirators and defibrillators, cardiac and pulmonary functions are now able to be sustained artificially, despite massive brain damage. That is, these technologies are able to separate loss of cardio-pulmonary function with the loss of all brain functions, whereas before one was quickly followed by the other. Currently, then, brain death is considered the legal point of death because this is what now constitutes the death of the human organism.

An embryo, however, is a biologically living entity, even without the possession of a functioning brain, or a heart or lungs for that matter. That is, at the blastocyst stage of development, neither brain activity nor cardio-pulmonary activity is necessary in order to sustain the embryo's life. Therefore, the two life-stages are not parallel. Whereas a more developed human being necessitates minimal brain activity in order to sustain organismic life, this is not the case for a human blastocyst, which sustains organismic life even prior to the commencement of brain activity (and even prior to the commencement of cardio-pulmonary activity). Therefore, if the possession of biological organismic life is sufficient for attributing personhood to human beings, a human blastocyst meets this criterion before the onset of brain activity.

Some philosophers have argued that moral status commences at the onset of the capacity for sentience. Sentience is important because it is at this time that a fetus can feel and perceive pain and pleasure and, therefore, it is here when it develops a conscious mind, albeit a rudimentary one. It is at this point that the fetus attains what Bonnie Steinbock (1992) calls a "biographical life" and the ability to be affected and, therefore, it is here, when the fetus attains an interest in continued existence. L. W. Sumner (1981) writes: "if morality has to do with the promotion and protection of interest of welfare, morality can concern itself only with beings who are conscious or sentient. No other beings can be beneficiaries or victims *in the morally relevant way* . . . there are no moral dimensions to [our] acts unless the interests or welfare of some sentient creature is at stake. Morality requires the existence of sentience in order to obtain a purchase on our actions" (pp. 136–137). Steinbock (1992) echoes Sumner in this regard: "We are not morally required to consider [a fetus's] interests because, prior to becoming conscious and sentient, fetuses do not *have* interests … Life is in a being's interest if the experiences that comprise its life are, on the whole, enjoyable ones. Such a life is a good to the being in question … By contrast, embryos and preconscious fetuses do not have lives that they value, lives that are good to them. Life is no more a good to an embryo than it is to a plant or a sperm" (pp. 45, 57–58).

According to this argument, then, only beings that are sentient are capable of being affected and possessing interests. In turn, only beings that have interests possess moral status because it is only then that they can be harmed (by experiencing pain or distress) or benefited (by experiencing pleasure or happiness). It is at this point, and only this point, that continued existence can be said to be in a being's interests, and therefore, it is only here when a being possesses a right to life. Because embryos are not conscious or sentient entities, they do not possess moral status and therefore do not possess a right to life. Steinbock (2006) applies this view, which she calls "the interest view," to hESCR when she writes: "Lacking interests, embryos do not have a welfare of their own. In this respect, they are like gametes. Gametes are alive and human, but this is not sufficient for moral status. To have moral status is to be the kind of being whose interests and welfare we moral agents are required to consider. Without interests, there is nothing to consider" (p. 30).

It should be briefly noted that gametes are unlike embryos in one very key, metaphysically important, manner: gametes are not numerically identical with the future person, whereas an embryo is. Gametes as individual entities go out of existence once sygmany is complete, and a new organism, the embryo, emerges. The embryo, by contrast, is a numerically continuous entity throughout implantation, gestation, and birth. This point has been debated in the literature. Many argue that a blastocyst-staged embryo is not numerically identical with the future fetus, infant, child, or adult because it possesses the capacity to cleave and give rise to multiple embryos. The fact that all blastocysts possess this capacity, regardless of whether it actually occurs, is reason to believe that blastocysts are not essentially human individuals. Many philosophers espouse this point of view (e.g., Ford, 1991; DeGrazia, 2005; Steinbock, 2006), though others have argued against it (Oderberg, 1997; George & Lee, 2005). Indeed, Marquis (2007) actually rejects the application of his future of value argument to blastocysts because of the metaphysical difficulties of establishing an identity relation between the blastocyst and a future human being.

Two Responses

There are two possible responses a detractor of hESCR can give to this conception of personhood. First, if sentience is a necessary condition for moral status, and a right to life, then individuals in a persistent vegetative state (PVS), who have lost the capacity for sentience and consciousness have no interests to consider, including an interest in continued existence, and therefore may be euthanized in order to harvest their organs. This, however, would be a violation of the Dead Donor Rule (DDR), the widely accepted ethical (and legal) norm in medicine that governs organ donation and transplantation. According to the DDR, vital organs may be removed only from antecedently dead patients, and the organ removal may not be the cause of death (Robertson, 1999). Individuals in a PVS are not regarded as dead, given that, although they may permanently lack the capacity for conscious awareness, they still exhibit brain activity.

However, if Steinbock and Sumner are correct, and sentience is a necessary condition for moral status and rights, the DDR is misapplied for individuals in a PVS, and there is nothing wrong with killing them and removing their vital organs for donation. Indeed, the case can be made that hESCR violates the DDR as well, since the cells that are removed (which can be seen as an embryo's "organs" in that they serve vital functions) are what causes the embryo's death. If one retorts that the DDR applies only to persons, then the onus is on them to argue how an embryo is different than a person in a PVS: both are biologically living human beings that lack the capacity for sentience and consciousness.

Second, a strong case can be made that embryos and preconscious fetuses have more of a stake in continued existence than a PVS patient, and therefore may possess interests regardless of their lack of conscious appreciation. If the embryo is implanted in the womb, that very same entity becomes a fetus, an infant, a child, and an adult. Given that the life of a typical human being is a great good, and given that this is what lies in an embryo's future if gestated and born, this future life is one that the embryo has an interest in realizing. This is what Don Marquis (1989) calls a *future of value*. According to Marquis, depriving a being of its future of value by killing it is morally wrong because "killing inflicts (one of) the greatest possible losses on the victim ... when I am killed, I am deprived both of what I now value which would have been part of my future personal life, but also what I would come to value. Therefore, when I die, I am deprived of all the value of my future. Inflicting this loss on me is ultimately what makes killing me wrong" (pp. 189–190). Even though an embryo may not possess the necessary neural apparatus in order to currently value its life and experiences, it nevertheless has a future ahead of it in which it will indeed possess those values. This future is *its* future, and so a case can be made that embryos have an interest in realizing the goods that lie in its future, even if they have no capacity for consciousness. This is utterly different than someone in a PVS who *irrevocably* has lost the capacity to consciously enjoy her life. Therefore, a case can be made that it is morally worse to disaggregate an embryo for its stem cells than to remove the organs of someone in a PVS; in the former case, a future of value is being compromised, whereas this is not the case in the latter. An opponent of hESCR can present Marquis's future of value argument against Sumner's and Steinbock's contention that conscious awareness is necessary for interests and thus moral status. If it is wrong to kill me or you because doing so deprives us of our respective futures, it is equally wrong to destroy embryos for the same reason. Steinbock and Marquis have continually dialogued about this issue (Marquis, 1994; Steinbock, 2006); anyone who wishes to possess full appreciation of these arguments should read these essays as well.

Warren, Singer, and Tooley

The final criterion for personhood we will consider is one proffered by philosophers Michael Tooley (1972, 1985), Mary Ann Warren (1973), and Peter Singer (1979). According to these philosophers, the term "human being" actually has two distinct, but frequently conflated, meanings: "human being" in the biological sense, a member of the species *Homo sapiens*, and "human being" in the moral sense, to denote a person. There are many examples of nonhuman persons. Fiction presents us with a host of characters who are regarded as moral subjects who are not biologically human: Spock and Data from *Star Trek*, E.T., and a variety of artificial life forms that possess thoughts and emotions like human beings (like the androids in *Blade Runner* or *A.I.*). The concept of a personal God in Western theism is yet another example of a nonhuman person. God is certainly not a biological entity, though He has a mind, uses reason, is self-conscious, and is capable of forming relationships. From this we can derive a list of characteristics that an entity ought to possess in order to qualify as a person: consciousness, reasoning abilities, self-motivated activity, self-consciousness, and communication skills (Warren, 1973, p. 55).

According to Warren, only beings who possess these traits are persons and members of the moral community. A being who possesses none of these attributes, like a human embryo, is not a person, not a member of the moral community, and thus they lack rights, including the right to life. According to Singer and Tooley, without self-consciousness, a being is unable to perceive itself as a distinct entity existing over time and, therefore, can have no interest in continued existence (however, according to Singer, if the being is sentient, it is still a member of the moral community to a certain extent, since it has an interest in avoiding pain that ought to be respected). According to Warren, Singer, and Tooley, then, only individuals with certain cognitive capacities are persons, and only persons have a right to life.

Warren, Singer, and Tooley have presented a good case for why possessing these cognitive capacities are *sufficient* for moral status and rights; if these capacities are ones that we consider valuable, then they are valuable for whatever being possesses them, regardless of that being's species membership. This may require that we expand the moral circle to include nonhuman animals—for example, nonhuman primates—that possess these capacities even to a rudimentary extent. However, it is quite different to insist that possessing these cognitive capacities is *necessary* in order to enjoy a moral right to life, and, indeed, this presents us with some disturbing results, since it would mean that certain beings that are typically regarded as having a moral right to life would not. Individuals at the advanced stages of Alzheimer's disease, who no longer possess self-consciousness, would lack a right to life, as well as severely mentally disabled individuals; indeed, Warren (1973, p. 56) even admits as much. Moreover, as all three philosophers admit, there would be nothing intrinsically morally wrong with killing an infant (although there may be extrinsic reasons, e.g., the pain it would cause its parents), even a perfectly healthy one, since infants, while conscious, lack self-consciousness, reasoning abilities, and self-motivated activity. As Singer (1979) writes: "no infant—disabled or not—has a strong claim to life as beings capable of seeing themselves as distinct entities existing over time" (p. 182). For these reasons, among others, many philosophers have rejected this view as a plausible one for determining the necessary conditions for moral rights (Benn, 1973; Marquis, 1989, 1997; Schwarz, 1990). The fact that an embryo does not possess these traits is no more a reason to deny it personhood, and hence moral rights, than it would be to deny an infant personhood.

These prominent counterarguments against denying personhood to a blastocyst-stage embryo have formidable flaws. Given these flaws, an opponent of hESCR would conclude that there exist excellent reasons for regarding an embryo as a person and, relying on Marquis' argument, an interest in continued existence. It is true, as Maienschein points out, that an embryo cannot fulfill this interest without the proper environment, a welcoming uterus. However, the same can be said about an infant, who also needs a nurturing environment in order to fulfill its interest in continued existence, and yet infants are nevertheless accorded a right to life despite their dependence. For all these reasons, embryos ought to be considered persons with rights. And, like Shimp and the men of the Tuskegee experiment, their rights should not be sacrificed even to benefit the common good.

The Nothing-Is-Lost Principle and the Principle of Waste Avoidance

When a couple undergoes IVF, a woman's ova are removed and fertilized with her partner's sperm in a Petri dish. After several embryos have been created, a few are transferred back into the uterus for expectant implantation, gestation, and birth. There are times when all the embryos perish, and none implant, in which case more embryos are implanted for another round. However, there are times when the embryos do implant, and the desired infant(s) is born. Many times, the leftover embryos will be stored for future family planning, but often the parents decide that they do not want any more children. As a result, the embryos remain cryogenically frozen and will never become infants and children. Although the exact numbers vary, there are hundreds of thousands of surplus IVF embryos in fertility clinics across the United States. While some of the embryos may be put up for adoption, this option is possible only if the genetic parents consent to it, and they oftentimes do not. Consequently, the vast majority of these thousands of embryos will be discarded.

Advocates of hESCR argue that, if these embryos are going to be discarded anyway, then why not use them, instead, for potentially life-saving research? That is, if death is the inevitable outcome for these embryos, it would be better to have them die in the hands of researchers who can potentially derive therapeutic benefit from their demise, rather than meeting their end in an incinerator or at the bottom of a drain. Philosophically, there are two principles often appealed to in order to justify this conclusion: *the nothing-is-lost principle* (NLP) and *the principle of waste avoidance* (PWA).

Gene Outka (2002), although decrying the creation of embryos solely for research purposes, supports hESCR on embryos left over from IVF treatments. He does so via appealing to the NLP. The principle, first introduced by Paul Ramsey (1961), holds that the intentional killing of an innocent person is categorically morally wrong, except when two situations hold: (1) the innocent person will die in any case, and (2) other innocent life will be saved. Outka argues that: "it is correct to view embryos in reproductive clinics who are bound either to be discarded or frozen in perpetuity as innocent lives who will die in any case, and those third parties with maladies such as Alzheimer's and Parkinson's as other innocent life who may be saved by virtue of research on such embryos" (p. 193).

The NLP makes good sense in some cases but is highly counterintuitive in others. For example, removing an embryo lodged in a woman's fallopian tube, an ectopic pregnancy, will inevitably result in its death. Not removing it, however, will result in its death *and* the death of the pregnant woman. Either way, the embryo will perish, and removing it from the fallopian tube will at least save the woman. In this situation, the NLP justifiably applies. However, consider using this same logic to justify fatal experiments on Holocaust victims who have been designated for death. If the experiments are performed, then perhaps new knowledge will be derived that can ultimately lead to curing life-threatening ailments in other innocent persons. An application of the NLP seems to yield the conclusion that the victims should be experimented on, since they will die in any case, and other innocent lives can be saved.

What seems to make a moral difference in these cases is the antecedent circumstances that led to the tragic situation where an innocent person is going to inevitably die. In the case of an ectopic pregnancy, the antecedent situation was simply a typical pregnancy gone awry; no moral wrongdoing caused the embryo to be in a situation where its life had to be sacrificed. This is obviously not the case when it comes to the Holocaust. Using Holocaust victims for research only adds horrible insult to horrible injury. The pertinent question, then, is: how did surplus IVF embryos get to be in the situation that they are in? Was it morally permissible to create embryos with such abandon so that it was foreseeable that some would end up discarded? No one denies that trying to relieve infertility is a noble goal; the pain of infertility is very real, and couples who desperately want to have biological children have a right to avail themselves of the technology available to them to meet their procreative goals. But there are ways to do so without creating more embryos than one is willing to implant. Even Outka acknowledges that he is "disquieted by the way *in vitro* fertilization is practiced in our culture ... Approximately 10,000 embryos are added each year in procedures and processes that are substantially free of society-wide oversight—a general circumstance I lamented previously—and in which the profit motive plays a large but ill-considered role. Although many embryos will be transferred, it is certain that many more embryos are generated than will be transferred" (pp. 193, 206).

Germany's 1991 Embryo Protection Law (Beier & Beckman, 1991), for instance, regulates IVF so as to minimize the number of surplus embryos; no more than three embryos can be created per cycle, and all three must be transferred into the womb. A case can be made, therefore, that the wanton use of IVF technology in a manner that leads to the foreseeable creation of more embryos than will be implanted is illegitimate, and, therefore, the NLP cannot apply here.

It is important that this point is emphasized because it illustrates an inconsistency within the anti-hESCR community: although many oppose destroying embryos for research, very few (although some do) make similar judgments about the reproductive technology that also destroys embryos. If it is morally wrong to destroy embryos to alleviate disease, it is equally wrong to destroy them to alleviate infertility. Both are worthy and benevolent goals, but if the embryo is a person, then neither warrants its destruction. That is, opponents of hESCR must, in order to remain consistent, be opposed to the way IVF is practiced in the United States, which routinely creates more embryos than are transferred into the womb (it is worth mentioning that the Catholic Church has remained consistent on this matter, objecting both to hESCR and to fertility treatments that destroy embryos). Detractors of hESCR need not oppose IVF *simpliciter*, for while not all embryos that are transferred for implantation successfully attach themselves to the uterine lining, resulting in their expulsion, this happens frequently in natural reproduction as well. A system like that of Germany's may be more aligned with the arguments and values held by opponents of destructive embryo research (although it is important to note that this method brings with it dangers for the woman, since ovarian stimulation and egg retrieval pose health risks that would be repeated every time a new cycle is conducted).

Along a similar vein, John Harris (2004) proposes the PWA in order to justify the use of surplus IVF embryos for research purposes: "This widely shared principle states that it is right to benefit people if we can, wrong to harm them and that faced with the opportunity to use resources for a beneficial purpose when the alternative is to have those resources wasted, we have powerful moral reasons to do good instead" (p. 142). If one accepts the PWA, the argument goes, then we have a strong moral incentive to use surplus embryos slated for destruction in order to benefit those afflicted with disease. To do otherwise is not simply a violation of the duty of beneficence; it is also a violation of the duty of nonmaleficence. That is, failing to use surplus embryos for research not only fails to benefit the diseased; it actively harms them.

A detractor of hESCR would reject the application of the PWA to embryos because, unlike what Harris seems to hold, embryos are persons, not mere resources. Applying the PWA to persons, rather than resources, yields very different results. It would seem to imply, for example, that terminally ill persons may be euthanized in order to obtain their organs for patients in need of immediate transplants. After all, if we can benefit these patients, we should. Moreover, since the terminally ill person is going to die anyway, why not view her organs as resources that should be used rather than wasted? Of course, such an argument should rightly make us recoil. This is because persons are not resources, they are not objects, and so they cannot be instrumentalized in this manner, even if their respective deaths are imminent and even if the intent is to save the lives of other persons. If embryos are persons, then the PWA is inapplicable to them as well; the fact that their deaths are imminent does not grant us a license to destroy them for our goals, benevolent as they may be, just as a terminal patient's imminent death does not justify killing her for her organs.

At its foundation, the principle that detractors of hESCR are appealing to when responding to these two arguments is a deeply respected principle in moral philosophy: Immanuel Kant's second formulation of the categorical imperative, the formula of humanity. According to Kant (1785/1998), in all our endeavors with each other, we should always "act in such a way that [we] treat humanity, whether in your own person or in the person of another, always at the same time as an end and never simply as a means." In other words, persons cannot be treated as mere instruments, dehumanized to the point that they exist only for the benefit of others. Admittedly, this principle may be difficult to apply to human embryos. Kantian scholars are divided concerning what Kant meant by the term "humanity"; did he mean it to denote any and all members of the species *Homo sapiens* (Kain, 2009), or did he mean to denote only individuals with certain capacities, i.e., the ability to reason, to exercise free will, and to legislate that will in accordance with the moral law (Wood, 2008)? There are strong reasons supporting either position, but to explore them is beyond our scope here. Nevertheless, because opponents of hESCR regard embryos as persons, they also regard them as falling under the reach of Kant's imperative, and, therefore, disaggregating them for research purposes, even if they face inevitable destruction, treats them as a mere means (Novak, 2001).

Conclusion: Adult Stem Cells

Embryonic stem cells are typically regarded as far more malleable, and thus wider in application, than their adult counterparts. Because embryonic stem cells are undifferentiated, they can be manipulated to become any cell in the human body. To say that there has been no evidence of successful treatment with embryonic stem cells, as detractors of hESCR often do, is incorrect. In 2005, mice paralyzed due to spinal cord injuries were injected with human-embryonic stem cells, and regained the ability to walk weeks later after new nerve cells grew (BioNews, 2005; Cummings et al., 2005). In 2008, researchers at Novocell Inc. (now ViaCyte) in San Diego were able to convert human-embryonic stem cells into insulin-producing cells (Novocell, 2008), which would prove useful in combating diabetes. Other examples abound, and this illustrates that embryonic (and fetal) stem cells do, indeed, show great therapeutic potential.

Although adult stem cells are not as versatile, they are becoming increasingly more so. The conventional wisdom is that adult stem cells, because they are more specialized (as Maienschein puts it, they are either unipotent or multipotent) could produce only the type of cell from the tissue where they reside. For example, adult stem cells found in blood can give rise only to blood cells and not to cardiac cells. This poses a difficulty because stem cells are not found in all tissues of the body, so, without the ability to program themselves into different kinds of cells, adult stem cells are more limited in their application. Recently, however, this is starting to change. In 2007, 15 patients in the UK with type 1 diabetes were treated with stem cells harvested from their own blood, and, three years later, 13 of them still do not require daily insulin injections (thereby illustrating that the blood cells were successfully converted to insulin-producing cells; de Oliveira et al., 2012). In 2010, scientists at the University of Connecticut Health Center successfully converted adult skin stem cells into nerve cells found in the brain and in the spinal cord (Bauman, 2010). That same year, scientists at Mount Sinai School of Medicine were able to convert cells found in amniotic fluid into undifferentiated stem cells (MSSM, 2010). Examples such as these abound as well, and this illustrates the increasing plasticity of adult stem cells.

Given this, opponents of hESCR will argue, the choice presented in the comic mocking George W. Bush's stem-cell policies, which seemingly pits opponents of hESCR against sick individuals, is a false dichotomy. Strides in adult stem-cell research have illustrated that we can take care of the sick without sacrificing human life in its nascent state. Vulnerable human life, indeed *all* human life, deserves equal respect in all stages of development.

Note

1 I would like to thank my friend and colleague, Dr Jack Mulder, Jr (Assistant Professor of Philosophy at Hope College), whose comments proved invaluable in ensuring that I presented the strongest possible argument against hECR.

References

Bauman, D. (2010). UConn scientists generate functional nerve cells from adult skin cells. *Health Center Today*, October 19. Retrieved from: http://today.uchc.edu/features/2010/oct10/nervecells.html

Beier, H. M., & Beckman, J. O. (1991). German Embryo Protection Act (October 24th, 1990): Gesetz zum Schutz von Embryonen (Embryonenschutzgesetz-ESchG). *Human Reproduction*, *6*, 605–606.

Benn, S. (1973). Abortion, infanticide, and respect for persons. In J. Feinberg (Ed.), *The problem of abortion* (pp. 92–103). Belmont, CA: Wadsworth.

Bhowmik, S., & Yong, L. (2011). Induced pluripotent stem cells. *Chinese Medical Journal*, *124*, 1897–1900.

BioNews. (2005). Paralysed mice walk after stem cell injections. *BioNews*, September 21. Retrieved from: http://www.bionews.org.uk/page_12509.asp

Brody, B. (1975). *Abortion and the sanctity of human life: A philosophical view*. Cambridge, MA: MIT Press.

Cummings, B., Uchida, N., Tamaki, S., Salazar, D., Hooshmand, M., Summers, R., Gage, F., & Anderson, A. (2005). Human neural stem cells differentiate and promote locomotor recovery in spinal cord-injured mice. *Proceedings of the National Academy of Sciences: USA*, *102*, 14069–14074.

DeGrazia, D. (2005). *Human identity and bioethics*. Cambridge: Cambridge University Press.

de Oliveira, G., Malmegrim, K., Ferreira, A., Tognon, R., Kashima, S., Couri, C ... de Castro, F. (2012). Up-regulation of fas and fasL pro-apoptotic genes expression in type 1 diabetes patients after autologous haematopoietic stem cell transplantation. *Clinical & Experimental Immunology*, *168*, 291–302.

Ford, N. (1991). *When did I begin? Conception of the human individual in history, philosophy and science*. Cambridge: Cambridge University Press.

George, R., & Lee, P. (2005). Acorns and embryos. *The New Atlantis*, 7, 90–100.

Harris, J. (2004). *On cloning*. London: Routledge.

JPII (John Paul II). (1995). *Evangelium vitae: To the bishops, priests, deacons, men and women religious, lay faithful, and all people of good will on the value and inviolability of human life*. Retrieved from: http://www.vatican.va/holy_father/john_paul_ii/encyclicals/documents/hf_jp-ii_enc_25031995_evangelium-vitae_en.html

Kain, P. (2009). Kant's defense of human moral status. *Journal of the History of Philosophy*, *47*, 59–101.

Kant, I. (1785/1998). *Groundwork of the metaphysics of morals* (M. Gregor, Trans.). (Section I: Transition from common rational to philosophic moral cognition). Cambridge: Cambridge University Press.

Lanza, R. (Ed.). (2009). *Essentials of stem cell biology*. London: Elsevier.

Lee, P., & George, R. (2008). *Body-self dualism in contemporary ethics and politics*. Cambridge: Cambridge University Press.

Manninen, B. A. (2007). Respecting embryos within stem cell research: Seeking harmony. *Metaphilosophy*, *38*, 226–244.

Manninen, B. A. (2008). Are human embryos Kantian persons?: Kantian considerations in favor of stem cell research. *Philosophy, Ethics, and Humanities in Medicine*, *3*, 4. Retrieved from http://www.peh-med.com/content/3/1/4

Marquis, D. (1989). Why abortion is immoral. *Journal of Philosophy*, *86*, 183–202.

Marquis, D. (1994). Justifying the rights of pregnancy: The interest view. *Criminal Justice Ethics*, *13*, 67–81.

Marquis, D. (1997). An argument that abortion is wrong. In H. LaFollette (Ed.), *Ethics in practice* (pp. 91–102). London: Blackwell Publishers.

Marquis, D. (2007). The moral-principle objection to human embryonic stem cell research. *Metaphilosophy, 38*, 190–206.

Mill, J. S. (1859/2008). *On liberty*. Oxford: Oxford University Press.

MSSM (Mount Sinai School of Medicine). (2010). Amniotic fluid cells more efficiently reprogrammed to pluripotency than adult cells. Press release, March 15. Retrieved from: http://www.mssm.edu/about-us/news-and-events/amniotic-fluid-cells-more-efficiently-reprogrammed-to-pluripotency-than-adult-cells

MvS (*McFall v. Shimp*). (1978). No. 78-177711, Tenth Pennsylvania District Court. Retrieved from: http://www.ucs.louisiana.edu/~ras2777/judpol/mcfall.html

NCCUSL (National Conference of Commissioners on Uniform State Laws). (1981). Uniform determination of death act. Retrieved from: http://www.law.upenn.edu/bll/archives/ulc/fnact99/1980s/udda80.htm

Novak, M. (2001). The principle's the thing: On George Bush and embryonic stem-cell research. Retrieved from http://old.nationalreview.com/contributors/novak081001.shtml

Novocell. (2008). Novocell reports successful use of stem cells to generate insulin in mice. *ViaCyte*, February 20. Retrieved from: http://www.viacyte.com/news/press/2008-2-20.html

Oderberg, D. (1997). Modal properties, moral status, and identity. *Philosophy and Public Affairs, 26*, 259–298.

Outka, G. (2002). The ethics of human stem cell research. *Kennedy Institute of Ethics, 12*, 175–213.

Reverby, S. (2009). *Examining Tuskegee: The infamous syphilis study and its legacy*. Chapel Hill: The University of North Carolina Press.

Robertson, J. (1999). The Dead Donor Rule. *Hastings Center Report, 29*, 6–14.

Schwarz, S. (1990). *The moral question of abortion*. Chicago: Loyola University Press.

Seki, T., Yuasa, S., & Fukuda, K. (2012). Generation of induced pluripotent stem cells from a small amount of human peripheral blood using a combination of activated T cells and Sendai virus. *Nature Protocols*, 7, 718–728.

Singer, P. (1979). *Practical ethics*. Cambridge: Cambridge University Press.

Stein, G., Borowski, M., Luong, M., Shi, M-J., Smith, K., & Vazquez, P. (Eds.). (2011). *Human stem cell technology and biology: A research guide and laboratory manual*. Malden, MA: Wiley-Blackwell.

Steinbock, B. (1992). *Life before birth: The moral and legal status of embryos and fetuses*. Oxford: Oxford University Press

Steinbock, B. (2006). The morality of killing human embryos. *The Journal of Law, Medicine, and Ethics, 34*, 26–34.

Sumner, L. W. (1981). *Abortion and moral theory*. Princeton, NJ: Princeton University Press.

Thomson, J. J. (1971). A defense of abortion. *Philosophy and Public Affairs, 1*, 47–66.

Tooley, M. (1972). Abortion and infanticide. *Philosophy and Public Affairs, 2*, 37–65.

Tooley, M. (1985). *Abortion and infanticide*. Oxford: Oxford University Press.

Warren, M. A. (1973). On the moral and legal status of abortion. *The Monist, 57*, 43–61.

Wood, A. (2008). *Kantian ethics*. Cambridge: Cambridge University Press.

Zhou, H., Wu, S., Joo, J., Zhu, S., Han, D., Lin, T ... Ding, S. (2009). Generation of induced pluripotent stem cells using recombinant proteins. *Cell Stem Cell, 4*, 1–4.

Joint Reply

Jane Maienschein and Bertha Alvarez Manninen

We have the good fortune to have had the opportunity to sit down and talk about the issues involved surrounding human-embryonic stem-cell research. We wish this could happen more often in our often divided and divisive world today. In fact, we largely agree on what is at issue and even on what ought to be done.

Yes, research on human-embryonic stem-cell research should be allowed. This does not mean that the research will lead to therapies, nor that we should rush to develop therapies or should put our emphasis on doing so. And, simply because no widespread therapy has yet to be developed, it does not mean that embryonic stem-cell research is fruitless and should be abandoned. Rather, there are overriding reasons to allow research and to discover what we can learn. Ideally, this research will lead us to discover alternative therapies so that we do not need human embryos for medical reasons. And it is important that any research to be done should be done in a well-thought-out regulatory context, with careful attention to the safety of all involved, and reflectively respecting the range of divergent views about embryos insofar as that is possible.

Moreover, we should remind ourselves that research on embryonic and fetal tissue is far from being a new phenomenon. The research needed to perfect IVF technology, which is responsible for providing thousands of babies to infertile couples, involved embryonic experimentation. Indeed, many of the common vaccines that we routinely use today, e.g., chicken pox, hepatitis A, polio, rabies, and rubella vaccines, were all cultured on tissue from aborted fetuses. We have all benefited from research on embryonic and fetal tissue, and, unless we are willing to eschew these vaccines, it seems inconsistent as best, hypocritical at worst, to deny those afflicted with spinal-cord injuries, Parkinson's disease, Alzheimer's disease, and diabetes a chance to be cured of their ailments, as we have been largely cured of those above-mentioned.

Given what we know now, and for the foreseeable future, research can be carried out with available "extra" embryos that are now being discarded. While there are arguments that such extra embryos ought not to be produced, it is a fact that they exist and that they are being discarded. Carrying out useful research on these extras seems defensible, given all the circumstances. The onus is on those who oppose their use to argue how incinerating embryos or flushing them down a drain does a better service to humanity than allowing the deaths of these embryos to contribute positively to the world.

Moreover, as long as society condones the use of certain fertility treatments, and, indeed, federally funds it to a limited extent through insurance coverage, there is no consistent basis for not endorsing embryonic stem-cell research as well; if embryo destruction is deemed acceptable for producing infants for the

Contemporary Debates in Bioethics, First Edition. Edited by Arthur L. Caplan and Robert Arp.

infertile, it should be deemed acceptable for producing therapy for the sick. One concern that some critics have is that the process will not stop there, however. From research with the otherwise-discarded extras, we will be tempted to continue to develop therapies that will require more and more embryos. We may even be tempted to generate embryos solely for research purposes, so the complaint goes.

Yet this is not obvious, and in fact it is very likely, given the history of biology, that the lessons learned from effective research will lead to therapies that are not what we predict now and that rely on new approaches. Indeed, there is already accumulating evidence that the knowledge researchers are gaining about development from study of human-embryonic stem cells is yielding the knowledge to develop alternatives. Induced pluripotent stem cells are one example, and so are other reprogramming strategies with so-called adult stem cells.

There are very likely many ways that will emerge that do not rely on either embryonic or fetal stem cells for therapeutic use. But we will not and cannot know that unless we carry out the research now. We have to learn what development can do and how it does work before we can develop the same capacities in other ways. And we can do this research in a respectful and responsible way, as by developing regulations and standards for embryo handling and prohibiting production of embryos solely for research purposes. That is what we need: thoughtful, reflective, balanced science in the context of informed understanding of social contexts.

Part 9

Should We Prohibit the Use of Chimpanzees and Other Great Apes in Biomedical Research?

Introduction

As was noted in the first paragraph of the general introduction to this book, Fritz Jahr was the first to use the term "bioethics" in his 1927 article, "Bio-Ethics: A Review of the Ethical Relationships of Humans to Animals and Plants" (Jahr, 1927; Sass, 2007; Goldim, 2009). In that article, Jahr used Immanuel Kant's second formulation of his categorical imperative (which dictates that we treat other humans with respect as ends in and of themselves) and argued for a "bioethical imperative" that extended to *all* forms of life, not just rational human life. Then, in 1971, 1988, and 1995, Van Rensselaer Potter also used "bioethics" in relation to a general concern for living and nonliving things in nature (Potter, 1971, 1988; Potter & Potter, 1995). It was also noted in the general introduction that, for Jahr and Potter, what they referred to as "bioethics" would be considered today to be *environmental ethics*, where a central issue concerns the extent to which morality extends beyond humans to animals, other living things, and the biosphere (Attfield, 2003; Keller, 2010). As the reader will see, this section of the book closely resembles the bioethics of Jahr and Potter, and indeed, issues surrounding animal rights and morality are routinely mentioned in today's environmental ethics classrooms, *as well as* in bioethics classrooms due to the fact that animal experimentation is essential to biomedical research and advances.

Although there are legitimate objections to thinking this way, people generally feel that the more consciously aware something is, the more it has rights and privileges and, therefore, the more it should be treated with dignity and respect. Put crudely in another way: more mental capacity means more moral status. We do not think we are doing anything immoral when we crush

Contemporary Debates in Bioethics, First Edition. Edited by Arthur L. Caplan and Robert Arp.

a rock, for example, but we do look back with regret on those poor ants that we burned to death in the sun with a magnifying glass when we were kids. Further, we do think that the people we read about at ASPCA.org or Pet-Abuse.com who are convicted of dragging cats, dogs, rabbits, or other animals to their deaths behind their cars or pickup trucks for the fun of it probably deserve more fines and jail time than what they in fact receive, while poaching a chimpanzee or a gorilla might cause some to think that the poacher should receive the death penalty. And, obviously, many think that murdering a person warrants an "eye for an eye" kind of moral response for the murderer.

While there are those thinkers who argue that minds do not really exist for one reason or another—for example, what we mean by *mind* is really just brain and brain processes or functions (Churchland, P.S., 1986; Ramsey et al., 1990; Churchland, P.M., 1993)—let us assume that minds do exist, at least in the form of mental capacities, the way most people in the world believe these capacities exist. What kinds of qualities (features, properties, or characteristics) can be found with respect to a mind? If we can describe different qualities of mind, then we will probably be able to distinguish different types of mind, too.

First, it seems that most anything nonliving that is natural or human-made would not have a mind. Planets, parks, pebbles, tornadoes, tables, and transistors, for example, do not seem to perceive, think about, feel, or experience anything and, so, are mind*less*. If you think that a basic stimulus–response mechanism in a living thing is enough to qualify as a mind, then an amoeba has a mind, since it is able to respond to light and dark, and move its little amoeba body accordingly (Rogers, 2011). However, most people think that an animal with a complex enough nervous system (made up of a basic central nervous system and a basic peripheral nervous system) has a mind of some kind, and plenty of neuroscientists, psychologists, and other mind researchers think this, too (Burghardt, 1985; Bekoff et al., 2002; Lund, 2002; Chandroo et al., 2004; Hurley & Nudds, 2006; Pearce, 2008; Crystal & Foote, 2009; Lurz, 2009). Vertebrates like bony fish, reptiles, amphibians, birds, and mammals fit this bill, and we can probably say that these animals have a mind of some type.

The following are typical qualities of a mind. There are more divisions and distinctions that can be made, for sure (Chalmers, 1996; Piggins & Phillips, 1998; Bekoff et al., 2002; Maslin, 2007; Blackmore, 2011; Lurz, 2011), and we are aware of the fact that these qualities are not exhaustive.

- *Perceptual awareness* (perceptual mind): the ability to recognize an object through some sense mechanism, as well as associate a stimulus with some memory, which requires a fairly small brain. For example, fishes, lizards, snakes, and frogs will move toward someone who is about to feed them because they seem to recognize, and/or remember, that it is feeding time.
- *Basic reasoning* (reasoning mind): the ability to perform a basic inference like "this is an animal that will eat me; therefore, I must get out of here," as well as the ability to solve a simple problem like using a stick to get at food just out of reach, which requires a bigger brain having more interconnected neural connections capable of storing more memories. For example, cats, dogs, aardvarks, orangutans, and all other mammals will fight or flee, as well as share food, given a set of circumstances that requires them to do a basic "I need to think this through."
- *Consciousness* (conscious mind): the ability to recognize oneself as an actor in some event, think about one as a self who is thinking, form beliefs about the past and future, imagine things that could not be directly experienced by the senses, and experience a range of emotions that are more than basic pleasures and pains, all of which require a brain with a fairly big frontal lobe. For example, John believes that he could be President of the USA one day; Judy stands at the edge of the Grand Canyon, takes in the experience, and feels small in comparison; Mary devises a new hypothesis that explains another hypothesis of quantum mechanics; Joan reads this book and starts thinking about her own belief regarding the existence of a god; or Chris expresses the emotions of hope, then fear, then regret, when remembering a past event.

Notice that these qualities make it such that we can distinguish different types of mind: there is a type of mind that has perceptual awareness, call it *perceptual mind*; there is a type of mind that can engage in basic reasoning, call it *reasoning mind*; and there is *conscious mind*.

If pressed, most people would say that if a thing has at least perceptual awareness, then that thing has a mind. Notice that an amoeba does not seem to have perceptual awareness (so, it probably does not have a mind), and the same goes for a lot of other species in the various biological kingdoms like bacteria, fungi, and plants. Insects could be considered a borderline case where they may or may not have a mind (Giurfa & Menzel, 1997). All vertebrates seem to have perceptual awareness, so they probably have minds. Pet fish, lizards, birds, mice, cats, and dogs, as well as little children, easily recognize when it is feeding time, for example, so these animals all seem to be perceptually aware of what is going on around them.

But, there seems to be a big difference between a marlin's mind, a mouse's mind, and a man's mind. Basic reasoning and consciousness are qualities of a mind, too, but most people would not say that a marlin, or even a mouse, is conscious the way a man is. The fact that humans are able to not only speak, write, theorize, and create works of art, but also solve quadratic equations, construct space shuttles, erect cities, and uphold civil and moral laws to benefit the weakest members of a society all seem to be evidence of the fact that humans are conscious (Searle, 1992, p. 109; Crick, 1994, p. 20; Arp, 2008).

Notice that one cannot say *for sure, with absolute certainty* that an animal does or does not have a mind because we cannot get inside of their heads, so to speak (the same goes for humans, for that matter; I know I am thinking, but I cannot know if you are thinking or not). Plus, most animals cannot tell us what they are thinking, if they are thinking at all. However, we can and do perform experiments based upon human mental capacities, and this enables us to say that some individual of a species in the biological kingdom *probably* has a mind or not and, if it does have a mind, how advanced the mind might be (Allen, 1997; Seth et al., 2005; cf. Povinelli & Giambrone, 2000). Having said this, one of the sharpest philosophers in the history of Western thought, Bertrand Russell, maintained the following in a short piece entitled, "If Animals Could Talk" (Russell, 1932/2009): "We value art and science and literature, because these are things in which we excel. But whales might value spouting, and donkeys might maintain that a good bray is more exquisite than the music of Bach. We cannot prove them wrong except by the exercise of arbitrary power."

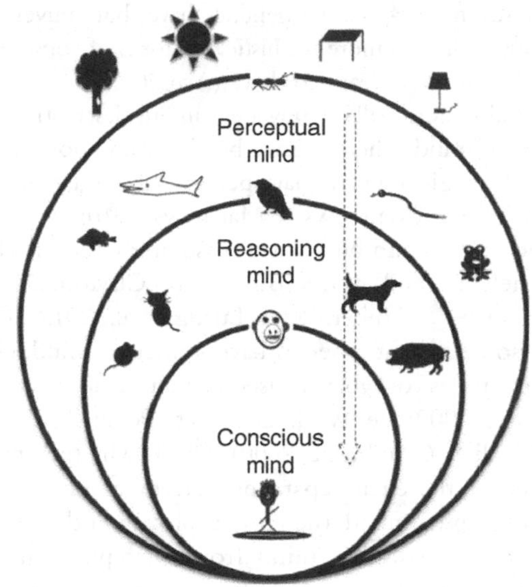

Figure P9.1 Types of mind

Figure P9.1 represents circles of the types of mind we have spoken about, as well as examples of vertebrates that exhibit that particular type of mind. There are things that we can all agree do not have minds—like tables, trees, and astronomical bodies—which are outside of the circles. We have drawn the figure in such a way that the dotted arrow represents a kind of hierarchy of less complex mind to more complex mind, with: perceptual mind being the least complex form of mind; reasoning mind building upon, and being more complex than, perceptual mind; and conscious mind building upon, and being more complex than both perceptual mind and reasoning mind. So, for example, humans have conscious, reasoning, and perceptual mind, while cats have reasoning and perceptual mind only, and fish have perceptual mind only.

Also, there are *varying degrees* within the types of mind. For example, it is probably the case that sharks have a less sophisticated form of perceptual mind than lizards, in general, have; but there are some species of amphibians that have a more sophisticated form of perceptual mind than most lizards have. It is probably the case that mice have a less sophisticated form of reasoning mind than dogs, in general, have; but many species of primates have a more sophisticated form of reasoning mind than most dogs have. It seems to be the case that infants have a less sophisticated form of conscious mind than seven-year-olds, in general, have; but university professors have a more sophisticated form of conscious mind than seven-year-olds have (Arp, 2007).

Finally, there will be gray areas in our description of types of mind where it may be that some nonvertebrate biological species have perceptual mind, perhaps some insects (Matthews & Matthews, 2010). Or, that some reptiles and birds have reasoning mind, maybe chameleons and crows (Emery & Clayton, 2004; Wantanabe & Huber, 2006; Lustig et al., 2012). Or, that some primate species have conscious mind, like chimpanzees or gorillas (see Gallup, Anderson, & Shillito, 2002; de Waal, 2002; cf. Povinelli, 1996; Povinelli & Giambrone, 2000). This is why the ant is placed on the circle separating perceptual mind from nonperceptual mind, the crow is placed on the circle separating reasoning mind from perceptual mind, and the chimpanzee is placed on the circle separating conscious mind from reasoning mind.

We noted above that there is a correlation between an advanced form of mind and robust moral rights and privileges. According to a family of moral theories that can be called *anthropocentric* (the Greek word *anthropos* means "human"), moral status derives from, and depends upon, complex forms of conscious rationality, including the ability to conceptualize the world in a mutually understandable way. This kind of view is one of the oldest in Western philosophy and has been advocated by almost every major philosopher (and other thinkers) in Western history. It also has enduring popularity for us humans, obviously, since we are the only kinds of things that can engage in complex forms of conscious rationality(!)—at least enough to be able to subjugate other species and dominate the planet. Also, this view of morality goes hand in hand with the view that humans are the most important, valuable, and/or sacred kinds of biggest-brained things in the universe.

Now, there are problems with anthropocentric versions of moral theory, but we will look at a significant one here. Any anthropocentric view—almost by definition—seems straightforwardly *biased* in favor of humans, which itself (the bias) could be considered immoral from the start. Peter Singer (1975/2009, 1979) referred to this biased thinking as a kind of *speciesism*, analogous to racism, sexism, or ageism. On the anthropocentric view, it makes sense that humans would not only deserve full rights and privileges, but also deserve to be treated "most morally"—so to speak—since humans are the ones with the biggest brains and the only kinds of things that can conceptualize the world in a mutually understandable way. Anything other than a human does not have interests or a *genuine* realization and concern for well-being, so these things simply do not count morally. Or, they count only insofar as they serve our interests as the big-brained bosses of this planet. In his famous book from 1974, *People or Penguins: The Case for Optimal Pollution*, William Baxter (1974) epitomizes the anthropocentric position as it still stands today: "Damage to penguins, or sugar pines, or geological marvels is ... simply irrelevant ... Penguins are important because people enjoy seeing them walk about rocks" (p. 15). There are also so-called *harder* and *softer* versions of anthropocentricism (Cohen & Regan, 2001; Scully, 2002; Nussbaum, 2005; Zamir, 2007).

So, certain anthropocentric moral theorists would have no problem: keeping some animal as a useful pet, say, as a means of protection of person or property; killing an animal outright for sport or just the fun of it; testing lethal drugs on an animal for the purposes of helping humans or just to see what happens; making animal-skinned briefcases to sell at the flea market.

Almost completely opposed to the anthropocentric view of morality is a set of moral views that can be called *utilitarian*. According to utilitarian views, moral status derives from, and depends upon, the capacity to feel pleasure and pain, and one should always and everywhere maximize pleasure and minimize pain as much as is possible. So, bringing the most pleasure to the majority of things that can experience pleasure is the moral thing to do, while anything else is immoral. Another way to think about this in this context is that there are certain living things that have an *interest* in merely living out their lives unbothered, unmolested, and unharmed, and the moral thing to do is to respect the interests of any living thing. This kind of view has not been popular with anthropocentricists, as you can imagine, since animals having a reasoning mind and a perceptual mind (if they experience pleasure and pain) would be considered on a par with humans having a conscious mind. Also, this view of morality goes hand in hand with the view that humans are *just as* important, valuable, and/or sacred as *any other* kind of living, self-interested, pleasure-and-pain-experiencing animal in the universe. Back in 1932, Bertrand Russell (1932/2009) maintained simply: "There is no impersonal reason for regarding the interests of human beings as more important than those of animals" (p. 118).

The most influential contemporary utilitarian arguments come from Princeton University philosophy professor, Peter Singer. Singer (1975/2009, 1979) argues for what he calls the *expanding circle*, which is basically the idea that morality ought to continue to expand ever wider according to utilitarian theory until all beings capable of experiencing pleasure and pain get the moral consideration they deserve (also Schweitzer, 1936; Taylor, 1986/2011). Singer is interesting because his suggestion almost always provokes a reaction: some think it goes too far, others think it does not go far enough. Those who think it goes too far think that there *is* something special about being human, something (like full consciousness) that we do not share with the animals that specifically entitles us to a kind of moral consideration that is cheapened if it included lesser forms of life. Such critics often mock these proposals by questioning why one stops at just animals (and usually the cute mammals, at that!). Why not give rights, privileges, and moral considerations to insects and trees, too?

Though the last question is intended to mock proponents of the expanding circle by questioning its boundaries (how far should it expand?), it is exactly the position taken by those who want to apply moral considerations to things beyond people and animals with more complex nervous systems. Aldo Leopold's (1887–1948) *land ethic*, for example, emphasizes the functional unity of ecosystems and attempts to give moral consideration to them in the interest of benefiting all the participants. This means that one ought to cultivate an almost spiritual reverence for forests, rivers, and even the ground itself (Callicott & Freyfogle, 2001). It is not as far-fetched as it sounds. People often care deeply about their homes and communities, and invest a great deal of energy into maintaining and beautifying them. If one thinks of one's environment as one's home, then the motivation carries over.

Of course, one might think, "I beautify my home because I live there"—the same regarding one's community, town, state, or country—with the land ethic turning out to be a covert form of anthropocentric self-interest. Indeed, there are interpretations of the land ethic that sound like this, and there are environmental arguments that take a similar line. This is not quite the right way to understand it, however, as the idea of caring for the land carries over to caring for ecosystems and the land *in general*. Consider how you might think and feel if you visited a friend who is renting a house in a different city from yours. You discover that the house is a poorly maintained hovel in a bad neighborhood. Though it does you no harm to stay there, you are still a bit bothered by it all. You feel that houses and neighborhoods (and towns, states, countries, if we want to keep extending the feeling) are the kinds of things that should be taken care of, even if they are not yours and even if the lack of maintenance has almost no impact on you whatsoever. So, goes the land ethic, should be your attitude towards your natural surroundings, including the animals, plants, and trees that live there.

A similar view, *deep ecology*, was advocated by the late Norwegian philosopher, Arne Naess (1912–2009). Deep ecology views the entire Earth as an organism, and questions the morality of a civilization that thinks of the Earth as a source of resources to use and exploit for its own benefit. Both deep ecology and the land ethic have reasons for extending moral consideration (though not always the same *kind* of moral consideration) to plants and inanimate objects, and both condemn the thoughtless exploitation of natural resources (Naess, 1973; Devall & Sessions, 2001; Ehrenfeld, 2009).

As you can imagine, plenty of utilitarians, land ethicists, and deep ecologists have a moral problem with killing animals for sport, killing animals to eat, and killing animals for experimentation. Singer's utilitarian arguments from the 1970s have been incredibly influential for animal-protection groups all around the world. There are even some utilitarians, land ethicists, and deep ecologists who have a moral problem with zoos, aquariums, and keeping animals as pets. So, no wild lions kept in zoos; no mindless killing-machine sharks kept in aquariums; no naturally wild, but tamed, kitties or doggies as pets either. For example, Tom Regan (1983, 1995) has argued against the usage of animals in rodeos and the confining of animals in zoos. Animals have an interest in merely living out their lives unbothered, unmolested, and unharmed, and the moral thing to do is to respect the interests of these living things.

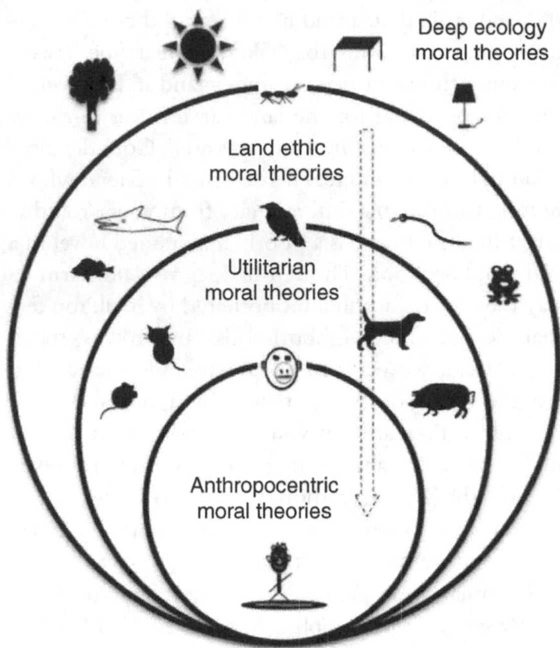

Figure P9.2 A modified version of the expanding circle

Based upon what we have said so far concerning types of minds, as well as anthropocentric, utilitarian, land ethic, and deep ecology versions of moral theory, Figure P9.2 represents a modified version of Singer's expanding circle of things deserving of moral status, rights, and privileges.

While deep ecologists and land ethicists are gaining recognition and moral traction with thinkers, organizations, institutions, companies, and lawmakers all over the world, it is really anthropocentric and utilitarian moral theories that not only are the most developed, but also have the most adherents and the most influence on law and policy-making in many countries of the world. With conceptual tools and arguments from thinkers such as Peter Singer and Tom Regan, groups such as People for the Ethical Treatment of Animals (PETA) have been championing the interests of animals from the utilitarian moral perspective since the early 1980s. In fact, PETA's slogan is: "Animals are not ours to eat, wear, experiment on, or use for entertainment." And, anthropocentricists of one stripe or another—emboldened by the ideas and arguments of numerous thinkers throughout the history of Western philosophy, such as Aristotle, St. Thomas Aquinas, René Descartes, and Immanuel Kant (narrowing Kant's notion of respect to include humans only, of course)—have been combatting PETA and other utilitarian animal-interest groups in response to what anthropocentricists see as the "mistake of placing children on equal footing with pigs" (Nordin, 2001, p. 11).

Probably because they closely resemble humans in numerous ways, utilitarian animal-rights arguments have been most convincing and effective concerning the nonharming of chimpanzees, gorillas, and orangutans. Figure P9.3 shows a simple classification of primates. Humans, chimpanzees, gorillas, and orangutans are generally classified as great apes based upon fairly extensive evolutionary, genetic, morphological, and behavioral data (Kelly, 1994; Groves, 2005, pp. 111–184; Dixson, 2012). And numerous researchers through the years have remarked something along the lines of what this commentator on The Science Forum has maintained, "Go to a zoo and look into the eyes of a primate, you'll see something very familiar staring back at you" (also Cavalieri & Singer, 1994). As the editors of *The Cambridge Encyclopedia of Human Evolution* note, we now have "confirmation from biochemical evidence" that "the difference between a human and a chimpanzee is only slightly less than that between a chimpanzee and a gorilla" (Jones et al., 1994, p. 7). It seems that humans share some 94–98% of their DNA with chimps (CSAS, 2005; Cohen, 2007).

Rather than looking behind the mirror for some other animal, or screaming at, hissing at, or attacking the image in the mirror, chimpanzees seem to recognize themselves in the mirror in numerous self-recognition tests that have been performed (Gallup et al., 2002). They also can be taught some sign language so as to communicate basic wants and needs in a way that is similar to the famous gorilla, Koko, who is able to understand some 1000 signs. A bonobo (a species of chimp) named Kanzi and an orangutan named Chantek have learned some sign language, too (Premack & Premack, 1984; Wallman, 1992). Given the fact that chimps live in small communities, rudimentary forms of justice as well as Machiavellian tactics have been observed by researchers, such as when chimp A takes too much food, and chimp B attacks him for

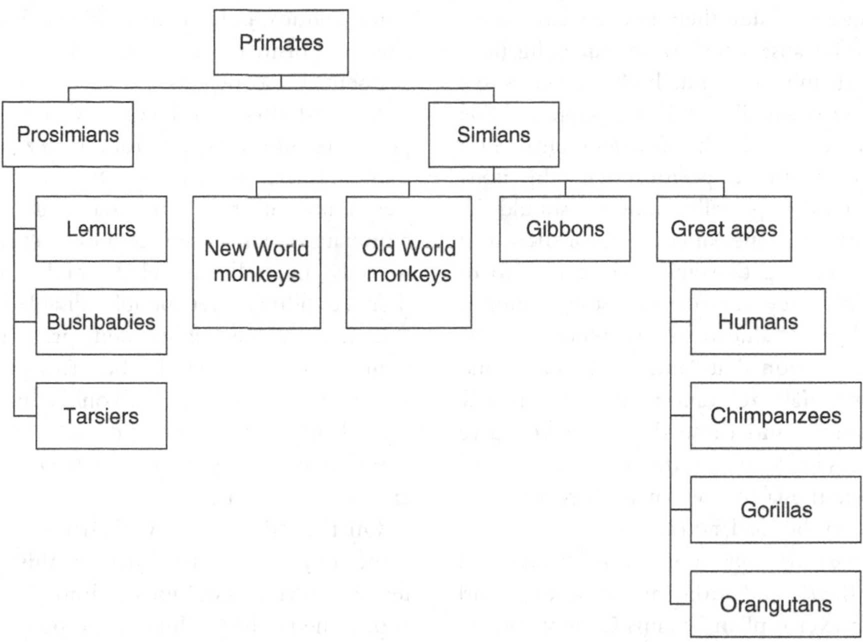

Figure P9.3 Primates

doing so, or when chimp C entices chimp D away from a female with food so that he can have sex with the female chimp D was wanting to have sex with (Lonsdorf et al., 2010; Whiten, 2010). And, for years, chimps in the wild have been observed performing fairly advanced forms of problem-solving, such as using a stick to get at food in a tree, climbing on one another to reach something high off the ground, and folding leaves like makeshift sacks to carry items, among many other human-like behaviors (Tomasello et al., 1987, 1993). Researchers have documented similar forms of problem-solving in gorillas and orangutans, too (Call & Tomasello, 1994; Miles et al., 1996; Parker, 1996; de Waal, 2002; Pearce, 2008).

Prosimians in general, gibbons, and especially Old World and New World monkeys (capuchins and macaques) have been used, and continue to be used, in experiments that include blood sampling, biopsies, surgeries, injections with various bacteria and viruses, and other procedures, many of which result in the death of the animal (Bennett et al., 1995; GRL, 2012). Although there is a history of using chimps, gorillas, and orangutans for research and testing in the United States and abroad, chimps are the only species remaining in laboratories today. In fact, the United States is the largest remaining user of chimpanzees in biomedical research in the world, while Australia, Austria, the Balearic Islands, Belgium, Japan, the Netherlands, New Zealand, Spain, Sweden, and the UK have banned or limited their use (PRR, 2012). Given the present climate whereby utilitarian moral theories have become convincing to numerous people—coupled with the recommendations of the US National Research Council of the Institute of Medicine that "most current use of chimpanzees for biomedical research is unnecessary" (NRC, 2011)—the Great Ape Protection and Cost Savings Act of 2011 (H.R. 1513) was introduced by Maryland representative Roscoe Bartlett to the 112th US Congress, 2011–2012. The goals of the Act include phasing out "invasive research on great apes and the use of Federal funding of such research, both within and outside of the United States" as well as prohibitions against breeding and transporting great apes (USGPO, 2011).

The first author in this section, Jean Kazez, suspects that "the US will join other nations and give full protection from invasive research to chimpanzees. This will not be because we are going to grant them full rights but because we value them as our nearest non-human kin; and because we abrogate our obligations when we consign animals so much like ourselves to a lifetime of being biomedical research subjects." She puts forward what she calls the *value-to-us argument*, a cautious and conservative position whereby non-human great apes—especially chimps—should be protected because of a "special concern for their own near and dear, allowing that apes may matter to us especially because they are our closest non-human kin." She couples the value-to-us argument with the common-sense position that "animals do suffer, and they have other morally relevant mental states as well, such as preferences; and these things directly give rise to obligations in us, such as the obligation to feed our pets, use anesthesia for veterinary surgery, avoid hitting animals on the road, and the like."

"Why do we use *any* animals in biomedical research?" asks the second author in this section, Carl Cohen. "The answer is plain," claims Cohen: "We do it because, using animal subjects, we can make progress in medicine that we could not otherwise make." Cohen is aware of the fact that animals can sense pain, no doubt—especially the great apes—and he is also sensitive to the moral imperative to prevent or minimize pain, if possible, in animal experimentation: "Caution is essential throughout; *primum non nocere*, first, do no harm." However, he argues from a straightforward anthropocentric perspective that for the sake of human health and progress, the great apes (orangutan, gorillas, and especially chimps) should be utilized in research and experimentation because they are the species closest to humans and thus act as the best models for biomedical research. Most importantly, Cohen claims that chimps can be afflicted with diseases, disorders, and syndromes that are similar to the afflictions of humans, but which cannot be induced in any other species. For example, he notes that polio was eradicated from the Western hemisphere through research performed on chimps, and, although numerous chimps died in polio experiments, "there are few among us who would not now agree that the gain for humankind in making possible the elimination of all poliomyelitis justified that use of chimpanzees. From a scientific and from a moral point of view it was entirely right." And he notes other biomedical advances related to meningitis, yersiniosis enterocolitica, and hepatitis where chimps, other great apes, and primates were, and continue to be, utilized as essential test subjects.

We end this introduction with two paraphrased points to ponder, one from Kazez and one from Cohen. Kazez notes in her chapter something along the lines of this: the standard, healthy adult chimpanzee has more cognitive capacities than a severely mentally disabled child—or even many disabled adults—yet people disabled in this way still have more rights and privileges than the chimpanzee. We would be hard-pressed to find anyone on the planet who would condone the use of severely mentally disabled people in AIDS or hepatitis experiments the way in which chimps have been, and continue to be, used.

On the other hand, Cohen notes in his chapter something along the lines of this: imagine if a female gorilla got loose from a zoo and she approached a little child while police officers with weapons were present. And imagine that the police decide to kill the gorilla, even if she appears to be pulling the child to her breast, as she would one of her own young ones. We would be hard-pressed to find anyone on the planet who would *not* condone the killing of the gorilla. Except, of course, for those who subscribe to The Great Ape Project's (GAP) *Declaration on Great Apes*, which begins, "We demand the extension of the community of equals to include all great apes: human beings, chimpanzees, gorillas and orang-utans" (GAP, 2012). By GAP's thinking, claims Cohen, the life of a human child is equal to that of a gorilla, so it would appear that the police have unlawfully, unjustly, and immorally murdered the gorilla.

References

Allen, C. (1997). Animal cognition and animal minds. In P. Machamer & M. Carrier (Eds.), *Philosophy and the sciences of the mind: Pittsburgh-Konstanz series in the philosophy and history of science* (pp. 227–243). Pittsburgh: Pittsburgh University Press.

Arp, R. (2007). Awareness and consciousness: Switched-on rheostats. *Journal of Consciousness Studies*, *14*, 101–106.

Arp, R. (2008). *Scenario visualization: An evolutionary account of creative problem solving*. Cambridge, MA: MIT Press.

Attfield, R. (2003). *Environmental ethics: An overview for the twenty-first century*. Cambridge: Polity Press.

Baxter, W. (1974). *People or penguins: The case for optimal pollution*. New York: Columbia University Press.

Bekoff, M., Allen, C., & Burghardt, G. (Eds.). (2002). *The cognitive animal: Empirical and theoretical perspectives on animal cognition*. Cambridge, MA: MIT Press.

Bennett, B., Abee, C., & Henrickson, R. (Eds.). (1995). *Nonhuman primates in biomedical research: Biology and management*. London: Academic Press.

Blackmore, S. (2011). *Consciousness: An introduction*. Oxford: Oxford University Press.

Burghardt, G. (1985). Animal awareness: Current perceptions and historical perspective. *American Psychologist, 40*, 905–919.

Call, J., & Tomasello, M. (1994). The social learning of tool use by orangutans (*Pan pygmaeus*). *Human Evolution, 9*, 297–313.

Callicott, J.B., & Freyfogle, E. (Eds.). (2001). *Aldo Leopold: For the health of the land, previously unpublished essays and other writings*. Washington, DC: Island Press.

Cavalieri, P., & Singer, P. (Ed.). (1994). *The great ape project: Equality beyond humanity*. New York: St. Martin's.

Chalmers, D. (1996). *The conscious mind*. Oxford: Oxford University Press.

Chandroo, K., Yue, S., & Moccia, R. (2004). An evaluation of current perspectives on consciousness and pain in fishes. *Fish and Fisheries, 5*, 281–295.

Churchland, P.M. (1993). Evaluating our self conception. *Mind and Language, 8*, 211–222.

Churchland, P.S. (1986). *Neurophilosophy: Toward a unified science of the mind/brain*. Cambridge, MA: MIT Press.

Cohen, J. (2007). Relative differences: The myth of 1%. *Science, 316*, 1836.

Cohen, C., & Regan, T. (2001). *The animal rights debate*. Lanham, MD: Rowman & Littlefield.

Crick, F. (1994). *The astonishing hypothesis*. New York: Simon & Schuster.

Crystal, J., & Foote, A. (2009). Metacognition in animals. *Comparative Cognition & Behavior Reviews, 4*, 1–16.

CSAS (The Chimpanzee Sequencing and Analysis Consortium). (2005). Initial sequence of the chimpanzee genome and comparison with the human genome. *Nature, 437*, 69–87.

Devall, B., & Sessions, G. (2001). *Deep ecology: Living as if nature mattered*. Layton, UT: Gibbs Smith Publishers.

De Waal, F. (Ed.). (2002). *Tree of origin: What primate behavior can tell us about human social evolution*. Cambridge, MA: Harvard University Press.

Dixson, A. (2012). *Primate sexuality: Comparative studies of the prosimians, monkeys, apes, and humans*. Oxford: Oxford University Press.

Ehrenfeld, J. (2009). Sustainability by design: A subversive strategy for transforming our consumer culture. New Haven, CT: Yale University Press.

Emery, N., & Clayton, N. (2004). The mentality of crows: Convergent evolution of intelligence in Corvids and apes. *Science, 306*, 1903–1907.

Gallup, G., Anderson, R., & Shilito, D. (2002). The mirror test. In M. Bekoff, C. Allen, & G. Burghardt (Eds.), *The cognitive animal* (pp. 325–333). Cambridge, MA: MIT Press.

GAP (The Great Ape Project). (2012). Declaration on great apes. Retrieved from: http://www.greatapeproject.org/en-US

Giurfa, M., & Menzel, R. (1997). Insect visual perception: complex abilities of simple nervous systems. *Current Opinion in Neurobiology*, 7, 505–513.

Goldim, J. (2009). Revisiting the beginning of bioethics: The contribution of Fritz Jahr (1927). *Perspectives in Biology and Medicine, 52*, 377–380.

GRL (Gibbon Research Lab). (2012). The gibbon research lab. Retrieved from: http://www.gibbons.de/main/index.html

Groves, (2005). Order primates. In D. Wilson & D. Reeder (Eds.), *Mammal species of the world: A taxonomic and geographic reference* (pp. 111–184). Baltimore, MD: Johns Hopkins University Press.

Hurley, S., & Nudds, M. (Eds.). (2006). *Rational animals?* Oxford: Oxford University Press.

Jahr, F. (1927). Bio-Ethik: Eine Umschau über die ethischen Beziehungen des Menschen zu Tier und Pflanze. *Kosmos: Handweiser für Naturfreunde, 24*, 2–4.

Jones, S., Martin, R., & Pilbeam, D. (1994). *The Cambridge encyclopedia of human evolution*. Cambridge: Cambridge University Press.

Keller, D. (Ed.). (2010). *Environmental ethics: The big questions*. Malden, MA: Wiley-Blackwell.

Kelly, J. (1994). Evolution of apes. In S. Jones, R. Martin, & D. Pilbeam (Eds.), *The Cambridge encyclopedia of human evolution* (pp. 223–230). Cambridge: Cambridge University Press.

Lonsdorf, E., Ross, S., & Matsuzawa, T. (Eds.). (2010). *The mind of the chimpanzee: Ecological and experimental perspectives*. Chicago: University of Chicago Press.

Lund, N. (2002). *Animal cognition*. London: Routledge.

Lurz, R. (Ed.). (2009). *The philosophy of animal minds*. Cambridge: Cambridge University Press.

Lurz, R. (2011). *Mindreading animals: The debate over what animals know about other minds*. Cambridge, MA: MIT Press.

Lustig, A., Keter-Katz, H., & Katzir, G. (2012). Threat perception in the chameleon (*Chamaeleo chameleon*): evidence for lateralized eye use. *Animal Cognition, 12*, 1–22.

Maslin, K. (2007). *An introduction to the philosophy of mind*. Malden, MA: Polity Press.

Matthews, R., & Matthews, J. (2010). *Insect behavior.* New York: Springer Science + Business Media.

Miles, H., Mitchell, R., & Harper, S. (1996). Simon says: The development of imitation in an enculturated orangutan. *Journal of Comparative Psychology, 105*, 145–160.

Naess, A. (1973). The shallow and the deep, long-range ecology movement: A summary. *Inquiry, 16*, 95–100.

Nordin, I. (2001). Animals don't have rights: A philosophical study. *Philosophical Notes, 62*, 1–14.

NRC (National Research Council of the Institute of Medicine of the National Academies). (2011). *Chimpanzees in biomedical and behavioral research: Assessing the Necessity.* Washington, DC: The National Academies Press.

Nussbaum, M. (2005). Beyond compassion and humanity: Justice for non-human animals. In C. Sunstein & M. Nussbaum (Eds.), *Animal rights: Current debates and new directions* (pp. 325–407). Oxford: Oxford University Press.

Parker, S. (1996). Apprenticeship in tool-mediated extractive foraging: The origins of imitation, teaching and self-awareness in great apes. *Journal of Comparative Psychology, 106*, 18–34.

Pearce, J. (2008). *Animal learning and cognition: An introduction.* New York: Psychology Press.

Piggins, D., & Phillips, C. (1998). Awareness in domesticated animals—concepts and definitions. *Applied Animal Behaviour Science, 57*, 181–200.

Potter, V.R. (1971). *Bioethics: Bridge to the future.* Englewood Cliffs, NJ: Prentice-Hall.

Potter, V.R. (1988). *Global bioethics: Building on the Leopold legacy.* East Lansing, MI: Michigan State University Press.

Potter, V.R., & Potter, L. (1995). Global bioethics: converting sustainable development to global survival. *Medicine and Global Survival, 2*, 185–190.

Povinelli, D. (1996). Chimpanzee theory of mind? In P. Carruthers & P. Smith (Eds.), *Theories of theories of mind* (pp. 293–329). Cambridge: Cambridge University Press.

Povinelli, D., & Giambrone, S. (2000). Inferring other minds: Failure of the argument by analogy. *Philosophical Topics, 27*, 161–201.

Premack, D., & Premack, A. (1984). *The mind of an ape.* New York: W.W. Norton.

PRR (Project R&R: Release and Restitution for Chimpanzees in US Laboratories). International bans. Retrieved from: http://www.releasechimps.org/mission/end-chimpanzee-research/country-bans/#axzz1tuWVFuZo

Ramsey, W., Stich, S., & Garon, J. (1990). Connectionism, eliminativism and the future of folk psychology. *Philosophical Perspectives, 4*, 499–533.

Regan, T. (1983). *The case for animal rights.* Berkeley: University of California Press.

Regan, T. (1995). Are zoos morally defensible? In B. Norton, M. Hutchins, E. Stevens, & T. Maple (Eds.), *Ethics on the ark: Zoos, animal welfare, and wildlife conservation* (pp. 38–51). Washington, DC: Smithsonian Books.

Rogers, K. (Ed.). (2011). *Fungi, algae, and protists.* New York: Britannica Educational Publications.

Russell, B. (1932/2009). If animals could talk. In J. Slater (Ed.), *Bertrand Russell: Mortals and others* (pp. 117–118). London: Routledge.

Sass, H-M. (2007). Fritz Jahr's 1927 concept of bioethics. *Kennedy Institute of Ethics Journal, 17*, 279–295.

Schweitzer, A. (1936). The ethics of reverence for life. *Christendom, 1*, 225–239.

Scully, M. (2002). *Dominion: The power of man, the suffering of animals, and the call to mercy.* New York: St. Martin's Press.

Searle, J. (1992). *The rediscovery of the mind.* Cambridge, MA: MIT Press.

Seth, A., Baars, B., & Edelman, D. (2005). Criteria for consciousness in humans and other mammals. *Consciousness and Cognition, 14*, 119–139.

Singer, P. (1975/2009). *Animal liberation.* New York: Random House.

Singer, P. (1979). *Practical ethics.* Cambridge: Cambridge University Press.

Taylor, P. (1986/2011). *Respect for nature: A theory of environmental ethics.* Princeton, NJ: Princeton University Press.

Tomasello, M., Davis-Dasilva, M., Camak, L., & Bard, K. (1987). Observational learning of tool use by young chimpanzees. *Human Evolution, 2*, 175–185.

Tomasello, M., Savage-Rumbaugh, S., & Kruger, A. (1993). Imitative learning of actions on objects by children, chimpanzees, and enculturated chimpanzees. *Child Development, 64*, 1688–1705.

USGPO (United States Government Printing Office). (2011). H.R. 1513: Great ape protection and cost savings act of 2011. Retrieved from: http://www.govtrack.us/congress/bills/112/hr1513/text

Wallman, J. (1992). *Aping language.* Cambridge: Cambridge University Press.

Watanabe, S., & and Huber, L. (2006). Animal logics: Decisions in the absence of human language. *Animal Cognition, 9*, 235–245.

Whiten, A. (2010). A coming of age for cultural panthropology. In E. Lonsdorf, S. Ross & T. Matsuzawa (Eds.), *The mind of the chimpanzee: Ecological and experimental perspectives* (pp. 87–100). Chicago: University of Chicago Press.

Zamir, T. (2007). *Ethics and the beast: A speciesist argument for animal liberation.* Princeton, NJ: Princeton University Press.

Chapter Seventeen

We Should Prohibit the Use of Chimpanzees and Other Great Apes in Biomedical Research

Jean Kazez

In this chapter, I argue that we should stop using chimpanzees (and other great apes) in biomedical research on two grounds. First, they have special value to us as our nearest nonhuman relatives. Second, due to systemic problems with the way chimpanzees are used in research, continuing to use them would be inconsistent with our obligations to these animals. Further, I claim that a third argument, appealing to animal rights, is unneeded and may not be available.

Models for Humans

In July 2010, the fate of 200 chimpanzees living on the Holloman Air Force base in Alamogordo, New Mexico, became a topic of heated US debate (Frosch, 2010). The primate facility was created in 2000 as a sanctuary for the chimp population of the Coulston Foundation, which had closed its labs after being charged with horrendous animal-welfare violations over a period of two decades. Now, 10 years later, the National Institutes of Health (NIH) wanted to transfer these animals to the Southwest National Primate Research Center in San Antonio, Texas, where they would once again be used in biomedical research.

These apes would join about 150 already in San Antonio, adding to roughly 1000 chimpanzees used for research in the US (NCRR, 2007). The facility's website explains that chimpanzees were "critical to the development of vaccines for hepatitis A and B" and are now used primarily in "developing and testing vaccines and drugs for hepatitis C" (SNPRF, 2012). According to a careful investigation conducted by Kathleen Conlee of the Humane Society of the United States (Conlee, 2007), chimpanzees in US labs are also used "as models for human reproduction, malaria, gene therapy, respiratory viruses, Crohn's disease, drug and vaccine testing, and other infectious diseases" (p. 114; also Kluger, 2005; Oshinsky, 2005). Despite the initial hopes of researchers in the 1980s and 1990s, chimpanzees are no longer considered viable models of AIDS, since HIV infection rarely progresses to AIDS in this species.

Hepatitis C research is not easy on chimpanzees, despite the video of frolicking apes displayed at the San Antonio facility's website (SNPRF, 2012). In the course of this research, the apes are injected with virus, watched for signs and symptoms, frequently biopsied (largely percutaneously, i.e., through the skin), and kept in isolation whenever they are being studied (Bettauer, 2010). Apes are not natural carriers of hepatitis C, which spreads between humans primarily by blood transfusion and when drug abusers share needles. But they can be infected, and they

Contemporary Debates in Bioethics, First Edition. Edited by Arthur L. Caplan and Robert Arp.

appear to be the only nonhuman species that can be infected—hence the San Antonio facility's interest in the Alamogordo chimpanzees.

The proposed transfer led to reintroduction of the Great Ape Protection Act (GAPA), which was initially introduced in Congress in 2009 with 160 cosponsors (HSUS, 2010). A descendant of the Great Ape Project, founded by Peter Singer and Paola Cavalieri in 1994 (Cavalieri & Singer, 1994), GAPA would phase out all invasive research on *Pan troglodytes* and (less important, since they are seldom used) the rest of the great apes—bonobos (the other species of chimp, *Pan paniscus*), orangutans, and gorillas. All primates (comprising about 20 species) already receive extra consideration under the federal Animal Welfare Act (originally passed by US Congress in 1966), which requires "a physical environment adequate to promote the psychological well-being of primates." (APHIS, 2012, §2143). Under the CHIMP act, passed in 2000, chimpanzees came to be favored in another way: if they survive research, and they are not useful for further research, they must be retired to a federally approved sanctuary, not killed (as other animals would be). GAPA takes the ultimate step: it prohibits all invasive research on the great apes. Passage would not put the US in the vanguard; in fact, just the opposite. Starting with the UK in 1997, many countries around the world have altogether prohibited using the great apes as research subjects or restricted researchers to studies that can benefit the research subject and/or the subject's species.

With the 200 chimpanzees bound for Texas, animal advocates focused on the plight of these animals. Meanwhile, pro-research organizations did their best to redirect attention to humans who could benefit from continued research. Opposition to GAPA is strenuous in the biomedical research community (Wolinetz, 2010). If we care about the human victims of diseases like hepatitis C (who include, potentially, ourselves and our own loved ones), then how could we *not* use the chimpanzees to find cures?

Apes, Art, Trees

Seldom discussed when animal research is in question, but obviously true, is that we forfeit medical advances all the time, with no special fanfare or debate. For example, the US funds art museums, instead of channeling every last tax dollar into medical research. We could raise more money for AIDS and hepatitis C research by selling off the treasures of the National Gallery, but nobody thinks we should do that. Nor is this just a matter of some unique importance possessed by art. The trees lining roads cast shadows that can befuddle drivers and turn highway runoffs into deadly crashes. Cutting them down would save some number of lives every year. Likewise, highway engineers know that by reducing speed limits, thousands of highway fatalities could be prevented. Yet few believe the trees must be cut down and the speed limits reduced. All these examples show that on the whole we reject the idea that saving the maximum number of human lives is our constant number one imperative. Other things are important, too—art, the natural world, the lifestyle we prefer—and we will continue giving them their due.

We value art, trees, and fast driving enough to let more people die so we can have them. Do we also care about chimpanzees to that degree? In fact, more and more people do. Of course, someone who knows nothing at all about the great apes will not have this reaction. But that is true of art, too. The artistically ignorant will want all money to go to medical research, none to art, but it makes sense to think funding priorities should be based on informed preferences, not ignorant preferences.

Why do so many informed people attach special value to chimpanzees? For one, they are our closest nonhuman relatives, historically speaking: chimpanzees and humans diverged from a common ancestor about 7 million years ago. They are also our closest non-human relatives genetically, sharing 94–98% of our genes, depending on research methodology (NIH News, 2005; Cohen, 2007). In fact, when we inform ourselves about the great apes, we learn that we are arguably great apes, too. Vanity makes us resist the classification, but many scientists think that genetically, and in terms of evolutionary history, it makes good sense for *Homo sapiens sapiens* and *Pan troglodytes* (the common chimpanzee), as well as *Pan paniscus* (pygmy chimpanzees or bonobos), to be grouped together (Diamond, 1992; Bjork et al., 2011; Reader et al., 2011).

Chimpanzees have a great deal in common with human beings psychologically. Like us, they have some level of self-awareness. We know they do because they pass the mirror self-recognition test, unlike the vast majority of species. They will examine their faces in a mirror, instead of searching behind the mirror for the "other" animal (Gallup et al., 2002). That alone is no huge accomplishment, but it suggests that chimps can be aware of their own plight in a deeper way than most other animals can. This is not to trivialize what other animals suffer—we can all tell what our own cats and dogs feel about being trapped in a small space, stepped on, or hungry. The point is that there are extra dimensions to chimpanzee experience, making it more like our own.

Chimpanzees can also be taught rudimentary sign languages (Wallman, 1992). An ape being injected or biopsied could, with sufficient training, literally *ask* the technician to stop, in contrast with other animals protesting inarticulately. Frans de Waal has shown that chimpanzees have some of the rudiments of morality (de Waal, 2006). Chimps can empathize with their troop mates, and will get angry when others get more than their fair share—they seem to grasp the concept of fairness. There are experiments that suggest chimps have a stronger awareness of the future than other species; they are more capable of planning and strategic thinking (Lonsdorf et al., 2010). As Jane Goodall (2002) famously discovered, they use tools and pass on local customs, so that chimpanzees in geographically separated troops have different "cultures." Their social interactions and way of life are different from our own, but similar enough that de Waal speaks of "chimpanzee politics."

We care about chimpanzees for all of the above reasons, but also because they are an endangered species (IUCN, 2012). Native to equatorial Africa, it has been estimated that their numbers will have been halved by the end of the 60-year period from 1970 to 2030, the result of habitat destruction, poaching (largely for the lucrative bush-meat trade), and disease. Now, chimpanzees can be preserved in zoos, and even in laboratories. So, merely preserving the genome does not require us to stop experimenting on chimpanzees; in fact, the more we breed them for research, the more the genome can be expected to survive. But what we value is not just the genome, or the existence of individual chimpanzees. We value there being communities of chimpanzees freely living their own lives, instead of being our captives, and living the very restricted lives we impose on them. The more they dwindle in Africa, the more it will become disturbing to think that the remaining animals are incarcerated in our labs and infected with our diseases.

Call the argument I have just made the *value-to-us argument*. It is the most cautious and conservative argument that can be made for the GAPA. It gives animals no new-fangled place in the order of things. It does not so much as assert that we have obligations to chimpanzees, let alone assert that they have rights. The argument does not lead in the direction of exempting all animals from research, because not all animals have as much value to us as the great apes do. The reasoning indulges human special concern for their own near and dear, allowing that apes may matter to us especially because they are our closest nonhuman kin. Even with all this caution and conservatism, we can still make a good case against further experimentation on chimpanzees.

The Moral Status of Animals

But is that all we can say? The argument so far ignores an important fact about apes. Unlike paintings, they can suffer; they have preferences. We can look into the eyes of chimpanzees and feel compelled to do things *on their behalf*. We seem to have obligations directly toward them, whereas we have no obligations directly toward paintings. Everything we do with respect to paintings is really for ourselves or other people.

The fact that apes can feel and want, and that we must do things *for their sake*, could strengthen the case I have made so far on behalf of the GAPA. And certainly, it is a case of strengthening, not replacing. There is no incompatibility between protecting apes because of their value to us *and* because we have duties to them directly. What we are contemplating is that there are two reasons to protect them, not just one.

At times there has been strong resistance to the idea that animals have feelings and preferences, and that we have obligations toward them. In the seventeenth century, renowned philosopher René Descartes (1632/1864) argued that animals have no feelings whatever—no conscious mental life at all. He thought consciousness required a soul; and you could not attribute souls to apes or dogs without starting down a slippery slope and finally attributing souls to insects—which to his mind would be patently absurd.

Periodically, even today, a philosopher steps up to the plate and tries to argue that animals see nothing, hear nothing, feel nothing—consciously, that is (see Macphail, 1998). Obviously, signals propagate through animal nervous systems just like they do through ours. The debate is only about the *feeling* aspect, or sometimes it is about whether animals really have beliefs and desires, as opposed to just having complicated neural mechanisms that register inputs from the world, and generate outputs in the form of behavior.

What about the idea that we have obligations to animals? Again, there have been philosophers who abjure the whole idea. Immanuel Kant, the great philosopher of the enlightenment, holds that we have no duty to feed a starving cat or relieve the pain of a suffering dog for the animal's sake, since dogs and cats are not (on his view) the sort of being to whom it is possible to have duties, however much they do suffer. He did worry that cruelty to animals might lead us to be cruel to other humans, so for that reason he did think we should feed our cats and help our dogs (Kant, 1762–1764/1997).

As much as they are philosophically interesting, I will set aside unusual positions that convince nearly nobody today (for further discussion, see Kazez, 2010, chs. 2–3). We will assume here the common-sense picture—animals do suffer, and they have other morally relevant mental states as well, such as preferences; and these things directly give rise to obligations in us, such as the obligation to feed our pets, use anesthesia for veterinary surgery, avoid hitting animals on the road, and the like.

Putting all of that in a nutshell, you might say what we are assuming is that animals have rights. But rights talk is open to many different interpretations. And the interpretation makes a huge difference to the sort of arguments you can make about the great apes. Ethicists who hold that animals have rights in a minimal sense think there are conditions in an animal (like pain) that give rise to obligations in us, obligations that are owed directly to the animal. These could be relatively limited obligations, like the obligation to ensure that animals used in research receive adequate food, housing, and pain relief. Or our obligations to animals could be quite strong, forcing us to make sweeping changes to our way of life (Singer, 1975/2009; Regan, 1983).

Ethicists who think animals have rights in a stronger sense have in mind what are often referred to as *human* rights. Consider how we condemn research on nonconsenting humans—like the Guatemalan prisoners infected with syphilis by American researchers in the 1940s (this only recently came to light; see McNeil, 2010). If someone asked how the researchers could have been expected to pass up medical progress on syphilis, we would simply say they *had* to, since human prisoners have rights, and the experiments violated them. If rights like this were extended to some animal species—and do not let the nomenclature make you think they absolutely could not be—experimentation on that species would have to be drastically curtailed or terminated.

To take these ideas seriously, we have to be aware of our own biases, and try to drop them or at least see beyond them. Clearly we do have biases. Even if we are attached to our pets, we are prone to think that animals are "just animals." Philosophers since the ancient Greeks have tried to capture what it is to be human in terms of a contrast between human excellences and animal deficiencies; recall Aristotle's famous characterization of humans as *rational* animals in his *Metaphysics* (Z.10–12) and *Nicomachean Ethics* (I.13). All cultures allow animals to be used for human benefit in myriad ways. On a visceral level, humans find some species more than inferior, and actually repellant. In short, we are *speciesists*—to use a term that entered English in the 1970s: we have a deep-seated bias in favor of the human species and against other species (Singer, 1975/2009; Regan, 1983).

Eliminating speciesist bias is an important step in rethinking animal ethics, but we need to be careful about what counts as speciesism and what does not. Clearly we should count blanket disparagement of animals as speciesist: distaste for fur, tails, feathers, scales, and the like is an obvious bias. If your gut feeling is "they're just animals," that is surely sheer prejudice. We should also count it as speciesist when one makes a moral distinction—"we can do X to apes, but not to humans"—and can back it up with nothing but sheer species: "They're apes, and we're humans, end of story." We ought to recognize that "human" is simply a biological category (it just means "member of *Homo sapiens sapiens*"). How could a mere biological category, in and of itself, be a status-conferring, ethics-changing honorific? On the other hand, we should not assume it is automatically speciesist to believe we can do X to apes, but not to humans, no matter how we arrive at that view. Overcoming speciesism does not mean we have to see animals and humans as interchangeable, no matter what the moral issue or context.

With all of that in mind, we can now look more closely at our obligations to animals and whether they allow us to use the great apes for research. Then, we will consider whether we ought to extend strong rights to animals.

Our Obligations to Animals

What obligations do we have to animals? Would it be consistent with those obligations for us to go on using the great apes in biomedical experiments? We will take the general question first.

Perhaps this is the predominant view of our obligations to animals: we may do just about anything to them that meets our own wholesome needs and desires, but we must not inflict more harm than is integral to meeting them. This ethic says, for example, that we are permitted to put animals in zoos, because wanting to view them is perfectly wholesome, and we cannot do so unless they are in cages. But keeping them in tiny cages is not integral to satisfying our desires—they must be in big enough cages. Raising animals for food and profit is permitted—what is wrong with enjoying the taste of meat and wanting to make money? To do both (the prevailing ethic says), we may castrate bulls, and dehorn and brand them, all without pain relief, and that is necessary for cattle ranching to be profitable and beef to be tasty. But flogging sick animals is not integral to the activity, so it is forbidden. Using animals in research is permitted, because the goal is to save human lives and alleviate health problems; but doing experiments without anesthesia is not allowed, because we can achieve our ends at lower cost to the animals. The general idea is that as long as we are aiming at legitimate goals (nutrition, entertainment, life, health, enjoying food, etc.), there is no problem with *what* we are doing to animals. At most, there are problems with *how*. We should be using animals for our bona fide purposes without imposing more harm on them than necessary.

In reality, I think a much more status quo-challenging ethic emerges, the minute we start taking it seriously that an animal's suffering and frustration, etc., do generate obligations in us (also Scully, 2002). It is actually incoherent to divide our thinking into an accommodating *what we do* stage and a critical *how we do it* stage. That combination of indifference and concern is simply inconsistent.

To answer questions about *what* we have to decide whether causing some sort of harm to an animal or group of animals is warranted and necessary, given the benefit to another individual or group (usually human). Our thinking about this should consider four issues:

1. *Severity of suffering*. Will the harm done to individual animals involve such devastating pain, impairment, loss of life, and degradation that going forward is intolerable, just about whatever the outcome? I say *just about* because we can all imagine thought experiments that juxtapose great suffering with fantastically large and certain benefits; one chimpanzee suffers horribly, but we know the result will be a cure for cancer. Rarely, in real life, do we actually confront such scenarios.
2. *Probable outcome*. Is there a high probability of future health benefits, or rather is the experiment most likely only going to advance academic careers, or make everyone look busy, or secure a bigger piece of the funding pie for a particular facility or institution? As cynical as it sounds, we must recognize motivations behind animal research besides the health-related ones that are worthy of respect (Singer, 1975/2009, ch. 2).
3. *Balance*. If the harm to animals will not be intolerable, then we still need to make a judgment of balance. Harming 10 dogs to benefit a million people is one thing; harming a million dogs to benefit 10 people is another. Even if the ratio is acceptable, there are still questions to be asked. We should be wary of benefits that look impressive only in the aggregate. Suppose you can extract Whiff (a heavenly perfume) only by torturing one dog for an hour. One hour of torture yields enough Whiff for

a trillion seconds of human pleasure. Thus, torturing the dog increases total pleasure in the world, despite the dog's suffering. Surely that impressive aggregate, a trillion seconds of pleasure, does *not* provide warrant for harming the dog. An aggregate that matters, morally, has to be an aggregate *of* benefits (or harms) that matter taken one by one.

4. *Subject species.* It is not wrong to see experimentation on some species as particularly disrespectful and cruel. In part, that is because the different psychology of different species makes for variation in impact. It is also not immaterial that death for some animals has a much higher cost than for others. A young chimp can lose 50–60 years of life by dying in an experiment, and a mouse (for example) up to 3 years.

It should be obvious that thinking along these lines is *close* to thinking like a utilitarian. A utilitarian says that an experiment on animals is permissible just in case it produces the greatest possible balance of benefits over costs, taking into account all affected (including sentient animals). The main difference lies with the question of balance. The utilitarian says we *should* aggregate the costs and benefits that will come from performing an experiment. Tiny benefits can add up and become sufficient, in the aggregate, to outweigh huge costs to individual animals. But the "Whiff" example mentioned above calls that into question.

Suppose, then, we evaluate experiments in this close-to-utilitarian manner. Each individual experiment will pass or fail based on these criteria. Many will fail, especially in light of the special vulnerability of apes—their richer, more human-like experience of captivity. Conceivably, though, some experiments will pass muster. Because of the latter, permissible (in principle) experiments, should we allow the continued use of apes in biomedical research after all? Should we reject GAPA?

As much as philosophers may like to focus on hypothetical *individual* experiments, in the real world approval has to be extended to a whole system of research or not at all. We should continue the system that permits research on chimpanzees only if the living conditions for the apes, and *all* of the experiments thereby sanctioned, are likely to pass muster. And that is extremely unlikely.

Why so unlikely? To begin with, there is no such thing as green-lighting *just* the rare justified experiment. If a primate facility owns chimpanzees, there is reason to think the experimentation will be relentless. Consider the staggering cost of maintaining chimps: \$300–500,000 over their 50–60-year life spans (NCRR, 2012). That, together with the paucity of available animals, gives labs an incentive to keep animals alive as long as possible, but also to use them in as many studies at they can. It is a fantasy to think animals will be housed indefinitely in leafy natural settings, and left alone until researchers design the rare, ethically unimpeachable experiment, with lost costs to animals, high probability of future benefits, and an impressive cost–benefit balance. Animals must be used, re-used, and used some more—as the controversial attempt to unretire the Alamogordo 200 made abundantly clear.

Furthermore, oversight and transparency are limited. The institutional animal care and use committees (IACUCs) that oversee animal research, as mandated by the US Animal Welfare Act, are made up of insiders, not neutral and autonomous judges. Furthermore, they do not judge by the criteria I have suggested. Their mandate is not to address *what* research is done using animals, but to regulate *how* it is done. As Larry Carbone, a lab veterinarian, writes in *What Animals Want* (Carbone, 2004), "The IACUC's focus is much more on reworking the details of a protocol than judging its ethical acceptability" (p. 183). In nearly 20 years of working on IACUCs, he has "rarely seen a protocol rejected," he writes. This does not mean the committees do nothing—far from it. They just do not make the sort of judgments of balance that are central to ethical permissibility. The balance question is out of bounds because the committees assume practically *any* benefits to humans are worth pursuing, even if the costs to animals are disproportionate. Their job is to see to it that, given a study *will* be done—possibly *despite* a gross cost–benefit imbalance—it is no worse for the animals than it absolutely has to be. Given what we know about the workings of these committees—that they are *not* full-fledged ethics committees—given what we know about past research on primates (see Singer, 1975/2009, ch. 2), and given what we can still see in recent undercover videos made by reputable animal protection organizations

(HSUS 2012), it would be unreasonable to trust that primates are being treated as they should be in US research labs.

And then there are worries about possible pointlessness. Much of the research done with chimpanzees in the last 20 years did not have the hoped-for medical benefit. Chimpanzees were used in fruitless AIDS research, many spending years living alone in sterile cages, as researchers waited for them to develop the disease (Diamond, 1992, ch. 1; Wise, 2001, ch. 1). They proved resistant, and their suffering was in vain. There is an ongoing debate about whether chimpanzees are likely to shed much light on hepatitis C (Bettauer, 2010; also Lee et al., 2010).

The value-to-us argument gives us one reason to support GAPA, and consideration of our obligations gives us a second reason. But are we thinking in the right terms? Instead of adopting a set of moral criteria close to utilitarianism, would it make more sense to extend full rights to apes?

Rights for Apes

So-called *human rights* give an individual a sort of inviolability that imposes enormous limits and obligations on others. Rights afford stronger protection than the close-to-utilitarian protection I have been discussing. In virtue of human rights, we do not infect healthy human beings with hepatitis C, even if their suffering would be balanced by huge benefits to a large number of people. Extending rights to animals would lead to a simple, straightforward defense of GAPA. But is this extension plausible?

Perhaps the most frequently made argument for the rights of animals is the *argument from marginal cases* (AMC). This argument takes different forms, but the common denominator is this insight: humans can have robust moral rights even if they are not well endowed with the capacities we prize most highly—reason, self-awareness, moral acuity, creativity, etc. Babies, elderly people with severe dementia, and people with cognitive impairments all surely have rights.

To make the rest of the argument vivid, think of a particular child with Down syndrome, call her Dawn. Dawn has strong rights just like anyone else—a right to life, a right not to be used in research without her informed consent, etc. Now, picture Chuck, a chimpanzee with the same mental abilities as Dawn—a fairly realistic assumption, given what we know about Down syndrome and chimpanzees. If Dawn has strong rights, then how can Chuck fail to have them, too?

If the AMC is sound, then we should no more use the great apes in research than we should use impaired children. By producing variations on the argument that match other animals to other atypical humans, with greater and greater impairments, we can generate arguments that rule out experimentation on many other species as well, including all the ones typically used in research labs.

Despite its initial appeal, I think the AMC is shaky. The problem is that it turns on a problematic implicit premise: rights proceed solely from an individual's mental abilities, so that if x and y have the same abilities (like Dawn and Chuck) they must have exactly the same rights. This premise can coherently be questioned (see Kazez, 2010, ch. 6).

A very different sort of argument for the rights of apes takes a direct approach, *first* explaining what gives rise to basic rights in typical, adult human beings, and leaving children and people with impairments out of the picture. Ethicists with this orientation tend to think along lines influenced by Kant, focusing not on elementary sentience, but on attributes like autonomy, self-awareness, rationality, and morality. But do animals really have "enough" of any of those attributes? Kant clearly thought not (see Kazez, 2010, ch. 2), but the neo-Kantian animal advocate points out that we do not think humans have stronger or weaker rights, the more or less they possess these attributes; rather, having rights is a question of meeting a threshold. The argument, then, is that the great apes meet the threshold too, even though they have much less of each critical "power" than a normal human being does. For example, Steven Wise (2002) has argued that the great apes and a number of other highly cerebral species have enough "practical autonomy" to be rights holders. Thomas White (2007) makes an argument along related lines on behalf of dolphins.

Do animals really meet the threshold for strong rights? At this point in time, it is hazy where that threshold lies, and we are also not so sure about the relevant abilities. For example, self-awareness is notoriously difficult to study and has many facets—it is not entirely a matter of recognizing your body as your own. Morality also has multiple facets. Do the great apes exemplify the right ones? Interestingly enough, Frans de Waal, a primatologist with great esteem for apes, rejects the rights approach (de Waal, 2006). "What if we drop all this talk of rights," he writes, "and instead advocate a sense of obligation?" (p. 77). You will recall that this is exactly what I did earlier. Drawing on our sense of obligation, and without rights talk, we can appreciate that we have good reason to stop experimenting on chimpanzees and other great apes.

The Great Apes Are Special

The value-to-us argument gives us a strong reason to support GAPA, and the close-to-utilitarian argument gives us a second and very different reason. Nothing here turns on grand assertions about animal rights, and as I have argued, that is a good thing—it is not clear that we can make a sound argument that animals have the sort of rights we do.

So, what happened to the Alamogordo chimpanzees? Fifteen of them were transferred to San Antonio in the summer of 2010. Once the NIH plan came to light, politicians of both parties, animal advocates, and celebrities protested. Even Governor Bill Richardson of New Mexico took a strong stand against the plan. On January 6, 2011, after six months of controversy, the NIH announced that the chimpanzees would remain in Alamogordo for another two years. The US National Research Council of the Institute of Medicine of the National Academies (NRC) was asked to study the scientific necessity of using chimpanzees in medical research.

In the fairly near future, I suspect the US will join other nations and give full protection from invasive research to chimpanzees. This will not be because we are going to grant them full rights but because we value them as our nearest nonhuman kin, and because we abrogate our obligations when we consign animals so much like ourselves to a lifetime of being biomedical research subjects.

On December 15, 2011, the NIH announced results of the study it had commissioned in January. The NRC wrote an advisory report guided by the conviction that the great apes are "special." Chimpanzees, they claim, "share biological, physiological, behavioral, and social characteristics with humans, and these commonalities may make chimpanzees a unique model for use in research. However, this relatedness—the closeness of chimpanzees to humans biologically and physiologically—is also the source of ethical concerns that are not as prominent when considering the use of other species in research" (NRC, 2011, p. 14). The panel's task was to advise the NIH about the "necessity" of using chimpanzees in the sort of research funded by that institution. Although they were not required to tackle ethical issues, the authors decided to define *necessary* in such a way as to give it ethical content (p. 14). On their definition, biomedical research involving chimpanzees is "necessary" just in case: "1. There is no other suitable model available, such as in vitro, nonhuman in vivo, or other models, for the research in question; 2. The research in question cannot be performed ethically on human subjects; 3. Chimpanzees are necessary to accelerate prevention, control, and/or treatment of potentially life-threatening or debilitating conditions" (NRC, 2011, p. 282).

In essence, the authors moved beyond AWA restrictions on *how* research is done, to regulating *what* is done. Balance has to be considered: acceptable research has to promise gains serious enough to outweigh the harm done to chimpanzees. It also has to be impossible to achieve the same gains using a nonanimal model, a different species, or an ethically designed human model. The authors also stipulate that necessary (and so permissible) research must be done "on animals maintained in an ethologically appropriate physical and social environment or in natural habitats" (p. 27).

The authors assessed current research involving chimpanzees using their criteria and concluded: "While the chimpanzee has been a valuable animal model in past research, most current use of chimpanzees for biomedical research is unnecessary, based on the criteria established by the committee, except potentially for two research uses." (NRC, 2011, pp. 66–67). They upheld certain types of research on monoclonal antibodies for now, but said they would become unnecessary in the future; rejected current research on RSV (respiratory syncytial virus); and were split on hepatitis C research.

The authors write, "The present trajectory indicates a decreasing scientific need for chimpanzee studies due to the emergence of nonchimpanzee models and technologies" (p. 67).

But they clearly rejected a ban, acknowledging the possibility of necessary research in the future. What they propose is that their criteria be used on a case-by-case basis to evaluate all future research proposals involving chimpanzees. Furthermore, they propose that the committees making these assessments need to be more independent than those currently tasked with reviewing proposals: "The committee believes that the assessment of potential future use of the chimpanzee would be strengthened and the process made more credible by establishing an independent oversight committee that uses the recommended criteria and includes public representatives as well as individuals with scientific expertise, both in the use of chimpanzees and alternative models, in areas of research that the potential for chimpanzee use" (NRC, 2011, p. 70).

Progress?

NIH chief Francis Collins accepted the advisory panel's recommendations and announced that while the NIH determines how to implement them, all US experimentation on chimpanzees will be suspended. The tussle over the Alamagordo chimps turned out to have enormous ramifications.

In my view, these developments represent progress, but is it enough progress? It remains to be seen just how the panel's recommendations are implemented. Will committees become truly independent? Will their members be as willing as the advisory panel to turn down research? If the recommendations are perfectly implemented, the changes will represent significant progress, but I (and many animal advocates) will still have to object. I believe the value-to-us argument warrants a total ban on chimpanzee research. As profoundly as we value human health, clearly we value much else besides—art, nature, historical monuments, endangered species. I believe it is inconsistent with our values to keep using our closest nonhuman relatives as models of human disease.

References

APHIS (Animal and Plant Health Inspection Service, US Department of Agriculture). (2012). Retrieved from: http://www.aphis.usda.gov/publications/animal_welfare/content/printable_version/fs_awawact.pdf; also see Animal welfare act. Retrieved from: http://www.aphis.usda.gov/animal_welfare/publications_and_reports.shtml

Bettauer, R. (2010). Chimpanzees in hepatitis C virus research: 1998–2007. *Journal of Medical Primatology, 39*, 9–23.

Bjork, A., Liu, W., Wertheim, J., Hahn, B., & Worobey, M. (2011). Evolutionary history of chimpanzees inferred from complete mitochondrial genomes. *Molecular Biology and Evolution, 28*, 615–623.

Carbone, L. (2004). *What animals want: Expertise and advocacy in laboratory animal policy*. Oxford: Oxford University Press.

Cavalieri, P., & Singer, P. (Ed.). (1994). *The great ape project: Equality beyond humanity*. New York: St. Martin's.

Cohen, J. (2007). Relative differences: The myth of 1%. *Science, 316*, 1836.

Conlee, K. (2007). Chimpanzees in research and testing worldwide: Overview, oversight and applicable laws. *Proceeding of the 6th World Congress on Alternatives & Animal Use in the Life Sciences: AATEX, 14*, 111–118.

Descartes, R. (1632/1864). Treatise on man. In C. Adam, P. Tannery, & N. Chaix (Eds.), *Oeuvres de Descartes* (vol. 11, pp. 301–488). Paris: N. Chaix.

de Waal, F. (2006). *Primates and philosophers: How morality evolved*. Princeton, NJ: Princeton University Press.

Diamond, J. (1992). *The third chimpanzee: The evolution and future of the human animal*. New York: Harper.

Frosch, D. (2010). Will aging chimps get to retire, or face medical research? *New York Times*, September 1. Retrieved from: http://www.nytimes.com/2010/09/02/us/02chimps.html

Gallup, G., Anderson, R., & Shilito, D. (2002). The mirror test. In M. Bekoff, C. Allen, & G. Burghardt (Eds.), *The cognitive animal* (pp. 325–333). Cambridge, MA: MIT Press.

Goodall, J. (2002). *My life with the primates: The fascinating story of one of the world's most celebrated naturalists*. New York: Simon & Schuster.

HSUS (The Humane Society of the United States). (2010). A history of advocating for chimpanzees used in research. Retrieved from: http://www.humanesociety.org/issues/chimpanzee_research/timelines/history.html

HSUS (The Humane Society of the United States). (2012). Video: Rescue from a research lab. Retrieved from: http://www.humanesociety.org/video/.

IUCN (International Union for Conservation of Nature and Natural Resources). (2012). Red list of threatened species: pan troglodytes. Retrieved from: http://www.iucnredlist.org/apps/redlist/details/15933/0

Kant, I. (1762–1764/1997). *Lectures on ethics* (P. Heath & J. B. Schneewind, Trans.). Cambridge: Cambridge University Press.

Kazez, J. (2010). *Animalkind: What we owe to animals.* Malden, MA: Wiley-Blackwell.

Kluger, J. (2005). *Splendid solution: Jonas Salk and the conquest of polio.* New York: G. P. Putnam.

Lee, R., Zola, S., VandeBerg, J., Rowell, T., & Abee, C. (2010). Letter to the editor: Regarding Bettauer. *Journal of Medical Primatology, 39*, 361–362.

Lonsdorf, E., Ross, S., & Matsuzawa, T. (Eds.). (2010). *The mind of the chimpanzee: Ecological and experimental perspectives.* Chicago: University of Chicago Press.

Macphail, E. (1998). *The evolution of consciousness.* Oxford: Oxford University Press.

McNeil, D. (2010). US apologizes for syphilis tests in Guatemala. *New York Times*, October 21. Retrieved from: http://www.nytimes.com/2010/10/02/health/research/02infect.html

NCRR (National Center for Research Resources). (2007). Report of the chimpanzee management plan working group. Retrieved from: http://www.ncrr.nih.gov/comparative_medicine/chimpanzee_management_program/ChimP05-22-2007.asp

NCRR (National Center for Research Resources) (2012). Chimpanzee management program. Retrieved from: http://www.ncrr.nih.gov/comparative_medicine/resource_directory/primates.asp

NIH News. (2005). New genome comparison finds chimps, humans very similar at the DNA level. *NIH News*, August 31. Retrieved from: http://www.genome.gov/15515096

NRC (National Research Council of the Institute of Medicine of the National Academies). (2011). *Chimpanzees in biomedical and behavioral research: Assessing the Necessity.* Washington, DC: The National Academies Press.

Oshinsky, D. (2005). *Polio: An American story.* Oxford: Oxford University Press.

Reader, S., Hager, Y., & Laland, K. (2011). The evolution of primate general and cultural intelligence. *Philosophical Transactions of the Royal Society, B: Biological Sciences, 366*, 1017–1027.

Regan T. (1983). *The case for animal rights.* Berkeley, CA: University of California Press.

Scully, M. (2002). *Dominion: The power of man, the suffering of animals, and the call to mercy.* New York: St. Martin's Press.

Singer, P. (1975/2009). *Animal liberation.* New York: Random House.

SNPRF (Southwest National Primate Research Facility) (2012). Chimpanzees. Retrieved from: http://www.sfbr.org/SNPRC/primates_chimpanzees.aspx

Wallman, J. (1992). *Aping language.* Cambridge: Cambridge University Press.

White, T. (2007). *In defense of dolphins: The new moral frontier.* Malden, MA: Wiley-Blackwell.

Wise, S. (2001). *Rattling the cage: Toward legal rights for animals.* Cambridge, MA: Perseus Publishing.

Wise, S. (2002). *Drawing the line: Science and the case for animal rights.* Cambridge, MA: Perseus Publishing.

Wolinetz, C. (2010). FASEB opposes great ape protection act. *American Society for Biochemistry and Molecular Biology Today*, January. Retrieved from: http://www.asbmb.org/asbmb today/asbmbtoday

Chapter Eighteen

We Should Not Prohibit the Use of Chimpanzees and Other Great Apes in Biomedical Research

Carl Cohen

In this chapter, given that chimpanzees can contract diseases that afflict humans but that cannot be induced in other animal species, I argue that their use in biomedical research must not be prohibited. What we learn from animal research permits the safe development of new and better treatments for human diseases and disorders. Further, the reality is that chimpanzees and other apes are not members of the human species, and so apes are not deserving of the same rights and privileges as humans; your daughter and the orangutan she watches in the zoo are not moral equals. Only zealotry on behalf of animals leads animal-rights activists to assert an equality whose unreality is perfectly evident to children at first blush, and equally evident to thoughtful adults upon reflection.

Introduction

Most medical researchers derive no satisfaction from the experimental use of chimpanzees, and would avoid it if the costs of that avoidance were not too high. There are good reasons to discourage the experimental use of chimpanzees. But ought their use be categorically prohibited? To that question, the answer is no.

It is helpful to begin with the more general question. Why do we use *any* animals in biomedical research? Animal subjects are sentient; investigators are keenly aware of their vulnerability and explicitly accept the obligation to treat their subjects humanely. But distress for those animals is often unavoidable, and sometimes they die. Knowing this, we continue to use them. Why?

The answer is plain. We do it because, using animal subjects, we can make progress in medicine that we could not otherwise make. What we learn from animal research permits the safe development of new and better treatments for human diseases and disorders. When it is possible to replace animals without hindering medical advance, replacement is rightly welcomed. But such replacement is possible only in limited spheres. Where the targets of research are new drugs, or vaccines, or surgical procedures, the use of animals is often not eliminable without imposing great risks, even intolerable risks, on humans. The evidence for this conclusion, in the history of medicine and in current scientific investigations, is overwhelming. The essential role of animal subjects in biomedical research is not here in dispute (ILAR, 1996).

Contemporary Debates in Bioethics, First Edition. Edited by Arthur L. Caplan and Robert Arp.

Biological Similarities

What accounts for this essential role is the biological fact that animals are *like* human beings in many important respects. Human life is the product of evolution; it is therefore to be expected that many of the features of our bodies—the human cardiovascular system, for example, or the human immune system, or the human gastrointestinal tract—are quite similar to the analogous systems found in mice, or pigs, or monkeys. All animate life is the outcome of an evolutionary process that has produced, in different species of animals, similar organs with very similar structures and functions.

These similarities underlie the role of animals in research as *models* of human beings. Investigators who hope to eliminate or cure some human disease will seek out animals in which that disease also arises, and will try alternative treatments of the disease in those models before testing those treatments in humans.

Animal research is critical because new drugs will have consequences for the organism not yet fully understood; the new stuff may be toxic, or dangerous in other ways. We hypothesize that some new pharmaceutical compound will alleviate some disorder—but does it in fact have that happy outcome? And what side effects of the new compound may be anticipated? The answers to such questions are not known. The only way to get those answers is to try the new stuff out, to experiment.

The ideal subjects of such experiments are humans, since it is human disorders that are the target. But experimenting directly on humans is in many contexts too fraught with danger. Imposing such risks on humans, even with their consent, is wrong if those risks can be avoided; laws and regulations governing research often forbid it. If the quest for the cure or the vaccine in question is to be advanced, it is often the case that the only alternative open to us is to try the new stuff on some subjects that are not human but very *similar* to the humans we aim to support.

Some species of animal, whose organic systems are well understood and known to be very much like analogous human systems, is taken to be a *model* for the investigation of that human disorder. When the efficacy of the new stuff has been repeatedly confirmed in the model (in the mouse or the guinea pig, for example), we can very cautiously devise the first phase of clinical trials with human volunteers. In that first phase, we seek only to learn whether the stuff under examination is *safe* for use in humans. Even testing of that preliminary sort imposes great risks on humans if we have no evidence that the stuff can be safely tolerated by some nonhuman animal model. Data showing both safety and efficacy in animals, often in more than one model species, may eventually justify the enlistment of human subjects (ILAR, 1996).

Animal data may prove deceptive. What is innocuous in a pig may be toxic in humans; what is toxic in a mouse may be innocuous in humans. Malaria is preventable in mice, but the vaccine that produces immunity in that species unfortunately does not have that happy result in humans. There is no avoiding all risk, but we do our best to minimize it, and even from failures much may be learned. Caution is essential throughout; primum non nocere, first, do no harm.

The human disease whose cure we seek often does not arise, and cannot even be induced, in any one of the species we had hoped to use as model. In that case, the essential preliminary task of investigators is that of *finding the model* upon which the needed testing can be done. This may prove to be an objective very difficult to achieve.

Chimpanzee as the Ideal Model

This brings us to the biomedical use of chimpanzees, *Pan troglodytes*, which we may reasonably take as representative of all the great apes. Chimpanzees have been maintained in captivity for many years for purposes of scientific research, during the first half of the twentieth century chiefly for research on behavior and cognition. The similarities of chimpanzees and humans came to support research on neurobiology and physiology (Bennett et al., 1995; Abee et al., 2012). Comparative medicine often relied on chimpanzees. When the exploration of space began in the latter decades of the twentieth century, the risks of space travel were very poorly understood; chimpanzees were used as human surrogates (NASA, 2012). The life of a chimpanzee is precious, but it is not a human life, and if one or the other must be risked, the choice is not hard for most of us to make.

The most valuable and irreplaceable uses of chimpanzees, however, have been those in which they have served as models for certain highly problematic diseases. *Chimpanzees can contract diseases that afflict humans but that cannot be induced in other animal species.* This is the key to all the argument that follows; it is the reason that their use must not be prohibited.

Chimpanzees seem to be almost human. They not only have an almost human form, but in some ways also act nearly as we do. They have a consciousness of self far greater than that of rodents or canines. They are quite intelligent and can learn things that most other animals can never possibly learn. By manipulating objects with their hands, which are strikingly similar to our own, they can *do* many of the things that humans can do. It is obvious that apes are much more similar to human beings than are mice or pigs, or other species commonly used as experimental models (Premack & Premack, 1984; Lund, 2002).

The similarity of chimpanzees to humans extends also to their genetic makeup. Every animal species is what it is by virtue of its gene pool. The human gene pool, we have learned, is largely shared with most other animal species (even fruit flies!) but is *very* largely shared by chimpanzees; approximately 94–98% of our genetic code is indistinguishable from that of the chimpanzee (CSAS, 2005).

Of course, humans and chimpanzees are also *dissimilar* in many very important ways. It is widely believed that human beings differ from all other animals in that each human has been blessed with a soul, a spiritual entity endowed by a supernatural creator. This claim I do not here address. It may be true, but support for it must come from beliefs and arguments beyond all scientific confirmation. Since our question concerns the use of chimpanzees in research, we are well advised to restrict ourselves to what can be empirically confirmed. I therefore put aside, as a justification of the distinction between humans and chimpanzees, all claims regarding supernatural endowments. We are dealing with two animal species, like in many ways, unlike in many other ways.

Similarity between *Pan troglodytes* and *Homo sapiens sapiens* bears upon chimpanzee use in two opposing ways. On the one hand, that likeness underlies the widespread desire to *protect* chimpanzees from harm, as we would protect humans. So similar are they (some contend) that chimpanzees are, with humans, members of a larger community of equals. If they are that, it would surely be wrong to use them as the subjects of medical experiments without their consent. But since chimpanzees are not competent to give or withhold consent, this view of the similarity of the two species entails the prohibition of the use of chimpanzees as biomedical subjects. I will return later to this claim.

On the other hand, it is the great similarities of humans and apes as organisms that cause many to conclude that chimpanzees are *irreplaceable models* in the investigation of some human diseases. If they are that, their complete exclusion from the pool of possible research subjects would come only at very great cost to human well-being.

A Bit of History

Consider first the importance of chimpanzees as models through which human diseases may be investigated. This is a long story; what follows is no more than summary. I begin with several backward glances. Long ago, a renowned anatomist at the University of London, Sir Solly Zuckerman (1933), wrote this: "Apes are chosen as experimental subjects largely because they are the only animals suitable for the investigation of certain diseases, for example, poliomyelitis, or for the analysis of physiological mechanisms such as the menstrual cycle." That was 1933.

Forty-three years later, the Nobel Prize for Physiology or Medicine was awarded to two researchers, Baruch Blumberg, an American, and D. Carleton Gajdusek, a Pole, for their work identifying new mechanisms for the spread of infectious diseases. About their discoveries, it will suffice to say this: (a) Blumberg proved that it is possible to develop a vaccine against a very serious human disease of the liver, hepatitis B. His proof was based entirely on his work with chimpanzees (Highfield, 2011; also Ganem & Prince, 2004); and (b) Gajdusek was able to determine the way in which some infectious diseases of the brain are communicated. He was able to do this only through his work with chimpanzees (Gajdusek et al., 1967).

In 2003, the Nobel prize in Physiology or Medicine was awarded to Paul Lauterbur and Sir Peter Mansfield for their discoveries concerning magnetic resonance imaging, a diagnostic technology now of the very greatest importance (Wade, 2003). Chimpanzees were among their principal subjects.

In the quest for a polio vaccine, research using chimpanzees has served humanity in a most wonderful way. In 1952, 58,000 people in the United States contracted polio. Thousands of these victims died; many more were sentenced to life imprisonment in the device known as the *iron lung*. To develop a vaccine that would prevent polio, it was essential to be able to culture the virus itself. Researchers were stymied by their inability to find some animal tissue that could serve as host. This extraordinarily difficult obstacle was finally overcome, in 1949, in the laboratory of Dr John Enders at Children's Hospital in Boston, where it was shown that the virus could be cultured employing a complicated process that relied on cells taken from the kidneys of primates (Kluger, 2005; Oshinsky, 2005).

But what would the polio vaccine itself be like? Two different types of vaccine were being pursued. One would use a killed virus administered by injection, which retains viral characteristics sufficient to produce protective antibodies in the recipient. A second type, administered by mouth, would use a live virus weakened in such a way that it would actually give the patient a polio infection, but one too weak to do damage.

Testing any such vaccines was a obviously a very dangerous enterprise. The reality of that danger had been shown by the fact that earlier efforts to test a polio vaccine on human children had resulted in their *contracting* the very disease whose prevention was the objective. In the end, the efficacy of any vaccine could only be proved by trials in humans; but before human children could be put at risk, strong evidence was needed that the vaccine really worked.

To gather such evidence, animals in which polio could be induced were needed. Chimpanzees were (and still are) the *only* animals known that might serve this vital function. Dr Hilary Koprowski, working in the Lederle Laboratories, a New York pharmaceutical firm, developed a live-virus vaccine in which he had confidence. He tested it on himself and on a lab assistant. Much more testing was essential. He gave the vaccine to nine chimpanzees. He then fed these chimpanzees strong doses of the same strain of poliovirus. None of the chimpanzees developed polio. Still more evidence was needed. In 1950, he gambled, testing the vaccine *in secret* on children in a state institution for youngsters with developmental disabilities. All of the children developed polio antibodies, and none of them contracted polio. This testing on human children, however, was severely criticized by the National Foundation for Infantile Paralysis for risking an epidemic by rushing to tests on humans before animal data gave adequate assurance of safety.

Testing vaccines is *always* dangerous; testing the polio vaccine on human children was particularly dangerous. If investigations were to advance, there would need to be a population of nonhuman subjects on which the vaccine might be tried. But those subjects had to be animal models that *could* indeed contract polio, for it is only by exhibiting the subsequent immunity of such subjects that the efficacy of the vaccine might be demonstrated. Such nonhuman subjects, who could contract the disease, and upon whom a vaccine could be tested without risk to human children, were chimpanzees.

With chimpanzees exhibiting immunity, the needed large-scale trials of the new vaccine on human children could go forward, and they did, with splendid success. On April 12, 1955, the first polio vaccine, devised by Dr Jonas Salk, was declared to be, after two years of trials, "safe, effective, and potent." This announcement came from the University of Michigan School of Public Health, only a few hundred meters from where I sit as I write this. Childhood vaccination against polio very quickly became routine, as it is still. By the close of the 1950s, the number of reported polio cases in the United States had been reduced to one dozen. Polio was totally eradicated from the Western Hemisphere not long after that, and it is now nearing eradication in other parts of the world as well. The development of a vaccine that gives complete protection against polio, said the chairman of the Board of Directors of the American Medical Association, "is one of the greatest events in the history of medicine." Indeed, it was that. It could not have happened had researchers been forbidden to use chimpanzees (Oshinsky, 2005; Kluger, 2005).

Our thankfulness for this development is tinged with regret. To test the vaccine on apes, there needed to be control populations whose members did *not* receive the vaccine; many splendid animals died. Still, there are few among us who would not now agree that the gain for humankind in making possible the elimination of all poliomyelitis justified that use of chimpanzees. From a scientific and moral point of view, it was entirely right.

We cannot know whether there will be in the future discoveries of similar magnitude made possible only with the use of chimpanzees. After animal research is done, testing on human populations is ultimately unavoidable. But there are diseases for which the essential, preliminary animal research cannot be done in any animals other than the apes. Polio is only one of these. In chimpanzees, the expression of those diseases is quite similar to their expression in humans. These diseases include meningitis, and yersiniosis enterocolitica (an infectious disease contracted most often by children from the ingestion of pork), hepatitis, and others. To find ways of combating these serious and widespread human disorders, chimpanzees are the most suitable models we know.

Other animal models may one day be found that are equally close to humans, although that is not likely. Other ways of testing vaccines for some especially problematic diseases may (or may not) be eventually discovered. These theoretical possibilities cannot justify the preclusion of animal subjects now whose use holds early promise of important scientific advance.

AIDS and Hepatitis

Consider the cases of two other widespread diseases. The first is acquired immunodeficiency syndrome (AIDS) and the HIV virus that causes it in humans, whose gravity is well understood. The second is hepatitis, liver disease, which has many forms that plague humanity around the world.

The quest for a vaccine for AIDS—the goal now most ardently pursued by virologists worldwide—has thus far been completely unsuccessful. Chimpanzees are the only animals other than humans in whom AIDS can be induced (Friedman et al., 2006). Their use in this sphere has declined, however, because they resist the disease in puzzling ways. But even failure can prove instructive. The near identity of some chimpanzee genes with their human analogs enables investigators to identify the genetic basis of the greater resistance to AIDS in the chimpanzee. This opens some investigative doors that may prove fruitful. When research in the sphere of immunodeficiencies was young, the role of the chimpanzee was very important. We cannot be sure about what can and cannot be learned from chimpanzees in the continuing battle against AIDS. Billions of dollars have been dedicated to the development of an AIDS vaccine over decades. The exact number of vaccines that have been tested is not known, but the US National Institute of Allergy and Infectious Diseases (NIAID, 2012) has reported more than 50 vaccines evaluated in more than 100 trials. No vaccine has yet been found that affects the progression of the disease; no vaccine has been approved for use.

In the 1990s a new disease, simian immunodeficiency virus (SIV), was discovered, and from that time the models of choice for human immunodeficiency have been other primates, mainly macaques, infected with SIV (Joag, 2000). Even optimistic researchers have predicted that an effective vaccine for *human* immunodeficiency is more than a decade away; others, despairing, predict that it will not come for half a century. It is not probable that the experimental use of chimpanzees will bring this long quest to fruition.

But *we cannot know* what the course of these investigations will reveal. Vaccines of very different kinds have been tried: some have used inactivated viruses, some have used DNA plasmids, and some have used recombinant proteins and recombinant viruses. Of all the candidate vaccines for AIDS, 88% have failed the first, safety phase of their investigation. This realm is replete with risk. A virus blending the simian and the human (called therefore *chimeric*) has also been tried, also without success. An animal model that will make possible the safe testing of candidate vaccines remains critical. We do not know what that ideal model will be, or even if one will ever be found.

Some AIDS researchers advocate a return to the use of chimpanzees. Whether that return is justifiable, or may one day become justifiable, is currently a matter of scientific dispute. Vaccine trials using chimpanzees have failed, and trials using other primates have also failed. We do not know what will succeed, or whether anything will ever succeed (Girard & Plotkin, 2012). The value of an AIDS vaccine, if ever it were found, would be incalculable. In our present state of ignorance, it would be presumptuous, and a serious moral mistake, to prohibit categorically now an animal model that *may* one day prove to contribute greatly to human well-being. At the very least, we must maintain the *availability* of chimpanzees as the search for an AIDS vaccine continues.

Hepatitis (a liver disease) presents a yet more compelling case. The disease is very serious, leading often to death. No effective treatment for hepatitis has been found. The only way to develop cures, and above all an effective hepatitis vaccine, is to experiment with an animal model in which hepatitis can be induced. There is no other way. Medical scientists have thus far found it impossible to induce this infection in mice, rabbits, pigs, or any other common animal model. *Chimpanzees are the only animal models in which hepatitis can be induced.*

Hepatitis takes many forms, commonly identified by letter: hepatitis A, hepatitis B, etc. Hepatitis C (called HVC), for which there is no vaccine yet, infects more than 100 million people worldwide. It often leads to liver cancer and death. It was *in* the chimpanzee that the hepatitis C virus was first discovered, not very long ago, by Dr Michael Houghton, a Canadian virologist at the University of Alberta. Research on the disease depended, after discovery, on the ability to develop infectious clones of HVC, and at first that could be done only by using chimpanzees. Chimpanzees are no longer needed for that purpose, because infected humans are available to supply these clones (Hanlon, 2012). But experimental *vaccines* can only be tested on *un*infected individuals, and so, if a vaccine is ever to be found for hepatitis C, it is essential that chimpanzees remain available (Bukh, 2004).

It has been learned, on one main line of inquiry using chimpanzees, that certain immune system cells, called T-cells, become exhausted in persons infected with hepatitis C. What is being sought is a compound that will reinvigorate those T-cells. The Bill and Melinda Gates Foundation is now supporting a five-year program aiming to develop a drug that will generate a positive response in those T-cells. Success in this remains very uncertain, but, as one hepatitis C researcher (at Nationwide Children's Hospital in Columbus, Ohio) put the matter very simply: "The chimpanzees were absolutely critical" (Wadman, 2011).

There are other immunotherapies to combat hepatitis C and also hepatitis B; they are very risky. We may not reasonably ask uninfected humans to serve as subjects in such studies. The number of humans who risk hepatitis is *very large*; the number of chimpanzees required to explore these possibilities is *very small*, probably less than a few hundred. If researchers take on the duty to do what they can to protect humans from that serious disease, would we be right to *forbid* them to use the one species, *Pan troglodytes*, that may lead to their success? Surely not.

There is yet another disease, malaria, perhaps the most terrible of all, which we understand better because of earlier research with chimpanzees. Here, the role of chimpanzees is of another kind. Chimpanzees do not now serve as the principal animal model in malaria research. Nevertheless, for those who battle malaria, the chimpanzee is of very great interest. Why? Malaria is a parasitic disease; when a malaria vaccine (now being sought desperately) is ultimately found, its use will be the first workable vaccine for the control of *parasitic* infection in humans. But the understanding of all parasitic diseases, including malaria, has been much advanced by research with chimpanzees. Apes, in their natural state, harbor species of parasites that are not distinguishable from parasites found in humans. There are four major kinds of malaria parasites, and they have all been found to infect chimpanzees (Coatney et al., 1971). Trials of malaria vaccines do not now rely on chimpanzees as subjects; one recent vaccine trial, partially successful, was never tested on chimpanzees at all. But it does not follow that the development of that vaccine did not depend in part on what had been earlier learned about parasitic diseases in chimpanzees.

There are other reasons we ought not categorically prohibit the biomedical uses of chimpanzees, reasons less weighty yet worthy of consideration. Here are two examples: First, oral contraceptives have an impact on the sexuality of human females that is not fully understood. Because chimpanzees are both like and unlike humans in responding to hormones, research using chimpanzees can advance the understanding of such impacts on sexuality (Nadler et al., 1986).

Also, terrorist attacks using biological weapons may someday come. We do not expect them, but we ought to be prepared for them. One day we may need to learn very quickly how infectious bio-weapons are *transmitted*. We may need to develop vaccines and therapies to combat those biological weapons. Under such awful circumstances, chimpanzee colonies, maintained in humane sanctuaries of course, may prove to be an irreplaceable resource.

In sum, we cannot know what biomedical resources will be needed in confronting the maladies and emergencies of an uncertain future. Chimpanzee research has proved extremely helpful to medical science in the past. It may prove helpful in the future. Knowledge is not so wide or so deep that we may be confident now that nothing of great importance can any longer be learned from chimpanzees.

The Continued Need for Chimpanzee Research

This conclusion, which plainly demands a negative answer to the question confronted in this chapter, is also exactly the conclusion reached by the very most knowledgeable and thoughtful scientific opinion of the present day. In December of 2011, a report was issued by the US Institute of Medicine, and the National Research Council, entitled *Chimpanzees in Biomedical and Behavioral Research: Assessing the Necessity* (NRC, 2011). The authors of this report are a committee of 12 of the most distinguished researchers in the country, who examined thoroughly the medical research that has been done, and the research that is now being done, using chimpanzees. Their conclusions parallel precisely the argument of the preceding sections of this chapter.

The report is lengthy and meticulously detailed. Merely the bibliography appended to that report—the studies and papers from around the world that were scrutinized and relied upon—is a small book. One who seeks a definitive answer to the question we confront here must attend to this report with greatest respect. I present below the central conclusions of this most authoritative body. Citations by page number refer to the report (CBBRAN) identified above.

CBBRAN flatly states: "Over many years scientific advances that have led directly to the development of preventive and therapeutic products for life-threatening or debilitating diseases and disorders have been dependent upon scientific knowledge obtained through experiments using the chimpanzee" (p. 64). Five specific instances are identified in which the chimpanzee is now in use to answer crucial questions about the treatment, prevention and/or control of infectious diseases that "*defy alternative experimental approaches, and that therefore may require the use of the chimpanzee*." The need for chimpanzees "cannot be discounted over the long term" (p. 65, emphasis added).

The Committee developed a set of highly restrictive criteria to determine, for any given case, whether the use of chimpanzees in that research is necessary, and concluded that very many uses of chimpanzees are not now necessary. However, the Committee concluded, there are two current fields of research, of great importance, in which the continuing use of chimpanzees ought not be foreclosed. One of these concerns the development of monoclonal antibodies (laboratory-engineered cells that attach themselves to defects in cancer cells, and thus may supplement the body's immune system); the other concerns the development of a prophylactic vaccine for hepatitis C. There was some disagreement within the Committee concerning the need for a pre-clinical "challenge study" of any HVC vaccine, and thus also about how much the use of chimpanzees might accelerate prophylactic vaccine development (p. 67).

Without qualification, the Committee did conclude that "A new, emerging, or reemerging disease or disorder may present challenges to treatment, prevention, and/or control that defy nonchimpanzee models and technologies and *therefore may require the future use of chimpanzees*" (p. 67, emphasis added).

Also, without qualification, the Committee concluded that "chimpanzees may be necessary for obtaining otherwise unattainable insights to support understanding of social, neurological, and behavioral factors that include the development, prevention, or treatment of disease" (p. 68).

The central thrust of this decisive and authoritative report is precisely the thrust of my argument in this chapter. However much chimpanzee use is declining, it remains, and it will remain for the indefinite future, an alternative in biomedical research that would be wrongheaded to foreclose by prohibition.

A Special Moral Category?

Finally, what reasons are given to put this group of animals, chimpanzees and other great apes, in a special moral category? It is widely understood and generally agreed that animal models are vitally important in biomedical research. Why are chimpanzees to be excluded?

Chimpanzees are different from other animals, say advocates of the prohibition of chimpanzee research, because the great apes are not merely similar to humans, but are in fact *of our kind*. With humans, they are (it is alleged) members of a community of equals.

It is reasonable to speak of a worldwide human community in which certain basic moral principles or rights are recognized as applicable to all. The advocates of what is called The Great Ape Project (GAP) assert flatly that chimpanzees and orangutans are, by nature, full members of this moral community. Their *Declaration on Great Apes* begins, "We demand the extension of the community of equals to include all great apes: human beings, chimpanzees, gorillas and orang-utans" (GAP, 2012). I contend that this demand is unwarranted, and that the moral equality it supposes is simply false.

The stark contrasts between humans and apes ought to be confronted honestly. Does an orangutan hanging from a tree in the zoo, however beautiful and admirable it may be, have a moral standing equal to that of the reader of this essay, or her father or her daughter? The great apes have natural features and limitations marking them as profoundly different from humans. Only zealotry on behalf of animals leads the authors of GAP to assert an equality whose unreality is perfectly evident to children at first blush, and equally evident to thoughtful adults upon reflection. To justify the prohibition of chimpanzee research that might lead to vast improvements in human well-being one would need to establish the absolute moral equality of humans and the great apes. I deny that moral equality.

"But then you are a *speciesist*," comes the reply. "You think that being a member of one species endows one with rights that members of other species do not have!" Yes, I am that, of course. Peter Singer, one of the principals of GAP, quite explicitly holds that species membership may not be used to justify the preferential treatment of humans. It is just like racism, he contends, and we all know how evil that is. Singer (1975/2009) puts it thus: "The racist violates the principle of equality by giving greater weight to the interests of members of his own race when there is a clash between their interests and the interests of those of another race. The sexist violates the principle of equality by favoring the interests of his own sex. Similarly, the speciesist allows the interests of his own species to override the greater interests of members of other species. The pattern is identical in each case" (p. 9).

This is a dreadful argument. It *assumes* the equality of animals and humans, which is the very point at issue. Moreover, it defends this equality using an insidious analogy that is rhetorically effective because of the nastiness of the vice to which speciesism is likened. Giving preference to one race over another is indeed unconscionable. Racism *is* despicable because we know that between the races there are no morally relevant differences. But between species of animals, as between apes and humans, there are enormous differences too obvious to catalog.

Differences among animal species are of the greatest *moral* importance. Refusing to attend to those differences would lead to grave moral error. It would be wrong to treat dogs as we treat mice, or mice as we treat cockroaches, because the *natures* of dogs, mice, and roaches are relevant in determining the care and treatment they deserve. This is obvious to any person of good sense. Being a speciesist, as Singer uses that term, is not only not a fault but a necessary condition for humane moral conduct.

Some chimpanzee behaviors are analogous to human behaviors, for which reason we pay far more attention (for example) to the psychological needs of apes than of cows. But primates are just like cows and unlike humans in many respects: they relieve themselves whenever so inclined, and cannot be toilet-trained. Apes are naturally aggressive when mature; they attack (and may kill) other apes and their caretakers. Like wolves, they are wild animals, nearly impossible to tame. They do exhibit much intelligence, but they are certainly not moral beings by nature. *Species differences count.* Apes are not members of the human species, and no declaration by GAP can make them so. Your daughter and the orangutan she watches in the zoo are not moral equals.

Do this simple thought experiment: Suppose a gorilla had escaped its cage and were now advancing toward a nearby human child. Zookeepers rushing to the scene fear for the life of the little girl. If it were necessary to wound, or perhaps even to kill the gorilla to protect that child, would we not think that justifiable? Of course we would. But the logic of the position of the GAP does not permit that response. It entails that the life of that escaped gorilla is as important, as morally worthy, as the life of any human being.

Who bears the burden of proof in this dispute? We begin with a huge set of obvious and very great differences between the species. Putting these differences aside, the sponsors of GAP *declare* the moral equality of humans and apes. Upon this supposed equality, they rest their demand for the categorical prohibition of the use of chimpanzees in biomedical research, no matter what benefits that research might provide. Even measures of enormous potential value to humans may not be contemplated (on that view) if the lives of apes were to be put at risk. This consequence ought be accepted only if that alleged "community of equals" could be conclusively proved. But the "demand" for the equal treatment of apes and humans is not proof, or even evidence, of that supposed equality.

I conclude, all things considered, that the use of chimpanzees and other great apes in biomedical research ought not to be prohibited.

References

Abee, C., Mansfield, K., Tardif, S., & Morris, T. (Eds.). (2012). *Nonhuman primates in biomedical research: Biology and management.* London: Academic Press.

Bennett, B., Abee, C., & Henrickson, R. (Eds.). (1995). *Nonhuman primates in biomedical research: Biology and management.* London: Academic Press.

Bukh, J. (2004). A critical role for the chimpanzee model in the study of hepatitis C. *Hepatology, 39,* 1469–1475.

Coatney, G., Collins, W., & Contcos, P. (1971). *The primate malarias.* Washington, DC: US National Institute of Allergy and Infectious Diseases.

CSAS (The Chimpanzee Sequencing and Analysis Consortium). (2005). Initial sequence of the chimpanzee genome and comparison with the human genome. *Nature, 437,* 69–87.

Friedman, H., Specter, S., & Bendinelli, M. (Eds.). (2006). *In vivo models of HIV disease and control.* New York: Springer Science + Business Media.

Gajdusek, D. C., Gibbs, C., & Alpers, M. (1967). Transmission and passage of experimenal "kuru" to chimpanzees. *Science, 155,* 212–214.

Ganem, D., & Prince, A. (2004). Hepatitis B virus infection—Natural history and clinical consequences. *The New England Journal of Medicine, 350,* 1118–1129.

GAP (The Great Ape Project). (2012). Declaration on great apes. Retrieved from: http://www.greatapeproject.org/en-US

Girard, M., & Plotkin, S. (2012). HIV vaccine development at the turn of the 21st century. *Current Opinion in HIV & AIDS,* 7, 4–9.

Hanlon, J. (2012). Vaccine discovered for hep C by Michael Houghton who discovered HCV in 1989. *Bioresearchonline,* February 21. Retrieved from: http://www.natap.org/2012/newsUpdates/022312_01.htm

Highfield, R. (2011). The life and times of a vaccine pioneer. *The New Scientist,* April 6. Retrieved from: http://www.newscientist.com/blogs/shortsharpscience/2011/04/obituary.html

ILAR (Institute of Laboratory Animal Resources of the Commision on Life Sciences of the National Research Council). (1996). *Guide for the care and use of laboratory animals.* Washington, DC: National Academy Press.

Joag, S. (2000). Primate models of AIDS. *Microbes and Infection, 2,* 223–229.

Kluger, J. (2005). *Splendid solution: Jonas Salk and the conquest of polio.* New York: G. P. Putnam.

Lund, N. (2002). *Animal cognition.* London: Routledge.

Nadler, R., Herndon, J., & Wallis, J. (1986). Adult sexual behavior: Hormones and reproduction. In G. Mitchell & J. Erwin (Eds.), *Comparative primate biology: Vol. 2a (behavior and ecology)* (pp. 363–407). New York: Alan R. Liss.

NASA (National Aeronatics and Space Administration). (2012). A brief history of animals in space. Retrieved from: http://history.nasa.gov/animals.html

NIAID (National Institute of Allergy and Infectious Diseases) (2012). NIAID research. Retrieved from: http://www.niaid.nih.gov/labsAndResources/pages/default.aspx?wt.ac=tnLabs

NRC (National Research Council of the Institute of Medicine of the National Academies). (2011). *Chimpanzees in biomedical and behavioral research:*

Assessing the Necessity. Washington, DC: The National Academies Press.

Oshinsky, D. (2005). *Polio: An American story*. Oxford: Oxford University Press.

Premack, D., & Premack, A. (1984). *The mind of an ape*. New York: W.W. Norton.

Singer, P. (1975/2009). *Animal liberation*. New York: Random House.

Wade, N. (2003). American and Briton win Nobel for using chemists' test for M.R.I.'s. *The New York Times*, October 7. Retrieved from: http://www.nytimes.com/2003/10/07/us/american-and-briton-win-nobel-for-using-chemists-test-for-mri-s.html

Wadman, M. (2011). Animal rights: Chimpanzee research on trial. *Nature*, *474*, 268–271.

Zuckerman, S. (1933). *Functional affinities of man, monkeys, and apes*. London: Kegan Paul.

Reply to Cohen

Jean Kazez

Carl Cohen and I agree on a number of important points. We see a special problem with research using the great apes; we think some animal experimentation can be justified; and we do not want to think about these issues in terms of animal rights. Nevertheless, we do disagree on whether research on the great apes should be prohibited.

Reading between the lines of Carl's paper, my impression is that for him, it almost goes without saying that we can use animals in research to the extent that we need to, in order to make medical progress. It is because of that background assumption that he thinks he makes a strong case by accumulating examples of fruitful medical research that involved chimpanzees. I think we should not treat it as a default that we can experiment on animals. The more complex and sensitive these animals are, the less it is a default.

Before leaving the topic of past and future medical research, I do have a few worries about Carl's overview. The National Research Council's report (NRC, 2011) states that we now have many alternatives to using chimpanzees in biomedical research. As a result, the authors flatly deny that the past is a reliable guide to the future. So, I think data from the heyday of animal research, like Carl presents, should be seen as a very weak indicator of what we will need to do in the future.

I am also worried about his example involving the polio vaccine. The discovery of the polio vaccine is one of the most spectacular successes in the history of medical research, so it has a lot of rhetorical clout to say that experimentation on chimpanzees was critical. In fact, chimpanzees played a very minor role in the development of the polio vaccine, and I have to quarrel with some of Carl's account. About 100,000 *monkeys* were involved in the development of the polio vaccine (Oshinsky, 2005, p. 17)—mostly rhesus and cynomolgus monkeys. Monkeys, of course, are not apes: they are very different in their genetics, evolutionary relationship with humans, and psychology. Polio virus can be induced in monkeys as well as in chimpanzees, if it is injected directly into their brains—which is just what researchers in Jonas Salk's laboratory did during the typing and vaccine testing phases of polio research (Kluger, 2005, pp. 115–17).

Carl points out that in 1947, Hilary Koprowski tested *live*-virus vaccine on nine chimpanzees before giving it to a group of impaired children at a home for the intellectually impaired, but it should not be thought that this was a pivotal stage in the development of the polio vaccine. Jonas Salk tested the *killed*-virus vaccine on hundreds of *monkeys* before he *also* tested it out on hundreds of impaired children at two institutions. It is his monkey-tested vaccine that was delivered to the general population starting in 1954 (for details, see Kluger, 2005; Oshinsky, 2005).

So much for science and medical history. The real issue here is ethics. The success of the search for a

Contemporary Debates in Bioethics, First Edition. Edited by Arthur L. Caplan and Robert Arp.

polio vaccine would not stop us from wondering if it was right to test vaccine on impaired children before offering it to the general population. By the same token, success does not foreclose questions about whether monkeys *or* chimpanzees should have been used. To think carefully about experimenting on apes, we must focus not only on successful research, but also on unsuccessful research; and on the exact cost to animals of both types of research. And of course, we must carefully craft ethical standards before we can reach any verdicts.

In the last section of his paper, Carl challenges the ethical standards commonly used to argue against animal research. He has in mind the sort of ethicist who wants to "expand the circle," to use Peter Singer's famous phrase. The case against using black men in syphilis studies without their consent (in the US, from 1932 to 1972) was made by saying that blacks and whites are equals, that they have the same rights. The case against using impaired children to test polio vaccine in the 1940s and 1950s takes the same form: we are all equals, we all have the same basic rights. For this sort of ethicist, prejudice against animals is just one more bias to be removed, leaving us with yet another member of the "community of equals."

For decades, this was in fact the tenor of much animal advocacy. Peter Singer (1975/2009) wrote that all animals are equal in *Animal Liberation*, and Tom Regan (1983) made "the case for animal rights," in the classic by that name. The Great Ape Project, founded by Singer and Paola Cavalieri in 1994 (Cavalieri & Singer, 1994), does proclaim that apes are persons, and call for recognition of their rights. But animal advocacy in another key has been proliferating in the last decade. There is Matthew Scully's (2002) superb book, *Dominion*, which both passionately champions animals and slams the idea that they are rights-bearing equals of human beings. Other animal advocates who maintain some distance from equality claims are philosophers David DeGrazia (1996), Martha Nussbaum (2005), Tzachi Zamir (2007), and animal scientist, Temple Grandin (Grandin & Johnson, 2010).

I made two arguments for prohibiting the use of the great apes in biomedical research. One focuses on the value to us of chimpanzees. If they matter enough to us, we will be willing to forfeit medical advances in order to protect them. This is not shocking or unusual. We forfeit medical advances every time we spend public funds on something else—whether it is promoting the arts, preserving historic monuments, or keeping national parks in pristine condition. This is obviously not an argument that involves attributing rights to apes or seeing them as our equals. The paintings we use public funds to produce or preserve do not (of course) have rights, and are not our equals.

I made a second argument as well. Chimpanzees are sentient beings, and probably sentient in some of the more complex ways we are, as a result of their high intelligence and self-awareness. So, we should cause them suffering only if a large enough balancing gain is at stake. My worry is that the system in which primates are used for research makes it unlikely these judgments of balance will be made scrupulously enough. After all, a primate facility has to pay the high costs of maintaining these animals, whether they are used in research or not. This gives decision-makers an incentive to approve as much research as possible. Again, this is not an argument that turns on any claim of strict equality. It only presupposes that animal suffering matters considerably, and that is something that has come to be a matter of consensus in our society.

I am impressed with the NIH advisory panel's report, and so is Carl, but it is clear he does not want to constrain animal researchers as strictly as the authors propose to do. The panel says a "necessary" (and so acceptable) study *must* be one that could not be performed ethically on human beings. In their scheme, experimenting on a consenting human being is preferable to experimenting on nonconsenting chimpanzees. Carl, on the other hand, says that research should be done on chimpanzees instead of humans, even when humans would consent to be research subjects. It is notable that he commends the panel, but is in fact more sanguine than they are about the usefulness of chimpanzees in future research, and more lenient about when they should be used.

Finally, a few words about Carl's reply to my paper (space does not permit a reply to all of his points). Carl imagines that the core of my case is my personal "care" and "affection" for chimpanzees. His stated reason for focusing on my feelings in this way is that I made what I called a value-to-us argument. It should be obvious, though, that there is a difference between valuing something and feeling care and affection. My analogy was with valuing trees and art. We do not emote over the trees that we decide to save, even knowing there will be more highway fatalities as a result. Some people may feel strong affection for chimpanzees—Jane Goodall comes to mind—but some do not. Whether I do or do not has no relevance to the arguments I have made.

Another problem is Carl's quip that I have merely really made a value-to-me argument, not a value-to-us argument. In the EU, Australia, and many other countries, experimentation on the great apes has already been prohibited, suggesting widespread special valuing of these animals. In the US, research on the great apes has been increasingly restricted over time, to the point that now the NIH has changed all of the rules, making future research much less likely. This happened as a result of public outcry over the Alamogordo chimps. In Congress, the Great Ape Protection Act, which would outright prohibit research on chimpanzees, had 160 cosponsors in 2009 (USGPO, 2011). A 2001 Zogby poll (Zogby, 2003) of the American public asked whether chimpanzees should be treated like property, like children, like adults, or "not sure"—and 51% said "like children." Supporters of prohibition include a wide array of philosophers, scientists, and politicians, many of them not generally involved in animal advocacy. So, the value-to-us argument is about at least a large number of us, and quite obviously not only about my values.

References

Cavalieri, P., & Singer, P. (Ed.). (1994). *The great ape project: Equality beyond humanity*. New York: St. Martin's.

DeGrazia, D. (1996). *Taking animals seriously: Mental life and moral status*. Cambridge: Cambridge University Press.

Grandin, T., & Johnson, C. (2010). *Animals make us human: Creating the best life for animals*. New York: Mariner Press.

Kluger, J. (2005). *Splendid solution: Jonas Salk and the conquest of polio*. New York: G. P. Putnam.

NRC (National Research Council of the Institute of Medicine of the National Academies). (2011). *Chimpanzees in biomedical and behavioral research: Assessing the necessity*. Washington, DC: The National Academies Press.

Nussbaum, M. (2005). Beyond compassion and humanity: Justice for non-human animals. In C. Sunstein & M. Nussbaum (Eds.), *Animal rights: Current debates and new directions* (pp. 325–407). Oxford: Oxford University Press.

Oshinsky, D. (2005). *Polio: An American story*. Oxford: Oxford University Press.

Regan, T. (1983). *The case for animal rights*. Berkeley: University of California Press.

Scully, M. (2002). *Dominion: The power of man, the suffering of animals, and the call to mercy*. New York: St. Martin's Press.

Singer, P. (1975/2009). *Animal liberation*. New York: Random House.

USGPO (United States Government Printing Office). (2011). H.R. 1513: Great ape protection and cost savings act of 2011. Retrieved from: http://www.govtrack.us/congress/bills/112/hr1513/text

Zamir, T. (2007). *Ethics and the beast: A speciesist argument for animal liberation*. Princeton, NJ: Princeton University Press.

Zogby, J. (2003). Poll: Current chimp retirement status. *American Anti-Vivisection Society Magazine*, February, p. 5.

Reply to Kazez

Carl Cohen

Jean Kazez presents an appealing case for the prohibition of research using chimpanzees. Her tone and spirit are moderate; she is not a zealot. She *cares* a great deal about chimpanzees, and understandably wants us to care about them as she does. Her caring is in fact the heart, the foundation of her principal argument, which she calls the value-to-us argument.

Many informed people attach special value to chimpanzees, she observes, for a variety of reasons. That is certainly true; I am among them. The genetic relations of *Homo sapiens sapiens* and *Pan troglodytes* are close; chimpanzees and humans have much in common; chimpanzee populations dwindle. Chimpanzees deserve *and receive* a good deal of special attention. We ought to do what we reasonably can to protect and preserve them. That far, there is no dispute between Jean and myself.

Can this understandable affection for chimpanzees serve as the premise of a sound argument whose conclusion is that we ought to *prohibit categorically* all research using chimpanzees? No. The wisdom of legal prohibition simply does not follow from the truth of her caring. Most of us care deeply for many things that we are nevertheless prepared to risk, pehaps even sacrifice, for the sake of objectives of very great importance. Jean thinks that we must avoid the use of chimpanzees even for what are likely to be life-saving results. She calls this her value-to-us argument, but she might more accurately have called it her *value-to-me* argument. The position she defends (until we get to her *close-to-utilitarian argument*, which we shortly will) is entirely *subjective*.

The persuasiveness of this subjective argument depends upon her ability to convince the rest of us to share her estimate of the relative value of chimpanzee and human lives. In that effort, I reckon she will not succeed with most folks. After all, she points out, we do permit things—fast cars, and tree-lined highways—that put humans at risk. But we do not have to permit those things, so it must be that saving human lives is not our "constant number one imperative." Do these observations convince us that, being genuinely concerned about chimpanzees, we must protect them from all invasive research, even if that entails our defeat in the quest for a live-saving vaccine? Of course not. We could sell off the treasures of our National Gallery, she notes, and channel every dollar into medical research, but we do not! Does this show that we care more about paintings than human lives? Of course not. Research institutes have many other sources of funds; more critical for them than additional money is the availability of an animal model with which to pursue, and test, the vaccines that will save human lives. This quest, I emphasize, is terribly important. Even as I write this response, *The Annals of Internal Medicine* reports (February 21, 2012) that death rates from hepatitis C are increasing and now exceed the death rate due to HIV–AIDS. Besides

Contemporary Debates in Bioethics, First Edition. Edited by Arthur L. Caplan and Robert Arp.

humans, the *only* animal on which a hepatitis C vaccine could be tested is the chimpanzee.

The principal argument upon which Jean relies is, in truth, hardly an argument at all. It is an earnest expression of her values, a gracious confession of her willingness to forgo medical advance (for example) in battling hepatitis, from which she probably does not suffer, for the sake of the comfort (not the lives) of chimpanzees.

Her second argument, which we may call utilitarian, concludes that continuing to use chimpanzees in medical research would be inconsistent with our obligations to them. Her premise, with which I fully agree, is that because animal subjects do feel pain and distress, researchers are constrained by serious moral limitations in what they do. How does her argument advance? Well, Jean is certainly not an opponent of all animal research. She understands that animal models have played, and do play, a central role in much biomedical research. What is called for, in her view (and in mine), is a thoughtful utilitarian evaluation of all animal research. What we may rightly do, she observes, as well as how we may do it, will be more wisely determined if we apply a very reasonable schema that she provides. She would have us weigh: (1) *severity of suffering*; (2) *probable outcome*; (3) *balance*; and (4) *subject species*. Let us apply Jean's schema to research using chimpanzees.

1. *Severity of suffering*. Chimpanzees can certainly suffer, but they do not suffer severely when used in research. Because of their very great value, they are cared for as assiduously as research needs permit. Every effort is made to assure them a long and healthy life. Their lives in captivity are, in fact, generally healthier and longer than the lives of chimpanzees in the wild. They do not suffer nearly as much as the humans who contract the diseases whose prevention is the target of the research in which they are involved. Very rarely do chimpanzees die as a consequence of their involvement in research, while humans all too frequently die from the diseases in question.
2. *Probable outcome*. Because chimpanzees have so many influential advocates, they are used almost exclusively in trials of importance. Because of their small number and central role, investigations in which chimpanzees are involved are almost certain to be *worthy*—worthy of greatest care and scrupulous review. Some animal research (but not much) may serve chiefly, as Jean suggests, to advance careers or make people look busy. That is most certainly not true about research with chimpanzees.
3. *Balance*. At this point her argument against chimpanzee research collapses completely. Her example of an unacceptable balance, "harming ten million dogs to benefit ten people," would indeed be outrageous, but it is nearly absurd. Chimpanzees are most certainly not going to be sacrificed in large numbers; very probably they will not be sacrificed at all. On the other hand, the number of human beings now alive who stand to benefit from research with chimpanzees is very great; a 2012 report from the Centers for Disease Control and Prevention tells us that more than *3.2 million people* are currently infected with hepatitis C. The potential beneficiaries of research with nonhuman primates are virtually uncountable. How many children would have contracted polio over this past half century had the polio vaccine not been devised in the 1950s? And here is the other side of the scale: there are *a grand total of 937 chimpanzees* now available for research in the United States. Balance indeed!
4. *Subject species*. Jean wisely joins me in insisting upon attention to the differences among species; we are both speciesists. Some species, she points out, deserve special attention because of their greater capacities, or special vulnerabilities. Chimpanzees are indeed among these, and therefore do receive, and must continue to receive, the most thoughtful attention and care.

We are speciesists because (as I argued earlier at length) we recognize that our obligation to any animal subject is a function of the species of which that animal is a member. Because that species (*Pan troglodytes*, for example) has certain biological features, certain known sensitivities, limitations, and needs, we ought to do (or refrain from doing) certain things with its members. Species membership is an important consideration, as Jean rightly insists when presenting her utilitarian schema. Elsewhere she contends that "eliminating speciesist bias" is something we must do. But attending to the special features of different species is most certainly not a bias—it is a demand of rational morality in the world of animal research.

Jean concludes her attack on chimpanzee research by asserting, without warrant, that the cost of maintaining chimpanzees would lead inevitably to their relentless, heartless exploitation. She contends that it would be impossible to "green light" only those experiments (of which she plainly admits there may be some) that can pass a reasonable utilitarian evaluation. In this despair, she is quite mistaken. When the Report of the Institute of Medicine to which we both refer (NRC, 2011) was issued, it was immediately accepted and applied by the Director of the National Institutes of Health, Francis Collins, to research at all of the Institutes. Chimpanzees, said Dr Collins, deserve "special consideration and respect." Henceforth the *only* research using chimpanzees that will be permitted is research critical for human health, research that cannot be advanced in other ways because the diseases in question "defy alternative experimental approaches" (Gorman, 2011). It is false to say, and misleading to suggest, that if we do not prohibit *all* chimpanzee research, many of the uses of chimpanzees will be needless and wasteful. The reverse is the case.

Jean's humane affection for the great apes—like so many others—leads to conclusions about what is worth what in medicine that most ordinary folks, and virtually all medical scientists, find quite unacceptable. These subjective judgments cannot serve as the justification of public policy.

She also proposes that we weigh, in a thoughtful utilitarian spirit, the costs and benefits of the prohibition of chimpanzee research. I agree that this should be done—and indeed it *has* been done very recently by some of the most knowledgeable medical scientists on the planet. We both agree that the *Chimpanzees in Biomedical and Behavioral Research* report, specifically addressing the necessity of chimpanzee research, deserves great respect. It concludes, as I conclude, that it would be a grave scientific mistake to forbid all uses of chimpanzees, and other great apes, in biomedical research. Putting the incalculable value of millions of human lives into the balance, we will conclude that such a prohibition would be a grave moral mistake as well.

References

Gorman, J. (2011). U.S. will not finance new research on chimps. *The New York Times*, December 15. Retrieved from: http://www.nytimes.com/2011/12/16/science/chimps-in-medical-research.html?_r=0

NRC (National Research Council of the Institute of Medicine of the National Academies). (2011). *Chimpanzees in biomedical and behavioral research: Assessing the necessity*. Washington, DC: The National Academies Press.

Part 10

Should the United States of America Adopt Universal Healthcare?

Introduction

"Everyone has the right to a standard of living adequate for the health and well-being of himself and of his family, including food, clothing, housing, and medical care and necessary social services, and the right to security in the event of unemployment, sickness, disability, widowhood, old age, or other lack of livelihood in circumstances beyond his control." So claims Article 25 of the Universal Declaration of Human Rights, which was adopted on December 10, 1948 by the United Nations General Assembly (UN, 2012). While there are those who would argue against certain people deserving and receiving basic needs—such as a dictator, or group of fanatics, zealots, or tyrants bent on oppressing a segment of the population—almost every person regardless of their nationality agrees that one's social circumstances *should* be such that the kinds of basic needs mentioned in Article 25 are provided. During a video message produced for the Prince Mahidol Award Conference in Bangkok at the end of January, 2012, United Nations Secretary-General, Ban Ki-moon, claimed: "Health care is a right, not a privilege. And universal health coverage can help make that possible. With it we can break barriers—the barriers of economic status, age, and gender—so that every child, every woman, and everyone has access to a healthy life" (UNSG, 2012). Of course, agreeing that some policy *ideally* should be instituted is different from actually instituting that policy, and this is certainly true with respect to universal healthcare. An often-heard lament from opponents as well as supporters in the United States and other nations who currently do not provide it is, "Who's going to pay for it?"

As the name implies, *universal healthcare* (UHC) refers to the medical coverage and services that are sanctioned and guaranteed by the government and provided to all the citizens of a country. UHC is usually funded primarily through taxation of the country's citizens. For citizens of Japan, the UK, Germany, and Canada who have been living with

Contemporary Debates in Bioethics, First Edition. Edited by Arthur L. Caplan and Robert Arp.

UHC for several generations now, being taxed for such a service is an accepted part of life. The question, "Who's going to pay for UHC?" can be answered—by taxation of citizens. Many Western European countries view universal access to healthcare as not only a legal right but also a moral right along the lines of Ban Ki-moon's thinking. And in other nations, UHC not only provides citizens with a basic right to healthcare but also, arguably, helps to control healthcare costs (Blendon et al., 2003; Lu & Hsiao, 2003).

However, the US has never had UHC, and only recently has begun the process of guaranteeing its citizens basic healthcare as a fundamental right. Of the estimated 313 million US citizens alive in 2012, it is probably the case that only about 275 million were covered by a health plan (this is conservative, actually; see DeNavas-Walt et al., 2011; USCB, 2011; Sommers & Wilson, 2012), and some 25 million did not have adequate coverage (Collins et al., 2008).

On June 28, 2012, the US Supreme Court ruled that the Patient Protection and Affordable Care Act (PPACA, often referred to as *Obamacare* because President Barack Obama signed this federal statute into law on March 23, 2010) does not violate the US Constitution (NFIB, 2012). The PPACA requires that all US citizens must purchase health insurance—whether from private (employer or otherwise), public (government), or nonprofit insurers—or face penalties in the form of fines and taxes, with exceptions made for religious beliefs or financial hardship.

This universal requirement placed upon citizens is known as the *individual* or *insurance mandate*, and already exists in nations such as Austria (since 1967), Belgium (since 1945), Germany (since 1941), Greece (since 1983), Luxembourg (since 1973), South Korea (since 1988), and Switzerland (since 1994). Chief Justice John Roberts wrote the ruling for the US Supreme Court and noted that although the "federal government does not have the power to order people to buy health insurance," it does have "the power to impose a tax on those without health insurance" (NFIB, 2012, Section D). Essentially, then, Roberts and the other assenting Justices would seem to view healthcare as a public necessity worth collecting taxes on, much like a nation's other public goods such as road infrastructure, education, or welfare programs. However, many see this landmark ruling as a hair-splitting move having the outcome of the US government violating the rights and freedoms of citizens by forcing healthcare on those who do not wish to purchase it. Ultra-conservative talk show host, Rush Limbaugh, makes a lot of money and does not have health insurance, since he can afford to pay out of pocket (TBS, 2012). By 2015, Limbaugh will be paying a tax—which he views as a fine/punishment—for choosing not to have health insurance. And he, as well as a great many other Americans, thinks this is unjust.

Besides the individual mandate, the PPACA purports to remove the annual and lifetime caps on coverage set by insurers, reduce co-pays as well as remove co-pays on certain services (such as health screenings), limit the ability of insurers to rescind policies, prevent sex and age discrimination by insurers, set up health-insurance exchanges whereby buyers could easily and readily compare price and coverage, require that adult children be insured into their mid 20s as part of family coverage, and offer tax credits to small businesses who provide employees with health insurance (PPACA, 2010; WP, 2010). Importantly, the PPACA is concerned with making sure that people with pre-existing medical conditions—such as cancer, advanced forms of diabetes, severe heart conditions, or mental illness—would be insured. There is popular support for universal availability of insurance. A 2009 poll of 1002 Americans (23% Republican, 34% Democrat, 32% Independent) conducted by Abt SRBI, Inc. noted that some 80% favor a healthcare system that requires healthcare insurance companies to offer coverage to anyone, even if they have a pre-existing condition (ASRBI, 2009).

In response to the question, "Who's going to pay for it?" given that the PPACA purports to enforce an individual mandate, part of the cost for US UHC will be absorbed through taxes, especially raising taxes on the fairly generous healthcare packages that are typically offered to senior executives and other corporate members. It is argued, then, that other sources of funding for US UHC include the money gained from penalizing (a) people who refuse to buy health insurance and (b) companies (mostly larger ones) that do not provide insurance for their employees, as well as utilizing the money saved as a result of cutting

Medicare and Medicaid spending through better reward structures, eliminating Medicare Advantage plans that give private insurers funding to sell private healthcare plans, and slowing the growth of Medicare provider payments. Finally, it has been argued that under Obamacare, there will be an increased emphasis on wellness and prevention such that the need for medical services and costs will be mitigated—on the whole, the American people will be more health-conscious with a UHC. Echoing the factors just mentioned (and others), Cutler et al. (2010), for example, estimated that from 2010 to 2019, the PPACA not only will have reduced total national health expenditures by 590 billion as well as lowered premiums by about $2000 per family, but also will likely slow national health expenditures from 6.3% to 5.7%.

US citizens actually already pay taxes for quasi-UHC for certain segments of its population. Although the US does not currently have full-blown UHC, it does offer what is known as *single-payer healthcare assistance* to active military and veterans and their families, certain American Indian tribes, Federal prisoners, as well as through Medicare, Medicaid, and the State Children's Health Insurance Program. The VA healthcare system is the largest, single-payer government-run health service in the world. In a single-payer healthcare system, the government provides insurance for all citizens and pays all healthcare expenses through a single source, which may be public, private, or a combination of both. In Canada, for example, the government contracts healthcare services from private organizations through its Medicare program, while healthcare services, resources, and personnel are provided by the government itself in the UK through its National Health Service. Other countries with single-payer healthcare assistance include Italy (since 1978), Japan (since 1938), Kuwait (since 1950), Norway (since 1912), Spain (since 1986), and Sweden (since 1955).

The intent of the PPACA, however, is to turn the US into what is known as a *two-tier healthcare system*. In such a system, the government provides a basic healthcare coverage to all its citizens (the first tier, which is the UHC part), while allowing people to choose additional coverage from private organizations if they want to (the second tier). As can be imagined, some countries with a two-tier system have publicly sanctioned UHC that is well funded, efficient, and of a high quality, so the private healthcare sector maintains a smaller presence. On the other hand, there are countries where the UHC is poorly funded, inefficient, and of a low quality, so the private system provides a better-quality service, but usually at a higher cost. Countries with a two-tier system include Australia (since 1975), Denmark (since 1973), France (since 1974), Ireland (since 1977), Israel (since 1995), New Zealand (since 1938), and Singapore (since 1993), among others. There can be an insurance mandate along with a single-payer or two-tier system. As was noted already, UHC with the PPACA in the US purports to be a two-tier system with an insurance mandate that is similar to Germany's healthcare system.

The reasons why Americans historically have resisted UHC are many (see Starr, 1982; Rothman, 1993; Cutler, 2004; Mayes, 2004; Quadagno, 2005; Altman & Shactman, 2011). A good introduction to the US healthcare system in its present state is *An Introduction to the US Health Care System*, by Jonas et al. (2007; also see the papers in Kovner & Knickman, 2011). From the founding of the US in 1776 to the early twentieth century, the overall thinking concerning healthcare services, personnel, and insurance essentially was that the federal government would leave these matters to the states, and the states would leave these matters to private and voluntary programs. In the early twentieth century, a reformer group called the American Association for Labor Legislation attempted to get members of the American Medical Association (AMA) and the American Federation of Labor (AFL) to support a bill drafted in 1915 called the Standard Bill, which was to be passed (hopefully) by the US Congress that would offer medical benefits, maternity benefits, sick pay, and a death benefit of $50.00 to all American manual workers and those earning less than $1200 a year.

The AMA initially supported the bill, but once disagreements regarding how doctors would be paid emerged, coupled with the idea that many medical services and procedures would be monitored and regulated, and have a capped charge, the AMA rejected it. Major unions like the AFL saw the bill as a compulsory, paternalistic reform that would create a system of state supervision over people's health—a concern about UHC that is still very prevalent in the US today with the often-heard rhetorical question, "Do you want the government controlling *your* health care decisions?" (see Brown, 2007)—as well as something that would weaken unions by taking over their role in providing social benefits. In later years, after collective bargaining was legally sanctioned, the AFL would reject attempts at UHC. They feared being cut out of healthcare bargaining—and the money gained from dues associated with this bargaining. Primarily because of the bill's $50.00 death benefit, the commercial insurance industry (consisting mainly of Prudential and Metropolitan insurance companies) and the Insurance Economic Society also opposed it because of the fact that their life-insurance business would likely have been taken away.

The first Red Scare after World War I and the second Red Scare after World War II seemed to cement UHC with communism and/or socialism in the minds of many Americans—these ideologies being perceived as straightforwardly evil, as they are to many Americans today—and insurance companies, unions, and many doctors bolstered this connection in a propaganda-like fashion at times. In fact, the AMA utilized this slippery slope in a 1945 pamphlet to scare Americans: "Would socialized medicine lead to socialization of other phases of life? Lenin thought so. He declared socialized medicine is the keystone to the arch of the socialist state" (Sharp, 2011, n. 10). Many congressmen and other US government personnel bought into the Red Scare associated with UHC and helped to forestall congressional decisions concerning the National Health Act of 1939 put forward by Franklin D. Roosevelt and the Wagner–Murray–Dingell Bills of 1943, 1944, 1945, 1946, 1947, 1948, 1949, 1950, 1951, 1952, 1953, 1954, 1955, and 1956. When he was president of the US from 1945 to 1953, Harry S Truman's versions of the Wagner–Murray–Dingell Bill even specified clearly that (a) there would be no death benefit and (b) doctors could choose their method of payment to try and win insurance companies and the AMA over to the idea of UHC.

Also, during World War II, the Office of Price Administration was established in 1941 by the US government to control the amount of money that private companies could charge for certain foods, rent, and other goods and services. Wage controls were imposed as well, so that companies could not lure employees away from government jobs that were thought to be essential during wartime so that the war against the Axis powers could be won. Now, here is the fascinating part. In order to attract employees without violating any laws, companies started offering potential employees health insurance. Thus, the link between private companies and health insurance was ratified and solidified in the minds of Americans during this time, and such a link persists to this day (Manning, 1960; Waslee, 1992). Ask any American on the street today why s/he needs a full-time job, and part of the answer will almost always be, "Because of the benefits."

In 1965, the US Congress and President Lyndon B. Johnson enacted Medicare under Title XVIII of the Social Security Act to provide health insurance to people age 65 and older, regardless of income or medical history. Under Title XIX of the Social Security Act Medicaid was also enacted, a program jointly funded by federal and state governments that is managed by the states, which provides medical and health-related services for low-income families and people with certain disabilities. Recall from the above that these two programs constitute a quasi-UHC in the form of single-payer healthcare assistance to certain segments of the American population.

Karen Palmer (1999) sums up the reasons why UHC has never been fully adopted in the US:

> interest group influence (code words for class), ideological differences, anti-communism, anti-socialism, fragmentation of public policy, the entrepreneurial character of American medicine, a tradition of American voluntarism, removing the middle class from the coalition of advocates for change through the alternative of Blue Cross private insurance plans, and the association of public programs with charity, dependence, personal failure, and the almshouses of years gone by.

Of course, we can add to these reasons (probably) the most important one, namely, the fact that certain people—doctors, the corporate members of insurance agencies, union bosses, and others—felt that they would lose money as a result of an American UHC system. For example, it is estimated (and this is a conservative estimate) that American corporate insurance profits have increased by some 230% over the past three decades (CEA, 2012).

"An obvious lesson from the last 50 years is that we can never get to UHC by incremental changes of our multi-payer private/public financing system." So claims John Geyman in the first chapter of this section. Geyman has written many books on the subject of UHC in America, and continuing, he maintains: "The private insurance industry in America, with its 1,300 insurers, is based on the business model of medical underwriting which excludes higher-risk people from coverage in the first place and denies many claims later to increase its financial bottom line ... Moreover, many of those who are 'covered' will find themselves with high-deductible, low-benefit policies that cover only 60 or 70% of their total health care costs." He argues that since healthcare is a fundamental right (not a privilege) existing for patients with medical needs, a healthcare system, therefore, should be a public service that is not based on an ability to pay for services rendered, nor should it be a commodity for sale in the marketplace, the ultimate goal of which is to line the pockets of corporate stakeholders. He also makes the interesting point that "programs that are not universal, such as Medicaid in America today, tend to be divisive and unpopular, since taxpayers feel they are paying for programs that do not benefit them." In the end, he points to the US's neighbor to the north, Canada, and their Medicaid program as a solid example of a healthy, functional, single-payer, government-funded—yet privately delivered—system that could work equally well in the United States. And importantly, this system will cost "no more and probably less than" Americans are paying now.

Much of Geyman's argument rests on the claim that the US healthcare system is a free market. The second author in this section, Glen Whitman, emphatically denies this. While it is true, claims Whitman, that a "panoply of federal and state interventions have made healthcare one of the most regulated industries in the economy," it is not a market in the way that other commodities and services are in the US, such as cars and gas (examples that Whitman utilizes throughout his chapter). And, even if healthcare is a right—a position that Whitman actually denies—then other so-called rights such as food, clothing, and shelter are just as market-based as healthcare, which at least calls into question the possibility of disentangling rights from the free market. Whitman's biggest problems with a UHC in the US as described by Geyman, however, can be stated succinctly: Under a single-payer UHC, "Americans' healthcare would be rationed by means of global budgets, caps on the availability of treatments and drugs, bureaucratic denials of service, and most of all, waiting." Waiting is a significant issue, since we all know that in many medical circumstances, quickly responding to diseases or disorders can literally mean the difference between life and death.

There are many other reasons why Whitman is against a single-payer UHC, but the following one resonates with most Americans,: "Socialized funding would also encourage government intrusion into personal lifestyle decisions." And, for better or for worse, Americans hold sacrosanct the idea of being able to make choices unimpeded by their own government.

References

Altman, S., & Shactman, D. (2011). *Power, politics, and universal health care: The inside story of a century-long battle.* Amherst, NY: Prometheus Books.

ASRBI (Abt SRBI, Inc.). (2009). Most Americans eager for healthcare reform; divided on potential solutions. Retrieved from: http://www.srbi.com/MostAmericansEagerforHealthcareReform.html

Blendon, R., Schoen, C., DesRoches, C., Osborn, R., & Zapert, K. (2003). Common concerns amid diverse systems: Health care experiences in five countries. *Health Affairs, 22,* 106–121

Brown, K. (2007). The freedom to spend your own money on medical care: A common casualty of universal coverage. *Cato Institute, Policy analysis no. 601,* 1–15.

CEA (Council of Economic Advisers). (2012). Economic report of the president: Statistical tables relating to income, employment, and production. Retrieved from: http://www.gpo.gov/fdsys/browse/collection.action?collectionCode=ERP

Collins, S., Kriss, J., Doty, M., & Rustgi, S. (2008). Losing ground: How the loss of adequate health insurance is burdening working families—findings from the Commonwealth Fund biennial health insurance surveys, 2001–2007. *Center for American Progress, The Commonwealth Fund, August, 2008 Issue Brief.* Retrieved from: http://www.commonwealthfund.org/Publications/Fund-Reports/2008/Aug/Losing-Ground--How-the-Loss-of-Adequate-

Health-Insurance-Is-Burdening-Working-Families--8212-Finding.aspx
Cutler, D. (2004). *Your money or your life: Strong medicine for America's health care system*. Oxford: Oxford University Press.
Cutler, D., Davis, D., & Stremikis, K. (2010). The impact of health reform on health system spending. *Center for American Progress, The Commonwealth Fund, May, 2010 Issue Brief.* Retrieved from: http://63.131.142.217/~/media/Files/Publications/Issue%20Brief/2010/May/1405_Cutler_impact_hlt_reform_on_hlt_sys_spending_ib_v4.pdf
DeNavas-Walt, C., Proctor, B., & Smith, J. (2011) *Census Bureau, current population reports, P60–239: Income, poverty, and health insurance coverage in the United States, 2010.* Washington, DC: Government Printing Office.
Jonas, S., Goldsteen, R., & Goldsteen, K. (2007). *An introduction to the US health care system*. London: Springer.
Kovner, A., & Knickman, J. (Eds.). (2011). *Health care delivery in the United States*. London: Springer.
Lu, J-F., & Hsiao, W. (2003). Does universal health insurance make health care unaffordable? Lessons from Taiwan. *Health Affairs, 22*, 77–88.
Manning, T. (1960). *The Office of Price Administration: A World War II agency of control*. New York: Henry Holt.
Mayes, R. (2004). *Universal coverage: The elusive quest for national health insurance*. Ann Arbor: University of Michigan Press.
NFIB (*National Federation of Independent Business v. Sebelius*). (2012). Retrieved from: http://www.supremecourt.gov/opinions/11pdf/11-393c3a2.pdf
Palmer, K. (1999). A brief history: Universal health care efforts in the US Talk at Physicians for a National Health Program Meeting. Retrieved from: http://www.sfu.ca/~mfs2/SUMMER%202010/HSCI%20305/MIDTERM/4_US%20and%20International%20HC%20Systems/A%20Brief%20History%20of%20US%20Medicare.pdf
PPACA (Patient Protection and Affordable Care Act). (2010). Retrieved from: http://democrats. senate.gov/reform/patient-protection-affordable-care-act.pdf
Quadagno, J. (2005). *One nation, uninsured*. Oxford: Oxford University Press.
Rothman, D. (1993). A century of failure: Health care reform in America. *Journal of Health Politics, Policy and Law, 18*, 271–286.
Sharp, E. (2011). CCF: Origins of Canadian socialism. Ludwig von Mises Institute of Canada Brief. Retrieved from: http://www.mises.ca/posts/articles/ccf-origins-of-canadian-socialism/comment-page-1/#to-ccf-origins-of-canadian-socialism-n-10
Sommers, B., & Wilson, L. (2012). Fifty-four million additional Americans are receiving preventive services coverage without cost-sharing under the Affordable Care Act. US Department of Health and Human Services ASPE Issue Brief. Retrieved from: http://aspe.hhs.gov/health/reports/2012/PreventiveServices/ib.pdf
Starr, P. (1982). *The social transformation of American medicine*. New York: Basic Books.
TBS (*The Baltimore Sun*). (2012). No 'Rush' to health insurance policy. *The Baltimore Sun*, July 1, Retrieved from: http://articles.baltimoresun.com/2012-07-01/news/bs-ed-limbaugh-letter-20120629_1_health-insurance-rush-limbaugh-policy
UN (The United Nations). (2012). Universal declaration of human rights. Retrieved from: http://www.un.org/en/documents/udhr/index.shtml
UNSG (The United Nations Secretary General). (2012). Universal coverage can make health care 'a right, not a privilege.' Retrieved from: http://www.un.org/News/Press/docs/2012/sgsm14077.doc.htm
USCB (US Census Bureau). (2011). Income, poverty and Health Insurance coverage in the United States: 2010. Retrieved from: http://www.census.gov/newsroom/releases/archives/income_wealth/cb11-157.html
Waslee, T. (1992). *What has government done to our health care?* Washington, DC: The Cato Institute.
WP (The Washington Post). (2010). *Landmark: The inside story of America's new health care law and what it means for us all*. New York: PublicAffairs.

Chapter Nineteen

The United States of America Should Adopt Universal Healthcare

John Geyman

Essential healthcare is not available to all Americans. Our market system is based largely on ability to pay, not medical need as it is in most advanced countries around the world. The business model of profitable financial bottom lines continues to drive costs beyond the reach of ordinary Americans. We are left with an increasing crisis of economic, social, and moral dimensions. This chapter makes the case for publicly financed universal healthcare that will increase access, affordability, value, quality, and equity of healthcare for all Americans.

Introduction

Whether we recognize it or not, healthcare is a moral matter. We all are born, live our lives confronting many healthcare problems and accidents requiring medical care, and die at the end of a journey involving extensive experience with our healthcare system. But necessary healthcare in the US is *not* available to everyone. There are many barriers to adequate healthcare for many millions of Americans, whether financial, geographic, or cultural. And since we live in a country that has still not accepted healthcare as a right and continues to debate whether it should be available to all Americans, universal healthcare (UHC) is both a timely and essential subject for this volume.

As we know from our own experience, the costs of healthcare are growing rapidly, far exceeding annual increases in the cost of living and rendering even basic care unaffordable for millions of people. In these days of budget cutting under the guise of fiscal austerity at both state and federal levels, financial barriers to care are becoming ever higher, leaving many Americans without essential care, increasing their suffering and resulting in worse health outcomes and, too often, earlier death.

After the 2008 national elections, we saw an intense debate over how healthcare should be financed and delivered in this country, culminating in the Patient Protection and Affordable Care Act (PPACA) of 2010 (PPACA, 2010). That debate was skewed by blatant deception and disinformation by those forces trying to exploit their own self-interest in our current maret-based system. The debate largely ignored the moral and medical dimensions of healthcare, diverted instead to the role of government vs. the unfettered marketplace. The resulting legislation will fall far short of its original goals—to provide universal access to affordable care of good quality for everyone—as fully described in my book, *Hijacked: The Road to Single Payer in the Aftermath of Stolen Health Care Reform* (Geyman, 2010).

Contemporary Debates in Bioethics, First Edition. Edited by Arthur L. Caplan and Robert Arp.

The debate we should have been having has still not taken place. These are some of the basic issues, which remain completely unresolved in this country (also see Geyman, 2008a, 2008b):

- Should healthcare be a human right or a privilege?
- Should we have a system of universal access, based on medical need, or the present one based on ability to pay?
- Who is the healthcare system for? Is it for patients and their families, or corporate stakeholders in the marketplace?
- Should healthcare be a public service, or a commodity for sale on an open market?

In order to make the case for UHC in this country, we will consider these four interrelated subjects: (1) historical and international perspectives; (2) the current unsustainable landscape in healthcare; (3) the rationale for UHC from moral, economic, social, and political viewpoints; and (4) how we can achieve UHC.

Historical and International Perspectives

This is not a new subject in this country. A century ago, Theodore Roosevelt ran as a progressive in the presidential campaign of 2012 on a platform of universal health insurance, an effort finally defeated five years later by an alliance between business and organized medicine. Since then, other presidents have supported UHC, including FDR in the mid-1930s (when he backed off fearing opposition from organized medicine) and Harry Truman during his administration. The passage of Medicare in 1965 was a landmark advance in assuring a defined set of medical benefits for all Americans age 65 and older, with Medicaid in the same year providing an important new safety net for low-income Americans. But most of the ensuing years have seen the continued growth of unrestrained markets in healthcare, based more on a business model than a service ethic (Quadagno, 2005).

One of the barriers to a reasoned debate over healthcare in this country is a strong undercurrent of belief among many in American exceptionalism—as if our problems are uniquely American, we are obvisly the best, and we have little to learn from other countries. This is an arrogant, shortsighted, and incorrect view. Other advanced countries have struggled with the same kinds of problems that we have with our healthcare system, including how to assure access and quality of care, contain costs, and steward limited resources for the common good.

Table 19.1 lists 15 advanced countries that achieved universal coverage for their entire populations between 1960 and 1980. And other countries have developed higher-performing healthcare systems at much less cost while assuring universal access (Davis et al., 2010), as shown by Table 19.2.

This is not to say that some of our leaders have not made strong efforts to bring common sense and a societal perspective to health policy. Representatives from the United States were part of an international working group of four countries convened in London in the late 1990s. Known as the Tavistock Group (1999), it included input from physicians, nurses, ethicists, academicians, healthcare executives, an economist, a jurist, and a philosopher. That group drafted these ethical principles that should underpin any country's healthcare system:

- Healthcare is a human right.
- The care of individuals is at the center of the healthcare delivery system but must be viewed and practiced within the overall context of continuing work to generate the greatest possible health gains for groups and populations.
- The responsibilities of the healthcare delivery system include the prevention of illness and the alleviation of disability.

Table 19.1 Countries achieving universal health-insurance coverage, 1960–1980

1960	*1970*	*1980*
Canada	Denmark	Australia
Czech Republic	Finland	Hungary
Iceland	Japan	Ireland
New Zealand		Italy
Norway		Portugal
Sweden		
UK		

Table 19.2 Seven-nation summary scores on health-system performance

1 is best; 7 is worst	*Australia*	*Canada*	*Germany*	*Netherlands*	*New Zealand*	*UK*	*USA*
OVERALL RANKING	3	6	4	1	5	2	7
Quality care	4	7	5	2	1	3	6
Effective care	2	7	6	3	5	1	4
Safe care	6	5	3	1	4	2	7
Coordinated care	4	5	7	2	1	3	6
Patient-centered care	2	5	3	6	1	7	4
Access	6.5	5	3	1	4	2	6.5
Cost-related access problems	6	3.5	3.5	2	5	1	7
Timeliness of care	6	7	2	1	3	4	5
Efficiency	2	6	5	3	4	1	7
Equity	4	5	3	1	6	2	7
Long, healthy, and productive lives	1	2	3	4	5	6	7

- Cooperation with each other and those served is imperative for those working within the healthcare delivery system.
- All individuals and groups involved in healthcare, whether they provide access or services, have the continuing responsibility to help improve its quality.

Despite the good work of many healthcare professionals and others dedicated to improving our healthcare system, however, their efforts have continued to fall by the wayside as corporate stakeholders, lobbyists, and willing politicians successfully fend off reform and prevail over the common good.

An obvious lesson from the last 50 years is that we can never get to UHC by incremental changes of our multi-payer private/public financing system. The private insurance industry in America, with its 1300 insurers, is based on the business model of medical underwriting which excludes higher-risk people from coverage in the first place and denies many claims later to increase its financial bottom line. The PPACA has bailed out this industry through extensive government subsidies (Goldman, 2009; cf. Mayhall, 2012), and even then at least 23 million Americans will remain uninsured by 2019. Moreover, many of those who are "covered" will find themselves with high-deductible, low-benefit policies that cover only 60 or 70% of their total healthcare costs. The various incremental attempts to gain universal coverage over the years through such mechanisms as mandating employers to provide coverage or requiring individuals to buy coverage have all failed to achieve universal coverage. As other countries have found—in particular, Canada, the UK, and New Zealand (see, for example, Goodman et al., 2004; ACP, 2008)—a single-payer public financing system is the most effective approach to meet that goal.

The Current Untenable Healthcare Landscape

The present healthcare delivery system in this country serves business interests much more than patients. Its costs are pricing healthcare beyond the reach of ordiary Americans. Though we pay much more than any other country for healthcare, we get less value in return (see, for example, Guyatt et al., 2007; Schoen et al., 2007). The "system" is dysfunctional, poorly coordinated, and inaccessible to a growing part of the population. It is cruel to many millions who have to forego needed care due to costs (Wilper et al., 2008). Too much unnecessary, even harmful, care is being provided to those who can pay, while too little care is provided for those without adequate insurance coverage. The system is unsustainable in the long run.

These are some of the markers of our failing healthcare system, as described in my book, *Breaking Point: How the Primary Care Crisis Endangers the Lives of Americans* (Geyman, 2011):

- The Great Recession since 2008 has been the biggest economic trauma since World War II, wiping out many jobs and wealth, diminishing hope for much of the population, and clouding the American Dream itself.
- During 2011, almost one in five working Americans was underemployed, while California, Michigan, and Oregon had underemployment rates over 20%.
- The middle class is quickly disappearing. For example, between 1980 and 2008, when tax cuts were extended to the rich as well as other benefits to corporations and Wall Street, the average annual income of the bottom 90% of Americans rose by only $303!
- The costs of private health insurance are growing at two or three times the cost-of-living rate, even as insurance covers a lesser share all the time of individuals' and families' total healthcare costs.
- While the median US annual household income is now about $50,000, the average annual total healthcare costs for a family of four are $19,393, an impossibility for middle-class families and more than double what it was 10 years ago.
- The number of patient visits to physicians has declined sharply since 2008 due to unaffordable costs.
- Two million cancer patients forego recommended care because of their costs.
- Fifty million people are uninsured, even including about 1.5 million veterans between the age of 18 and 64.
- Forty-five thousand Americans die each year—one every 12 min—for lack of health insurance; those deaths even include more than 2200 uninsured veterans under the age of 65.
- The US has the highest number of preventable deaths compared to other advanced nations.
- In cross-national studies, the US ranks 37th for health outcomes and 54th for fairness of financing.
- Since the 2010 mid-term elections and the gains made by Republicans in state capitols and Congress, draconian budget cuts are hollowing out an already-tattered safety net of public programs such as Medicaid.

In short, we are in the midst of a healthcare meltdown with no solution on the short-term horizon. Figure 19.1 shows the extent of runaway healthcare costs in this country since 1970 compared to other advanced countries around the world. These costs are driven by many factors, including technological advances, uncontrolled prices, and perverse incentives throughout our market-based system that encourage unnecessary and inappropriate services, and a financing and payment system that rewards increased volume of services (see Linden, 2010). Already one-sixth of the nation's GDP—and headed for 20% in another few years—healthcare costs threaten to bankrupt the current system, perhaps even the country, unless we can make fundamental reforms of our financing and payment system.

The Case for UHC

Given our failures over the last many decades in trying to gain UHC through multi-payer financing, it is now clear that the only way to achieve that goal is through single-payer public financing, or an improved Medicare-for-all program. The employer-based system of health insurance, begun during the World War II years, declines every year, and now covers less than 60% of American workers, often with inadequate coverage at that. Many workers are locked into jobs they would like to leave but for the loss of this coverage. Our population is much more mobile than in past generations. States are highly variable in terms of their regulations of private insurance and in their Medicaid programs, so UHC will be required. This will be the only reliable and sustainable way to reform US healthcare, achieving universal coverage while containing costs and establishing mechanisms to monitor quality and outcomes of care.

Healthcare and healing should not be commodities for sale on a market where the business ethic prevails—maximize profits and avoid expensive risks.

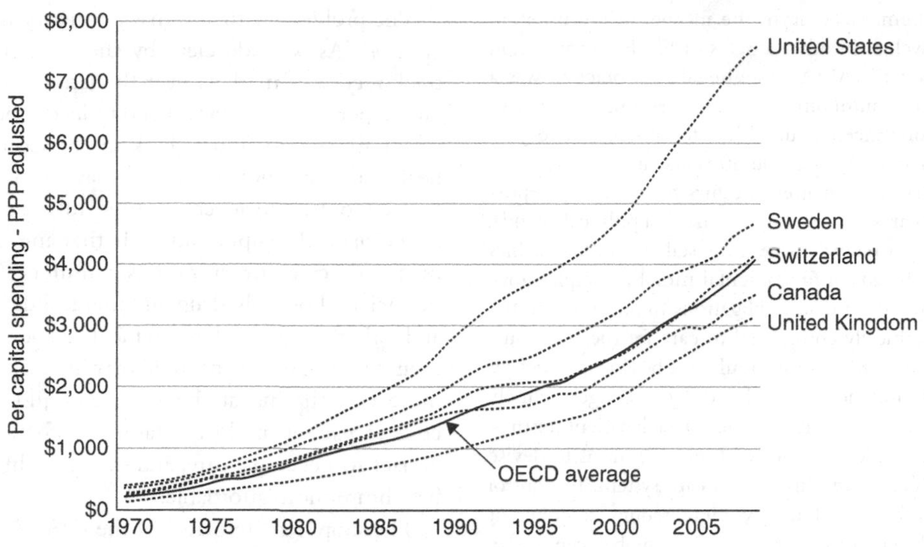

Figure 19.1 Growth in total health expenditures per capita, US and selected countries, 1970–2008

About 20% of patients (mostly older and those with chronic disease) account for 80% of the nation's annual healthcare costs (CSG, 2006; SSAB, 2009). None of us can know what our own future health problems will be, and many cannot be avoided. When we have an accident or develop chest pain in the middle of the night, we should be able to expect accessible, affordable, and competent care regardless of our age, employment status, class, income, or net worth. What we need as a nation is a way to provide such care in the most efficient, reliable, fair, and sustainable way. Thus, healthcare has more in common with fire and police protection than markets oriented to making the most money from patients' and families' medical problems.

We are in the midst in a battle for the soul of medicine and healthcare between the market "ethic" and a professional service ethic. This results in a moral challenge to the medical profession. Compared to 150 years ago, Dr Edmund Pellegrino, a leading medical ethicist at Georgetown University's Center for Clinical Bioethics, sums up this challenge this way:

> Today, we face another; but far more complicated, moral crisis. The enormous power of medical technology, couled with the legitimization of the market ethos in healthcare, threatens to overshadow both physician and patient. What will our moral response be? What place in that response should and will the moral guideposts of the Hippocratic Oath, and the AMA Code of Ethics play? Should professional codes of ethics be abandoned entirely in an autonomy-obsessed society? Should the traditional medical ethos be replaced entirely by a new code, one modified to suit current economic and political realities? Is a universal code even possible in our multicultural, morally pluralistic, democratic society? (Pellegrino, 1999, pp. 107–108)

With the growth of managed care in the 1990s, physicians were employed by managed care organizations and rewarded for restricting services to patients. In the jargon of the industry, "covered lives" of plan enrollees were traded within the managed care market. Today, most physicians are employed by hospitals or one or various kinds of managed care organizations, and are under pressure to meet their employers' expectations for profits. As the old adage goes "he who pays the piper calls the tune."

Dr Marcia Angell, former editor of the *New England Journal of Medicine*, has identified the ethical problem for physicians working under these circumstances with divided loyalties to their patients and employers. She describes the physician's ethical problem with this "double agent" role in these perceptive terms:

> History shows us that ethics in practice are often highly malleable, *justifying* political decisions rather than

informng them. Necessity is the mother of invention, in ethics as well as in other aspects of life. For example, in 1912, when the AMA thought salaried practice was a threat to the autonomy of the profession, its Code of Ethics pronounced it unethical for physicians to join group practices. Now, some 80 years later, we are again hearing that it is a matter of ethics for the medical profession to carry out essentially what is a political agenda. But ethics should be a little more stable than that. Ethics should be based on fundamental moral principles governing our behavior and obligations to one another. If a doctor is ethically committed to care for the individual patient, that commitment should not be abridged lightly. And it should not be nullified by a budget crunch. Doctors should continue to care for each patient unstintingly, even while they join with other citizens to devise a more efficient and just health care system. To control costs effectively will in my view require a coherent national health care system, with a global cap and a single payer. Only in this way can we have an affordable health care system that does not require doctors to be double agents. (Angell, 1993, pp. 285–286)

The Market

We have seen a continued drumbeat over the last 40 years promoting the magic of competition and markets in healthcare as the answer to our system problems of access, costs, and quality. Market advocates also preach the priority of "choice" and irresponsibility of consumers (a bad word—they mean patients!) in making decisions about their own healthcare. Many conservatives also argue (often only in code words) that the crux of healthcare inflation is bad decisions by consumers. Hence, the trend over the last 20 years has been toward "consumer-driven healthcare" (see, for example, Goodman, 2006), based on the premise that patients with "more skin in the game" (i.e., more cost-sharing) will make better decisions (i.e., use less healthcare, whether necessary or not). The implication is that patients make bad choices and over-utilize healthcare services indiscriminately. Variants of this view include "if you can't afford care, you don't deserve it" and "you don't deserve care for bad lifestyle choices." And of course, market advocates never mention the bigger problem of perverse incentives within the market-based system with *over*-utilization of healthcare services for which the supply side is responsible.

The problem with this market theory is that *it does not work*. As is made clear by the foregoing and the track record of markets over the last 40 years, market failure pervades the system and indeed itself is a priary reason for system failure (Park, 2008). Competition in healthcare does not work as it may for other areas of the economy. Instead, competitive markets lead to *consolidation* on the supply side, whether among hospitals, managed care organizations, insurers, or others. Physicians, hospitals, drug and medical device makers, and other suppliers have wide latitude to set their own prices. And consumer-driven healthcare, with more cost-sharing at the front end, just shifts more costs to patients and their families, often becoming a barrier to necessary care, and doing nothing to make healthcare more affordable.

The supposed "reforms" of the PPACA, claimed by supporters to help contain costs in coming years, are also likely to be ineffective. Instead, they are more cororate than patient-friendly. As just two examples, the drug industry avoided any provisions in the legislation to control their prices or to import prescription drugs from other countries. As another example, the "accountable care organizations" called for by the PPACA by 2014 are already leading to further consolidation in many markets.

As is fully described in my 2008 book, *Do Not Resuscitate: Why the Health Insurance Industry is Dying and How We Must Replace It*, the insurance industry plays a major role in perpetuating uncontrolled healthcare inflation in this country. The largest insurers are investor-owned, with a fiduciary responsibility to their shareholders and little accountability to their enrollees. They siphon off at least 20% (in some cases much more) of the premium dollar for various administrative and marketing costs as well as profits and sky-high CEO compensation. They seek out the healthiest enrollees, avoid the sick if possible, limit benefits to maximize their potential markets, deny claims whenever possible, and fight against any restraint of their rate-setting prerogatives. Wendell Potter, an insider with a long career in the insurance industry, blew the whistle on the industry's egregious practices in his important 2010 book, *Deadly Spin: An Insurance Company Insider Speaks Out on How Corporate PR is Killing Health Care and Deceiving Americans* (Potter, 2010). Meanwhile, of course, the industry lobbies and fights against any regulation by government at both federal and state levels, but welomes intervention by government in handing it 32 million new enrollees under the PPACA, many with federal subsidies.

In spite of the "reforms" of insurers' bad practices promised by backers of the PPACA, the industry and Wall Street have already weighed in on the industry's future. After the first quarter of 2011, the industry was starting to cash in on a bonanza from the new law. When UnitedHealth Group, the largest insurer in terms of revenue and market value, reported a 13% increase in profits, its stock prices soared to a 52-week high; the five other largest insurers had similar gains the next day. Stephen Hemsley, UnitedHealth Group's CEO, "earned" almost $102 million in 2010; his stock options are now estimated at about $1 billion (Potter, 2011).

Social Basis for UHC

The societal unity that characterized the World War II years and the 1950s in the US has long since disappeared. Today, the country is beset with larger gaps in income and opportunity than at any time in the nation's history. As one example, the richest Americans in 2009 accounted for 63.5% of the nation's wealth, while the bottom 80% collectively held just 12.8% (Geyman, 2009). As the middle class falls apart, a large underclass is growing, including those who are unemployed, are underemployed, and have just one job within a family, seniors, and retirees. All of these people on Main Street have great difficulty affording and gaining access to necessary healthcare. They are being left behind as corporate wealth increases and Wall Street prospers.

Demographic trends accelerate these socioeconomic differences. The numbers are already striking. There are 20 Americans aged 65 and older today for every 100 between 20 and 64, the usual working age group. That number is projected to increase to almost one-third of the working age population by 2025. The first members of the Baby Boomer generation, 79 million strong, are turning 65, and many have not been able to accumulate adequate funds for their retirement years (DHHS, 2012). Less than one-half of American adults now believe that their children will have a higher standard of living than theirs, and more than one-quarter believe that it will be lower.

A UHC program for our entire population of more than 300 million Americans would bring our people together regardless of age, income, occupation, or class. Countries with single-payer UHC have demonstrated this kind of social solidarity for many years. Conversely, programs that are not universal, such as Medicaid in America today, tend to be divisive and unpopular, since taxpayers feel they are paying for programs that do not benefit them.

Healthcare is a classic example of all of us being in the same boat—we are all born, get sick from one time to another, and die at the end of the road. So, we all need assurance that healthcare will be available and affordable when we need it, and will not bankrupt us. Markets can never provide that security.

Canada, our neighbor to the north, offers a good example of societal strength resulting from its Medicare program, a publicly financed, national, single-payer program coupled with a private delivery system. Though denigrated by its critics (especially on the American side of the border) and by some Canadians wanting to privatize it, public support for the program continues so strong that even a conservative government treats it as a third rail of politics. As recently as 2007, surveys showed that only 12% of Canadians wanted to completely rebuild their system (compared to 34% of respondents in the US; see Guyatt et al., 2007).

Political Basis for UHC

National surveys over the past 70 years have consistently shown strong public support for a system of national health insurance. This has ranged from more than one-half to two-thirds of Americans, and was even at the 74% level during the 1940s. An analysis by the Pew Research Center after the 2008 elections found that conservatives were evenly split concerning a guarantee by the federal government of UHC, even if that involved increasing taxes.

The AMA and many medical organizations still fight against UHC as "socialized medicine." This is an erroneous and disingenuous claim, since traditional

Medicare and the Veterans Administration are single-payer programs, and they would not eliminate either. Recent studies of physicians' attitudes have actually shown that three of five US physicians support UHC, so most of their organizations do not represent their constituencies on this issue. And some physicians' organizations, such as Physicians for a National Health Program (PNHP), are gaining larger membership and momentum all the time in their advocacy for UHC.

If we had a real democracy, we would have had UHC by now. Instead, powerful corporate stakeholders in the very profitable medical–industrial complex have been able to perpetuate the market-based system through many election cycles despite the increasingly adverse impacts of this system on ordinary Americans. These stakeholders and their lobbyists have successfully bought off politicians in both major parties. They have used a revolving door of influence between industry, lobbying groups, and government, even extending to staffs of Congressional committees drafting actual legislation. The PPACA is an excellent example of political compromises that serve industry more than patients and their families. Without effective mechanisms for cost containent, affordability of healthcare will remain an urgent problem for many Americans, government subsidies will become unsustainable, and our unaccountable profit-driven system will continue on with large amounts of unnecessary and inappropriate care servng the interests of providers on the supply side more than patients.

As the 2012 election cycle got under way, the GOP over-reached on its healthcare proposals and had a hard time explaining its proposed policies to the public. While trying to posture as defenders of Medicare, Republicans have long been in favor of converting Medicare into a smaller welfare-like program through vouchers. The objective of the Newt Gingrich-led 1994 Contract with America actually sought to see Medicare "wither on the vine." Today, under the banner of wanting smaller government and fiscal austerity, with more "choice" and personal responsibility on the part of patients (read more cost-sharing, and lesser use of care!), it is playing a game of deception and disinformation. While offering no real alternative to address access, cost, and quality problems of our failing healthcare system, Rep Paul Ryan (R-WI), as chairman of the House Budget Committee, has put forth a proposal that would introduce means-testing to the Medicare program, together with further privatization and contraction of future funding without any cost containment on the supply side. House Majority Leader Eric Cantor (R-VA) acknowledges that not all patients will get optimal healthcare with private insurance, saying further that "we're not for everyone having the same outcome guaranteed" (Pequet, 2011).

When the growing population of seniors 65 years and older, plus the oncoming wave of Baby Boomers, realize that they will be spending *much* more for healthcare in the future, with access even more of a problem, we can anticipate a major revolt within the electorate. We have only to remember the power of seniors in 1989, when they forced Congress to repeal its 1988 Medicare Catastrophic Care Act, which called on 40% of beneficiaries to pay more than 80% of the costs of catastrophic coverage.

If we can cut through the smoke and mirrors of the right's stance on healthcare to widely accepted principles of conservatives, we can find a mountain of potential support among conservatives for UHC. Dr Donald Light, a Fellow at the University of Pennsylvania's Center for Bioethics and co-author of *Benchmarks of Fairness for Health Care Reform* (Daniels et al., 1996) has observed that conservatives in every other industrialized county have supported universal access to necessary healthcare on the basis of these four conservative moral principles: *anti-free riding, personal integrity, equal opportunity, and just sharing*. He proposes these guidelines for conservatives to stay true to these principles:

1. Everyone is covered, and everyone contributes in proportion to his or her income.
2. Decisions about all matters are open and publicly debated. Accountability for costs, quality and value of providers, suppliers, and administrators is public.
3. Contributions do not discriminate by type of illess or ability to pay.
4. Coverage does not discriminate by type of illness or ability to pay.
5. Coverage responds first to medical need and suffering.

6. Nonfinancial barriers by class, language, education, and geography are to be minimized.
7. Providers are paid fairly and equitably, taking into account their local circumstances.
8. Clinical waste is minimized through public health, self-care, prevention, strong primary care, and identification of unnecessary procedures.
9. Financial waste is minimized through simplified administrative arrangements and strong bargaining for good value.
10. Choice is maximized in a common playing field where 90–95% of payments go toward necessary and efficient healthcare services and only 5–10% to administration. (Light, 2002, pp. 4–6)

UHC: A Real Alternative

UHC will provide healthcare access to all Americans from the first day on after such a bill is passed and implemented by Congress. Every citizen, regardless of age, income, or health status, will have a Medicare card assuring access to physicians, other licensed providers, and hospitals of their choice for all necessary care from birth to death. There will no cost-sharing at the front end or other barriers to a comprehensive set of defined benefits, including dental care and mental-healthcare with parity.

All Americans will be in one large risk group—all 300-plus million of us—so that the risks of accidents and illness can be shared broadly. UHC will reverse the current approach by private insurers to slice and dice populations of enrollees into ever-smaller risk pools—those younger and healthier than most of us who will have the lowest use of healthcare services. The private health-insurance industry will be banned from covering benefits offered through UHC; any continued role it might have would be for additional supplemental healthcare services (cf. Baker et al., 2008).

At least $400 billion a year will be saved by eliminating the profits, subsidies, tax benefits, and administrative and marketing costs of private insurers (Geyman, 2008b, 2009; Kaplan & Rodgers, 2009). The massive administrative waste of some 1300 private insurers in our present multi-payer system will be eliminated in a simplified single-payer system. These savings can be re-channeled to direct patient care. Annual global budgets will be negotiated with hospitals and other facilities, as well as negotiated arrangements of payment to physicians and other providers. They will have less administrative burden and hassle now imposed by third-party payers, and have more time and energy to devote themselves to patient care.

Traditional Medicare operates with administrative overhead of about 3%, compared to an average of 18% for commercial insurance and as much as 26% for investor-owned Blues (PNHP, 2012). Monopsony or bulk purchasing of drugs, medical devices, and supplies is another way that money will be saved under UHC.

By eliminating administrative waste and reducing perverse incentives leading to volume-based overutilization of inappropriate and unnecessary services, costs can be contained to a sustainable level. Studies have found that public financing of healthcare is much more efficient and less expensive than private financing. The Congressional Budget Office has also determined that a single-payer system can provide universal coverage and still save money due to administrative simplification.

UHC can be financed through a progressive tax system that will cost individuals, families, and employers no more and probably less than they are paying now. Citizens will have the dignity of paying patients, while physicians, other healthcare professionals, hospitals, and other facilities will compete in the old-fashioned way—by availability, quality, and effectiveness of care (see the papers in O'Brien & Livingston, 2008).

Traditional publicly financed and administered Medicare gives us a good model upon which to build UHC. It has demonstrated its efficiency and reliability as a defined-benefit program over the last 45 years. Even at that, however, it is not a perfect program. Improvements under UHC should include mechanisms for coverage and reimbursement policies based on scientific evidence, not subject to political influence from industry or interest groups. Medicare-for-all should also introduce price controls that are fair to patients, providers, facilities, and industry alike. We will also have to address as a society the limits of healthcare and the need to steward limited resources

Table 19.3 Alternate futures based on paradigm

Financing	*Single-payer*	*Multi-payer*
Access	Universal access, one tier	Decreasing acess, multi-tier
Costs	Manageable	Uncontrolled inflation
System quality	Improved	Degraded
Health disparities	Diminished	Aggravated
Equity	Improved	Worse
System efficiency	Improved	Decreased
Bureaucracy	Simplified	Increased and more fragmented
Sustainability	Improved	Imploding on itself
Social fabric	Strengthened	Further frayed
US workforce	More competitive	Less competitive
Population health	Improved	Declining
Public satisfaction	Increased	Decreased

for the common good. Table 19.3 summarizes alternate futures for the US based on a financing system (Geyman, 2009).

Conclusion

As is clear from the foregoing, the US healthcare system is a shambles. It is falling apart, imploding on the basis of limited access, uncontrolled inflation of unaffordable costs, and mediocre quality comparing poorly with other advanced nations that pay only one-half what we pay in this country. All incremental efforts to reform our market-based system over the last 40 years have failed to resolve its problems of access, costs, quality, and equity. This failing system cannot and should not be sustained. For as Herbert Stein, well-known economist, reminds us in what has become know as Stein's Law: "If something cannot go on forever, it will stop."

Single-payer UHC is not a new or unproven idea and has been proven effective for decades in many advanced countries around the world (Glaser, 1991, 2012). We must also remember that whatever healthcare system evolves in response to future reform attempts will be an ethical statement about what kind of people we are in what kind of country.

References

ACP (American College of Physicians). (2008). Achieving a high-performance health care system with universal access: What the United States can learn from other countries. *Annals of Internal Medicine, 148*, 55–75.

Angell, M. (1993). The doctor as double agent. *Kennedy Institute of Ethics Journal, 3*, 287–292.

Baker, C., Caplan, A., Davis, K., Dentzer, S., Epstein, A., Frist, B . . . Tuckson, R. (2008). Health of the nation—coverage of all Americans. *The New England Journal of Medicine, 359*, 777–780.

CSG (The Council of State Governments of the USA). (2006). Costs of chronic diseases: What are states facing? Retrieved from: http://www.healthystates.csg.org/NR/rdonlyres/E42141D1-4D47-4119-BFF4-A2E7FE81C698/0/Trends_Alert.pdf

Daniels, N., Light, D.W., & Caplan, R. L. (1996). *Benchmarks of fairness for health care reform*. New York: Oxford University Press.

Davis, K., Schoen, C., & Stremikis, K. (2010). *Mirror, mirror on the wall: How the performance of the US health care system compares internationally, 2010 update*. New York: The Commonwealth Fund.

DHHS (Department of Health and Human Services) (2012). Aging statistics. Retrieved from: http://www.aoa.gov/aoaroot/aging_statistics/index.aspx

Geyman, J.P. (2008a). *The corrosion of medicine: Can the profession reclaim its moral legacy?* Monroe, ME: Common Courage Press.

Geyman, J.P. (2008b). *Do not resuscitate: Why the health insurance industry is dying and how we must replace it*. Monroe, ME: Common Courage Press.

Geyman, J.P. (2009). *The cancer generation: Baby boomers facing a perfect storm*. Monroe, ME: Common Courage Press.

Geyman, J.P. (2010). *Hijacked: The road to single payer in the aftermath of stolen health care reform*. Monroe, ME: Common Courage Press.

Geyman, J.P. (2011). *Breaking point: How the primary care crisis endangers the lives of Americans*. Monroe, ME: Common Courage Press.

Glaser, W. (1991). *Health insurance in practice: International varations in financing, benefits, and problems*. London: Jossey-Bass.

Glaser, W. (2012). Universal health care in other countries. *HealthPac Online*. Retrieved from: http://www.healthpaconline.net/rekindling/Articles/Glasser.htm

Goodman, J. (2006). Consumer directed health care. *Networks Financial Institute Policy, Brief No. 2006-PB-20*. Retrieved from: http://papers.ssrn.com/sol3/papers.cfm?abstract_id=985572#PaperDownload

Goodman, J., Musgrave, G., & Herrick, D. (2004). *Lives at risk: Single-payer health insurance around the world*. Oxford: Rowman & Littlefield.

Guyatt, G., Devereaux, P., Lexchin, J., Stone, S., Yalnizyan, A., Himmelstein, D . . . Bhatnagar, N. (2007). A systematic review of studies comparing health outcomes in Canada and the United States. *Open Medicine, 1*. Retrieved from: http://www.openmedicine.ca/article/view/8/1

Kaplan, E., & Rodgers, M. (2009). The costs and benefits of a public option in health care reform: An economic analysis. Berkeley Center on Health, Economic & Family Security. Retrieved from: http://www.google.com/url?sa=t&rct=j&q=&esrc=s&frm=1&source=web&cd=3&ved=0CFoQFjAC&url=http%3A%2F%2Fwww.law.berkeley.edu%2Ffiles%2Fchefs%2FPublic_Option_Economic_Analysis.pdf&ei=runVT97gC5GJ2AXd9KmZDw&usg=AFQjCNF_9jt_-PrBHaVNdqQpfjU4w66j2Q&sig2=c6lj____V7k4UeN4tO8nDA

Light, D. (2002). A conservative call for universal access to health care. *PennBioethics: University of Pennsylvania Center for Bioethics Newsletter, 9*, 1–15.

Linden, R. (2010). *Rise and fall of the American medical empire: A trench doctor's view of the past, present, and future of the US healthcare system*. North Branch, MN: Sunrise River Press.

Mayhall, V. (2012). The insurance industry and the great recession, part II: Did the federal government rescue the insurance industry during the financial crisis? Breazeale, Sachse, & Wilson's blog, March 26. Retrieved from: http://www.insuranceregulatorylaw.com/2012_03_01_archive.html

O'Brien, M., & Livingston, M. (Eds.). (2008). *10 excellent reasons for national health care*. New York: The New Press.

Park, A. (2008). America's health checkup. *Time*, November 19. Retrieved from: http://www.time.com/time/speials/2007/printout/0,29239,1860289_1860561_1860562,00.html

Pellegrino, E. (1999). One hundred fifty years later: The moral status and relevance of the AMA code of ethics. In R. Baker, A. Caplan, L. Emanuel, & S. Lathan (Eds.), *The American medical ethics revolution: How the AMA's code of ethics has transormed physician's relationships to patients, profesionals, and society* (pp. 107–123). Baltimore, MD: Johns Hopkins Press.

Pequet, J. (2011). Cantor: Private health care rationing is better than government's. *The Hill*, May. Retrieved from: http://thehill.com/blogs/healthwatch/health-reform-implementation/158979-cantor-private-healthcare-rationing-better-than-governments

PNHP (Physicians for a National Health Program). (2012). Single-payer FAQ. Retrieved from: http://www.pnhp.org/facts/single-payer-faq

Potter, W. (2010). *Deadly spin: An insurance company insider speaks out on how corporate PR is killing health care and deceiving Americans*. New York: Bloomsbury Press.

Potter, W. (2011). Insurers getting rich by not paying for care. *PR Watch*, April 29. Retrieved from: http://prwatch.org/news/2011/04/10665/insurers-getting-rich-not-paying-care

PPACA (Patient Protection and Affordable Care Act). (2010). Retrieved from: http://democrats. senate.gov/reform/patient-protection-affordable-care-act.pdf

Quadagno, J. (2005). *One nation, uninsured*. Oxford: Oxford University Press.

Schoen, C., Osborn, R., Doty, M. Bishop, M., Peugh, J., & Murukutla, N. (2007). Toward higher-performance health systems: Adults' health care experiences in seven countries, 2007. *Health Affairs, 26*, w717–w734.

SSAB (The Social Security Advisory Borad of the USA). (2009). The unsustainable cost of health care. Retrieved from: http://www.ssab.gov/documents/TheUnsustainableCostofHealthCare_508.pdf

Tavistock Group. (1999). A shared statement of ethical principles for those who shape and give health care: A working draft. *Effective Clinical Practice, 2*, 143–155.

Wilper, A., Woolhandler, S., Lasser, K., McCormick, D., Bor, D., & Himmelstein, D. (2008). A national study of chronic illess disease prevention and access to care in uninsured US adults. *Annals of Internal Medicine, 149*, 170–176.

Chapter Twenty

The United States of America Should Not Adopt Universal Healthcare

Let's Try Freedom Instead

Glen Whitman

The US healthcare system is not a free market, and its worst problems are attributable to existing government interventions. Implementing a single-payer system would do little to solve those problems and much to make them worse. Under single-payer, Americans' healthcare would be rationed by means of global budgets, caps on the availability of treatments and drugs, bureaucratic denials of service, and, most of all, waiting. Socialized funding would also encourage government intrusion into personal lifestyle decisions. Instead of embracing a flawed solution based on coercion and government interference in healthcare decisions, Americans should embrace a system based on voluntarism, freedom of choice, and personal responsibility.

Introduction

Support for adopting a single-payer healthcare system in the United States is driven largely by the belief that the US currently has a free-market healthcare system, and that system has failed. In truth, the US has nothing close to a truly free market in healthcare, and most problems of the US system derive from perverse incentives created by state and federal interventions in the healthcare system.

I will not defend the existing US healthcare system, though I will defend certain aspects of it. Instead, I will make the case for a different system—one based on freedom of choice with individual, family, and community responsibility. I will show how the US has strayed far from that ideal in several ways, resulting in predictably poor outcomes. Then, I will address the proposed alternative, the single-payer system, and explain why it cannot deliver on its promises; at least, not without unjustified sacrifices in terms of both healthcare performance and personal freedom.

The "Right" to Healthcare vs. Freedom of Choice

Advocates of single-payer proposals, and others aimed at producing universal coverage, often speak of healthcare as a "right." Why? Most likely because they regard healthcare as a necessity. But that cannot be the whole answer, as many other necessities are provided largely by the market, including food, shelter, and clothing. Government does regulate these markets to guarantee safety and prevent fraud. And sometimes the government provides targeted financial assistance to

Contemporary Debates in Bioethics, First Edition. Edited by Arthur L. Caplan and Robert Arp.

help people in need; for instance, food stamps help the poor buy food, and Section 8 vouchers help the poor get housing. But no one seriously proposes single-payer food, single-payer housing, or single-payer clothing. There is no movement for collectivized farms and national cafeterias. What makes healthcare different?

Because many people believe (incorrectly) that our current system is a free market that has failed, they embrace the alternative of having the government treat healthcare as a right. The fact that current policy has not manifestly failed in other areas, such as food and clothing, explains the absence of "rights" language on those areas. But as we will see later from the performance of actual single-payer systems, declaring something a right does not mean that everyone will have it.

Healthcare differs fundamentally from other things we regard as rights, such as freedom of speech and religion. These are often called "negative" rights because the only obligation they place on others is to *refrain* from certain acts such as censoring your speech or burning your church. Healthcare, however, refers to goods and services. As such, a right to healthcare would constitute a "positive" right, meaning a right that requires people to use resources and labor to satisfy it. Positive rights have economic implications that negative rights do not.

Although some philosophers argue that *only* negative rights are valid (Jordan, 1991; Narveson, 2001), I will not argue that here. My point is narrower: as a matter of both logic and practice, enforcing positive rights usually means invading negative rights. It involves restricting the choices of people about how to use their own labor and property. Single-payer systems *by definition* restrict people's ability to buy and sell health services without the state's involvement and permission. They also restrict the terms on which people can trade—by, for instance, setting maximum prices at which doctors can sell their services.

In Canada, for instance, the provincial governments prohibit people from buying private insurance to cover services promised by the public healthcare system. In 2005, the Canadian Supreme Court struck down Quebec's prohibition on private insurance as a violation of human rights (*Chaoulli v. Quebec*, 2005), although the ramifications of that ruling remain unclear. Other nominally single-payer systems, despite the misleading name, do permit varying levels of private provision. (For simplicity, I will continue to call these systems "single-payer.") But even when single-payer systems permit some private alternatives, they still restrict personal choice through their dominant influence on the industry, which crowds out options that would otherwise have been available from the private sector. For most citizens, opting out of the public system entirely—with a corresponding tax break—is not possible.

In choosing among policies, we should favor voluntarism over coercion and diversity over one-size-fits-all solutions whenever possible. That means allowing people to choose for themselves which health services to buy and sell, which mutually agreeable prices to pay for them, what kinds of insurance to cover the payments with, and how to balance health against other life goals.

People have different values and preferences. For some, good health and longevity supersede all other goals, leading them to demand more comprehensive and generous healthcare plans. For others, extending lifespan is less important than enjoying one's earlier years; for them, less generous healthcare plans could make sense. For those who distrust Western medicine in favor of nontraditional forms of healthcare, bare-bones traditional coverage may suffice. And for some people, such as Christian Scientists, modern healthcare does not seem valuable at all. The point is not that these people are correct—I, for one, trust Western medicine and would like plenty of it—but that they are individuals whose preferences deserve to be respected. Some state healthcare policies, such as the recently passed PPACA in the US, make exceptions for Christian Scientists. The proper response from non-Christian Scientists is to ask, "Where's *my* exception? Why should I have to join an obscure religion to exercise freedom of choice?"

Government health systems often rely on the notion of "medical necessity" to define what the state guarantees. This term implies the existence of an *objective* standard of care that everyone should receive. But objectivity is an illusion here. Medical science may be able to give us objective, factual information about survival rates, risk factors, side effects, etc. But it cannot tell us what values and preferences we should have, how to weigh risk against reward, how to weigh health against other life goals, or which services are worth their cost in money or discomfort. These are value-laden matters without objective answers. In practice, "medical necessity" is defined politically by bureaucrats, committees, and lobbyists.

Of course, freedom does imply responsibility. A society cannot give people a blank check to impose the costs of more expensive decisions—such as having a less nutritious diet, or always selecting name-brand over generic drugs—on their fellow citizens. For that reason, a free system will always expect individuals to bear much of the burden of their medical decisions.

Respecting freedom does not mean people never need a helping hand. It simply means individuals have *primary* responsibility for their own health. The next level of responsibility is family and community, especially in the form of private charity and mutual aid. Community efforts are preferable to state action for two reasons. First, they are voluntary, which is valuable in itself. Second, community providers have more personal information and "local knowledge" (Hayek, 1945) than civil servants, and thus a better chance of understanding the specific needs of the people they help.

Contrary to popular belief, mutual aid is a viable alternative to the state in providing care to the needy. David Beito (2000), for instance, has documented the prevalence of mutual-aid societies in the late nineteenth and early twentieth century. Such societies provided various services to their members, including early forms of health insurance, but were eventually crowded out by the growth of the welfare state, among other factors.

When individual and community responsibility fall short, there can be a legitimate role for government; but even then, there are many alternatives short of single-payer systems. Minimal and targeted government interventions, such as subsidies for the worst off, can fill in the gaps without trampling freedom of choice.

Individual rights may sometimes be overridden for the sake of other goals, but the bar should be high. At a minimum, before adopting a single-payer system, we should check to see if the goal of providing good healthcare can be met in other ways that are more compatible with freedom. As it turns out, it can.

What Is Wrong with US Healthcare?

Critics of US healthcare often charge that it produces worse health outcomes at much higher cost than other countries. They are half-right: the US system does cost a lot. But is it true that the US system produces worse outcomes? The statistics allegedly showing inferior performance in the US cannot be taken at face value.

Life Expectancy and Other Aggregate Measures

The most commonly cited statistic is life expectancy. At 78.3, the US ranks 36th among UN member nations; Japan is first at 82.6 (UN, 2007). But numerous factors besides healthcare affect life expectancy, including nutrition, exercise, obesity, tobacco use, alcohol use, genetics, racial diversity, geography, violent crime, and highway accidents. It turns out that several of these factors contribute to the shorter US lifespan. Specifically:

- The US suffers a high rate of death rate due to injuries—including homicide, suicide, and traffic accidents—relative to other Organization for Economic Co-operation and Development (OECD) countries, with the highest injury mortality rate among the original 20 OECD members (WHO, 2010, pp. 59–68).
- The US also has the highest obesity rate among OECD nations, at 32.2% for men and 35.5% for women (IOTF, 2012).
- While the US no longer leads the developed world in smoking, it did from the 1930s to the mid-1980s (Forey et al., 2002). Because the effects of smoking can appear decades after the fact, smoking during this earlier period has lingering effects on mortality today. One study shows that if smoking deaths were eliminated, the US life expectancy for men at age 50 would rise from 15th place to 12th among 21 OECD nations, and for women it would rise from 17th to 9th (Preston et al., 2011, p. 119).

Factors that are harder to quantify also matter. Nutrition and exercise matter, independent of their impact upon obesity, and anecdotal evidence suggests the US does worse than other countries in these areas. Genetics also apparently plays a meaningful role in determining longevity (Day, 1998). For instance, one gene associated with longevity (found in mitochondrial rather than nuclear DNA) is more prevalent in people of Japanese origin (*Science Daily*, 2009). Results like these suggest the US's relatively high level of racial diversity may contribute to its lower life expectancy.

Taken together, these considerations demonstrate that simple life-expectancy figures do not demonstrate poor US healthcare performance. Other aggregate measures, such as infant mortality and disease-specific mortality rates, suffer from similar problems. And index statistics designed to take into account multiple factors, like the World Health Organization's famous ranking of world healthcare systems, are even more misleading because they place weight on factors that are both logically incoherent and indicative of the authors' underlying biases (Whitman, 2008).

Direct Measures of Healthcare Performance

More direct measures of healthcare performance indicate that the US does better than other countries in some important areas. For most types of cancer, studies show better relative survival rates in the US than in most developed countries, including Europe, Australia, and Canada (Coleman et al., 2008). A study of patients diagnosed with cancer between 1996 and 2002 looked at five-year survival rates for 16 categories of cancer, and found that relative survival rates were higher in the US than in Europe for 14 of 16 categories, with no significant difference for the remaining two (Verdecchia et al., 2007).

A problem with five-year survival rates is that they can be artificially boosted by earlier diagnosis; treatment aside, people with an earlier stage of cancer have longer left to live. But other statistics support the claim that US cancer treatment is superior. The US breast-cancer mortality ratio (deaths due to breast cancer divided by incidence of breast cancer) is lower than that of other developed nations; the same is true of prostate cancer (Anderson & Hussey, 2000, p. 20). Note that if the early-diagnosis criticism is correct, it means the US does a better job of early screening for cancer.

The US performs well in other categories as well. Its HIV/AIDS mortality ratio is lower than that of other developed nations (Anderson & Hussey, 2000, p. 21). Studies indicate that Americans with hypertension are more likely to take medication for the condition and more likely to get increased doses when their blood pressure is not under control (Wolf-Maier et al., 2003, 2004; Wang et al., 2007).

The US also makes greater use of high-tech medical equipment. The US has more MRIs and CT scanners per capita than every OECD nation except Japan, and (though the data here are less complete) appears to deliver more actual scans to patients (OECD, 2010). It would be better to measure outcomes instead of inputs, because there are questions about how much difference the equipment makes in terms of mortality. Nevertheless, it is clear the US does not skimp in this area.

The US has low-performing areas as well, kidney disease being a notable example (Kim et al., 2006). In many areas, reliable comparative evidence simply is not available. But based on the existing evidence on specific conditions, US healthcare performance appears at least on par with other developed nations.

The Real Problem: Cost

If performance is not what is wrong with US healthcare, then what is? In a word, *cost*. US health expenditures do dramatically exceed those of other countries. In 2007, we spent $7289 per capita on healthcare; the next closest competitor was Norway at $4763 (Anderson & Markovich, 2009).

Of course, some of the factors that explain lower US life expectancy also help explain higher expenditures. Given that Americans have a higher prevalence of certain conditions, such as heart disease, they should be expected to spend more. Sicker people need more healthcare.

Furthermore, there is a strong correlation between per-capita GDP and healthcare spending—put simply, richer countries spend more on healthcare (Reinhardt et al., 2004, p. 11). The United States' high per-capita GDP accounts for 47% of the difference between US per capita healthcare spending and the OECD median (Cannon & Tanner, 2005, p. 20).

But the healthcare spending gap is too large to be blamed entirely on differing health needs and higher income. To understand why US health spending is so massive, we need to consider the undesirable effects of US healthcare policy.

The True Story of US Healthcare

The US healthcare system is not a free market. A panoply of federal and state interventions have made healthcare one of the most regulated industries in the economy. But no intervention has had such far-reaching effects as a seemingly innocuous provision of the tax code written over 60 years ago.

The Tax Preference for Employer-Provided Health Insurance

During World War II, the federal government imposed wage and price controls throughout the economy. Companies that wanted to attract more employees could not legally offer higher wages. But some employers hit upon an alternative strategy: offer potential employees health insurance instead. The War Labor Board approved this approach, and the IRS followed suit by not classifying health benefits as taxable income (Waslee, 1992, p. 55).

This quirk of the tax code—adopted for reasons having nothing to do with healthcare policy—remains in place to this day. The favorable tax treatment of employer-provided insurance has caused several major distortions in the healthcare market.

First, the tax break favors employer-provided insurance over insurance acquired in other ways, such as the individual market or groups like churches and mutual-aid societies. As a result, people who lose their jobs often lose their health insurance, too.

Second, the tax break favors healthcare spending over spending on other goods and services, because most other goods and services must be paid for with after-tax dollars. People respond to this incentive by funneling more money into the health sector than they otherwise would.

Third, the tax break favors health *insurance* over health*care*, because out-of-pocket expenditures on medical services must be covered with after-tax dollars. People therefore have an incentive to get as much of their healthcare in the form of health insurance as possible. The result is bloated health-insurance policies that cover all manner of services, including those it would make more sense to pay for directly.

All of this stands in sharp contrast to other forms of insurance, such as auto insurance. Hardly anyone gets auto insurance through their employer. Nobody buys auto insurance that covers gas fill-ups, oil changes, and car washes. Car owners understand that these are routine and expected costs of having a car. Insuring them would not make them any cheaper; on the contrary, it would make them more expensive. Imagine if you filed a claim with your auto-insurance company every time you filled up your tank. Both the gasoline and the added bureaucracy would drive up your insurance premiums.

The economic function of insurance is to prepare for *large* and *uncertain* expenses (Little, 1937; Zeckhauser, 1993), such as collisions that cause major damage to a vehicle. But with health insurance, Americans regularly hold policies with coverage for all kinds of medical expenses, including routine doctor visits, monthly prescriptions, and sometimes optional services as well. This is akin to buying auto insurance for gas fill-ups and car washes, and its primary effect is to raise costs.

To take just one example, birth control pills are often covered by health insurance. If you are using the pill correctly, you need a new package every month; there is no real uncertainty here. Insurance coverage does not make the cost of birth control disappear—it is just included in the insurance premium, which rises by the cost of birth control pills plus the bureaucratic cost. Costs also rise because the insurance encourages additional usage. If insurance companies are not allowed to charge different premiums based on gender, some of the cost may be shifted from women to men. But the overall cost to society of providing birth control does not go down; it goes *up* from the unnecessary bureaucracy and increased usage.

The peculiar tax treatment of healthcare has contributed to an unfortunate confusion between health insurance and healthcare. Uninsured people are often characterized as having "no healthcare," because the

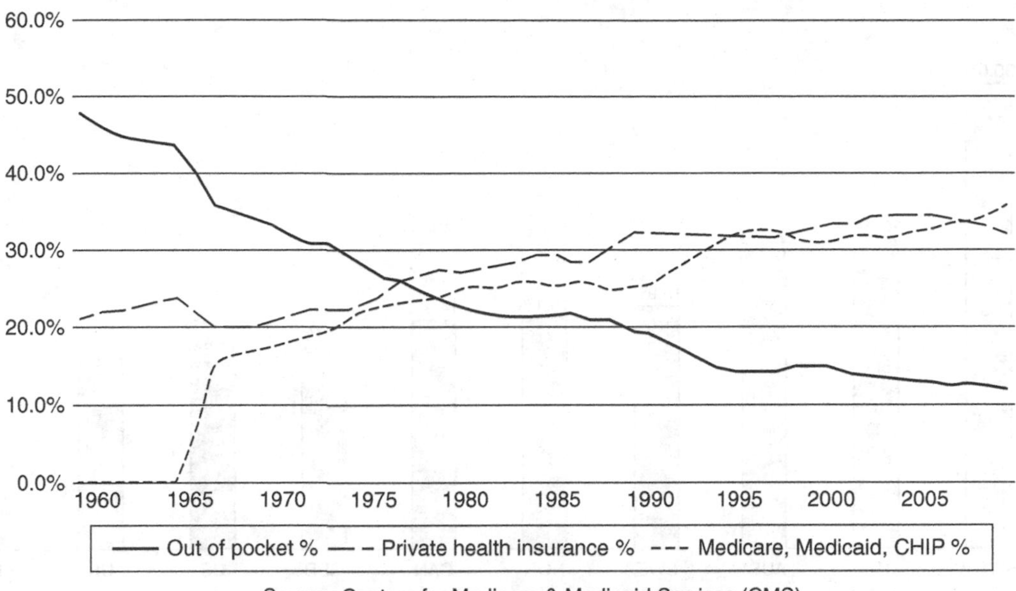

Figure 20.1 Sources of funding as a percentage of total US health expenditures, 1960–2009

notion of paying for services out-of-pocket seems bizarre. Yet that is exactly what we should be doing: paying for a much larger portion of medical services directly, and using insurance primarily for catastrophic health events. That does not mean routine medical expenses are unimportant. They are just as important as food, shelter, and clothing. But we do not pay our rent and grocery bills with insurance.

The Third-Party Buyer Problem

The tax-code-driven expansion of employer-provided private insurance has occurred alongside a massive expansion of public insurance programs, most notably Medicare and Medicaid. In 1965, the actuary for Medicare predicted it would cost $9 billion by 1990; in actuality, it had ballooned to $66 billion (Blevins, 2003). Now, its annual cost is $452 billion and rising. Medicare, Medicaid, and the Children's Health Insurance Program (CHIP) together constitute more than a fifth of the federal budget (see Figure 20.1; CBPP, 2011). Public insurance and tax-subsidized private insurance have combined to create a massive *third-party buyer problem*—meaning the tendency of people to purchase more services at higher prices when someone else is paying the bill.

In 2007, Americans paid only 12.2% of per-capita health expenditures out of pocket. The entire remaining 87.8% was covered by third-party buyers, either public (45.3%) or private (42.4%). The US out-of-pocket percentage is actually *lower* than that of many other countries, including many with nominally single-payer systems. Canadians paid 14.9% out of pocket; the UK, 11.5%; Norway, 15.1%; Sweden, 15.9%; and Australia, 18.2%. Of the countries in the study, only the French paid less out of pocket, at 6.8% (Anderson & Markovich, 2009, p. 5); see Figure 20.2.

What is wrong with third-party buyers? To understand, it is useful to return to the auto-insurance example. Imagine if, for some reason, you did buy auto insurance for gas fill-ups and car washes. Under the policy, you pay nothing for these services at the point of sale; they are effectively free. Or maybe you make a small copayment of $10 per fill-up, $5 per carwash. Either way, you would probably increase your demand for those services. Why not take a little joyride, or wash the car a bit more often? If it is covered, why not get the car fully detailed?

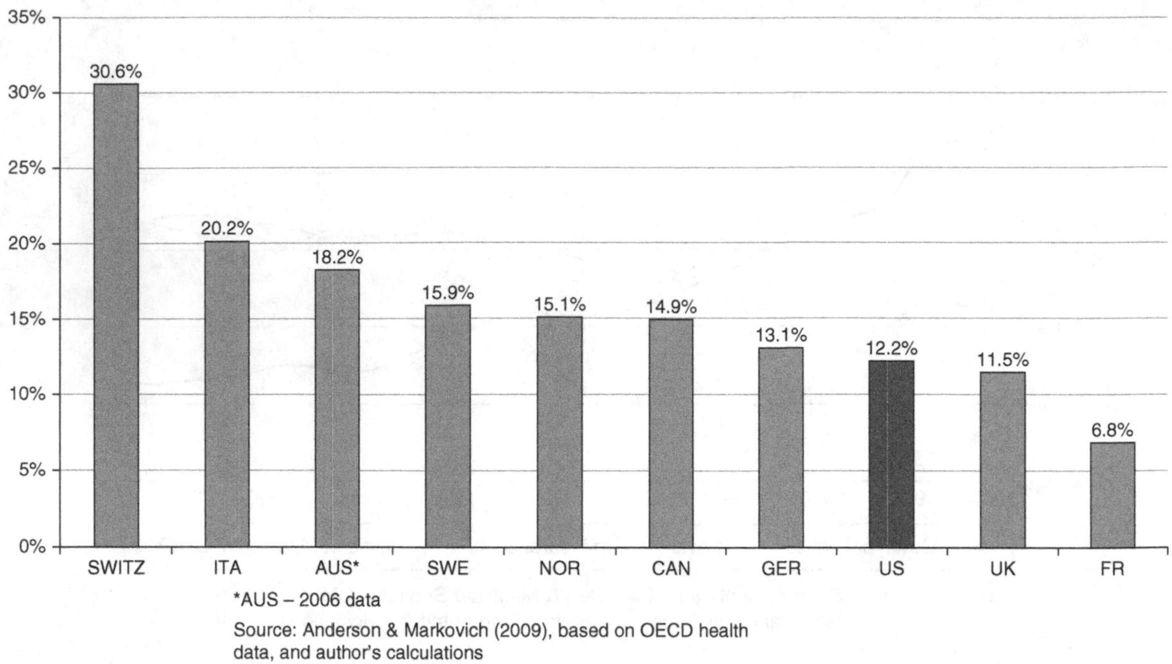

Figure 20.2 Percentage of total health expenditures paid out of pocket, by country (2007)

More importantly, you would probably pay less attention to price. If you were paying for gas directly, you might drive an extra couple of blocks to the cheaper gas station. But with insurance, you are shielded from price differences. If enough people had this kind of auto insurance, maybe gas stations would stop posting prices. Gas prices would be negotiated with the auto-insurance companies, and drivers would mostly be unaware of them. Drivers would, however, have to pay much higher auto-insurance premiums.

As strange as these practices may sound, they are commonplace in the market for healthcare. Insured patients rarely ask about prices, and doctors almost never post them. When a patient does ask for a price, the doctor usually must consult the hidden price schedule that the practice has worked out with the patient's insurance provider. For the most part, patients are encouraged to make healthcare choices without regard to cost.

But the costs of care are still there. Behind the scenes, prices continue rising because neither doctors nor patients have a strong incentive to keep them down. High prices and inflated usage manifest themselves in higher insurance premiums. For those with employer-provided insurance, the higher premiums result in lower wages or fewer wage increases (Baicker & Chandra, 2006).

Further evidence that third-party payments contribute to healthcare cost growth is provided by cosmetic surgery, a field where most payments are made out of pocket. Devon Herrick (2010, p. 2) shows that from 1992 to 2010, while prices of medical care and physician services grew almost twice as much as prices in general (as measured by the CPI), cosmetic surgery prices grew only half as much as prices in general—meaning the inflation-adjusted price of cosmetic surgery actually fell.

State-Level Regulations

State-level policies have also contributed to the rising cost of healthcare. State legislatures have enacted a hodgepodge of regulations that reduce insurance coverage for catastrophic events while encouraging people to buy services they do not want or need.

Community rating laws limit the ability of insurance companies to charge differential rates based on customers' cost-related characteristics. *Guaranteed issue* laws require insurance companies to offer coverage to anyone. Although springing from good intentions, community rating and guaranteed issue both tend to raise premiums (especially for the young and healthy) and thus to reduce overall coverage (Herring & Pauly, 2006; Wachenheim & Leida, 2007).

But more significant than either of these are *mandated benefits*. A mandated benefit is a healthcare product or service that any health-insurance policy must include by law. In total, the 50 states have passed over 2100 such laws, or more than 40 per state (Bunce & Wieske, 2010), a testament to the lobbying efforts of medical specialties that benefit from having more customers. Existing mandates include a wide variety of services, including acupuncture, chiropractic, hair transplantation, in vitro fertilization, and so forth.

The point is not that these are not valid services, but that not everyone wants them. More importantly, mandated benefits have driven up premiums by 20% or more, depending on the state (Bunce & Wieske, 2010). In essence, mandated benefits laws force customers to buy "Lexus coverage" when they might prefer "Honda coverage." Those who cannot afford the higher price join the ranks of the uninsured.

And insurance regulations are just the beginning. A web of immigration restrictions, residency requirements, and qualifying exams limit the number of foreign doctors who can enter US medical practice, despite physician shortages in inner-city and rural areas (AP, 2007), and despite evidence that foreign doctors are no worse at performing their duties (Goodwin, 2010). A majority of States prohibit nurse practitioners from practicing independently of physicians, despite no evidence of worse outcomes (Christian et al., 2007). In general, licensure laws restrict the ability of midwifes, pharmacists, and other substitute providers to compete with physicians (Blevins, 1995).

What about Single-Payer?

The supposed alternative to the US system is to adopt a single-payer system, similar to those in Canada and elsewhere, in which the government acts as a monopoly buyer of medical services. Would such a system work here?

A single-payer is just another kind of third-party buyer. As discussed earlier, third-party payments encourage patients to consume more medical services while ignoring their cost. In this sense, the US and other developed countries are quite similar. The difference lies in how we have responded to the problem. The US has responded by placing few limits on care and letting costs run wild. The single-payer countries have responded by limiting care through bureaucratic means.

The single-payer countries ration access to healthcare in various ways. They impose global budgets on hospitals, which cap total spending for the year, regardless of whether demand has been met (Anderson & Hussey, 2004). They limit introduction of new drugs, procedures, and technologies while resisting the diffusion of older ones (Robinson, 1999, p. 5). They issue centralized rulings to deny treatments based on patient characteristics, including age, severity of condition, and smoking and obesity status (Smith, 2008; Donnelly, 2010a, 2010b).

And most importantly, they make people wait. Waiting lengthy periods of time for care, whether specialist consultations or surgeries, is simply a fact of life in single-payer countries. In Canada, patients wait an average of 18.2 weeks, or over four months, between being referred by a general practitioner and getting an elective surgery or treatment. For some procedures, the wait is much longer; the longest wait is 35.2 months, or almost three years, for orthopedic surgery (Barua et al., 2010, p. 5).

The Canadian experience is not unique. Waiting times are a "main health policy concern" in about half of OECD countries, and a "serious health policy concern" for 12 (Siciliani & Hurst, 2003, p. 7). The US was one of only three countries (along with Germany and France) classified as having no waiting-time problem.

A study of five English-speaking countries found the US had only 5% of patients reporting a wait longer than four months for surgery, as compared to 23% in Australia, 26% in New Zealand, 27% in Canada, and 38% in the UK (Blendon et al., 2002, p. 188). A study focusing on elective coronary bypass surgery found the percentage of patients who waited longer than three months to be "88.9% in the UK, 46.7% in Canada, 18.2% in Sweden and 0% in the US. For elective coronary angiography, the percentage was 22.8% in the UK, 16.1% in Canada, 15.4% in Sweden and 0% in the US" (Siciliani & Hurst, 2003).

Waiting times should rightfully be considered a price—a price paid in time rather than money. Some patients are in pain or discomfort while they wait. Others die on the waiting list. John Goodman reports, "During one 12-month period in Ontario, Canada, 71 patients died waiting for coronary bypass surgery while 121 patients were removed from the list because they had become too sick to undergo surgery with a reasonable chance of survival" (Goodman, 2005, p. 3).

US patients sometimes wait, too. But they typically do not wait as long or as often. There is, however, one context where waiting is common in the US—the Health Maintenance Organization (HMO), also known as managed care. HMOs control costs by empowering managers to make decisions about care and to limit usage. The expansion of HMOs helped to keep healthcare spending growth low during the 1990s. But dissatisfaction with that system led to a decline in HMOs—total enrollment peaked in 2000 (KFF, 2011, Exhibit 2.13)—and the resumption of healthcare spending growth in the 2000s.

If you want to know what single-payer is like, imagine one giant HMO—without even the option of choosing a different one. As the HMO experience shows, Americans dislike having their choices made for them. Will they be any more likely to tolerate it under a single-payer system? If they do, we can expect rationing by waiting. If they do not, then single-payer will not really push down costs. A US single-payer system could easily turn out to be just a variation on the status quo: open access with bloated spending.

Indeed, it is questionable whether existing single-payer systems can successfully control growth in health spending. All modern economies have a problem with expansion in their healthcare sectors. From 1996 to 2006, the median OECD country's healthcare spending grew at an average annual rate of 3.9%. The US average annual growth rate of 3.6% fell *below* the median. For Canada, the growth rate was 3.7%; for the UK, 4.8%; for New Zealand, 4.3%; for Australia, 4.1% (Anderson & Markovich, 2008, p. 5). Other countries, including France, Germany, and Switzerland, had somewhat lower growth rates. But there is no reason to think the US would mimic the slower-growing rather than faster-growing single-payer systems. Note that Australia, France, and Ireland are generally regarded as two-tier systems—where a basic healthcare coverage is provided by the government to all its citizens, while also allowing for additional coverage from private companies—whereas Canada, Japan, and the UK have more pure single-payer systems.

Assuming the US under single-payer would experience about the same growth rate as other single-payer systems, any cost savings from switching to single-payer would have to result from a one-time "level shift" to a lower base level of spending. This seems highly unlikely given historical experience. Although the Canadian single-payer system was implemented piecemeal in the provinces, the key jumps in federal involvement occurred in 1966 (Medical Care Act) and 1984 (Health Canada Act). In neither of those years, nor the years just following, did Canada experience a drop in health expenditures (SC, 1983; CIHI, 2010, p. 2).

There is one possible route for pushing down costs in a single-payer system, but only with damaging side effects: pharmaceutical price controls. The United States accounts for 45% of the world's spending on pharmaceuticals, as compared to Europe's 27–31% and Japan's 9–12% (Northrup, 2005, p. 29; IMS Health, 2008). These revenues provide the incentive to engage in research and development of new drugs. By paying more, the US effectively subsidizes the development of new drugs that improve health worldwide, while the rest of the world gets a comparatively free ride. The effect of the US market's support for innovation is evidenced by the disproportionate number of innovations and discoveries made by Americans and US-based firms (Whitman & Raad, 2009).

If a US single-payer system forced down drug prices, we could expect fewer life-saving and life-improving drugs in the future. This is recognized even by advocates of government-run systems. Robert Reich, Labor Secretary under President Bill Clinton, for example, said this: "us[ing] the bargaining leverage of the federal government in terms of Medicare, Medicaid … to force drug companies and insurance companies and medical suppliers to reduce their costs ... means less innovation, and that means less new products and less new drugs on the market, which means you are probably not going to live that much longer than your parents" (Taranto, 2009).

Everybody's Business: Socialized Costs vs. Personal Freedom

Single-payer systems force everyone to buy into a one-size-fits-all healthcare package, as though the same choices would be right for everyone. But how do other matters of personal choice fare under a system of socialized costs? Sadly, we already know the answer to this question. In the US, every instance in which a government program has covered healthcare expenditures with tax dollars has resulted in demands—often successful—to restrict personal choice.

The most obvious and controversial example is abortion. In 1976, the so-called "Hyde Amendment" restricted and defined the circumstances under which Medicaid would pay for abortion, and with various changes, the Hyde amendment has been with us ever since (NAF, 2006). Fortunately, for women who want abortions, Medicaid is not the only way to get one. But what happens when all healthcare spending is covered by a single-payer?

Pro-choice advocates often respond to abortion opponents by saying, "Don't like abortion? Then don't have one." And that response makes sense when nobody else is involved. But with public funding, the argument no longer works. Everyone who pays taxes is involved.

The same goes for any other lifestyle choice affecting, or affected by, healthcare. When smoking is purely a personal matter, smokers can rightly say, "It's my body, my choice." But when taxpayers have to pay the resulting medical bills, that position weakens. Smokers and the companies who supply them arguably impose costs on the rest of us. This is precisely the argument that allowed state attorneys general to sue tobacco companies for costs incurred by Medicaid (Levy, 2000). Similarly, riding a motorcycle might seem to be a personal choice. But the fact that injured motorcyclists turn up in publicly funded emergency rooms has repeatedly been used to justify laws requiring helmets (Max et al., 1998). Other lifestyle restrictions loom on the horizon; for instance, fat taxes, trans-fat bans, and food-marketing restrictions have been advocated on grounds that overweight and obese people are a burden on the public purse (for example, Ruiz, 2009).

And these are just proposals that have occurred under the present US system, in which health costs are only partially socialized. What would happen if they were fully, or near-fully, socialized under a single-payer system? The most likely answer is growing intrusion into people's private choices because, in an important sense, *they will no longer be private*. Sexual behavior? Fair game, because sexual choices undoubtedly affect personal health. Exercise, nutrition, risky sports, and recreational activities? The argument is the same: what the public funds, the public may control. Some people will push for greater restrictions on personal liberty from a purely financial motive. Others will use socialized costs as cover for advancing a moralistic agenda they probably already held (as in the case of abortion). Together, these groups will provide the added political weight needed to impose ever greater restrictions on personal liberty.

The Alternative

It is a truism of economics that when consumers face lower prices, they demand more goods and services. As the price approaches zero, demand shoots through the roof. This is not just an American phenomenon; it is true everywhere, including countries with single-payer systems. If left unconstrained, burgeoning demand leads to exploding costs. Given these facts, there are essentially only three options:

- Option #1: Leave demand unchecked and let costs run wild. The US has unwittingly chosen this option. Existing policies encourage most Americans to consume health services without attention to cost, with predictable results. As a side effect, the decisions made by the insured population have made care unaffordable for much of the remaining population.
- Option #2: Constrain demand by means of centralized bureaucracy. That is the option embraced

by single-payer countries, where government agencies decide for everyone what kinds of healthcare to fund. These countries do not face the massive costs of the US, but they do face increasing public dismay at the resulting waiting lists and denials of service.

- Option #3: Give people the freedom to make their own healthcare decisions, but also confront them with a greater portion of the costs of their choices. This is the only system with the potential to constrain costs *without* centralized control, and it is the system Americans should strive to achieve.

To be sure, some people will not be happy with this system, because they would prefer to get everything they want for free. But everything-for-free is simply not an option—not in the US, and not anywhere else. Costs and benefits of healthcare services must be compared, and trade-offs must be made; the real question is who should make them. Rather than empowering government agents and distant bureaucracies to make health decisions for everyone, Americans should take the reins for themselves.

References

Anderson, G., & Hussey, P. (2000). *Multinational comparisons of health systems data.* New York: The Commonwealth Fund.

Anderson, G., & Hussey, P. (2004). *Special issues with single-payer health insurance systems.* HNP Discussion Paper. Washington, DC: The World Bank.

Anderson, G., & Markovich, M. (2008). *Multinational comparisons of health systems data.* New York: The Commonwealth Fund.

Anderson, G., & Markovich, M. (2009). *Multinational comparisons of health systems data.* New York: The Commonwealth Fund.

AP (The Associated Press). (2007). Foreign doctors rebuffed by new US barriers. *The Associated Press*, July 20. Retrieved from: http://www.msnbc.msn.com/id/19873847/ns/health-health_care/

Baicker, K., & Chandra, A. (2006). The labor market effects of rising health insurance premiums. *Journal of Labor Economics, 24*, 609–634.

Barua, B., Rovere, M., & Skinner, B. (2010). *Waiting your turn: Wait times for health care in Canada, 2010 report.* Studies in Health Care Policy. Vancouver, BC: Fraser Institute.

Beito, D. (2000). *From mutual aid to the welfare state: Fraternal societies and social services, 1890–1967.* Chapel Hill, NC: The University of North Carolina Press.

Blendon, R., Schoen, C., DesRoches, C., Osborn, R., Scoles, K., & Zapert, K. (2002). Inequities in health care: A five-country survey. *Health Affairs, 21*, 182–191.

Blevins, S. (1995). The medical monopoly: Protecting consumers or limiting competition? Cato Institute Policy Analysis, No. 246. Washington, DC: The Cato Institute.

Blevins, S. (2003). *Universal health care won't work—witness Medicare.* Washington, DC: The Cato Institute.

Bunce, V., & Wieske, J. (2010). *Health insurance mandates in the states 2010.* Alexandria, VA: Council for Affordable Health Insurance.

Cannon, M., & Tanner, M. (2005). *Healthy competition: What's holding back health care and how to free it.* Washington, DC: The Cato Institute.

CBPP (The Center on Budget and Policy Priorities). (2011). *Where do our federal tax dollars go? Policy basics.* Washington, DC: The Center on Budget and Policy Priorities.

Chaoulli v. Quebec. (2005). 2005 SCC 35, 1 S.C.R. 791.

Christian, S., Dower, C., & O'Neil, E. (2007). *Overview of nurse practitioner scopes of practice in the United States—discussion.* San Francisco, CA: The Center for the Health Professions.

CIHI (Canadian Institute for Health Information). (2010). *National health expenditure trends.* Ottawa, ON: Canadian Institute for Health Information.

Coleman, M., Quaresma, M., Berrino, F., Lutz, J-M., De Angelis, R., Capocaccia, R ... Young, J. (2008). Cancer survival in five continents: A worldwide population-based study (CONCORD). *Lancet Oncology, 9*, 730–756.

Day, M. (1998). You'll end up just like mum. *The New Scientist*, January 31. Retrieved from: http://www.newscientist.com/article/mg15721192.300-youll-end-up-just-like-mum.html

Donnelly, L. (2010a). Patients denied hip surgery and fertility treatment amid NHS cash crisis. *The Telegraph*, December 4. Retrieved from: http://www.telegraph.co.uk/health/healthnews/8181390/Patients-denied-hip-surgery-and-fertility-treatment-amid-NHS-cash-crisis.html

Donnelly, L. (2010b). Smokers and fat patients thrown off NHS waiting lists. *The Telegraph*, December 18. Retrieved from: http://www.telegraph.co.uk/health/healthnews/8211626/Smokers-and-fat-patients-thrown-off-NHS-waiting-lists.html

Forey, B., Hamling, J., Lee, P., & Wald, N. (Eds.). (2002). *International smoking statistics: A collection of historical data from 30 economically developed countries.* Oxford: Oxford University Press.

Goodman, J. (2005). *Health care in a free society: Rebutting the myths of national health insurance.* Cato Institute Policy Analysis, No. 532. Washington, DC: The Cato Institute.

Goodwin, J. (2010). Study: Foreign-trained doctors as good as those trained in USA. *USA Today*, August 8. Retrieved from: http://www.usatoday.com/news/health/2010-08-08-doctors-foreign-training_N.htm

Hayek, F. (1945). The use of knowledge in society. *American Economic Review, 35*, 519–530.

Herrick, D. (2010). *Why health costs are still rising. Brief analysis, No. 731.* Dallas, TX: National Center for Policy Analysis.

Herring, B., & Pauly, M. (2006). The effect of state community rating regulations on premiums and coverage in the individual health insurance market. NBER Working Paper, No. 12504. Cambridge, MA: National Bureau of Economic Research.

IMS Health (2008). *Global pharmaceutical sales by region—2007.* IMS Health. Retrieved from: http://www.imshealth.com/deployedfiles/imshealth/Global/Content/StaticFile/Top_Line_Data/GlobalSalesbyRegion.pdf

IOTF (International Obesity Task Force). (2012). *Obesity prevalence worldwide.* Retrieved from: http://www.iaso.org/iotf/obesity/

Jordan, J. (1991). Why negative rights only? *The Southern Journal of Philosophy, 29*, 245–255.

KFF (Kaiser Family Foundation). (2011). *Trends and indicators in the changing health care marketplace.* Kaiser Family Foundation. Retrieved from: http://www.kff.org/insurance/7031/index.cfm

Kim, S., Schaubel, D., Fenton, S., Leichtman, A., & Port, F. (2006). Mortality after kidney transplantation: A comparison between the United States and Canada. *American Journal of Transplantation, 6*, 109–114.

Levy, R. (2000). *Larger implications of the tobacco settlement.* Washington, DC: The Cato Institute.

Little, L. (1937). Economics and insurance. *The Review of Economic Studies, 5*, 32–52.

Max, W., Stark, B., & Root, S. (1998). Putting a lid on injury costs: The economic impact of the California motorcycle helmet law. *Journal of Trauma: Injury, Infection & Critical Care, 45*, 550–556.

NAF (National Abortion Federation). (2006). *Public funding for abortion: Medicaid and the Hyde Amendment.* Washington, DC: National Abortion Federation.

Narveson, J. (2001). *The libertarian idea.* Peterborough, Ontario: Broadview Press.

Northrup, J. (2005). The pharmaceutical sector. In L. Burns (Ed.), *The business of health care innovation* (pp. 27–102). Cambridge: Cambridge University Press.

OECD (Organization for Economic Cooperation and Development). (2010). OECD health data 2010; Frequently requested data. Retrieved from: http://www.oecd.org/document/16/0,3343,en_2649_34631_2085200_1_1_1_1,00.html

Preston, S., Glei, D., & Wilmoth, J. (2011). Contribution of smoking to international differences in life expectancy. In E. Crimmins, S. Preston, & B. Cohen (Eds.), *International differences in mortality at older ages* (pp. 105–131). Washington, DC: The National Academies Press.

Reinhardt, U., Hussey, P., & Anderson, G. (2004). US health care spending in an international context. *Health Affairs, 23*, 10–25.

Robinson, J. (1999). *The corporate practice of medicine.* London: University of California Press.

Ruiz, R. (2009). Commentary: A fat tax is a healthy idea. *CNN Politics*, October 9. Retrieved from: http://articles.cnn.com/2009-10-05/politics/ruiz.obesity.tax_1_obesity-epidemic-unhealthy-corn-farmers?_s=PM:POLITICS

Siciliani, L., & Hurst, J. (2003). *Explaining waiting times variations for elective surgery across OECD countries. OECD Health Working Paper, No. 7.* Washington, DC: OECD Publishing.

SC (Statistics Canada). (1983). *Historical statistics of Canada.* Statistics Canada. Retrieved from: http://www.statcan.gc.ca/pub/11-516-x/11-516-x1983001-eng.htm

Science Daily (2009). "Longevity gene" common among people living to 100 years old and beyond. *Science Daily*, February 4. Retrieved from: http://www.sciencedaily.com/releases/2009/02/090203081624.htm

Smith, R. (2008). Anger over NHS restrictions for osteoporosis treatment. *The Telegraph*, May 3. Retrieved from: http://www.telegraph.co.uk/health/3269270/Anger-over-restrictions-on-NHS-treatment-for-osteoporosis.html

Taranto, J. (2009). "We're going to let you die"; who said it? Hint: It wasn't Sarah Palin. *Wall Street Journal*, October 14. Retrieved from: http://bit.ly/2rppny

UN (The United Nations). (2007). *World population prospects: The 2006 revision.* New York: United Nations.

Verdecchia, A., Francisci, S., Brenner, H., Gatta, G., Micheli, A., Mangone, L., & Kunkler, I. (2007). Recent cancer survival in Europe: A 2000–02 period analysis of EUROCARE-4 data. *Lancet Oncology, 8*, 784–796.

Wachenheim, L., & Leida, H. (2007). *The impact of guaranteed issue and community rating reforms on individual insurance markets.* Seattle, WA: Milliman.

Wang, Y., Alexander, G., & Stafford, R. (2007). Outpatient hypertension treatment, treatment intensification, and control in Western Europe and the United States. *Archives of Internal Medicine, 167*, 141–147.

Waslee, T. (1992). *What has government done to our health care?* Washington, DC: The Cato Institute.

Whitman, G. (2008). *WHO's fooling who?: The World Health Organization's problematic ranking of health care systems. Cato*

Institute Briefing Papers, No. 101. Washington, DC: The Cato Institute.

Whitman, G., & Raad, R. (2009). *Bending the productivity curve: Why the US leads the world in medical innovation. Cato Institute Policy Analysis, No. 654*. Washington, DC: The Cato Institute.

WHO (World Health Organization). (2010). *World health statistics: 2010*. Geneva: World Health Organization.

Wolf-Maier, K., Cooper, R., Banegas, J., Giampaoli, S., Hense, H., Joffres, M … Vescio, F. (2003). Hypertension prevalence and blood pressure levels in 6 European countries, Canada, and the United States. *Journal of the American Medical Association, 289*, 2363–2369.

Wolf-Maier, K., Cooper, R., Kramer, H., Banegas, J., Giampaoli, S., Joffres, M … Thamm, M. (2004). Hypertension treatment and control in five European Countries, Canada, and the United States. *Hypertension, 43*, 10–17.

Zeckhauser, R. (1993). Insurance. In D. Henderson (Ed.), *The Fortune encyclopedia of economics*. New York: Warner Books.

Reply to Whitman

John Geyman

Looking over the citations in Dr Whitman's well-crafted paper extolling the claimed virtues of freedom and personal responsibility of individuals as the way to reform US healthcare, I am not surprised by these recommendations. Many of the references are to right-wing think tanks, including the Cato Institute and the National Center for Policy Analysis (NCPA). Their "research" studies are promulgated through a biased ideological perspective encompassed in their published mission statements. They selectively cull the literature for reports supporting their position, and do not meet scholarly criteria of independent evidence-based research. The well-funded NCPA, for example, announces this goal on its website: "to develop and promote private alternative to government regulation and control, solving problems by relying on the strength of the competitive, entrepreneurial private sector." Its 2002, 135-page report countered 20 "myths" about single-payer national health insurance (NHI) using distorted evidence and unproven claims (Goodman & Herrick, 2002). I rebutted those "myths" elsewhere under eight categories: access, cost containment, quality, efficiency, single-payer as solution, control of drug prices, ability for business to compete abroad, and public support for single-payer NHI (Geyman, 2005).

Dr Whitman and I do agree on some things: that uncontrolled healthcare costs are a critical problem needing containment, that patients should have maximal choice in gaining the healthcare that they need, that our healthcare system should be efficient and responsive to their individual preferences, and that there is an urgent need to reform our system. But we are looking at the elephant of healthcare from such widely divergent perspectives that we disagree on what the real problems are and how to reform US healthcare.

For openers, we disagree on the causation of the cost problem. Dr Whitman puts forward the time-worn conservative mantra of consumer-directed healthcare (CDHC) that places the burden on controlling healthcare costs on the patient. This is the concept of "moral hazard," which assumes that patients will over-utilize healthcare services if given free rein. He blames any system of third-party payment, whether private employer-sponsored insurance (ESI) or public coverage such as Medicare and Medicaid, as opening up Pandora's box. But he ignores the responsibility of the supplier side of healthcare in driving up prices and costs, a major flaw in his argument, since physicians order most healthcare services that are delivered, and they and other providers profit from them whether necessary or not.

It is not possible in this limited space to counter all the ungrounded assertions in Dr Whitman's argument that freedom trumps the need for universal healthcare in America. But these points can be made based on

Contemporary Debates in Bioethics, First Edition. Edited by Arthur L. Caplan and Robert Arp.

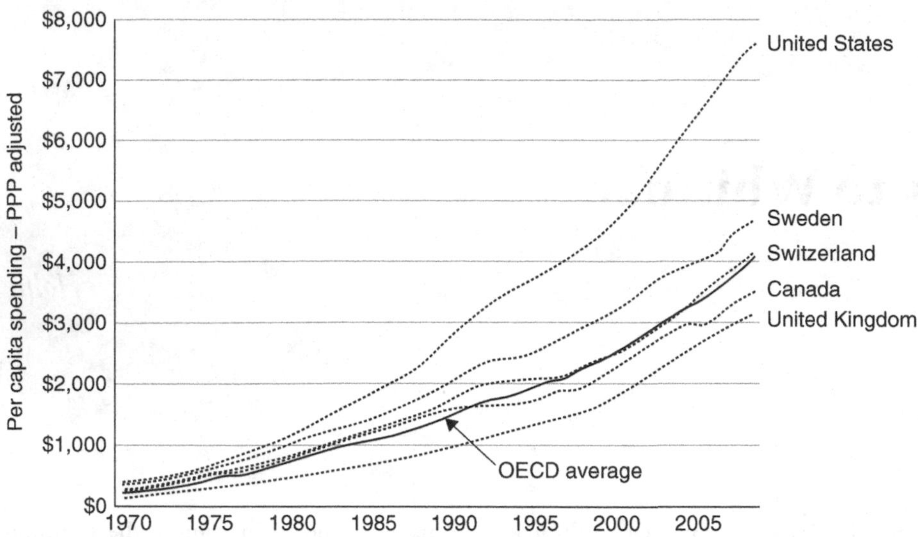

Figure cmp19.1 Growth in total health expenditures per capita, US and selected countries, 1970–2008

objective experience, national and international studies that refute some of the claims made above.

1. *CDHC and markets, after many years of trial, have failed to contain healthcare costs.* The theory of moral hazard goes back to the late 1960s (Pauly, 1968). It has provided the conceptual underpinning of the conventional theory of private health insurance since then. It holds that when patients have more "skin in the game" through such cost-sharing requirements as co-payments and deductibles, the more prudent and careful they will be in making decisions about their own healthcare. Many traditional insurance plans cover about 80% of healthcare costs (though that proportion is declining rapidly with the development of high-deductible, low-benefit plans). This theory of cost containment has been fully tested over many years, and has failed, as my Figure cmp19.1 conclusively shows (KFF, 2011).

2. *Public financing systems control costs better than privately financed healthcare.* Note my Figure cmp19.1 for growth in total health expenditures per capita comparing experience in the US from 1970 to 2008 with other advanced countries that have one or another form of universal coverage. Figure cmp19.2 shows that medical costs financed by private commercial insurance plans are considerably higher than those funded by Medicare (Blitzer, 2011). Moreover, a 2012 report on annual national health expenditures found that we are paying private insurers more than four times as much in administrative costs and profits as we are spending on government administration of health-insurance programs (Keehan et al., 2012). Case closed!

3. *Single-payer systems achieve better access, quality of care, and patient outcomes than multi-payer systems with little or no cost sharing.* Note again my table (Table 10.2), based on research by the Commonwealth Fund, comparing the US with six other advanced nations. Here are other markers that buttress this point: First, single-payer systems in most other advanced countries have minimal cost sharing (e.g., no deductibles). Patients with chronic disease are often exempted from cost sharing. A cross-national study by the National Bureau of Economic Research found in 2010 that Americans pay by far the highest out-of-pocket costs for healthcare, yet are two to five times more likely to those in other countries to reduce their use of healthcare (Lusardi et al., 2010).

Second, a comprehensive analysis of the effects of cost sharing by the Robert Wood Johnson Foundation drew this conclusion:

> Cost sharing is not well-targeted to low-value service … Caution should be used when increasing cost-sharing or low-income populations or the chronically ill. Not only

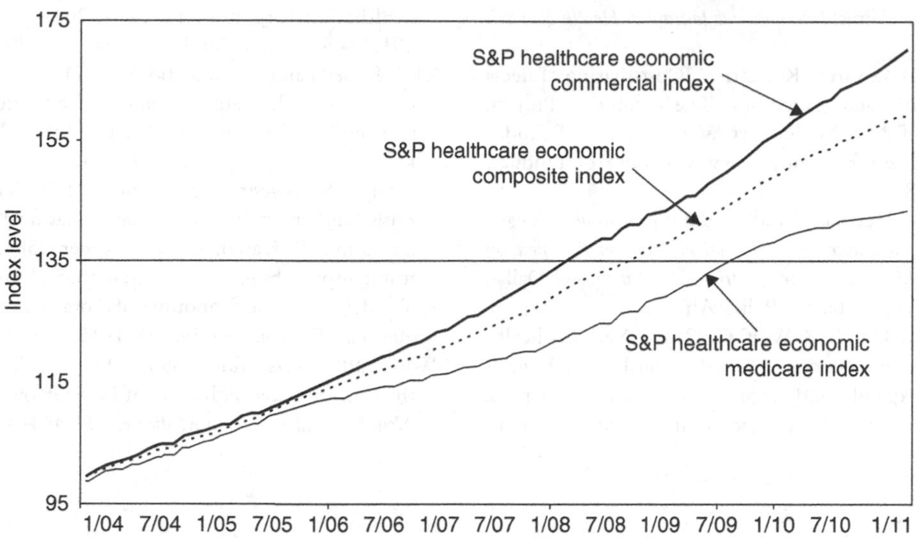

Figure cmp19.2 S&P healthcare economic indices, 12-month averages

are low-income populations disproportionately affected by increased cost sharing, but they are also more price sensitive than other income groups ... Increased cost sharing for people with chronic conditions may result in higher expenditures for hospitalizations and other adverse outcomes if necessary care is reduced. (Goodell & Swartz, 2010)

4. *The private sector restricts choice more than the public sector.* Traditional Medicare, as a single-payer program, offers patients full choice of physician and hospital wherever they are in the country. It has served as a reliable source of affordable comprehensive healthcare for 45 years. Where would we be today without this important program, which has been strongly supported by the public throughout those years? Dr Whitman's plea to eliminate health insurance and third-party payers as the enemy seems to lack any valid theoretical basis as well as any political support.

Granted, Medicare beneficiaries have restricted choice to the extent that many physicians (in the *private* sector!) will not accept new patients because of lower reimbursement under Medicare. But there are many ways in which the supposedly more efficient private sector restricts choice for patients, including changes of in-network providers and hospitals, lock-in rules preventing enrollees from making changes they desire, and withdrawal of plans from the area.

5. *Healthcare is not a commodity; unlike buying a car, it is a basic human need, regardless of ability to pay.* This quotation by Drs Steffie Woolhandler and David Himmelstein, general internists at Harvard Medical School and co-founders in the late 1980s of Physicians for a National Health Program (PNHP), makes the case in this compelling way: "In our society, some aspects of life are off-limits to commerce. We prohibit the selling of children and the buying of wives, juries, and kidneys. Tainted blood is an inevitable consequence of paying blood donors; even sophisticated laboratory tests cannot supplant the gift-giving relationship as a safeguard of the purity of blood. Like blood, healthcare is too precious, intimate, and corruptible to entrust to the market" (Woolhandler & Himmelstein, 1999).

References

Blitzer, D. (2011). US healthcare costs continue to rise, but at declining rates according to A&P Healthcare Economic Indices. *S&P Indices*, May 19. Retrieved from: http://www.standardandpoors.com/indices/sp-healthcare-economic-indices/en/us/?indexId=sp-healthcare-economic-indices

Geyman, J. (2005). Myths and memes about single-payer health insurance in the United States: A rebuttal to conservative claims. *International Journal of Health Services, 35*, 63–90.

Goodell, S., & Swartz, K. (2010). Cost-sharing: Effects on spending and outcomes. The Synthesis Project, Policy Brief No. 20, Robert Wood Johnson Foundation. Retrieved from: http://www.rwjf.org/pr/product.jsp?id=71583

Goodman, J., & Herrick, D. (2002). *Twenty myths about single-payer health insurance: International evidence on the effects of national health insurance in countries around the world*. Dallas, TX: National Center for Policy Analysis.

Keehan, S., Cuckler, F., & Wolf, C. (2012). National health expenditure projections: Modest annual growth until coverage expands and economic growth accelerates. *Health Affairs*, July 31. Retrieved from: http://content.healthaffairs.org/content/early/2012/06/11/hlthaff.2012.0404.full.pdf+html

KFF (Kaiser Family Foundation). (2011). Snapshot: Health care costs, health care spending in the United States and selected OECD countries. Retrieved from: http://www.kff.org/insurance/snapshot/oecd042111.cf

Lusardi, A., Schneider, D., & Tufano, P. (2010). The economic crisis and medical care usage. National Bureau of Economic Research, Working Paper 15843. Retrieved from: http://hbswk.hbs.edu/item/6350.html

Pauly, M. (1968). The economics of moral hazard: Comment. *American Economics Review, 58*, 1–15.

Woolhandler, S., & Himmelstein, D. (1999). When money is the mission—the high costs of investor-owned care. *The New England Journal of Medicine, 341*, 444–446.

Reply to Geyman

Glen Whitman

In general, Dr Geyman's essay confirms my fears about single-payer healthcare. Geyman affirms that his preferred system would implement global budgets and price controls, empower government bureaucrats to decide which kinds of care will and will not be covered, mandate a one-size-fits-all healthcare package for all Americans, and ban people from seeking private alternatives when the public system fails to meet their needs.

We do agree on some things. The current US system has unnecessarily high costs, is afflicted with perverse incentives that often lead to wasteful care, and suffers from a serious lack of proper cost containment. But we differ on the source of these problems and their solution.

Mischaracterization of the US System

Geyman sees the US healthcare system as a free market. He claims our "current market-based system" is supported by advocates of the "unfettered market." He says the years since 1965 "have seen the continued growth of unrestrained markets in healthcare."

This is just not true by any reasonable measure. The US has a profoundly mixed system. Healthcare markets are riddled with government intervention. The percentage of health expenditures covered by government insurance has increased steadily from 1965 onward. The percentage covered by private insurance—which, in its current form, is largely a creation of tax subsidies—has also grown significantly. Meanwhile, the percentage covered out of pocket has steadily dwindled. The number of state-level mandated benefits has increased every year, from a handful in the 1960s to over 2000 today, and continues rising by about 50 per year (CAHI, 2010).

Given a mixed system, it is a non sequitur to blame every problem on markets. My chapter discusses the economic reasons to blame government instead.

Hostility to Markets

Geyman's essay evinces a general mistrust of markets. He repeatedly points to profit-seeking as the malevolent force behind US healthcare problems. If his diagnosis were correct, then his argument should apply more broadly; we should want single-payer for everything. But when we look at other goods and services, we find that profit-seeking enterprises frequently provide high-quality output at falling prices. Walmart and other warehouse stores have succeeded in providing low-income people with clothing and other goods at affordable prices (see, e.g., Basker, 2005). Grain prices have trended downward for the better part of a century, recent spikes notwithstanding (Sumner,

Contemporary Debates in Bioethics, First Edition. Edited by Arthur L. Caplan and Robert Arp.

2009). High-tech products, such as computers and audio equipment, commonly start with high prices and then rapidly become affordable to almost anyone—for instance, a DVD player in the mid-1990s would have cost $500 or more; now you can get one for $50 or less.

These examples illustrate a general principle: in a competitive market, profits provide firms with an incentive to perform better. To avoid losing business to their rivals, they must offer price–value combinations that customers prefer. Cost-cutting efforts that reduce quality must usually be accompanied by compensating price reductions. If these market processes are not functioning well in healthcare, we should ask what specific factors are impeding them; blaming "profit" is not a satisfying answer. Geyman mentions "market failure," but he does not elaborate. Some healthcare analysts point to adverse selection and moral hazard as sources of market failure in insurance, but these problems have largely been solved in other insurance markets. In healthcare, regulations have stymied the usual market solutions.

Geyman repeats the common assertion that government programs like Medicare have lower administrative costs than market firms. Again, if this argument were generally true, then we should prefer single-payer systems in every industry. Why don't we? Because administration serves important functions, like monitoring wasteful usage and searching for quality improvements. The bloated budgets of government agencies, like the Department of Defense, can be traced in part to ineffective administration. As Michael Cannon puts it, "Medicare keeps its measured administrative-cost ratio relatively low by avoiding important administrative activities (which shrinks the numerator) and tolerating vast amounts of wasteful and fraudulent claims (which inflates the denominator). That is a vice, yet advocates of a new government program praise it as a virtue" (Cannon, 2009, p. 4).

Geyman's aversion to markets is so great that he even calls "consumer" a "bad word." This is simply bizarre. Under any system, patients consume medical goods and services. Therefore, they are consumers, by definition. Pretending they are not does not repeal the laws of economics.

Misplaced Concern with Inequality

When Geyman says, "In cross-national studies, the US ranks 37th for health outcomes and 54th for fairness of financing," he is referring to the WHO's ranking of healthcare systems, which I briefly criticized in my chapter. I will expand on that critique here.

The WHO ranking system is based on five factors. Three of them, accounting for 62.5% of the index's total weight, are "disparity" measures (including a financial-fairness measure). Disparity measures do not measure actual healthcare performance; they measure *differences* in performance. To see why this does not make sense, imagine two countries: country A, where healthcare is *mediocre* for everyone; and country B, where half the population has *good* healthcare, and the other half has *great* healthcare. Any reasonable person would prefer country B's system—but on a disparity measure, country A would get a better score because it is more equal.

Put differently, disparity measures measure *relative* quality: do the rich get better care than the poor? But what we should care about is *absolute* quality: are the poor getting good care? Disparity measures are the wrong way to answer that question.

The financial-fairness measure is flawed in an additional way. Given how it is calculated, a country gets a worse financial-fairness score if some households spend an especially large fraction of their income on healthcare. But a country also gets a worse score if some households spend an especially *small* fraction of their income on healthcare. In other words, the US is penalized because Bill Gates spends too little of his income on healthcare. Note also that the 37th place rank for "health outcomes" is not independent of the 54th place rank for "financial fairness," because the latter is included when calculating the former. The WHO rankings are flawed in other ways as well, documented in my extended essay on the subject (Whitman, 2008).

Rose-Colored Single-Payer Glasses

For all the warts Geyman spies on the status quo, he sees few if any flaws with single-payer. He paints a something-for-nothing picture of single-payer as simple, high-quality, and low-cost. The realistic picture of single-payer is not so pretty.

To the extent single-payer systems control costs, they do so by denying care through global budgets, price controls, bureaucratic rulings, and long lines. If their citizens have a "right" to healthcare, it is a right to only as much care as the government decides to provide, and no more. Some systems, including Geyman's ideal, prohibit people from arranging to get covered services outside the system.

The assumption of greater fairness and equality under single-payer is questionable. Single-payer systems also display disparities in the care provided to ethnic minorities, for instance (Goodman, 2010). This should be no surprise: higher-status citizens have greater odds of working the system to get what they want. Contrary to the claim that single-payer systems reduce the correlation between income and health, a recent study shows that "the health-income gradient is slightly steeper in Canada than it is in the US" (O'Neill & O'Neill, 2007). In 2010, an estimated 44,794 Canadians, or 1% of all Canadian patients, traveled to another country for treatment (Esmail, 2010)—an option available mainly to the well-to-do.

Geyman rails against the involvement of special interests in shaping current policy, but special interests would continue to have their say in a single-payer system. Our single-payer Department of Defense does not curb the lobbying efforts of defense contractors; indeed, it was the entanglement of Defense with its contractors that led President Eisenhower to coin the term "military–industrial complex." A single-payer healthcare system could further engorge the growing "medical–industrial complex."

According to Geyman, there would be no "cost-sharing" with patients in his system. Yet cost-sharing is the *only* means of controlling costs that still permits individual choice. His hostility to HMOs is ironic, given that single-payer systems share all the same problems. The doctor's conflict of interest—between the patient on one hand and the payer on the other—is not avoided by substituting one payer for another. The government health administration, too, would be under pressure to control costs. And its monopoly position would prevent patients from choosing another insurance provider if its cost-control measures were too strict.

Geyman approvingly cites medical ethicist Edmund Pellegrino, who asks, "Is a universal code even possible in our multicultural, morally pluralistic, democratic society?" That is an excellent question—one that poses a far greater dilemma for a single-payer system than a decentralized one. Geyman does not seem to recognize this.

I will conclude by citing one more thing upon which Geyman and I agree. He repeats the adage, "He who pays the piper calls the tune." Exactly. So, the relevant question is: Whom do you want calling the tune in personal healthcare decisions: patients or the government?

References

Basker, E. (2005). Selling a cheaper mousetrap: Wal-Mart's effect on retail prices. *Journal of Urban Economics, 58*, 203–229.

CAHI (The Council for Affordable Health Insurance). (2010). *Trends in state-mandated benefits, 2010.* Alexandria, VA: The Council for Affordable Health Insurance.

Cannon, M. (2009). *Fannie Med? Why a 'public option' is hazardous to your health. Cato Institute Policy Analysis, No. 6.* Washington, DC: The Cato Institute.

Esmail, N. (2010). Leaving Canada for medical care. *Fraser Forum, 3/4*, 19–21.

Goodman, J. (2010). Health care for profit. National Center for Policy Analysis. Retrieved from: http://healthblog.ncpa.org/health-care-for-profit/

O'Neill, J., & O'Neill, D. (2007). Health status, health care and inequality: Canada vs. the US The National Bureau of Economic Research, Working Paper No. 13429. Retrieved from: http://www.nber.org/papers/w13429

Sumner, D. (2009). Recent commodity price movements in historical perspective. *American Journal of Agricultural Economics, 91*, 1250–1256.

Whitman, G. (2008). *WHO's fooling who?: The World Health Organization's problematic ranking of health care systems. Cato Institute Briefing Papers, No. 101.* Washington, DC: The Cato Institute.

Part 11

Is There a Legitimate Place for Human Genetic Enhancement?

Introduction

In August of 2011, Dr Carl June and his team of researchers at the University of Pennsylvania Abramson Cancer Center reported that they had genetically engineered T cells to recognize and attack the protein CD19 located on the surface of cancerous cells. They then injected these T cells into three patients suffering from chronic lymphocytic leukemia, and, after a year's time, two of the patients were completely cancer-free, while the third was 70% cancer-free (Bazell, 2011; Porter et al., 2011). This was a clear case of *somatic gene therapy*, which aims at the treatment or prevention of a disease by isolating a segment of DNA containing a gene sequence from the somatic cell of one organism—called a *transgene*—and introducing it into the genome of a different organism. Cases of successful somatic gene therapy in various species of organisms other than humans are legion (see the references in Giacca, 2010). Other cases of somatic gene therapy in humans that indicate varied levels of success include Francesca Simonelli et al.'s (2010) treatment of subjects suffering from Leber's congenital amaurosis (a disease causing blindness) who improved their sight, as well as more than 20 subjects suffering from adenosine deaminase-deficient severe combined immunodeficiency (ADA-SCID, also called *bubble boy disease* because of the fact that many people suffering from the disease have had to live in a plastic enclosed environment) whose immune systems improved in treatments documented between 2000 and 2010 (Ferrua et al., 2010; also Sheridan, 2011).

Whereas, in somatic gene therapy, it is the individual organism's genome that is changed, and any effects are restricted to that individual, the goal of *germ-line gene therapy* is to engineer the individual organism's germ cells (sperm cells or egg cells) in such a way that the modification is inherited by the individual's offspring. One can imagine the benefits of this kind of therapy—the primary one being that it would prevent the inheritance of some genetically based diseases, even

Contemporary Debates in Bioethics, First Edition. Edited by Arthur L. Caplan and Robert Arp.

wiping some disease out of the gene pool altogether (Zimmerman, 1991; Walters & Palmer, 1997). There are countless examples of germ-line gene therapy success stories dealing with bacteria, plants, and numerous animal species (see, for example, the references in Elias & Annas, 1992 and Nielson, 1997; also Akhtar et al., 2011; Beltran et al., 2011). However, there is a general worldwide ban on germ-line gene therapy for humans and the other ape species for many reasons, a primary one articulated in a report prepared by members of a working group for the American Association for the Advancement of Science in 2000 which still holds true today:

> Members of the working group concluded that it is not now possible to undertake inheritable genetic modification (IGM) safely and responsibly. For IGM technologies to meet safety standards, there must be evidence that the procedures used do not cause unacceptable short-term or long-term consequences either for the treated individual or succeeding generations of offspring. This means that an altered embryo must be able to transit all human developments without a mishap due to the induced intervention. And for those techniques that add foreign material, there must be multigenerational data showing that the modification or improvement of a specific genetically determined trait is stable and effective and does not interfere with the functioning of other genes. (Frankel & Chapman, 2000, p. 23; also Marshall, 2000)

And apparently, stable and safe conditions analogous to those mentioned above have not even been met satisfactorily in animal germ-line gene therapies (Woods et al., 2006; Stein et al., 2010; Aronovich et al., 2011). So, it is no wonder that there is concern about such therapies for humans. Also, many methods of developing and creating materials to be used in germ-line animal therapy involve the destruction of embryos, so a ban on human-embryo experimentation—including reproductive human cloning—is tantamount to a ban on human germ-line gene therapy (see the language in UNDHC, 2005; Johnson & Williams, 2006; NCSL, 2011; Public Agenda, 2011).

Yet, there are plenty of thinkers who argue that germ-line gene therapy ought to be pursued for the nonhuman great apes, and eventually humans, too (Neel, 1993; Resnik, 1994; Schneider & Coutelle, 1999; Núñez-Mujica, 2006; cf. Schatten & Mitalipov, 2009; Cornetta & Meslin, 2011). Fritz Allhoff (2005), for example, asks us:

> Consider Huntington's chorea, which results from a single defective gene. In this particular case, the problem stems from a single gene—on chromosome 4—that issues excessive calls for glutamine production, and deletion of an appropriate string of the gene would wholly preclude this terrible affliction. In such cases, and presupposing safe and effective procedures, it would be entirely unreasonable to deny the moral legitimacy of the therapy. Even those who stand somewhat opposed to genetic interventions would grant that "it would be cruel, if not stupid, to suggest that we ought never to use genetic technology to heal the sick. (p. 27; Allhoff's quotation from Parens, 1995, p. 151)

Regardless of ideology—be it secular or religious—most people would agree that (1) doing away with unnecessary suffering, (2) eradicating disease, and (3) extending human life are all good things that should be pursued. In fact, in many ways, (1)–(3) form the basis for the human pursuit of gene therapy, as well as medicine in general. But what about using genetic engineering and advanced medical technologies to make a person taller, faster, stronger, or smarter? After all, the striving for human perfection of body and mind is as old as the early hominins who began to conceive of such a striving. A parent of a short, big-eared, somewhat feeble, emotionally immature child, for example, knows the headaches and heartaches of that child's interactions in grade school. And to save that child from painful interactions—including name-calling, bullying, manipulating, and others—what parent would not wish that her/his child had better (or at least statistically normal) physical, intellectual, and emotional capacities to at least level the social playing field, so to speak?

While the goal of genetic therapy is the treatment or prevention of a disease, disorder, or disability in an organism, the goal of *genetic enhancement* is the augmentation, increase, magnification, or enhancement of some capability or trait in an organism. For example, scientists have been able to genetically enhance mice to create "mighty mice" and "smart mice" that have enhanced strength and mental abilities. A second copy of the gene NR2B that makes the NMDA neuroreceptor—which is central to memory function—was added to these smart mice, causing them to remember and learn faster as they negotiated complex mazes more easily than their nonenhanced rodent counterparts. The smart mice were also able to retain these mental abilities into their latest stages of life, rivaling the intelligence of much younger mice. Interestingly enough, humans also have the same NR2B gene, fueling speculation that it is possible to create smart humans (Tang et al., 1999). Genetic enhancement has yielded super-bacteria, flies, mosquitoes, fish, rats, cows, dogs, cats, and monkeys, among other species of animals and plants (see the references in LeVine, 2006; also Melo et al., 2007). If you are an American, the trout or pork you eat may soon be from genetically enhanced animals, while there is almost no doubt that some of the corn- or soy-based products you ingest this week will be from genetically enhanced seeds (Parekh, 2004; Hillstrom, 2012).

It is important to draw attention to the distinction between therapy and enhancement, since there are cases where the same procedure, process, activity, or treatment regimen will be an instance of therapy for one person, but enhancement for another. For example, beta blockers are a class of drugs used regularly to treat heart arrhythmias, hypertension, and other cardiac diseases; but they also have the side effect of steadying one's hands. Einer Elhauge (2011) recounts the story of a sharpshooter in the 2008 Olympics who was stripped of his silver medal after it was discovered that he had taken beta blockers to help steady his aim in the 50 m free pistol competition. In 2007, Parvin Hakimi and researchers created "mighty mice" who could run 3½ miles for 6 h straight through over expression of the gene for the enzyme, phosphoenolypyruvate carboxykinases (PEPCK-C) (Hakimi et al., 2007). This gene is also found in humans. We can conceive of a person who lacks PEPCK-C benefitting from an overexpression of PEPCK-C to make up for the lack. We can also conceive of some nation trying to breed the ultimate warrior class of people by overexpressing—and hence enhancing—an already-normal level of PEPCK-C.

Genetic enhancement has been equated with *eugenics*, a term coined by the evolutionary biologist, Sir Francis Galton, in a footnote in his 1883 work, *Inquiries into Human Faculty and its Development* (Galton, 1883): "We greatly want a brief word to express the science of improving stock, which is by no means confined to questions of judicious mating, but which, especially in the case of man, takes cognisance of all influences that tend in however remote a degree to give to the more suitable races or strains of blood a better chance of prevailing speedily over the less suitable than they otherwise would have had. The word *eugenics* would sufficiently express the idea ..." And this idea had already been debated and discussed throughout the nineteenth century by Darwin (1871) and Thomas Malthus (1798/1959) in *An Essay on the Principle of Population*: "It does not ... seem impossible," claimed Malthus, "that by an attention to breed, a certain degree of improvement, similar to that among animals, might take place among men. Whether intellect could be communicated may be a matter of doubt; but size, strength, beauty, complexion, and perhaps longevity are in a degree transmissible" (p. 60).

Unfortunately, this "science of improving stock" idea—coupled with uninformed manipulations of Darwin's notion of natural selection, Herbert Spencer's notion of survival of the fittest, and the German idealist's notions of will—led to forced sterilization and racial cleansing in many parts of the world during the early part of the twentieth century (Proctor, 1988; Caplan, 1992), as well as to human experimentation, compulsory abortions and euthanasia, forced relocation, and the murder of millions of people deemed *Untermensch* ("under/sub human" or "undesirable") by the Nazis in the Final Solution and other *Rassenreinheit*—"racial purity"—programs of the Third Reich. "He who talks of the German people as having a mission to fulfill on this earth," claimed Hitler (1925–1926/1939) in *Mein Kampf*, "must know that this cannot be fulfilled except by the building up of a State whose highest purpose is to preserve and promote those nobler elements of our race and of the whole of mankind that have remained unimpaired" (p. 341). And Hitler definitely agreed with the philosopher Arthur Schopenhauer (1851/1970) that the "highest civilization and culture ... are found exclusively among the white races; and even with many dark peoples, the ruling caste or race is fairer in color than the rest" (p. 154).

In 1907, Indiana in the US passed the first sterilization law in the world meant to prevent "imbeciles" primarily in mental institutions from continuing to have children. Several countries around the world and another 30 US states would be enforcing sterilization laws by 1920. Even though the sterilization law in Indiana was overturned in 1921 by the Indiana Supreme Court, in 1927 the US Supreme Court upheld the State's right to forced sterilization in *Buck v. Bell* (274 US 200). By the early 1960s, well over 60,000 American men and women deemed to be "defective" because they were criminals, mentally ill, or mentally disabled had been sterilized. And it was the research and theories associated with eugenics—both scientific and religious—that provided the justification for sterilization to purge "impurities" that were considered detrimental to the "racial purity" of American society (Rosen, 2004; Lombardo, 2008, 2011; Bashford & Levine, 2010).

Hitler was aware of the US's eugenics position codified in *Buck v. Bell* when he wrote *Mein Kampf* (Kuhl, 1994; Lifton, 2000). And numerous nations by the mid-twentieth century adopted eugenics-based policies based upon the writings, ideas, and funding of Charles P. Davenport, Henry H. Goddard, Madison Grant, Harry H. Laughlin, and J. H. Kellogg of breakfast cereal fame (Carlson, 2001; Selden, 2005; Turda, 2010). Kyle Munkittrick rightly notes that "the phrase 'human enhancement' conjures *Gattaca*, Frankenstein's creature, and the social engineering of Huxley's *Brave New World*. The religious have their hells and their demons, while those of us with a more scientific disposition have our dystopias and Big Brothers." Eugenics-based ideas of racial purity were part and parcel to totalitarian regimes of the mid-twentieth century, where the so-called goods of the state trampled on the rights and freedoms of the individual (Caplan, 1992; Spitz, 2005). Note here how Hitler (1925–6/1939) prefers the dim-witted Superman to the critically thinking individual:

> Accordingly the State which is grounded on the racial idea must start with the principle that a person whose formal education in the sciences is relatively small but who is physically sound and robust, of a steadfast and honest character, ready and able to make decisions and endowed with strength of will, is a more useful member of the national community than a weakling who is scholarly and refined. A nation composed of learned men who are physical weaklings, hesitant about decisions of the will, and timid pacifists, is not capable of assuring even its own existence on this earth. (p. 349)

Genetic enhancement need not necessarily be equated with the negativity and atrocities of Hitler and Huxley, however (Caplan et al., 1998). For instance, *transhumanism* profoundly rejects the historical practices associated with eugenics, yet preserves the idea that "we can become better than human through technology. Unguided, natural evolution has done all it could hope to do. Transhumanists believe that from here on out, humans should take up the reins and craft the evolution of our species using nanotech, genetics, pharmaceuticals, and augmentations to go above and beyond our biology" (Munkittrick, 2011). And the final point of the Transhumanist Declaration from Humanity+ is the furthest thing from the slavery and injustice associated with fascist or communist totalitarianism, noting that people should have "wide personal choice over how they enable their lives. This includes use of techniques that may be developed to assist memory, concentration, and mental energy; life extension therapies; reproductive choice technologies; cryonics procedures; and many other possible human modification and enhancement technologies" (TD, 2012).

The concept, methodologies, and implementation of genetic enhancement can be separated from the now-debunked, pseudo-science of eugenics and its associated injustices and atrocities. The first author in this section, Nicholas Agar, is well aware of this distinction. Setting aside issues of eugenics, then, human genetic enhancement still presents us with two major concerns, which Agar addresses in his chapter. The first is the genetically enhanced "haves" being in an advantaged position over the nongenetically enhanced "have nots," or, as Princeton biologist Lee Silver puts it, given the close connection between genetic enhancement and the amount of money to *pay for* enhancements, "GenRich" versus the "GenPoor" (Silver, 1997). Agar offers a commonsense response, noting that issues of fairness concerning the rich and poor in a society transcend the human genetic enhancement debate; genetic enhancement opportunities, like any other opportunity, are subject to issues of fairness, but that does not mean that one should not genetically enhance *because* the rich have greater access to such an opportunity.

A second major concern with genetic enhancement has to do with the fact that when you genetically enhance human, you are changing the genes of potential future persons without their consent (see the papers in Savulescu & Bostrom, 2009). And such an action seems, prima facie, to be a violation of one's autonomy. Agar's response to this is to note that the majority of one's traits and abilities are a combination of genetic *and* environmental factors—a position he calls *interactionism*—and even if one's abilities have been genetically enhanced, it is still possible to counteract the enhancement so that it never comes to full fruition. As Agar notes, someone with an Einstein-like intellectual enhancement might choose to be a "feckless computer hacker or a sporadically employed laborer."

Agar makes a distinction between what he calls *radical enhancement* and *moderate enhancement*: "Radical enhancement is enhancement of a degree incompatible with values associated with being human. Moderate enhancements are of a lesser degree and, as such, are not incompatible with these values." Echoing what is known as the "yuck" argument, a term coined by Arthur Caplan (Schmidt, 2008) used by various thinkers to object to the cloning of humans, Agar rejects radical enhancement on the intuitive ground that we "sense a moral intrusion into nature's way of making things" when we engage in such practices. On the other hand, moderate enhancements are on a par with environmental enhancements, according to Agar, so that it makes no difference, for example, whether one's nutrition is improved in one's life genetically or through eating according to the World Health Organization's official diet. In this sense, the intuition that people have concerning the morality of genetic therapy, which is aimed at the treatment or prevention of a disease, would seem to be on a par with the intuition regarding *moderate* genetic enhancement, which is aimed at the augmentation or magnification of some capability or trait.

The second author in this section, Edwin Black, thinks that Agar's argument is a slippery slope. While mindful of Agar's distinction between moderate and radical enhancement, Black still thinks that: "Despite the magniloquent anti-cloning and anti-enhancement declarations of multilateral and multinational bodies, there is no law in any land on earth that can be invoked to stop the genetic trespass that will begin with cloning the cutest pets and proceed predictably into the mindset of the Third Reich." Black knows that humans continually strive to better their bodies and minds: "Certainly, the concept of improving human existence through modification of the environment is as old as humankind itself." However, he also knows that history has been rife with Frankensteins and Führers "playing God" and causing innocent people deemed to be abnormal, non-Aryan, ugly, or unworthy to suffer and die.

After detailing key moments in Western history dealing with racial purity and eugenics—including the positions of Plato and Aristotle—Black's argument is intuitive, but straightforward: "Now, the urge to improve mankind has again reared its head, this time based not on race but ona sense of real, engineered genetic superiority." But, as Black notes, this kind of genetic engineering "has already been tried—more than once. It culminated in a War Against the Weak."

However, as Agar notes in his reply to Black: "There are (very) many differences between Hitler's eugenics and a program of genetic enhancement that might be acceptable to the citizens of a culturally diverse, early twenty-first century, liberal democracy." Agar cautions against any slippery slope kind of argument, as the temptation oftentimes is to conclude erroneously that one will wind up at the bottom of the slope just because it is slippery all throughout. It is possible to *conceptually* divorce genetic enhancement from eugenics, for sure; but any human-enhancement programs of the future will undoubtedly be informed by the eugenics of days gone by, with the hope that none of the injustices and atrocities associated with eugenics will be repeated. Whether that hope is warranted remains to be seen.

References

Akhtar, N., Akram, M., Asif, H., Usmanghani, K., Shah, S . . ., & Ahmad, K. (2011). Gene therapy: A review article. *Journal of Medicinal Plants Research*, *5*, 1812–1817.

Allhoff, F. (2005). Germ-line genetic enhancement and Rawlsian primary goods. *Kennedy Institute of Ethics Journal*, *15*, 26–33.

Aronovich, E., McIvor, R., & Hackett, P. (2011). The Sleeping Beauty transposon system: A non-viral vector for gene therapy. *Human Molecular Genetics*, *20*, R14–R20.

Bashford, A., & Levine, P. (Ed.). (2010). *The Oxford handbook of the history of eugenics*. Oxford: Oxford University Press.

Bazell, R. (2011). New leukemia treatment exceeds "wildest expectations." *MSNBC*, August 10. Retrieved from:

http://www.msnbc.msn.com/id/44090512/#.TkLfM2GsCCU

Beltran, W., Cideciyan, A., Lewin, A., Iwabe, S., Khanna, H ..., & Aguirre, G. (2011). Gene therapy rescues photoreceptor blindness in dogs and paves the way for treating human X-linked retinitis pigmentosa. *Proceedings of the National Academy of the Sciences: USA*, *109*, 2132–2137.

Caplan, A. (Ed.). (1992). *When medicine went mad: Bioethics and the Holocaust.* Totowa, NJ: Humana Press.

Caplan, A., McGee, G., & Magnus, D. (1998). What is immoral about Eugenics? *American Journal of Public Health*, *319*, 184–185.

Carlson, E. (2001). *The unfit: A history of a bad idea.* Cold Spring Harbor NY: Cold Spring Harbor Press.

Cornetta, K., & Meslin, E. (2011). Ethical and scientific issues in gene therapy and stem cell research. In R. Chadwick, H. ten Have, & E. Meslin (Eds.), *The SAGE handbook of health care ethics* (pp. 356–367). London: Sage Publications.

Darwin, C. (1871). *The descent of man and selection in relation to sex.* London: D. Appleton and Company.

Elhauge, E. (2011). A little lower than God: What should limit our effort to redesign humans? Petrie-Flom Center for Health Law Policy, Biotechnology and Bioethics Reports. Retrieved from: http://www.law.yale.edu/documents/pdf/LEO/LEO_Elhauge_Little LowerThan God.pdf

Elias, S., & Annas, G. (1992). Somatic and germline gene therapy. In G. Annas & S. Elias (Eds.), *Gene mapping: Using law and ethics as guides* (pp. 142–154). Oxford: Oxford University Press.

Ferrua, F., Brigida, I., & Aiuti, A. (2010). Update on gene therapy for adenosine deaminase-deficient severe combined immunodeficiency. *Current Opinion in Allergy and Clinical Immunology*, *10*(6), 551–556.

Frankel, M., & Chapman, A. (2000). Human inheritable genetic modifications: Assessing scientific, ethical, religious, and policy issues. Retrieved from: http://www.aaas.org/spp/sfrl/projects/germline/report.pdf

Galton, F. (1883). *Inquiries into human faculty and its development.* New York: Macmillan and Company.

Giacca, M. (2010). *Gene therapy.* New York: Springer.

Hakimi, P., Yang, J., Casadesus, G., Massillon, D., Tolentino-Silva, F ... Hanson, R. (2007). Over expression of the cytosolic form of phosphoenolpyruvate carboxykinase (GTP) in skeletal muscle repatterns energy metabolism in the mouse. *The Journal of Biological Chemistry*, *282*, 32844–32845.

Hillstrom, K. (2012). *Genetically modified foods.* Farmington Hills, MI: Lucent Books.

Hitler, A. (1925–1926/1939). *Mein kampf.* J. Murphy (Trans.). London: Hurst and Blackette.

Johnson, J., & Williams, E. (2006). CRS report for Congress: Human cloning. Retrieved from: http://www.fas.org/sgp/crs/misc/RL31358.pdf

Kuhl, S. (1994). *The Nazi connection: Eugenics, American racism, and German national socialism.* Oxford: Oxford University Press.

LeVine, H. (2006). *Genetic engineering.* Santa Barbara, CA: ABC-CLIO.

Lifton, R. (2000). *The Nazi doctors: Medical killing and the psychology of genocide.* New York: Basic Books.

Lombardo, P. (2008). *Three generations, no imbeciles: Eugenics, the Supreme Court, and Buck v. Bell.* Baltimore, MD: Johns Hopkins University Press.

Lombardo, P. (Ed.). (2011). *A century of eugenics in America: From the Indiana experiment to the genome era.* Bloomington: Indiana University Press.

Malthus, T. (1798/1959). *An essay on the principle of population.* Ann Arbor, MI: University of Michigan Press.

Marshall, E. (2000). Moratorium urged on germ line gene therapy. *Science*, *289*, 2023.

Munkittrick, K. (2011). Debating extreme human enhancement. *Slate*, September 13. Retrieved from: http://www.slate.com/articles/technology/future_tense/features/2011/debating_extreme_human_enhancement/should_we_use_nanotech_genetics_pharmaceuticals_and_augmentations_to_go_above_and_beyond_our_biology.html

Melo, E., Canavessi, A., Franco, M., & Rumpf, R. (2007). Animal transgenesis: State of the art and applications. *Journal of Applied Genetics*, *48*, 47–61.

NCSL (National Conference of State Legislatures). (2011). Human cloning laws. Retrieved from: http://www.ncsl.org/default.aspx?tabid=14284

Neel, J. (1993). Germ-line gene therapy: Another view. *Human Gene Therapy*, *4*, 127–128.

Nielson, T. (1997). Human germline gene therapy. *McGill Journal of Medicine*, *3*, 126–132.

Núñez-Mujica, G. (2006). The ethics of enhancing animals, specifically the great apes. *The Jounral of Personal Cyberconsciousness*, *1*, 1–15.

Parekh, S. (Ed.). (2004). *The GMO handbook: genetically modified animals, microbes, and plants in biotechnology.* Totowa, NJ: Humana Press.

Parens, E. (1995). The goodness of fragility: On the prospect of genetic technologies aimed at the enhancement of human capacities. *Kennedy Institute of Ethics Journal*, *5*, 141–153.

Porter, D., Levine, B., Kalos, M., Bagg, A., & June, C. (2011). Chimeric antigen receptor-modified T cells in chronic lymphoid leukemia. *The New England Journal of Medicine*, *365*, 725–733.

Proctor, R. (1988). *Racial hygiene: medicine under the Nazis.* Cambridge, MA: Harvard University Press.

Public Agenda. (2011). Countries with bans on human cloning and/or genetic engineering. Retrieved from: http://www.publicagenda.org/charts/countries-bans-human-cloning-andor-genetic-engineering

Resnik, D. (1994). Debunking the slippery slope argument against human germ-line gene therapy. *The Journal of Medicine & Philosophy*, *19*, 23–40.

Rosen, C. (2004). *Preaching eugenics: Religious leaders and the American eugenics movement*. Oxford: Oxford University Press.

Savulescu, J., & Bostrom, N. (Eds.). (2009). *Human enhancement*. Oxford: Oxford University Press.

Schatten, G., & Mitalipov, S. (2009). Developmental biology: Transgenic primate offsrping. *Nature*, *459*, 515–516.

Schmidt, C. (2008). The yuck factor: When disgust meets discovery. *Environmental Health Perspectives*, *116*, A524–A527.

Schneider, H., & Coutelle, C. (1999). In utero gene therapy: The case for. *Nature Medicine*, *5*, 256–257.

Schopenhauer, A. (1851/1970). *Essays and aphorisms* (R. J. Hollingdale, Trans.). London: Penguin Books.

Selden, S. (2005). Transforming better babies into fitter families: Archival resources and the history of the American eugenics movement, 1908–1930. *American Philosophical Society*, *149*, 199–225.

Sheridan, C. (2011). Gene therapy finds its niche. *Nature Biotechnology*, *29*, 121–128.

Silver, L. (1997). *Remaking Eden: Cloning and beyond in a brave new world*. New York: Harper Perennial.

Simonelli, F., Maguire, A., Testa, F., Pierce, E., Mingozzi, F ..., & Auricchio, A. (2010). Gene therapy for Leber's congenital amaurosis is safe and effective through 1.5 years after vector administration. *Molecular Therapy*, *18*(3), 643–650.

Spitz, V. (2005). *Doctors from hell: The horrific account of Nazi experiments on humans*. Boulder, CO: Sentient Publications.

Stein S., Ott, M., Schultze-Strasser, S., Jauch, A., Burwinkel, B ..., & Grez, M. (2010). Genomic instability and myelodysplasia with monosomy 7 consequent to EVI1 activation after gene therapy for chronic granulomatous disease. *Nature Medicine*, *16*, 198–204.

Tang, Y-P., Shimizu, E., Dube, G., Rampon, C., Kerchner, G ... Tsien, J. (1999). Genetic enhancement of learning and memory in mice. *Nature*, *401*, 63–69.

TD (Transhumanist Declaration of Humanity+). (2012). Retrieved from: http://humanityplus.org/philosophy/transhumanist-declaration/

Turda, M. (2010). Race, science and eugenics in the twentieth century. In A. Bashford & P. Levine (Eds.), *The Oxford handbook of the history of eugenics* (pp. 62–80). Oxford: Oxford University Press.

UNDHC (United Nations Declaration on Human Cloning). (2005). Retrieved from: http://www.bioeticaweb.com/content/view/1267/765/lang,es/

Walters, L., & Palmer, J. (1997). *The ethics of human gene therapy*. Oxford: Oxford University Press.

Woods, N., Bottero, V., Schmidt, M., von Kalle, C., & Verma, I. (2006). Gene therapy: Therapeutic gene causing lymphoma. *Nature*, *440*, 1123.

Zimmerman, B. (1991). Human germ-line therapy: The case for its development and use. *The Journal of Medicine and Philosophy*, *16*, 593–612.

Chapter Twenty One

There Is a Legitimate Place for Human Genetic Enhancement

Nicholas Agar

In this chapter, I argue for a limited prerogative to genetically enhance human abilities. Genetic enhancements, considered as a category, should not be morally distinguished from environmental enhancements, considered as a category. We recognize some educational enhancements as morally acceptable, and so too we should recognize some genetic enhancements as morally acceptable. On the way to this conclusion, I reject five ways in which genetic enhancements might be systematically more morally problematic than environmental enhancements. I do not endorse all genetic enhancements, drawing a distinction between moderate and radical enhancements. I conclude with an argument that one difference between good and bad enhancements is of degree—enhancement is something that one can have too much of.

Introduction

This chapter defends the genetic enhancement of some human abilities. These abilities include mental traits such as intelligence and physical traits such as athletic endurance. The first step in this defense is to reject the idea that an enhancement's being genetic matters morally. The technologies of genetic selection or modification are some among many ways in which human characteristics may be enhanced. I will argue that there is no principled moral difference between enhancing intelligence by selecting or modifying genes and achieving the same end by selecting or modifying environmental influences.

We should not conclude from enhancement's ubiquity that it is morally unproblematic. Indeed, there are limits on a moral permission to genetically enhance. Enhancements of a degree that I shall call *moderate* are compatible with human values. These include boosting one's IQ by a few points or extending one's life span by a small number of years. More extreme enhancements, those that I shall label *radical*, conflict with human values. What marks off radical enhancements from moderate enhancements is that the former improve significant attributes and abilities to levels that *greatly exceed* what is currently possible for human beings. They include 100-fold enhancements of normal human intelligence and millennial life spans. I indicate how this appeal to human values can be made principled and to show how it helps to sort morally acceptable from unacceptable genetic enhancements. The degree of human enhancement is a more appropriate focus for our concerns than is the distinction between enhancements resulting from the manipulation of human genes and those resulting from the manipulation of human environments.

Contemporary Debates in Bioethics, First Edition. Edited by Arthur L. Caplan and Robert Arp.

Defining Genetic Enhancement

A first task in understanding genetic enhancement is to define the concept of enhancement. Enhancement is best understood by reference to biological norms. A typical contrast is with therapy, which includes measures designed to restore or preserve normal levels of biological functioning. The category of enhancement encompasses interventions whose purpose is to boost levels of functioning beyond biological norms. It also includes interventions whose purpose is to shift someone already enjoying a normal level of biological functioning, and therefore not a candidate for therapy, to a higher point on the spectrum of functioning properly considered normal. A particular drug can serve as a therapy in some contexts and enhance in others. Using synthetic erythropoietin (EPO) to counter the anemia resulting from chronic kidney disease has the purpose of restoring a patient's red blood cells to normal levels. Used in this way, it is a therapy. EPO can grant competitive advantages to Tour de France cyclists who enter the event with normal levels of red blood cells. For them, EPO is a means of enhancement.

Human biological norms are, depending on your views about how we were created, fixed either by evolutionary history or by God's plans. Hearts must pump blood with a certain level of efficiency to promote biological fitness, or to achieve God's purposes. On either reading, cardiomyopathy prevents a heart from functioning at the requisite level and is therefore an uncontroversial target of therapy. Those who aspire to enhance cardiac function seek improvements to hearts that already meet nature's or God's requirements.

Now that we have defined enhancement, it is straightforward to identify *genetic* enhancements: they are enhancements achieved by the selection or modification of genetic material. It is likely that at least some of the causes of Albert Einstein's exceptional scientific achievements resided in his genome. Suppose you could identify the specific genetic variants that contributed to Einstein's scientific genius and then introduce them into a very early embryo. All of the cells in the body of the resulting person would carry the Einsteinian genetic variants. There is certainly no guarantee that someone brought into existence in this fashion would achieve scientific genius. Perhaps he or she would be a feckless computer hacker or a sporadically employed laborer. But, if we have identified the hereditary factors relevant to Einstein's achievements then a child whose genome bears these factors should at least be viewed as having a head-start on the way to success as a scientist.

The Interactionist View of Human Development

The defense of genetic enhancement that follows assumes a view about how human beings are made. This *interactionist view* is opposed both to the genetic determinism, according to which human beings are shaped almost exclusively by genes, and to the environmental determinism that says that we are made by our cultures, educations, diets, and a host of other environmental factors (see Ridley, 2003; Nisbett, 2009). According to interactionism, we result from the complex interaction of tens of thousands of genes and uncountable environmental influences. There is no point in venturing guesses about which category of influence is more important. Genes acting alone cannot make a human being. But nor can environments. Identifying yourself with your genetic material is as ludicrous as literally, rather than metaphorically, identifying yourself with your school's educational philosophy. Both our environments and our genes are at least one causal remove from the properties—our memories, conscious thoughts, etc.—that constitute us.

This assertion of the parity of genetic and environmental influences may seem to be at odds with the oft-presented message that certain human traits are largely genetic, while others are largely environmental. For example, human eye color is often presented as a genetic trait. Height is, in contrast, partially genetic and partially environmental. Any apparent contradiction resolves after clearly separating two questions about the relationship between genes and environment. The statement that eye color is principally genetic addresses variation in human populations. It is the claim that most of the observed variation in eye color in human populations corresponds with variation in genes. When we compare groups of humans with brown eyes with groups made up of blue-eyed humans, the relevant differences lie largely in DNA.

A focus on the development of individuals exposes a different relationship between genes and environment. Here we are not interested so much in variation in current human populations, but instead in a particular developmental story, namely, the specific causal contributions genes and environment make toward a given individual's traits. I have brown eyes. Suppose the tape of my life were to be rewound to conception and restarted. It is likely that certain changes to my environment—the introduction of certain viruses or specific dietary modifications—would change my eye color. The sum of these counterfactual changes corresponds with the parts of my environment that are causally relevant to my eyes' brownness.

Parity is not identity. To say that genes are not more developmentally significant than the environment, and vice versa, is not to say that they make identical contributions. Their contributions are very different, and these differences must be understood by anyone hoping to enhance human performance. A given culture's understanding of human development and how to manipulate it determines what enhancements are available to its members. For example, it is relatively easy to imagine Roger Federer discovering a new training regime—an environmental modification—capable of improving his already-excellent tennis forehand. We have, in contrast, few clues about any genetic modifications that might produce the same result. This is certainly not to say that we will not discover them at some point in our future. It is possible that there are yet-to-be discovered genetic variants that, once introduced into Federer's genome, would enhance his visual system, allowing speedier analysis of the angle and velocity of balls coming to his forehand. At the very least, their possibility should not be ruled out in advance of investigation.

Potential Problems

Interactionism leads to the rejection of in principle moral differences between genetic and environmental enhancements. The lack of an in principle difference leaves plenty of room for differences in practice. Two physically identical guns should prompt different reactions if one is used exclusively for shooting targets, and the other exclusively for shooting people. In what follows, I explore five ways in which genetic enhancements might turn out to be more morally problematic then environmental enhancements.

Are genetic enhancements more morally problematic because they are of greater magnitude than environmental enhancements?

Perhaps genetic enhancements belong in a different moral category from environmental enhancements because their effects are (always or potentially) of greater magnitude. We know that there are environmental modifications—improvements to diet and education—that influence human intelligence. But there are limits on how smart such modifications can make us. Even the most enthusiastic advocates of omega-3 think that a diet rich in oily fish can boost intelligence only to a modest extent. It is not a way to turn an average achiever into a genius. In popular presentations at least, limits such as these appear not to constrain genetic engineers who are free to supplement existing intelligence genes with additional copies or to invent intelligence genes with novel modes of action.

Some of the apparent power of genetic enhancement comes from the fact that the chief venue for its presentation is science fiction. Suppose your story's central character has intellectual powers beyond those of any past or present human being. Readers will more readily attribute this trait to the unknown future (and therefore more Sci Fi) technology of genetic enhancement than they will to measures with which we are familiar, such as diets rich in oily fish.

It is possible that genetic enhancement could produce significant increases in intelligence. At least, it is dangerous for moral philosophers to proceed on the assumption that they will not. But it is also far from true that a few millennia of experiments in educating humans have exhausted ways in which human intelligence might be boosted. For example, the psychologist Anders Ericsson has done a great deal of work on the acquisition of skills by "deliberate practice" (Ericsson et al., 1993). Deliberate practice is more than just practicing hard; it involves sequences of activities carefully selected with the purpose of extending skills. Done right, deliberate practice seems capable of producing quite remarkable results. Ericsson cites the case of the Hungarian child psychologists, László and Klara Polgár, whose program of *extended* deliberate practice—tens of thousands of hours of learning from failures and not resting content with successes—turned their three daughters into some of the world's strongest chess players. The Polgárs' particular way of implementing deliberate practice satisfies our definition of enhancement, since the sisters' chess talents were well beyond human norms. László and Klara certainly did not cease their program of deliberate practice when their daughters achieved a level of competence in chess that might be considered normal for humans.

Some of the more radical advocates of enhancement see genetic modification as almost old hat. For example, Ray Kurzweil (2005) advocates grafting a variety of cybernetic implants and neuroprostheses to our bodies and brains. He imagines electronic neuroprostheses that will dramatically enhance our mental powers. There will be a gradual merger of human with machine. In its early stages, this merger will be motivated by a desire to fix parts of our brains that have become diseased. Cochlear implants already help profoundly deaf people to hear by directly stimulating their auditory nerves. Soon, prosthetic hippocampuses could be restoring the memories of people with Alzheimer's disease. Once we install the implants, we will face a choice about how to program them. We hope that they can at least match the performance of the parts of the brain they replace; we hope, for example, that prosthetic hippocampuses will be as good at making and retrieving memories as healthy biological human hippocampuses. But if you have gone to all the trouble of installing a prosthetic hippocampus, then why would you rest content with a human level of performance when you could have so much more? From a technological perspective, there is nothing sacred or special about our present intellectual powers. This attitude to the machinery of thought will lead, in the end, to a complete mechanization of the human mind. Kurzweil presents the resulting massively intelligent machine minds as, at one and the same time, completely nonbiological and fully human. The procedures that will introduce these devices into human brains do not modify genes. They are environmental.

To summarize, then, there is no reason to believe that environmental and genetic enhancements must differ in degree. Perhaps the tools of genetic enhancement available at a given time to a given culture will be more powerful than their tools of environmental enhancement. But it could just as easily be the other way around.

Are genetic enhancements more morally problematic than environmental enhancements because they pose a greater threat to our humanity?

We know that environmental modifications can produce all sorts of weird and wonderful effects on humans ranging from extended directed practice in chess to full body tattoos. Strange though these modifications are, they leave their subjects recognizably human. No one denies the humanity of the Polgár sisters or of Erik Sprague, a.k.a. the Lizardman, who has pursued his own personal enhancement agenda, tattooing his entire body with green scales, splitting his tongue, and making plans to acquire a tail transplant. Modifying human DNA differs in potentially pushing us beyond the genetic boundaries of the human species. Perhaps it will transform us and our descendants into a new biological species of posthumans.

The view of species as having definite genetic boundaries is challenged by new work on the relationship between development and evolution. According to the picture emerging from evolutionary developmental biology (the so called *evo-devo* approach) the novel traits of a new species do not emerge from the invention of a host of new genes (Carroll, 2005). They result largely from alterations to the regulation of elements in a shared genetic tool kit. On this view, birds evolved from theropod dinosaurs by modifications of switches regulating the expression of genes that have themselves been conserved.

Therapod dinosaurs did not lose tail genes and gain wing genes. They lost their tails and gained wings by differently regulating the genes that had produced tails and directed the development of arm bones. The paleontologist Jack Horner presents a vision of a Jurassic Park in which Tyrannosaurs are restored to life not by the cloning of preserved T-Rex cells, but instead by altering the timing of the relevant genes in the chicken genome (Horner & Gorman, 2010). On the evo-devo view, it is possible that a human genome could yield something that was manifestly nonhuman by altering the timing of a few key genes. This could be achieved by the insertion of new genetic regulatory sequences. But the fact that many regulatory signals originate from the environment opens the possibility of growing a posthuman from a human embryo by manipulating its early environment so as to achieve a different sequence of gene expression.

The possibility of cybernetic enhancements provides conceptually clearer cases of genetically human nonhumans. It is wrong to think that because they do not modify genes, they leave their subjects' humanity intact. The malevolent cyborgs that give their names to the *Terminator* movies are constructed by grafting a human epidermis over machine body. To the extent that these cyborgs are genetically anything, they are genetically human. But it is perverse to think of them as human. The cyborgs seem more properly viewed as genetically human nonhumans.

In the second half of this chapter, I present an argument for the claim that certain enhancements do in fact threaten our membership of the human species and, by implication, our connection with distinctive human values. This threat does not arise from the means by which these enhancements are engineered. There is no reason to think that genetic modification is intrinsically more likely to turn us into posthumans or into any other kind of nonhuman than is environmental modification.

Is genetic enhancement less fair than environmental enhancement?

If genetic enhancements follow the pattern set by other new technologies, they are likely to be very expensive when first introduced and therefore available only to the wealthiest among us. The rich will, as a consequence, supplement their existing environmental advantages with genetic ones.

This concern should not be minimized. But it attaches both to environmental enhancement and to genetic enhancement. There is no reason to predict that a superefficient electronic hippocampus capable of enhancing human memory will be cheaper than a genetic enhancement with this effect.

Concerns about fairness apply to techniques of environmental enhancement that exist now. Take the homeschooling program that turned Polgár girls into chess masters. Now consider the same technique directed at attributes more directly connected with economic success. Imagine a program of extended directed practice constructed on the basis of what was learned about the financial system in the wake of the 2008 financial crisis. Children schooled this way might acquire the capacity to identify stocks and bonds that should be sold short that would be mistakenly described by observers as signs of inborn financial genius. One could imagine that the very wealthy who find their time too valuable to homeschool their kids will have the option of hiring experts to give their children 10,000 h of directed practice at manipulating financial markets, an option unavailable to the poor. There is a danger that the rich will supplement their already-existing environmental advantages with even more powerful, very expensive environmental enhancements.

The factors that rightly prompt concerns about fairness are price, and other barriers to access are neither genetic nor environmental. They arise in connection with the broader category of enhancement. Presenting unfairness as a consequence of specifically genetic enhancements leaves us less able to anticipate and respond to inequalities and injustices brought by environmental enhancements.

Are genetic enhancements more morally problematic than environmental enhancements because they tend to conflict with recipients' autonomy?

The best opportunity to genetically enhance an organism arises at the very beginning of its life. A gene successfully introduced into a single-cell human embryo should be transported, by successive cell divisions, into every cell in the body of the resulting human being. This ideal opportunity arises before there has been any opportunity to consult the recipient of the enhancement.

Concerns about the timing of genetic enhancement are provocatively expressed by the German philosopher, Jürgen Habermas (2003). He argues against parental genetic enhancement of children on the grounds that a genetic enhancer "makes himself the co-author of the life of another, he intrudes—from the interior ... into the other's consciousness of her own autonomy." Habermas continues to note that the "programming intentions of parents who are ambitious and given to experimentation ... have the peculiar status of a one-sided and unchallengeable expectation" (Habermas, 2003, p. 51). He proposes that this distinguishes genetic from environmental enhancements. The purported asymmetry between genetic enhancer and genetically enhanced undermines the equality characteristic of liberal societies. Habermas portrays the future generations of a society practicing genetic enhancement as "defenseless objects of prior choices made by the planners of today ... The other side of the power of today is the future bondage of the living to the dead" (Habermas, 2003, p. 48).

Habermas has identified a danger from enhancement that arises whether the means of enhancement is environmental or genetic. For example, the earlier one begins a program of deliberate enhancement the sooner one becomes a world-beater. Eight-year-old chess players who have accumulated 10,000 h of deliberate practice are likely to beat 10-year-olds with a mere 5000 h. Those who wait for children to achieve the capacity to make autonomous choices about the direction their lives will take will almost certainly lose out to parents whose educational programs have commenced earlier.

The Polgár girls speak of their enjoyment of chess. Even so, it is not as if they had much input into their educational program. László Polgár chose to give chess lessons to his daughters not because he sensed in them some incipient interest in games of strategy, but because he judged chess to be the best way to demonstrate the efficacy of directed practice. He considered and rejected art and writing on the grounds that achievements in these areas tend to be more open to question. What some critics call a painting of genius others pronounce an ugly mess. If you checkmate your opponent in a game of chess, you are a winner regardless of the opinions of any spectator.

Even very ambitious programs of directed practice may seem to give their human objects an option of resistance unavailable to the prenatally genetically enhanced. Had the Polgár girls insisted on hurling any proffered chess pieces across the room, then László and Klara might have abandoned their plan to turn their daughters into world-beating chess players. Yet it is too late for a child to make it the case that her genome was never genetically altered.

This response overlooks an option of resistance available to the prenatally enhanced. While you in early adulthood may be too late to make it the case that the DNA of your embryo was never altered, you can prevent the alterations from having the effects your enhancer was hoping for. This opportunity is a consequence of the interactionist view of development according to which significant traits emerge not from the action of genes alone, but from the interactions of genes and environment. You can refuse to place the modified gene or genes in the environment necessary for them to have their intended effect. Suppose that you learn that your genome was altered with the intention of turning you into a brilliant mathematician. You are unlikely to become one if you refuse to study mathematics beyond grade-school level. The mere act of genetically enhancing mathematical aptitude in no way prevents this choice.

Are genetic enhancements more morally problematic than environmental enhancements because they are riskier?

The techniques that László and Klara Polgár used to enhance their daughters are novel. But these educational innovations should be acknowledged as significantly less novel than genetic modifications. Intensive homeschooling of the type described by Ericsson may lead to resentment, but it is unlikely to cause sudden death. When directed at an early embryo, genetic enhancement intervenes in processes that are foundational in human development. Our very preliminary understanding of how genes influence development should make us cautious about any alterations.

Genetic enhancement as it presents to us in the early twentieth century is riskier than the available methods of environmental enhancement. But this may not be true of the near future in which we achieve a better understanding of the technologies of genetic modification, and we confront new techniques of environmental enhancement. These environmental methods may include augmenting human brains with electronic neuroprostheses and injecting self-replicating nanobots into human bloodstreams. When these enhancement technologies become available, environmental enhancements, considered collectively, could be more dangerous than genetic enhancements.

This section does not pretend to be exhaustive. My prediction, based on the parallel contributions of genes and environment to the construction of human beings, is that any purported moral differences will disappear when subjected to closer examination. We should be morally consistent in respect of enhancements. This consistency is one of *moral evaluation* and not of *moral conclusion*. We are not obligated to arrive at the same moral conclusion about a list of proposed genetic and environmental enhancements any more than someone selecting a sports team is required to choose equal numbers of black and white players. At a given time in the history of a given society, a specific collection of enhancements, genetic and environmental, will be available to its members. It is entirely possible the genetic enhancements available in the industrialized world of the early twenty-first century conflict more strongly with autonomy, open up more significant social divisions, or are associated with greater risks than available environmental enhancements. But this does not show that the epithets "genetic" or "environmental" pick out morally relevant properties. To return to the sporting analogy—a team that includes mainly black players may draw allegations of racially biased selection practices, but this pattern could arise simply because the particular black players who present themselves happen to be superior to the white ones. The pattern should reverse if next year's white candidates are better.

Early twenty-first-century commentators make much of the potential for genetic technologies to radically recast human beings. If Kurzweil's (2005) predictions about the future of technology are accurate, then the attention of enhancers will soon turn to electronic enhancements presaged by current work in artificial intelligence. At this time, environmental enhancements should be the chief focus of moral investigation. They will be the chief category of changes interfering with autonomous choice or fracturing the human species into haves and have-nots.

Exploring Enhancement's Moral Limits

If morally problematic enhancements cannot be identified in terms of their provenance, then how are they to be identified? In what follows, I present enhancement as a way of treating human beings that can be good if practiced in moderation but is dangerous if taken to extremes. Many of the influences humans direct at themselves or each other fall into this category, such as drinking alcohol, exposure to direct sunlight, exercising, consuming saturated fats, and so on. Too much sun substantially elevates the risk of skin cancer. A moderate amount furnishes the body with requisite vitamin D. Alcoholism is a disease that destroys lives. But moderate drinking offers enjoyable experiences, promotes certain forms of sociability, and may reduce the risk of heart disease. Advocates of moderation face a practical difficulty dodged by abolitionists. There is an ongoing debate about what constitutes safe levels of sun tanning or drinking. The advocates of moderation must decide, in a principled fashion, what levels of exposure or consumption constitute enough but not too much. Zero is, in contrast, a level of exposure or consumption that is easily specified.

There is a moral difference between *moderate* and *radical enhancement*. This difference exists whether enhancements are produced by manipulating genes or by manipulating environments. Radical enhancement is enhancement of a degree incompatible with values associated with being human. Moderate enhancements are of a lesser degree and, as such, are not incompatible with these values. The threat to human values from radical enhancement is a danger additional to those canvassed in the previous section. It can suffice to make objectionable otherwise unproblematic enhancements.

The Inhumanity of Radical Enhancement

The following discussion borrows and adapts an argument from one of enhancement's fiercest critics, the conservative social critic Leon Kass. Kass (1997) deploys what has come to be called the "yuck" argument. In a version of the argument directed against human cloning, he appeals to an intuitive repugnance elicited by the practice. Our untutored response to human cloning is one of disgust, something that Kass presents as "the emotional expression of deep wisdom, beyond reason's power fully to articulate it" (p. 22). He finds genetic enhancement repellent for the same reason. According to Kass, we sense an immoral intrusion into nature's way of making human beings.

The "yuck" argument is mocked by some bioethicists (Harris, 2007, chapter 8). They find it uncomfortably close to the unreasoned reactions of racists to people whose skin color differs from their own. Racists are typically embarrassed by the poor quality of their moral reasoning. It would be bad—indeed "yucky"—if we empowered them to defend their views as the "emotional expression of deep wisdom, beyond reason's power fully to articulate."

I think the "yuck" argument is best understood not as a challenge to reason itself, but instead to superficial and simplistic uses of reason. The values that connect us with our humanity are hugely complex and mostly implicitly known. They can be made explicit only with great difficulty and even then only incompletely. Emotional reactions are useful but fallible indicators that these values have been infringed. They are often more reliable than are rational investigations of these values.

For a model of the implicit valuing of our humanity, consider the example of chicken sexing. Professional chicken sexers can reliably distinguish male from female chickens well before there are any differences detectable by the rest of us. They are clueless when it comes to explaining how they make their discriminations. This does not mean that chicken sexing is magic. Expert sexers have implicit knowledge of the distinguishing characteristics of very young male and female chickens, knowledge that can be made explicit only incompletely and with great difficulty.

The discriminatory powers of chicken sexers come from a long exposure to young chickens. I propose that some of our valuing fits this pattern. Prime examples are the attachments we feel with things with which we have longstanding, multifaceted associations. Suppose you were asked to give an account of the value you place on your hometown. There are many things that you might talk about: the town's fine but inexpensive Malaysian restaurants, its many off-road running tracks, the distinctive view of the harbor afforded by the town's hilly central suburbs, and so on. These could all be genuine facets of your valuing. But the basis of your valuing of your hometown is likely to resist succinct summary. Any list that you might give is bound to omit values borne out of your long association with it.

The valuing of a hometown is not rationally or morally compulsory. Values characteristic of a longstanding association will not be shared by someone who has never lived there, nor by someone whose experience of growing up there has been particularly unhappy. The scope of hometown values is relatively confined. They may justify resistance to developers' large-scale enhancement projects, for example, your objection to the placement of a monorail in its historic district even if it would be straightforward enhancement of the town's transport network and excellent for time-pressed tourists.

Our commitment to our humanity is a bit like our commitment to our hometowns. It is implicit, emerging from our multidimensional experience of being human. It comprises all of the very many ways in which human experiences are valuable.

Some very unusual humans might truthfully declare that they are unmoved by human values. This seems to be the view of some transhumanists who follow Julian Huxley in viewing humanity as "a wretched makeshift, rooted in ignorance." Most often, I suspect, these transhumanists are tricked into false and hasty renunciation of their human values. They are like chicken sexers, fooled into accepting a checklist compiled by a Ph.D. in biology as a more reliable guide to chick gender than their implicit knowledge.

A bias toward straightforwardly expressible values can cast doubt on necessarily amorphous and ambiguous human values. This may happen in much the same way as overemphasis on a few straightforwardly quantifiable things—efficiency of the transport network, proximity of hotels to tourist attractions, quality of housing stock—fools people into failing to give proper place to the less easily stated and quantified things that actually bind them to their hometowns. Familiar values may sometimes be outweighed. The gains from a new superefficient monorail network may be so great that a city's venerable trams should be scrapped. But we should not conclude from difficulties in stating and quantifying implicit hometown values that they should count for zero.

I offer the following sketch of one cluster of implicit human values, values that lead us to place a reduced value on the objectively more significant achievements enabled by radical enhancement. We humans have a privileged access to the achievements of other humans. This gives us a special reason to care about them. For example, we take greater pleasure in Usain Bolt's covering 100 in 9.58 s than we do in a second-hand Toyota Corolla covering the same distance faster. Einstein's discoveries matter to us more than the objectively greater discoveries of a future machine intelligence. Why is this? Natural selection has endowed us with insight into the endeavors, triumphs, and failures of other human beings. These psychological commonalities are part of what make humanity a single biological species. Nature has endowed us with insight into the psychologies of potential mates or hunt partners. This capacity connects us with humans with whom we have no plans to mate or go hunting. There is something universal and shareable about human experience in spite of the efforts by racists to create boundaries between groups of humans. It creates a shared human story, something under threat from radical enhancement.

Compare the manner of access that we have to nonhuman achievements. For example, humans are only inferentially impressed by the exploits of a dung beetle that finally manages to roll a dung ball up a slope, something we could do easily with a single pinkie. We must take into account facts about the relative sizes of beetle and ball to be properly impressed. This could be the attitude that radically enhanced intellects take to Einstein's achievement or athletically enhanced posthumans take to Bolt's sprints. They might be impressed only after they take into account the pathetic intellectual and athletic limitations of humans. We can, in contrast, be non-inferentially impressed. The limitations pertinent to Einstein's or Bolt's achievements are also pertinent to our own.

Comparing Moderate and Radical Enhancement

The moral calculus for moderate enhancement is more straightforward than is that for radical enhancement. We have a wealth of experience of moderate enhancement. It is appropriate for us to worry about the sacrifices Zsuzsa, Zsófia, or Judit had to make on the way to chess stardom. We might worry about the social consequences of unequal access to László and Klara's educational techniques. Although we recognize that there are dangers in the variety of enhancement practiced by László and Klara Polgár, we understand that moderate enhancement is frequently worth it. Zsuzsa, Zsófia, and Judit are, at the time of writing, happy, successful, and still in love with chess as they enter early middle age. Suppose we were to discover that László's and Klara's story about their program of extended deliberate practice was an elaborate fraud. Instead, their daughters' DNA had been secretly manipulated at some shady Eastern European genetics lab. This should not change our view about how their lives had turned out. No one is denying the humanity of Zsuzsa, Zsófia, or Judit. The version of reality in which they are genetically altered should not change this assessment.

The radical enhancements potentially offered by advances in genetics and artificial intelligence are significantly more morally vexed. They may bring us more dramatic benefits than those brought by moderate enhancement—greater extensions of our life spans and enlargements of our intellects. But we must balance these gains against losses sustained as we become disconnected from human values. These losses are not incurred in moderate enhancement. Compare the application of human values to proposed radical enhancements with the relevance of Parisian hometown values to proposals for urban renewal. The benefits bought by new shopping malls and public transport hubs would have to be massive to justify the bulldozing of "functionless" buildings such as the Tour Eiffel and the Arc de Triomphe, with the consequent severing to ties to the city's past. More moderate urban enhancements are, in contrast, likely to keep these historic buildings in place.

Posthumans, Martians, or machine intelligences are unlikely to be moved by specifically human values. We would be right to say that they miss out on experiences that we find valuable. But we should not presume that posthuman lives should be reconfigured so as to conform with our human values. It is likely that distinct posthuman, Martian, or android values will serve as guiding lights for them. This is how we locate the justificatory limits of implicit values. Merely implicit values can be appealed to in defending a connection with something. But they do not justify ill treatment of those who fail to share that connection. Values invoked to justify various ways of inflicting harm—killing or imprisoning sentient beings, for example—must be made explicit. The values that connect us to our humanity explain why we may want to forgo radical enhancement so as to remain human. However, they cannot justify ill treatment of nonhumans.

I have argued that the protection of human values can justify rejecting some of the more dramatic enhancements of our capacities. The flipside of this claim is that more moderate enhancements should be embraced as fully compatible with human values. It makes no difference whether these moderate enhancements are achieved by improving our diets or modifying our genomes.

References

Ericsson, A., Krampe, R., & Tesch-Romer, C. (1993). The role of deliberate practice in the acquisition of expert performance. *Psychological Review, 100*, 363–406.

Carroll, S. (2005). *Endless forms most beautiful: The new science of evo devo and the making of the animal kingdom*. New York: Norton.

Habermas, J. (2003). *The future of human nature*. Cambridge: Polity.

Harris, J. (2007). *Enhancing evolution: The ethical case for making better people*. Princeton, NJ: Princeton University Press.

Horner, J., & Gorman, J. (2010). *How to build a dinosaur: The new science of reverse evolution*. New York: Plume.

Kass, L. (1997). The wisdom of repugnance: Why we should ban the cloning of human beings. *The New Republic, 216*, 17–26.

Kurzweil, R. (2005). *The singularity is near: When humans transcend biology*. London: Penguin.

Nisbett, R. (2009). *Intelligence and how to get it: Why schools and cultures count*. New York: Norton.

Ridley, M. (2003). *Nature via nurture: Genes, experience, and what makes us human*. New York: Fourth Estate.

Chapter Twenty Two

There Is No Legitimate Place for Human Genetic Enhancement

The Slippery Slope to Genocide

Edwin Black

This chapter argues that, despite the magniloquent anti-cloning and anti-enhancement declarations of multilateral and multinational bodies, there is no law in any land on earth that can be invoked to stop the genetic trespass that will begin with cloning the cutest pets and proceed predictably into the mindset of the Third Reich. In other words, human genetic enhancement is a slippery slope leading to genocide, as history—much of which is recounted in this chapter—has demonstrated time and time again.

Introduction

Nicholas Agar's chapter endorsing some limited genetic enhancement in certain circumstances struck me as a very long philosophical discourse to explain why traversing down the slippery slope of genetic enhancement can become acceptable—so long as we apply the brakes on the decline. In other words, the chapter invites society to build on-ramps to a genetic autobahn that we will gradually help pave, mile by mile, with the hope that some speed limits will be observed.

But in truth, there will be no way to monitor the superhighway of genetic transformation. No traffic cops will patrol. It will be a biological free-for-all.

Despite the magniloquent anti-cloning and anti-enhancement declarations of multilateral and multinational bodies, there is no law in any land on earth that can be invoked to stop the genetic trespass that will begin with cloning the cutest pets and proceed predictably into the mindset of the Third Reich. Even if some protective laws, such as anti-cloning statutes, were to be adopted in one jurisdiction or another, many eugenic or genetic projects can be easily segmented into fractions until combined in a series of bio-assembly lines easily located in China, North Korea, Iran, Hong Kong, or a luxury yacht sailing in international waters.

When a human clone is created, be it an adorable child or a mutant monster, whether in Manhattan or the Cocos Islands (which enjoyed more than a century of slave breeding), the world will be confronted with an enhanced human Dolly which it cannot persecute, shun, or disallow any more than it can outlaw naturally born infants with birth defects or unwanted pregnancies. A measure of proportionality is needed here. History proves that compensating for man's frailty or weaknesses is genuine progress. Whether through environmental adjustments or genetics, enhancements to bring us closer to that elusive,

Contemporary Debates in Bioethics, First Edition. Edited by Arthur L. Caplan and Robert Arp.

ill-defined, and dangerous concept of "normal" are as craved as they are Promethean. As Agar points out, just enough sunlight gives one his daily dose of Vitamin D; too much causes skin cancer. Or, using the original Promethean storyline, fire can warm a person or incinerate his body.

Certainly, the concept of improving human existence through modification of the environment is as old as humankind itself. Prehistoric societies acquired warm clothing, walking sticks, tools, and weapons to enhance and extend their existence. Ancient civilizations going back to and preceding the Pharaohs developed concepts of hygiene, medicine, and even skull surgery. It is a natural inclination to strive to live longer, better, and survive unforgiving environments (Breasted, 1930, pp. 12–13, 33–37, 62–63).

At the same time, humanity has constantly reminded itself of the lessons of reaching too far too fast and, indeed, of the inherent curse of playing God. The Bible and other ancient books tell us that men were inspired to build temples—some quite grand. But those same tales tell of vainglorious man's effort to challenge the gods by building a tower tall enough to touch the heavens. The construction site was at Babel. That effort was met with doom, the story tells us. In the centuries since, every time humans have tried to play or outwit God, or natural forces, the cautionary tales always spell failure. The reason for Frankenstein's enduring nature is that it teaches that genius can only go so far, and playing God—or self-directing biology—can only result in disaster. Countless twentieth-century dramatic escalations on the Frankenstein theme have taken root into our collective consciousness: from the 1921 Czech play RUR, which introduced the word *robot*, to a world gone macabre in the 1927 film *Metropolis*, to a long list of Hollywood A and B apocalyptic productions.

The Philosophers

Flights of solipsistic eugenic fancy have been food for thought among philosophers throughout the ages. Indeed, eugenic-style killing, all too often, has been inspired by, perpetuated by, or justified by the philosophers. Although unarmed, philosophers and great thinkers have weaponized the dreams of many mass murderers with eugenicidal rationales and imperatives.

Spartan warriors practiced deadly ancient eugenics. It was said that their newborns were scrutinized in bizarre tests, such as bathing them in wine looking for signs of puniness, or inspecting them for telltale traits of infirmity. Those deemed unsuitable were thrown over the cliff or left to starve to death (Michell, 1964; Pomeroy, 2002).

Several centuries later, a thinker as enlightened as Plato sought to perpetuate and justify eugenic infanticide. In the *Republic*, Plato (1888) advised: "You have in your house hunting dogs and a number of pedigree cocks ... Do you then breed from all indiscriminately, or are you careful to breed from the best?" Plato's solution: "The offspring of the inferior, and any of those of the other sort who are born defective, they [the rulers] will properly dispose of them in secret, so that no one will know what has become of them." Plato's words, and histories of infant-killing regimens, set shining examples for eugenic murders centuries later.

After Plato, it was Aristotle (1885). He argued against fetal abortion, unless necessary for population control, or violated the rules of society. He wrote, "let there be a law that no deformed child shall live," adding, "but when couples have children in excess, let abortion be procured before sense and life have begun; what may or may not be lawfully done in these cases depends on the question of life and sensation."

In 1798, philosopher Thomas Malthus (1798/1959) picked up the torch, founding an enormously influential school of thought with *An Essay on the Principle of Population*. Malthus cried out for population control as the only way to outwit Earth's limited resources. He suggested "It does not ... by any means seem impossible that by an attention to breed, a certain degree of improvement, similar to that among animals, might take place among men. Whether intellect could be communicated may be a matter of doubt; but size, strength, beauty, complexion, and perhaps longevity are in a degree transmissible." He bemoaned the reluctance to implement forced procedures, writing, "As the human race, however, could not be improved in this way without condemning all the bad specimens to celibacy, it is not probable that an attention to breed should ever become general" (ch. 9).

In the mid-nineteenth century, the German philosopher, Arthur Schopenhauer (1851/1970), propounded proto-eugenic ideas, writing:

> With our knowledge of the complete unalterability both of character and of mental faculties, we are led to the view that a real and thorough improvement of the human race might be reached not so much from outside as from within, not so much by theory and instruction as rather by the path of generation. Plato had something of the kind in mind when, in the fifth book of his *Republic*, he explained his plan for increasing and improving his warrior caste. If we could castrate all scoundrels and stick all stupid geese in a convent, and give men of noble character a whole harem, and procure men, and indeed thorough men, for all girls of intellect and understanding, then a generation would soon arise which would produce a better age than that of Pericles. (p. 154)

Schopenhauer argued again, citing Plato, "If you want Utopian plans, I would say: the only solution to the problem is the despotism of the wise and noble members of a genuine aristocracy, a genuine nobility, achieved by mating the most magnanimous men with the cleverest and most gifted women." Schopenhauer's choice for the best stock was clear, "The highest civilization and culture ... are found exclusively among the white races; and even with many dark peoples, the ruling caste or race is fairer in color than the rest" (p. 154, §92).

In 1863, Francis J. Galton, a quizzical observer and inveterate counter of patterns, began turning his sharp eye on the teeming masses of poverty that plagued London society. He was the half-cousin of Charles Darwin. In a series of publications, Galton tried to predict how to direct the hereditary path of mankind, who should marry to bestow more of their noble quality, and who should not for fear of multiplying their wretchedness. In this way, society could combat poverty and its attached diseases. Together, poverty and disease constituted a drain on the British Empire's best protoplasm and, as a result of the mounting taxes to support charitable relief, a drain on the national fiscal budget. Galton tried in his own quirky way to elevate this utopian wondering into an organized set of rules (Black, 2003, ch. 2).

In 1883, Galton published Inquiries into Human Faculty and Development (Galton, 1883) and created a new term for his discipline. He played with many names for his new science. Finally, he scrawled Greek letters on a hand-sized scrap of paper, and next to them the two transliterated English fragments. The two rendered pieces were sewn together like found limbs. The Greek word for *well* was patched to the Greek word for *born*. In a flourish and with a jolt of mental electricity, the concept achieved animation. Galton's new term would tantalize his contemporaries, inspire his disciples, obsess his later followers, and eventually slash through the twentieth century like a sword. The finest and the fiendish would adopt the new term as their driving mantra. Families would be shattered, generations would be wiped away, and whole peoples would be nearly erased—all in the name of Galton's new word, brought into life from inert linguistic scavenging. The word he wrote on that small piece of paper was *eugenics* (Black, 2003, ch. 2). In a roar, it became alive. The newly awakened concept suddenly opened its irresistible eyes and hypnotized a gullible world.

Shortly after Galton's new data-less protoscience exploded into European thought, the towering German philosopher, Friedrich Nietzsche, found himself more than receptive to the notion. He took it to the next level. In the recovered notes of *The Will to Power*, Nietzsche (1906/1968) declared, "Society, the great trustee of life, is responsible to life itself for every miscarried life—it also has to pay for such lives: consequently, it ought to prevent them. In numerous cases, society ought to prevent procreation: to this end, it may hold in readiness, without regard to descent, rank, or spirit, the most rigorous means of constraint, deprivation of freedom, in certain circumstances castration." In that work, Nietzsche damned the Biblical injunction "Thou shall not kill" in favor of a new mandate for the decadent and supposedly degenerate bloodlines: "Thou shall not procreate." He railed, "Life itself recognizes no solidarity, no 'equal right,' between the healthy and the degenerate parts of an organism ... Sympathy for the decadents, equal rights for the ill-constituted—that would be the profoundest immorality, that would be anti-nature itself as morality!" (Book 3, §734).

American Eugenics

As we have seen, the philosophical firebreaks are easily jumped. These philosophical exercises are not mere historical curiosities, and were reinvented in America in the first years of the twentieth century as a quest to create a blonde, blue-eyed Nordic master race to rule the United States. At the time, America's elite were consternated with a nation rapidly shifting its socioeconomic fulcrums, absorbing millions of East Europeans and Jews from the East, Chinese indentured workers from the West, Mexicans from the recently conquered Southwest, Reconstruction-era freed slaves, and Indians off the reservation. The elite thinkers who adopted eugenic ideas were the moneyed gentlemen of the day with hands-on experience in livestock, that is, ranchers, breeders, farmers, and horse-racing enthusiasts. They fused their parlor-room banter, burnished racism, sense of innate superiority, and their progressive quest with Mendel's recently rediscovered Principles of Hereditary. The striped pea and the smooth pea will always yield a partially "defective" lineage. Voilà, their racial thought and utopian obsession gave birth to the pseudoscience of American eugenics. They were Utopians. As those who know Greek will discern, Utopia means "nowhere." But the race to this unreachable destination was a murderous gallop led by titans that mowed down helpless millions and subtracted millions more who were never born.

The truest victims of eugenicide were in fact the generations who never existed. They were the actual targets.

Dissecting exactly how the dark force of eugenics leaped from philosophical chants to genocide in action requires a journey through the hellish part of progressivism. Self-fulfilling philosophy became a self-fulfilling prophecy once it became entrenched in academia. The campus has been the historical breeding ground for genocide in the past several centuries. And all it required in the case of eugenics was the enzyme of money. Big money. Prestigious money. To be more specific: the philanthropic largess of America's greatest criminal corporations (Black, 2003, ch. 3).

Here we speak of the Harriman fortune, the Carnegie Institution, and the Rockefeller Foundation—respectively, the railroad robber baron, the ruthless coal and steel manipulator, and the much-prosecuted fraud king of oil. These men and their successors took the spoils of vast corporate criminal enterprises and laundered them through prodigious, ostensibly philanthropic charities. True, much of their mission was uplifting and helpful to humanity in the realms of arts and letters and science. But these fortunes were also capable of murderous social engineering. Andrew Carnegie rejected "indiscriminate charity . . . spent as to encourage the slothful, the drunken, the unworthy," in favor of "fixing" the social factors underlying the traits. John D. Rockefeller plowed his money into more than just good works but, to use his words, "a search for cause, an attempt to cure evils at their source" (Fosdick, 1952, p. 22; Carnegie, 1962, p. 29; Black, 2003, ch. 4). Their search for a remedy was to excise the problems—that is, excise them from the Earth. This led the philanthropies to eugenics, where the quest to do immeasurable good led them down the path of immeasurable evil.

The philanthropies invested millions in the development of eugenics, establishing in 1904 a scientific nerve center at bucolic Cold Spring Harbor on Long Island. In a compound nestled between the trees and the placid shore, eugenicists methodically used those fortunes to establish the Station for Experimental Evolution devoted to pinpointing the science, plus a Eugenics Record Office to keep track of potential individuals and family lines to eliminate, and numerous eugenic advocacy organizations to lobby the campus for academic acceptance and the state house for legislative action.

In essence, these raceologists took Mendel's rediscovered rules of raising peas, and felt they could apply the same principles to improving mankind. Indeed, because many eugenic pioneers and supporters were also ranchers, farmers, and breeders, they were convinced they could improve generations of human beings the same way one raises a better herd of cattle or field of wheat, by eliminating the bad stock and proliferating the good stock.

With little data—but plenty of bias—they concluded that striped peas or troubled people would spawn generations that were biologically determined to inherit the troubling social characteristic. In this bizarre Social Lamarckianism, you were not born into prostitution; prostitution was born into you. You were not thrown in criminality; you were a "born criminal." Poverty was an inherited trait. Therefore, one could eliminate any number of social ills by merely eliminating the people, as you would eliminate a black sheep from the flock.

Through their pseudoscientific journals and conferences, they adopted a variety of measures designed to protect society and the future inhabitants of the planet, and calculated to create a race of enhanced humans who would inherit a world better than the one before it because they would self-direct the course of human nature. They would pick and choose who would live and continue their lineage—and who would not. The ones selected for life were the white, blond, blue-eyed, Nordic types that exemplified their own parentage; the undesired ones: everyone else. Not even white people with brown hair—considered mongrel Caucasians—were to be tolerated. Hence, Appalachian "hillbillies" were targeted just as vigorously as Blacks, American Indians, southern Europeans, Jews, Asians, Hispanics, and all admixtures thereof.

To achieve this culling, the eugenicists wanted to systematically eliminate what they derisively labeled "the bottom tenth." In the first decade of the twentieth century, that meant 14 million Americans were to be subtracted at a swipe. When those 14 million were gone, eugenicists intended to subtract the bottom tenth of the remaining population. Slice after slice, the millions of unwanted humans and their bloodlines would be excised by eugenicists until there was no one left except those who resembled themselves: white, blond, blue-eyed, Nordic types (Black, 2003, chs. 3–6).

What methods would be used? Marriage prohibition and marriage nullification were implemented for those deemed racially or socially undesirable. Such laws were enacted from coast to coast. Criminal sanctions for interracial marriage were not completely negated until 1967 when *Loving v. Virginia* had such laws struck down. Eugenicists also advocated detention or confinement camps—some would call them concentration camps. These were established throughout Connecticut, Massachusetts, New York, New Jersey, Virginia, North Carolina, and many other states to quarantine those considered otherwise unsuited to exist in society, especially the so-called "feeble-minded," a never-defined and widely abused intelligence caste. Among the confinement centers shrouded behind high-sounding names were The Vineland Training School in New Jersey and the Virginia Colony for the Epileptic and the Feebleminded. Dozens of such detention centers were established.

Forced surgical sterilization of the undesired was imposed in jurisdictions across America. Some 60,000 individuals in 27 states, mostly young women, were forcibly sterilized, many without their knowledge, often by the use of trickery using misidentified medical procedures. Untold additional thousands were coercively or stealthily sterilized under federal programs. Indeed, enlightened California led the Union in forced sterilizations, performing nearly all sterilization procedures with little or no due process. In its first 25 years of eugenic legislation, California sterilized 9782 individuals, mostly women. Many were "diagnosed" as "bad girls," "passionate," "oversexed," or "sexually wayward." In 1933 alone, at least 1278 coercive sterilizations were performed, 700 of which were on women. The state's two leading sterilization mills in 1933 were Sonoma State Home, with 388 operations, and Patton State Hospital, with 363 operations. Other sterilization centers dotted the state in the state hospitals at Mendocino, Napa, Norwalk, Stockton, and Pacific Colony, among others. Coercive sterilization continued in some states, such as North Carolina, into the 1970s (Black, 2003; Lombardo, 2012).

Marriage restriction, confinement camps, and forced sterilization were always Plan B. But for American eugenics, Plan A was mass murder. Eugenicide was widely favored. The most favored, albeit debated, method was the "lethal chamber" or locally operated public gas chamber (Black, 2003, chs. 13–14).

In 1903, a committee of the National Conference on Charities and Correction conceded that it was as yet undecided whether "science may conquer sentiment" and ultimately elect to systematically kill the unfit. In 1904, the superintendent of New Jersey's Vineland Training School, E. R. Johnstone, raised the issue during his presidential address to the Association of Medical Officers of American Institutions for Idiotic and Feebleminded Persons. "Many plans for the elimination [of the feebleminded] have been proposed," Johnstone said as he referred to numerous recently published suggestions of a "painless death." That same year, the notion of executing habitual criminals and the incurably insane was offered to the National Prison Association (Black, 2003, chs. 13–14).

In 1905, the British eugenicist and birth-control advocate, H. G. Wells, published *A Modern Utopia.*

"There would be no killing, no lethal chambers," Wells wrote (Wells, 1905, pp. 143–144). Another birth-control advocate, the socialist writer Eden Paul (1917), differed with Wells and declared that society must protect itself from "begetters of anti-social stocks which would injure generations to come. If it [society] reject the lethal chamber, what other alternative can the socialist state devise?" (pp. 145–146).

Some US lawmakers considered similar ideas. Two years later in 1906, the Ohio legislature considered a bill empowering physicians to chloroform permanently diseased and mentally incapacitated persons. In reporting this, one eugenicist told his British colleagues that it was Ohio's attempt to "murder certain persons suffering from incurable disease." Iowa considered a similar measure.

In 1910, the eugenic extremist, George Bernard Shaw, lectured at London's Eugenics Education Society about mass murder in lethal chambers. Shaw proclaimed, "A part of eugenic politics would finally land us in an extensive use of the lethal chamber. A great many people would have to be put out of existence, simply because it wastes other people's time to look after them" (Shaw, 1910). Several British newspapers excoriated Shaw and eugenics under such headlines as "Lethal Chamber Essential to Eugenics" (also Stone, 2002, pp. 127–128).

In 1911, E. B. Sherlock's book, *The Feebleminded: A Guide to Study and Practice*, acknowledged that "glib suggestions of the erection of lethal chambers are common enough" (Sherlock, 1911). Like others, Sherlock rejected execution in favor of eugenic termination of bloodlines. "Apart from the difficulty that the provision of lethal chambers is impracticable in the existing state law," he continued, "... the removal of them [the feebleminded] would do practically nothing toward solving the chief problem with the mentally defective set ... the persistence of the obnoxious stock" (p. 267; also Elks, 1993, p. 203).

Despite the reluctance of many, a solid core of eugenicists was amenable to the idea. The eminent psychologist and eugenicist, Henry H. Goddard, seemed almost to express regret that such proposals had not already been implemented. In his infamous 1912 study, *The Kallikak Family*, Goddard commented, "For the low-grade idiot, the loathsome unfortunate that may be seen in our institutions, some have proposed the lethal chamber. But humanity is steadily tending away from the possibility of that method, and there is no probability that it will ever be practiced" (Goddard, 1912, pp. 101, 105–108). Goddard pointed to family-wide castration, sterilization, and segregation as better solutions because they would more broadly address the genetic sources.

In 1918, Paul Popenoe, an Army venereal disease specialist during World War I, co-wrote with Roswell Johnson the widely used textbook, *Applied Eugenics*, which argued, "From an historical point of view, the first method which presents itself is execution ... Its value in keeping up the standard of the race should not be underestimated" (Popenoe & Johnson, 1918, p. 194).

Despite the proponents among them, eugenic breeders concluded that American society was not ready to implement an organized lethal solution. Even still, many mental institutions and doctors practiced improvised medical lethality and passive euthanasia on their own. One institution in Lincoln, Illinois fed its incoming patients milk from tubercular cows, believing a eugenically strong individual would be immune. Thirty to 40% annual death rates resulted at Lincoln. Some doctors practiced passive eugenicide one newborn infant at a time. Other doctors at mental institutions engaged in systematic lethal neglect.

Real progress in eugenics took hold once eugenics, backed by philanthropic millions, seeded the greatest universities with raceology as a settled science. True, this science was devoid of reliable data, and thrived only on racist conclusions. But cyclonic self-certification, academic cross-referencing, and echo logic entrenched the fake science into the hallowed halls of Harvard, Princeton, Yale, Stanford, and many others. Racist lawmakers could wave the flag of scientific verity and its accompanying social imperative to justify their unjust biological persecution of minorities. In practice, we see Virginia's pseudoscientifically justified Eugenic Sterilization Act and its outright segregation mandate, the Racial Integrity Act, both passed within hours on the same day, March 24, 1920. The same sort of junk science was used in state after state to rationalize the unthinkable (Carlson, 2001; Black, 2003, chs. 13–16).

Even the United States Supreme Court endorsed aspects of eugenics. In its infamous 1927 *Buck v. Bell*

(274 US 200) decision, Supreme Court Justice Oliver Wendell Holmes wrote, "It is better for all the world, if instead of waiting to execute degenerate offspring for crime, or to let them starve for their imbecility, society can prevent those who are manifestly unfit from continuing their kind ... Three generations of imbeciles are enough." This decision opened the floodgates for thousands to be coercively sterilized or otherwise persecuted as subhuman (Lombardo, 2008, 2011). Years later, the Nazis at the Nuremberg trials quoted Holmes's words in their own defense.

The Final Solution

Only after eugenics became entrenched in the United States was the campaign transplanted into Germany, largely through the financial and pseudoscientific support of the Rockefeller Foundation, the Carnegie Institution, and the collective eugenic community in America.

Hitler studied American eugenics laws. He tried to legitimize his anti-Semitism by medicalizing it, and wrapping it in the more palatable pseudoscientific facade of eugenics. Hitler was able to recruit more followers among reasonable Germans by claiming that science was on his side. While Hitler's race hatred sprang from his own mind and a tradition of German superiority, the biological intellectual outlines of the eugenics Hitler adopted were made in America. In *Mein Kampf*, published in 1924, Hitler quoted American eugenic ideology and openly displayed a thorough knowledge of American eugenics. "There is today one state," wrote Hitler, "in which at least weak beginnings toward a better conception [of immigration] are noticeable. Of course, it is not our model German Republic, but the United States" (Hitler, 1943, pp. 439–440). Hitler proudly told his comrades just how closely he followed the progress of the American eugenics movement. "I have studied with great interest," he told a fellow Nazi, "the laws of several American states concerning prevention of reproduction by people whose progeny would, in all probability, be of no value or be injurious to the racial stock" (Wagener, 1987, pp. 145–146; Black, 2003, ch. 14).

Hitler even wrote a fan letter to a virulent American racist eugenic leader, Madison Grant, calling his race-based eugenics book, *The Passing of the Great Race*—Der Untergang der grossen Rasse—his "bible." Grant, an eminent naturalist, was a cofounder of the Bronx Zoo and a trustee of the American Museum of Natural History (Grant, 1936; Whitney, 1973).

Hitler's struggle for a superior race would be a mad crusade for a master race. Now, the American term "Nordic" was freely interchanged with "Germanic" or "Aryan." Race science, racial purity, and racial dominance became the driving force behind Hitler's Nazism. Nazi eugenics would ultimately dictate who would be persecuted in a Reich-dominated Europe, how people would live, and how they would die. Nazi doctors would become the unseen generals in Hitler's war against the Jews and other Europeans deemed inferior. Doctors would create the science, devise the eugenic formulae, and even hand-select the victims for sterilization, euthanasia, and extermination (Lifton, 2000).

In 1934, as Germany's sterilizations were accelerating beyond 5000 per month, California eugenics leader, C. M. Goethe, upon returning from Germany, ebulliently bragged to a key colleague, "You will be interested to know, that your work has played a powerful part in shaping the opinions of the group of intellectuals who are behind Hitler in this epoch-making program. Everywhere I sensed that their opinions have been tremendously stimulated by American thought ... I want you, my dear friend, to carry this thought with you for the rest of your life, that you have really jolted into action a great government of 60 million people" (Black, 2003, ch. 14). That same year, 10 years after Virginia passed its sterilization act, Joseph DeJarnette, superintendent of Virginia's Western State Hospital, complained in the Richmond Times-Dispatch, "The Germans are beating us at our own game."

More than just providing the scientific roadmap, America funded Germany's eugenic institutions. By 1926, Rockefeller had donated some $410,000—almost $4 million in today's dollars—to hundreds of German researchers. In May 1926, Rockefeller awarded $250,000 to the German Psychiatric Institute of the Kaiser Wilhelm Institute, later to become the Kaiser Wilhelm Institute for Psychiatry. Among the leading psychiatrists at the German Psychiatric Institute was Ernst Rüdin.

Another in the Kaiser Wilhelm Institute's eugenic complex of institutions was the Institute for Brain Research. Since 1915, it had operated out of a single room. Everything changed when Rockefeller money arrived in 1929. A grant of $317,000 allowed the Institute to construct a major building and take center stage in German race biology. The Institute received additional grants from the Rockefeller Foundation during the next several years. Leading the Institute, once again, was Hitler's medical henchman, Ernst Rüdin. Rüdin's organization became a prime director and recipient of the murderous experimentation and research conducted on Jews, Gypsies, and other "undesirables" (Black, 2003, ch. 15).

Beginning in 1940, thousands of Germans taken from old-age homes, mental institutions, and other custodial facilities were systematically gassed. Between 50,000 and 100,000 were eventually killed.

Leon Whitney, executive secretary of the American Eugenics Society, declared of Nazism, "While we were pussy-footing around ... the Germans were calling a spade a spade."

A special recipient of Rockefeller funding was the Kaiser Wilhelm Institute for Anthropology, Human Heredity, and Eugenics in Berlin. For decades, American eugenicists had craved twins to advance their research into heredity. The Institute was now prepared to undertake such research on an unprecedented level. On May 13, 1932, the Rockefeller Foundation in New York dispatched a radiogram to its Paris office: JUNE MEETING EXECUTIVE COMMITTEE NINE THOUSAND DOLLARS OVER THREE YEAR PERIOD TO KWG INSTITUTE ANTHROPOLOGY FOR RESEARCH ON TWINS AND EFFECTS ON LATER GENERATIONS OF SUBSTANCES TOXIC FOR GERM PLASM.

At the time of Rockefeller's endowment, Otmar Freiherr von Verschuer, a hero in American eugenics circles, headed the Institute for Anthropology, Human Heredity and Eugenics. Rockefeller's funding of that Institute continued both directly and through other research conduits during Verschuer's early tenure. In 1935, Verschuer left the Institute to form a rival eugenics facility in Frankfurt that was much heralded in the American eugenic press. Research on twins in the Third Reich exploded, backed up by government decrees. Von Verschuer wrote in Der Erbarzt, a eugenic doctor's journal he edited, that Germany's war would yield a "total solution to the Jewish problem" (Black, 2003, ch. 17).

Von Verschuer had a long-time assistant. His name was Josef Mengele. On May 30, 1943, Mengele arrived at Auschwitz. Von Verschuer notified the German Research Society, "My assistant, Dr Josef Mengele (M.D., Ph.D.) joined me in this branch of research. He is presently employed as Hauptsturmführer [captain] and camp physician in the Auschwitz concentration camp. Anthropological testing of the most diverse racial groups in this concentration camp is being carried out with permission of the SS Reichsführer [Himmler]."

Mengele began searching the boxcar arrivals for twins. When he found them, he performed beastly experiments, scrupulously wrote up the reports, and sent the paperwork back to von Verschuer's institute for evaluation. Often, cadavers, eyes, and other body parts were also dispatched to Berlin's eugenic institutes.

Rockefeller executives never knew of Mengele. With few exceptions, the foundation had ceased all eugenic studies in Nazi-occupied Europe before the war erupted in 1939. But by that time, the die had been cast. The talented men Rockefeller and Carnegie financed, the institutions they helped found, and the science they helped create had taken on a scientific momentum of their own in Nazi Europe.

Since World War II

After the war, eugenics was declared a crime against humanity—an act of genocide. Article 2 of the Genocide Treaty defines five acts of genocide including the effort to "impose measures intended to prevent birth within the group." At Nuremburg, Germans were tried, and they cited US laws and court decisions in their defense—to no avail. They were found guilty (Lemkin, 1945; CPPCG, 1948; Black, 2003, ch. 19).

Von Verschuer escaped prosecution and once again became a respected scientist in Germany and around the world. In 1949, he became a corresponding member of the newly formed American Society of

Human Genetics, organized by American eugenicists and geneticists. In the fall of 1950, the University of Münster offered von Verschuer a position at its new Institute of Human Genetics, where he later became a dean. In the early and mid-1950s, von Verschuer became an honorary member of numerous prestigious societies, including the Italian Society of Genetics, the Anthropological Society of Vienna, and the Japanese Society for Human Genetics.

Despite the genocide treaty, American states such as North Carolina continued to practice eugenic and coercively sterilize thousands for decades after the war. Ironically, the concept of genocide was cobbled together and written by Rafael Lemkin at Duke University in North Carolina beginning in about 1941.

Now, the urge to improve mankind has again reared its head, this time based not on race but a sense of real, engineered genetic superiority. Lee Silver of Princeton, a leading exponent of transhumanism, is among a group of intellectuals calling for self-managed genetic enhancement. Silver's book *Remaking Eden* declares that in the unstoppable transhumanist future, the human species will separate into two branches, the "gen-rich" and the "naturals." Silver predicted that the gen-rich would eventually dominate the planet and will be "as different from humans as humans are from the primitive worms with tiny brains that first crawled along the earth's surface" (Silver, 1997, epilogue). Criticism has caused him to back-pedal a bit, but that approach is still representative of an energetic, always-lobbying core of transhumanists whose aim is to make a better human.

In the end, the question of what biological or cultural measure is to be imposed upon the group is to be decided from within—not from above. That decision is not ours to make. Once we do, we begin to play God. That has already been tried—more than once. It culminated in a war against the weak.

References

Aristotle. (1885). *Politics*, B. Jowett (Trans.). Oxford: Oxford University Press.

Black, E. (2003). *War against the weak*. Washington, DC: Dialog Press.

Breasted, J. (Ed.). (1930). *The Edwin Smith surgical papyrus: Hieroglyphic transliteration, translation, and commentary*. Chicago: University of Chicago Oriental Institute Publications.

Carlson, E. (2001). *The unfit: A history of a bad idea*. Cold Spring Harbor, NY: Cold Spring Harbor Press.

Carnegie, A. (1962). *The gospel of wealth and other timely essays* (E. Kirkland, Ed.). Cambridge, MA: Harvard University Press.

CPPCG (Convention on the Prevention and Punishment of the Crime of Genocide). (1948). Retrieved from: www.hrweb.org/legal/genocide.html

Elks, M. (1993). The "lethal chamber": Further evidence for the euthanasia option. *Mental Retardation, 31*, 202–212.

Fosdick, R. (1952). *The story of the Rockefeller Foundation*. New York: Harper & Brothers.

Galton, F. (1883). *Inquiries into human faculty and its development*. London: J. M. Dent & Co.

Goddard, H. (1912). *The Kallikak family: A study in the heredity of feeble-mindedness*. New York: Macmillan.

Grant, M. (1936). *The passing of the great race*. New York: Charles Scribner's Sons.

Hitler, A. (1943). *Mein kampf* (R. Manheim, Trans.). Boston: Houghton Mifflin Company.

Lemkin, R. (1945). Genocide: A modern crime. *Free World, 4*, 39–43.

Lifton, R. (2000). *The Nazi doctors: Medical killing and the psychology of genocide*. New York: Basic Books.

Lombardo, P. (2008). *Three generations, no imbeciles: Eugenics, the Supreme Court, and Buck v. Bell*. Baltimore, MD: Johns Hopkins University Press.

Lombardo, P. (Ed.). (2011). *A century of eugenics in America: From the Indiana experiment to the genome era*. Bloomington: Indiana University Press.

Lombardo, P. (Ed.). (2012). *Against their will: North Carolina's sterilization program and the campaign for reparations*. Apalachicola, FL: Gray Oak Books.

Malthus, T. (1798/1959). *An essay on the principle of population*. Ann Arbor, MI: University of Michigan Press.

Michell, H. (1964). *Sparta*. Cambridge: Cambridge University Press, 1964).

Nietzsche, F. (1906/1968). *The will to power* (W. Kaufmann, Trans.). New York: Random House.

Paul, E. (1917). *Population and birth-control: A symposium*. New York: Critic and Guide.

Plato. (1888). *Republic*, B. Jowett (Trans.). Oxford: Oxford University Press.

Pomeroy, S. (2002). *Spartan women*. Oxford: Oxford University Press.

Popenoe, P., & Johnson, R. (1918). *Applied eugenics*. New York: Macmillan.

Schopenhauer, A. (1851/1970). *Essays and aphorisms* (R. J. Hollingdale, Trans.). London: Penguin.

Shaw, G. (1910). Lecture to the Eugenics Education Society, reported by *Daily Mail*, Mar. 4.

Sherlock, E. B. (1911). *The feeble-minded: A guide to study and practice*. New York: Macmillan.

Silver, L. (1997). *Remaking Eden: Cloning and beyond in a brave new world*. New York: Harper Perennial.

Stone, D. (2002). *Breeding superman: Nietzsche, race and eugenics in Edwardian and interwar Britain*. Liverpool, UK: Liverpool University Press.

Wagener, O. (1987). *Hitler: Memoirs of a confidant* (H. Turner, Trans.). New Haven, CT: Yale University Press.

Wells, H. G. (1905). *A modern utopia*. London: Chapman & Hall.

Whitney, L. (1973). *Autobiography of Leon F. Whitney*, unpublished manuscript circa 1973.

Reply to Black

Nicholas Agar

Edwin Black tells us much about the history of attempts to enhance humans by selecting hereditary material. He pleads that we beware of "on-ramps to a genetic Autobahn that we will gradually help pave, mile by mile, with the hope that some speed limits will be observed." Black offers a condensed history of the horrors of eugenics to justify rejecting of all forms of genetic enhancement or modification.

What should we make of this? It is a slippery-slope argument and thus belongs to a category of argumentation that philosophers are taught to be suspicious of. At the top of Black's slope is "cloning the cutest pets." At its bottom is "the mindset of the Third Reich." Philosophers learn that a slippery-slope argument can be refuted by invoking a principle that clearly distinguishes the practices at the top of the slope from those at its bottom. There are (very) many differences between Hitler's eugenics and a program of genetic enhancement that might be acceptable to the citizens of a culturally diverse, early-twenty-first-century, liberal democracy. The former was driven by a hodgepodge of unscientific prejudices; the latter would be informed by the understanding of human heredity brought by modern genetics (Kitcher, 1996). The former imposed a monolithic view about human flourishing; the latter would acknowledge a plurality of views about the good life. The former used murder as a tool of human improvement; the latter would insist on strict moral limits on individuals' enhancement plans. One can accuse contemporary advocates of genetic enhancement of making too much of these differences, but the very existence of the differences cannot be denied.

Too Many Slippery Slopes

Perhaps this response is a bit glib. It assumes that if there is a moral distinction, people will respect it. People with the mindset of the Third Reich may want to use the tools of genetic enhancement for purposes that they should recognize as wrong.

The real problem with Black's chapter is that it vastly oversimplifies the complexity of the modern world. To be alive and aware in the early twenty-first century is to find yourself simultaneously at or near the top of many slippery slopes. The Internet has brought Facebook bullying, cyber-stalking, social isolation, and lots and lots of porn. It is reasonable to ask where all of this is taking us. An emotionally satisfying response is to insist that the Internet be shut down. A better response is to recognize that much that it provides is good. We should preserve this while striving to eliminate or minimize the bad. To use Black's preferred metaphor, we should not abruptly apply the handbrake. But we should maintain a foot above the brake pedal, so that we can slow down and change direction if necessary.

Genetic enhancers should proceed with caution. But this caution should be informed by relevant probabilities.

Contemporary Debates in Bioethics, First Edition. Edited by Arthur L. Caplan and Robert Arp.

The frightening thing about catastrophic global warming is not that it is a *possible* consequence of industrial civilization; according to current climate models, it is a *probable* consequence. In the wealthy, culturally diverse liberal democracies that might consider implementing limited programs of genetic enhancement, Nazi-style doctrines of racial superiority are mainly the province of angry, socially marginal types. They may perpetrate the occasional massacre, but they are unlikely to find themselves in charge. It is possible that geneticists will forget all they have learned about the universality of the human genetic code and dedicate themselves to spreading the few comparatively trivial racially specific fragments of DNA. But it is unlikely.

There is a biotechnological slippery slope leading to the mindset of the Third Reich that scares me more than Black's. This is a slippery slope that leads to medical experiments on human subjects of the type conducted in concentration camps by Nazi doctors. Nazi experiments prompted an elaborate assemblage of protections for human subjects of medical research. These are potentially under threat from new developments in biotechnology. Recently, there has been a move to recast aging as a disease (de Grey & Rae, 2007). Wealthy people are being enticed by a vision of millennial life spans. These life spans will be available to them only if research proceeds quickly. Anti-aging therapies will require human trials. Here is the problem. Rejuvenation research potentially changes the relationship between the human subjects of research and its beneficiaries. Currently sick people test new therapies for themselves and for other sick people. As a person with insulin-dependent diabetes, I have participated in a (seemingly inconclusive) trial of a new therapy for the disease. How likely are rich people, who are in conventional terms perfectly healthy but who find themselves suffering from diseases defined into existence by a redefinition of normal aging, to want to test a new anti-aging therapy that may manipulate parts of their bodies at the cellular level? Will the poor be financially coerced into clinical trials by the rich who want rejuvenation therapies as soon as possible?

I find these terrifying prospects because I can see how they might come to pass in liberal democracies such as ours—societies cursed with an ever-widening gap between rich and poor. They certainly are not inevitable. The correct response to their possibility is not to ban medical research on human subjects. It is to be vigilant.

Genetic Enhancement vs. Eugenics

There is an apparent disconnect between Black's chapter and mine. I defend some forms of genetic enhancement. He attacks eugenics. It is easy to see why defenders of genetic enhancement would want to avoid being linked with the crimes described by Black. But I think defenders of genetic enhancement should accept that some of what they want to do is eugenics. It conforms with the original 1883 definition of eugenics offered by Francis Galton. Galton characterized eugenics as "the science of improving stock" (Galton, 1883/1973, p. 17, fn 1).

Galton wrongly thought that the poor-quality hereditary material collected in the bodies of the poor. The fact that someone writing in the late 1800s had false beliefs about human biology is not surprising. We are, after all, talking about an age in which the application of leeches was a preferred treatment for diabetes. It is not surprising that scientific advances would radically change the practice of eugenics. Of particular relevance is the interactionist picture of development that I discussed in my chapter. Genes make human beings only in combination with environmental influences. Public-health campaigns that seek to improve the children's diets can be seen as part of the campaign for human improvement described by Galton. Galton criticized social welfare programs because he saw them as preventing natural selection from eliminating the bad hereditary material that had accumulated in the lower social classes. But the mapping of the human genome and scientific investigation of human genetic variation show this to be a mistake. Social hierarchies do not sort genetic material according to quality. This improved understanding of heredity allows latter-day eugenicists to look to social welfare programs to improve the expression of hereditary factors rather than aiming to delete them.

Retaining the term "eugenics" prevents a dangerous forgetting. Genetic modification—like medical research on human subjects—is inherently risky. One reason Soviet nuclear engineers operated the

Chernobyl reactor in such a reckless fashion is that the state's propaganda ministries denied them information about past nuclear accidents. They were prevented from learning of the dangers accompanying the operation of their type of reactor. If we ditch the word "eugenics," we risk leaving current practitioners of human biotechnology in a position analogous to that of the Soviet nuclear engineers. Those practicing genetic enhancement should inform themselves about the ugly side of the history of human improvement.

Slippery Slopes and Slip-Proof Ladders

It is interesting to compare Black's slippery slope with a contrary line that has gained some currency of late. For example, Matt Ridley's (2010) book, *The Rational Optimist*, offers a synthesis of evolutionary theory and economics that reveals a future with more of everything good and less of everything bad. Steven Pinker's (2011) book, *The Better Angels of Our Nature*, points to a dramatic ongoing decline in violence, war, and other acts of nastiness. We might call philosophical appeals to this continuing trend of improvement the *slip-proof ladder*.

Ridley's and Pinker's books may be factually correct but motivationally dangerous. The new optimism ignores a key fact about human psychology. The good trends Pinker and Ridley report on demand sustained effort. This effort often requires an exaggerated, literally false picture of potential dangers. For example, my country has seen, over the past years, a decline in the numbers of injuries caused by drink driving. Research places much of the credit for this decline on television campaigns. These did not convey the literally true message "If you drink and drive there is real but very small increased likelihood that you will be involved in an accident that will cause a serious injury to you or someone else." Instead they gave the false impression of a world in which there were breathalyzer-equipped police at every second intersection and inattentive preschoolers crossing at every third. This false impression dramatically reduced road deaths.

Sometimes the truth can set you free, but other times it just makes you complacent. A sad fact about people is that we often require fires under our behinds to do the right thing. There is a danger that Ridley's possibly true statement that our environmental problems are *soluble* will be interpreted as the false claim that they are *solved*. Perhaps this is where we need Black's emotive language. It is useful for geneticists to have a false impression of the proximity of Nazi eugenics so they can maintain a safe distance from it.

References

De Grey, A., & Rae, M. (2007). *Ending aging: The rejuvenation breakthroughs that could reverse human aging in our lifetime*. New York: St Martin's Press.

Galton, F. (1883/1973). *Inquiries into human faculty and its development*. New York: AMS Press.

Kitcher, P. (1996). *The lives to come: The genetic revolution and human possibilities*. New York: Simon & Schuster.

Pinker, S. (2011). *The better angels of our nature: Why violence has declined*. New York: Viking.

Ridley. M. (2010). *The rational optimist: How prosperity evolves*. New York: Harper Collins.

Reply to Agar

Edwin Black

The first response from Agar would be to wave a rhetorical halt to any comparisons between his call for limited enhancement and eugenics together with its dark legacy and potential gruesome future. Ethnic groups are even now targets for extinction. Will it be possible to tolerate the inferior in a genetically enhanced world? Will it be possible in Iran? In China? In Brazil? In an economically convulsive United States? The slope we are being asked to navigate is uncharted. Surely, the rationales will be incremental, and written by the proponents in power, not the recipients of any such action. First, society will move on what seems like the most obvious cases: the criminal, the chronically indolent, and the disabled.

Ironically, at least one group would protest right this moment that Agar advocates a viewpoint that they consider an open eugenic genocidal act against their group. Go back and read Agar's essay, and you will see the justification sentence: "Cochlear implants already help profoundly deaf people to hear by directly stimulating their auditory nerves." Says who? One only need Google "Deaf" and "eugenics" and "cochlear implants" to discover a raging protest movement that now exists in the deaf community. The deaf assert that their culture and identity are defined by their language, which is American Sign Language. In this way, they are similar to those who communicate chiefly in Yiddish, Arabic, or French, and who define their very culture by the use of those languages. The deaf are now fighting with all their might against the well-oiled campaign to legislate mandatory cochlear implants for newborns. Ironically, this campaign is the successor war waged against the deaf by Alexander Graham Bell, one of America's pioneer eugenicists and one of the earliest stalwarts of the American eugenics. Bell served as a scientific advisor to the Eugenics Record Office and the international eugenic conferences that propounded compulsory sterilization and euthanasia as solutions to the existence of the unfit—including the deaf. But the deaf consider their culture to be one of vibrant and animated communication, even if they employ visual—not spoken—language. Implants, the deaf vigorously argue, would separate the deaf from their children and transfer them out of the "deaf group" into the "hearing group." Article Two of the Genocide Treaty defines five acts of genocide, and the fifth one is "Forcibly transferring children of the group to another group" (Levy, 2002; Lane, 2005). Some Little People have made the same argument as they struggle to retain the genetic character of their small-statured community, generation to generation (Taussig et al., 2008).

Here is a good place to mention that in 1904, a highly intelligent African pygmy named Ota Benga was incarcerated in a cage at the Monkey House for public display by the Bronx Zoo. For years, he was

Contemporary Debates in Bioethics, First Edition. Edited by Arthur L. Caplan and Robert Arp.

living proof for high and mighty eugenicists of the evolutionary process. Public outrage finally forced Benga's release. His right to exist outside the cage he was thrown into by the high-minded, well-published anthropologists and eugenicists of the American Museum of Natural History and the Bronx Zoo was finally, if begrudgingly, acknowledged. Upon his release, he became an educated tobacco industry worker. He ultimately committed suicide in Virginia in 1916 (NYT, 1916). It seems the definition of normalcy depends upon whether you are looking down or looking up.

References

Lane, H. (2005). Ethnicity, ethics, and the deaf-world. *Journal of Deaf Studies and Deaf Education, 10*, 291–310.

Levy, N. (2002). Reconsidering cochlear implants: The lessons of Martha's Vineyard. *Bioethics, 16*, 134–153.

NYT (*New York Times*). (1916). Ota Benga, pygmy, tired of America. *New York Times*, Jul. 16, p. 12.

Taussig, K-S., Rapp, R., & Heath, D. (2008). Flexible eugenics: Technologies of the self in the age of genetics. In J. Inda (Ed.), *Anthropologies of modernity: Foucault, governmentality, and life politics* (pp. 215–235). Oxford: Blackwell Publishing.

Part 12

Can There Be Agreement as to What Constitutes Human Death?

Introduction

In the spring of 2012, in the town of Beiliu, China, a 95-year-old woman named Li Xiufeng was discovered by her neighbor one morning in bed showing no signs of breathing or a heartbeat. She was placed in a coffin in the den of her home so that friends and relatives could pay their respects for the next week, as is Chinese custom. Six days later, the day before her funeral, neighbors returned to Li's home to prepare her body for the funeral. What they discovered was an empty coffin—the lid overturned and lying on the floor—and Li preparing dinner in her kitchen! "I felt so hungry, I wanted something to eat," claimed Li, "I pushed the lid for a long time to climb out" (Evans, 2012; Garland, 2012). There are countless other stories similar to this one, where folks hop out of coffins, or pound on morgue fridges from the inside. And, unfortunately, exhumed coffins throughout the nineteenth century and early twentieth have been found to have scratch marks on the inside, or the corpses' lungs to contain dirt, indicating that someone was actually buried alive (Hartmann, 1895; Bondeson, 2002). What we want to emphasize in these mistaken-for-dead stories is the fact that a person is often considered to be dead when s/he stops breathing, which then leads to the heart ceasing to function. This is a commonsense, layperson's approach to human death; when we come upon someone lying unconscious on the ground, we check for breathing and a pulse, and if s/he shows no signs of these, then we assume s/he is dead.

Because of the vital roles that the respiratory and circulatory systems play in the body, this is an assumption that *most* of the time turns out to be true, but—as in the case of Li Xiufeng and countless others in human history—is not *always* true. In their 1905 work, *Premature Burial and How It May Be Prevented, with Special Reference to Trance, Catalepsy and Other Forms of Suspended Animation* (Tebb & Vollum, 1905), William Tebb and Col. Edward Vollum quote something noted by the nineteenth-century physician,

Contemporary Debates in Bioethics, First Edition. Edited by Arthur L. Caplan and Robert Arp.

Sir Henry Thomas, which still holds true today: "It should never be forgotten that there is but one really trustworthy proof that death has occurred in any given instance, viz., the presence of a manifest sign of commencing decomposition." And decomposition has been observed to be taking place soon after the systemic shutdown of all of the parts and processes of a body, so many have held that death occurs, then, when there is a permanent cessation of all biological functions of an organism (Shewmon, 2001, 2004). This is known as the *systemic view of death*. In the case of Li Xiufeng, doctors and researchers speculate that (1) the neighbors were mistaken in thinking that her breathing and heartbeat had stopped altogether, and/or (2) her breathing and heartbeat may have stopped altogether for a time, or even slowed down for a time, but her brain and other parts of her nervous system were still operating along with the major systems of her body to keep her alive and quasi-asleep for nearly a week. Thus, in her case, there was not a permanent cessation of all vital biological functions, so she was not dead.

Given the integral connection between the cardiovascular and the nervous system in one's body, humans are routinely declared dead around the world in emergency rooms and operating rooms when it is determined that there is no way to achieve cardiopulmonary resuscitation. In fact, one of the criteria for determining death from the US's Uniform Determination of Death Act of 1981 is an "irreversible cessation of circulatory and respiratory functions." This is known as the *cardiopulmonary view of death*. Some 10 s after cardiac arrest in a person, there is the start of cessation of brain electrical activity, brain oxygen levels are depleted after 2 min, and brain cells start to die; and after 10 min, there are the beginnings of a systemic cell death in the body (Mullins, 2005). It is still possible to harvest various body parts and other organs such as corneas, bones, skin, kidneys, liver, pancreas, and lungs for donation after someone suffers cardiac arrest and, this occurs all the time in all parts of the world (Talbot & D'Allessandro, 2009; Manara et al., 2012).

We can think about what constitutes death in the same way we think about meeting the criteria for what in logic are known as *necessary* and *sufficient* conditions. A necessary condition refers to a condition, state of affairs, or logical construct whereby, given A and B, to say that A is a *necessary condition* for B is to say that it is impossible to have B without A. In other words, the absence of A guarantees the absence of B. So, for example, let A be "clouds" and B be "rain." Clouds (A) are a necessary condition for rain (B), or, put another way, the absence of clouds (A) guarantees the absence of rain (B). Notice that there are other necessary conditions for rain, too, like the temperature being a certain degree, atmospheric pressure being just right, etc. Other examples of necessary conditions include:

- A fuel and an oxidant are each necessary conditions for combustion—you cannot have combustion without fuel and an oxidant.
- The existence of a point is a necessary condition for the existence of a line—a line, by definition, is made up of an infinite number of points.
- In a certain school, taking PHIL 100: Introduction to Philosophy is a necessary condition for taking PHIL 300: Philosophy of Mind—you will not be able to take PHIL 300 unless you have taken PHIL 100.
- Breathing air, lactating, being endothermic, having a backbone, and possessing hair and three middle ear bones are all necessary conditions for being considered a mammal—it is not a mammal if it does not meet all of these conditions.
- Referencing Thomas's claim above, death of the body is a necessary condition for the total decomposition of the body—you are not going to completely decompose (hopefully!) if you are not dead.

A sufficient condition, on the other hand, refers to a condition, state of affairs, or logical construct whereby, given A and B, to say that A is a *sufficient condition* for B is to say that if A is the case, then B must also be the case. In other words, the presence of A guarantees the presence of B. So, for example, let A be "placing one's bare hand in a gallon of water" and B be "one's hand getting wet." Placing one's bare hand in a gallon of water (A) is a sufficient condition (that is all that *suffices*) for one's hand getting wet (B), or, put another way, the presence of one's bare hand in a gallon of water (A) guarantees the presence of one's hand getting wet (B). Notice that there may be other events that act as a sufficient condition for one's hand getting wet, including placing it in a pool, or in the ocean, or in a pot of cold chicken soup, etc. Other examples include:

- Being a cat is sufficient (condition) for being a mammal.
- Receiving a grade of D is sufficient for passing the class.
- Being an 18-year-old American is sufficient to vote in America.
- Breathing air, lactating, being endothermic, having a backbone, and possessing hair and three middle ear bones *taken together* comprise the total sufficient condition for being considered a mammal—if an animal has the set of the conditions just mentioned, then it is definitely a mammal.
- Again, referencing Thomas, being dead for many weeks suffices for being in a state of decomposition.

A *complete and accurate* explanation, account of an event, or definition will be understood in terms of meeting *both* necessary and sufficient conditions in what is known as a *bi-conditional relationship* that can be expressed as "claim X if and only if claim Y," where X is the *total sufficient condition* for a complete and accurate explanation, account, etc., and Y is the *totality of the necessary conditions* for a complete and accurate explanation, account, etc. A vitally important point to mention is that if there is a necessary condition missing, or if one or more of the necessary conditions or the sufficient condition is not accurate, then the explanation, account, or definition is not complete and accurate. Consider these examples.

First, think of rain and the conditions for rain to occur. "It rains *if and only if* there are clouds, the temperature is a certain degree, and barometric pressure is of a certain level" is equivalent to the expression of the totality of necessary conditions "If it rains, *then* there are clouds, the temperature is a certain degree, and barometric pressure is of a certain level (all necessary conditions)" *and* the total sufficient condition "If there are clouds, the temperature is a certain degree, and barometric pressure is of a certain level (the sufficient condition expressed as the totality of necessary conditions), *then* it rains," or in symbolic notation: $(R <-> C \& T \& B) \equiv (R -> C \& T \& B) \& (C \& T \& B -> R)$. Note that if someone claimed that wind was necessary for rain, then s/he would be wrong about a *necessary* condition for rain, and the explanation for rain would be incomplete and inaccurate; while if someone omitted clouds, then s/he would be missing a necessary condition for rain *and* would be wrong about the *sufficient* condition for rain, and, again, the explanation for rain would be incomplete and inaccurate.

We can see how it is important to get the necessary and sufficient conditions of a definition correct, so that we are labeling instances or examples of things correctly, or making accurate judgments or decisions. You might think that being a mammal is all that suffices for being a cat, and that would be incorrect, since there are other feline properties that specify a mammal as being a cat. Or, you might think that antibiotics kill viruses, and so, you take a regimen of antibiotics thinking that the antibiotics are a necessary condition for your ability to combat the virus you have; however, you would be wrong.

Now, we can apply what we know so far to the definition of, and conditions for, death. According to the *systemic view of death* we noted above—which is commonsensical and noncontroversial—"Some organism is dead if and only if there is a permanent cessation of all biological functions of an organism." This being the case, then we can see how Li Xiufeng clearly was not dead, since she did not meet the totality of necessary conditions for death—her heart and breathing may have ceased, but (a) they obviously did not cease *permanently*, and (b) *all* of her biological functions did not cease permanently, as her brain (apparently) and other parts of her nervous system were still operating along with the major systems of her body. So, her neighbors *mistakenly* thought Li had met all of the necessary conditions and the sufficient condition for her being dead, when they discovered her with no apparent breathing and heartbeat.

Especially since the emergence of ventilating machines in the twentieth century, along with recent developments in neuroscience, thinking about what constitutes death has shifted away from cardiopulmonary functioning and the cardiac view of death and toward an understanding of the brain and the degree to which it is functioning fully and properly. The main reasons for this shift include the fact that (1) there may be little or no *discernible* cardiopulmonary functioning, yet the brain may still be functioning (as in the Li Xiufeng case) and, especially, (2) it is now possible to help keep the brain functioning with the assistance of ventilating machines that maintain cardiopulmonary functioning. There are countless cases of people who have been hooked up to ventilators and feeding tubes for an extended period of time (days, months, even years) and actually live through such an ordeal with their brains—including memories, experiences, sensations, and other psychological states—intact (Richardson, 1997; Raisin, 2007; Lean, 2009; Eccles, 2012).

These cases of people waking up from comas—a state of temporary unconsciousness—coupled with the idea that consciousness in terms of self-awareness and subjective experience is what makes us specifically and uniquely human—has caused many to argue that a human is considered dead when the whole brain or a certain part of the brain (the higher, more advanced, part or parts associated with the neocortex) permanently ceases to function. According to the *whole-brain view of human death*, one is considered dead if and only if the entire brain permanently ceases to function. So, if Li Xiufeng's neighbors had the ability to perform an electroencephalography (EEG) test for electrical impulses from neurons functioning in the brain, they would have discovered that Li was still alive.

According to the *higher-brain view of human death*, one is considered dead if and only if the higher parts of the brain responsible for consciousness in terms of self-awareness and subjective experience located in the neocortex permanently cease to function (Gervais, 1986; Veatch, 1993; Lizza, 1999, 2009). Notice that a human in a persistent vegetative state (PVS) who lacks conscious awareness would be considered dead, on this definition (McKeown et al., 2012; also the articles in BJA, 2012). There is also the *brainstem view of human death* (also known as the *lower-brain view*) that entails the permanent cessation of brainstem function, which includes basic autonomic functions such as respiration, body-temperature regulation, and the control of heartbeat waking and sleep. If the brainstem stops working, so must the heart, unless a mechanical, artificial heart is available.

In order to understand the higher-brain and brainstem views of human death, it is necessary to describe the parts of the human brain in brief. There are a few standard ways to categorize the human brain (Bear et al., 2006; Kandel et al., 2012), but for our purposes here it may be best to offer an evolutionary description that comports with contemporary neuroscience and accentuates the distinction between higher and lower parts of the human brain. The human brain itself can be envisioned as a three-part brain (MacLean, 1991; Kaas, 1993, 1995, 1996, 2008; Streidter, 2005) having evolved the *neocortex*, but retaining the *limbic system* found in mammals and the *brainstem core* found only in reptiles:

- The base of the human brain is shared with reptiles and mammals, and consists of the brainstem, reticular formation, and striate cortex. These areas are where the necessary command centers for living are located, namely, the control of sleep and waking, respiration, body temperature, basic automatic movements, and the primary way stations for sensory input.
- The *paleomammalian* cortex evolved on top of the reptilian brainstem, allowing for more modules to develop: the thalamus, allowing sight, smell, and hearing to be used together; the amygdala and hippocampus, apparatuses for memory and emotions; and the hypothalamus, making it possible for the organism to react to more stimuli by refining, amending, and coordinating movements. The functioning of the paleomammalian and reptilian cortices are somewhat analogous to the functioning of a heart, pancreas, or kidney, since they are organized for automatic action and response. This makes sense from an evolutionary perspective, as reptiles, amphibians, and mammals out in the wild share the common problems of having to respond quickly to environmental stimuli so as to know whether to fight, flee, forage, or procreate in order to survive.
- Finally, in the evolutionary history of primates, the *neomammalian* cortex (or neocortex) evolved on top of the paleomammalian and reptilian brains. This area consists of the outer layer of the cerebral hemispheres—made up of six layers standardly labeled I, II, III, IV, V, and VI—and is responsible for (a) the fine tuning of lower functions, (b) complex multi-modular sensory associations, (c) voluntary motor control, (d) abstract thinking, (e) planning abilities, (f) responsiveness to novel challenges, and (g) consciousness in terms of self-awareness and subjective experience (also see Kandel et al., 2012).

Humans are unique among the primates in having (d)–(g) to the greatest extent, and according to advocates of the higher-brain standard of human death, it is these abilities that have permanently ceased when someone dies (Gervais, 1986; Veatch, 1993; Lizza, 1999, 2009). Note that the brainstem core and paleomammalian cortex may still be functioning to maintain the autonomic processes of the human body—for example, in someone in a PVS—but a human nonetheless is still dead on the higher-brain standard (BJA, 2012).

The whole-brain standard of death, where brainstem core (brainstem, reticular formation, and striate cortex), paleomammalian cortex (thalamus, amygdala, hippocampus, hypothalamus), and neomammalian cortex cease to function permanently, has been accepted as public policy by most governments of the world (Gardiner et al., 2012; also Wijdicks, 2002), while most states of the US follow the definition of death found in the Uniform Determination of Death Act, approved by the National Conference of Commissioners on Uniform State Laws in 1981: "§ 1. [Determination of Death]. An individual who has sustained either (1) irreversible cessation of circulatory and respiratory functions, or (2) irreversible cessation of all functions of the entire brain, including the brain stem, is dead. A determination of death must be made in accordance with accepted medical standards."

The higher-brain standard of death, as one can imagine, is highly controversial and definitely a hot-button issue in many parts of the world, probably due to the fact that so-called "lower" parts of the brain are still functioning, and so there are still basic bodily functions such as a beating heart and certain reflex behaviors still present. Consider the widely publicized cases of Karen Ann Quinlan, who lived with a feeding tube in a PVS from 1975 to 1985, and Terri Schiavo, who lived with a feeding tube in a PVS from 1990 to 2005. In both of those cases, it was medically determined that the higher brain parts—ones associated with abstract thinking, planning abilities, responsiveness to novel challenges, sentience and consciousness in terms of self-awareness and subjective experience—were not functioning (Rich, 1997; Baker, 2000; McMahan, 2002; Laureys et al., 2004; Thogmartin, 2005; Caplan et al., 2006; Machado & Korein, 2011; Schnakers & Laureys, 2012).

Table P12.1 represents the views concerning death we have discussed thus far.

Like most researchers, the first author in this section, James Bernat, sees the systemic standard of death as noncontroversial and trivially true, really—a

Table P12.1 Views of human death

Systemic view of human death	*Cardiopulmonary view of human death*	*Whole-brain view of human death*	*Brainstem view of human death*	*Higher-brain view of human death*
Permanent cessation of all biological functions	Permanent cessation of cardiac and respiratory functions	Permanent cessation of entire brain	Permanent cessation of brainstem	Permanent cessation of higher parts of brain
Holds for any animal with a brain	Holds for any animal with a heart	Holds for any animal with a brain	It is possible to assist cardiovascular, respiratory, and digestive functions with ventilator and feeding tube	Holds for humans, normally considered to be in a PVS
Decomposition occurs as a natural consequence indicating clearly that death has occurred		It is possible to assist cardiovascular, respiratory, and digestive functions with ventilator and feeding tube		It is possible to assist cardiovascular, respiratory, and digestive functions with ventilator and feeding tube
	For the four views above, it is possible to harvest body parts or organs for donation and/or transplantation			

decomposing human body is an obvious and reliable indicator of permanent cessation of all biological functions of that body, and no one seriously doubts that the body is dead. However, concerning the cardiopulmonary, whole-brain, brainstem, and higher-brain standards, Bernat holds to the whole-brain standard: "the irreversible cessation of brain functions serves as a criterion of death because it is a necessary and sufficient condition for the cessation of the organism as a whole." What is his basic reason for this position? Reiterating some basic neurobiology—to include brief descriptions of the functions of the parts of the brainstem core, paleomammalian cortex, and neomammalian cortex—it is because a "brain dead patient whose visceral organ functions are maintained only as a consequence of technological support has lost the functions of the organism as a whole and is only a living component part of a dead organism, analogous in type though not extent to a technologically supported isolated living organ or limb. The irreversible loss of the functions of the brain responsible for the emergent functions of the organism as a whole indicates that the brain dead patient is a mechanically supported, living component part of a human organism who has already died."

In the process of surveying some of the standard positions concerning death—to include quasi-religious, soul-based, substance dualist positions—Bernat underscores the importance of defining death. In fact, more than 30 years ago, Bernat devised what he calls a *biophilosophical analytic method* for determining death with his colleagues (Bernat et al., 1981). This method is widely used by doctors around the world, actually (Shewmon, 2010), and consists of: (1) setting the rules and terms of the shared paradigmatic world-view concerning death; (2) explicitly stating the necessary and sufficient conditions for the definition of death; (3) identifying the measurable criterion that will show that a particular person has met the necessary and sufficient conditions for death; (4) finally, creating tests "whose goal is to demonstrate that the criterion of death has been fulfilled with no false-positive and minimal false-negative determinations."

The second author in this section, Winston Chiong, thinks that it is misguided to place so much emphasis on the definition of death, especially a definition that requires an explicit statement of necessary and sufficient conditions a priori. He utilizes, in part, Wittgenstein's (1958) idea that there exist certain terms related to natural kinds that resist an essential, unified, form-like (in the objective, Platonic sense) definition. Instead, according to Wittgenstein, these natural types of terms derive a common understanding and meaning from a nonessential shared meaning based in an "interrelated cluster of features, which may be present or absent in different cases." Sharing Wittgenstein's analysis, Chiong thinks that there is no essential feature associated with the term *death*—as there might be with more conventionally based, naming terms like *bachelor, vixen,* or *railroad engineer*—so even attempting to get at the necessary and sufficient conditions for *death* is futile (the same holds for the term *life*). Rather, death might be all or a significant number of a cluster of features—Wittgensteinian *family resemblances*—including the absence of consciousness, the cessation of vital functions, nongrowth, and decay and putrefication, to name just a few.

The implication would seem to be that any one of the views of death described thus far—systemic, cardiopulmonary, whole-brain, brainstem, or higher-brain—may be appropriate to use in a given context with the evidence at hand. In his response to Chiong, Bernat notes that Chiong's cluster of features has a problem: it is "even more vague in its capacity to provide specific criteria that physicians can use to determine life or death in the tough cases." One could imagine a Chiong-inspired response to Bernat that goes something like this: "It is precisely the tough cases, however, that should cause doctors to pause and consider whether an a priori set of conditions should be used to determine life or death."

References

Baker, L. (2000). *Persons and bodies*. Cambridge: Cambridge University Press.

Bear, M., Connors, B., & Paradiso, M. (2006). *Neuroscience: Exploring the brain*. New York: Lippincott Williams & Wilkins.

Bernat, J., Culver, C., & Gert, B. (1981). On the definition and criterion of death. *Annals of Internal Medicine, 94*, 389–394.

BJA (*British Journal of Anaesthesia*). (2012). Supplemental issue: Diagnosis of death and organ donation (Vol. 108, suppl. 1).

Bondeson, J. (2002). *Buried alive: The terrifying history of our most primal fear*. New York: W.W. Norton.

Caplan, A., McCartney, J., & Sisti, D. (Eds.). (2006). *The case of Terri Schiavo: Ethics at the end of life*. Amherst, NY: Prometheus Books.

Eccles, L. (2012). The boy who came back from the dead: Experts said car crash teen was beyond hope. His parents disagreed. *MailOnLine*, April 24. Retrieved from: http://www.dailymail.co.uk/health/article-2134346/Steven-Thorpe-Teenager-declared-brain-dead-FOUR-doctors-makes-miracle-recovery.html

Evans, N. (2012). Zombie gran: 95-year-old Chinese woman terrifies neighbours by climbing out of her coffin six days after she "died." *Mirror*, February 26. Retrieved from:http://www.mirror.co.uk/news/weird-news/zombie-gran-95-year-old-chinese-woman-746295

Gardiner, D., Shemie, S., Manara, A., & Opdam, H. (2012). International perspective on the diagnosis of death. *British Journal of Anaesthesia, 108*, i14–i28.

Garland, I. (2012). Mourners left stunned when "dead" waiter, 28, wakes up at his own FUNERAL *Mail*, May 12. Retrieved from: http://www.dailymail.co.uk/news/article-2143513/Hamdi-Hafez-al-Nubi-Dead-waiter-28-wakes-FUNERAL.html#ixzz26rMLptrp

Gervais, K. (1986). *Redefining death*. New Haven, CT: Yale University Press.

Hartmann, F. (1895). *Buried alive: An examination into the occult causes of apparent death, trance and catalepsy*. Boston: Occult Publishing.

Kaas, J. (1993). Evolution of the multiple areas and modules within neocortex. *Perspectives in Developmental Neurobiology, 1*, 101–107.

Kaas, J. (1995). The evolution of isocortex. *Brain, Behavior, and Evolution, 46*, 187–196.

Kaas, J. (1996). What comparative studies of neocortex tell us about the human brain. *Revista Brasileira de Biologia, 56*, 315–322.

Kaas, J. (2008). Evolution of the brain in mammals. In M. Binder, N. Hirokawa, & U. Windhorst (Eds.), *Encyclopedia of neuroscience, vol. 1* (pp. 721–723). London: Springer.

Kandel, E., Schwartz, J., Jessel, T., Siegelbaum, S., & Hudspeth, A. (2012). *Principles of neural science*. New York: McGraw-Hill.

Laureys, S., Faymonville, M-E., De Tiege, X., Peigneux, P., Berre, J. . . . Maquet, P. (2004). Brain function in the vegetative state. In C. Machado & D.A. Shewmon (Eds.), *Brain death and disorders of consciousness* (pp. 229–238). New York: Kluwer Academic Publishers.

Lean, G. (2009). "Locked in a coma, I could hear people talking around me." *The Telegraph*, November 24. Retrieved from: http://www.telegraph.co.uk/health/6638155/Locked-in-a-coma-I-could-hear-people-talking-around-me.html

Lizza, J. (1999). Defining death for persons and human organisms. *Theoretical Medicine and Bioethics, 20*, 439–453.

Lizza, J. (Ed.). (2009). *Defining the beginning and end of life: Readings on personal identity and bioethics*. Baltimore, MD: Johns Hopkins University Press.

Machado, C., & Korein, J. (2011). Irreversibility: Cardiac death versus brain death. *Reviews in the Neurosciences, 20*, 199–202.

MacLean, P. (1991). *The triune brain in evolution*. Dordrecht: Kluwer Academic Publishers.

Manara, A., Murphy, P., & O'Callaghan, G. (2012). Donation after circulatory death. *British Journal of Anaesthesia, 108*, i108–i121.

McKeown, D., Bonser, R., & Kellum, J. (2012). Management of the heartbeating brain-dead organ donor. *British Journal of Anaesthesia, 108*, i96–i107.

McMahan, J. (2002). *The ethics of killings: Problems at the margins of life*. Oxford: Oxford University Press.

Mullins, D. (2005). *Pathology and microbiology for mortuary science*. Independence, KY: Delmar Cengage Learning.

Raisin, S. (2007). *Tour de life: From coma to competition*. New York: Three Story Press.

Rich, B. (1997). Postmodern personhood: A matter of consciousness. *Bioethics, 11*, 206–216.

Richardson, L. (1997). No miracles in coma cases, doctors say. *Los Angeles Times*, August 22. Retrieved from: http://articles.latimes.com/1997/aug/22/news/mn-24900

Schnakers, C., & Laureys, S. (Eds.). (2012). *Coma and disorders of consciousness*. London: Springer.

Shewmon, D. (2001). The brain and somatic integration: Insights into the standard biological rationale for equating "brain death" with death. *Journal of Medicine and Philosophy, 26*, 457–478.

Shewmon, D. (2004). The "critical organ" for the organism as a whole: lessons from the lowly spinal cord. *Advances in Experimental Medicine and Biology, 550*, 23–42.

Shewmon, D. (2010). Constructing the death elephant: a synthetic paradigm shift for the definition, criteria, and tests for death. *Journal of Medicine and Philosophy, 35*, 256–298.

Streidter, G. (2005). *Principles of brain evolution*. Sunderland, MA: Sinauer Associates.

Talbot, D., & D'Allessandro, A. (Ed.). (2009). *Organ donation and transplantation after cardiac death*. Oxford: Oxford University Press.

Tebb, W., & Vollum, E. (1905). *Premature burial and how it may be prevented, with special reference to trance, catalepsy and other forms of suspended animation*. London: Swan Sonnenschein.

Thogmartin, J. (2005). Autopsy report of Theresa Marie ("Terri") Schiavo: Case # 5050439. Retrieved from: http://www.abstractappeal.com/schiavo/autopsyreport.pdf

Veatch, R. (1993). The impending collapse of the whole-brain definition of death. *Hastings Center Report*, *23*, 18–24.

Wijdicks, E. (2002). Brain death worldwide: Accepted fact but no global consensus in diagnostic criteria. *Neurology*, *58*, 20–25.

Wittgenstein, L. (1958). *Philosophical investigations* (G. E. M. Anscombe, Trans.). New York: Macmillan.

Chapter Twenty Three

There Can Be Agreement as to What Constitutes Human Death

James L. Bernat

The persisting controversies over the definition of human death cannot be resolved unless scholars accept a four-step sequential analysis: (1) the *paradigm* stating the conditions and assumptions that frame the argument; (2) the *definition* making explicit our ordinary usage of the word "death;" (3) the *criterion* identifying the measurable general condition that shows that the definition has been fulfilled by being both necessary and sufficient conditions for death; and (4) the *tests* that demonstrate that the criterion of death has been fulfilled. Although the breadth of controversy on the definition and criterion of death makes it unlikely that scholarly consensus can be achieved, it may not matter if societies can establish publicly and professionally acceptable guidelines for physicians to determine death.

Statement of the Problem

The definition of human death was among the first topics debated by scholars in the early era of biomedical ethics and biophilosophy (Jonsen, 2008). For example, it was one of the first projects of the Institute of Society, Ethics, and the Life Sciences, later called the Hastings Center (Task Force on Death and Dying, 1972), and the first project of the President's Commission for the Study of Ethical Problems in Medicine and Biomedical and Behavioral Research (1981). Yet, despite several decades of further discussion and analysis, it stubbornly remains a source of scholarly fascination and contention.

This controversy was absent in the pre-technological era—roughly corresponding to before 1950—because in that era, death always was a unitary phenomenon. Because of the innate interdependency of respiratory, circulatory, and brain functions, when one function stopped, the others stopped within minutes. Thus, a person suffering cardiac arrest always also suffered respiratory arrest and vice versa. When brainstem function failed and spontaneous respiration ceased as a result, cessation of circulation followed rapidly and inevitably. No one had to consider whether a patient was dead or alive who had completely lost all brain functions while maintaining circulatory and respiratory functions because such cases were technologically impossible.

The introduction of the positive-pressure mechanical ventilator into medical practice in the 1950s permanently altered this interdependent relationship. For the first time, patients with irreversible cessation of all brain functions (including spontaneous respiration) could have their absent respiratory function successfully supported by tracheal positive-pressure mechanical ventilators, thereby preventing the development of immediate circulatory arrest. This

Contemporary Debates in Bioethics, First Edition. Edited by Arthur L. Caplan and Robert Arp.

"artificial" maintenance of respiration and circulation permitted the continued functioning of bodily organs, other than the brain, at least temporarily. The technological breakthrough of positive-pressure mechanical ventilators marvelously saved the lives of otherwise-healthy patients suffering temporary respiratory failure, but by supporting the respiration of patients who had lost all brain functions, it spelled the end of human death as a unitary phenomenon.

Once death ceased to be a unitary phenomenon, the question arose: were patients alive or dead who lacked all brain functions, but whose absent spontaneous respiratory and circulatory functions were mechanically supported? Their precise biological status became ambiguous. They shared some features associated with living patients because their autonomously beating hearts circulated blood oxygenated by the mechanical ventilator allowing their organs (except the brain) to remain functioning. But they also shared some features of dead patients in that they could not breathe or move at all, and showed no behavioral or reflex response to any stimulus.

The first physicians who described such patients intuited that they differed in an essential way from all other patients in coma who had ever been examined. A committee of Harvard University physicians and scholars coined the unfortunately misleading term *brain death* to describe them, and asserted that, because of the irreversible absence of their brain functions and despite the continued presence of their circulation and heartbeat, these patients were actually dead (Ad Hoc Committee, 1968). But, despite their pioneering insights, the Ad Hoc Committee provided no coherent philosophical analysis to prove their intuitive assertion.

The technological advance of the positive-pressure ventilator did not require a change in the definition of human death. Rather, by creating an example of a previously unanticipated biological situation, the new technology showed that formerly we lacked an explicit definition of death. Scholars therefore had to conduct the conceptual task of defining death by making explicit the meaning implicit in our ordinary use of the word *death* that had been rendered ambiguous by technological developments.

The question I consider here is whether scholars ever can agree on such a definition of death. Current disagreement extends beyond the content of a definition itself. Some scholars have argued that defining death is impossible (Halevy & Brody, 1993), unnecessary (Chiong, 2005), unimportant (Fost, 1999), culturally determined (Veatch, 1999), or innately dual (McMahan, 1995; Lizza, 1999). Even among scholars who agree on a definition, there is disagreement on the criterion of death that is necessary and sufficient to satisfy the definition. Some scholars advocate the whole-brain criterion (President's Commission, 1981; Chiong, 2005), the higher-brain criterion (Gervais, 1986; Veatch, 1993), the brainstem criterion (Pallis, 1995), or the circulatory criterion (Shewmon, 2001). To identify the sources of disagreement, I rely on the biophilosophical analytic method that my Dartmouth colleagues, Bernard Gert and Charles Culver, and I developed, that generally is regarded as the standard model of death analysis by other scholars in this field (Bernat et al., 1981).

Two important caveats are in order. First, although the definition and criterion of death remain a source of philosophical debate within the academy, standards for the bedside determination of death have been firmly settled within the medical community. This consensus has led to the acceptance of standardized clinical practice guidelines and reasonably uniform death statutes enacted in jurisdictions throughout the United States, Canada, and much of the developed and developing world. Thus, the ongoing academic debate over the definition and criterion of death has produced no more than a negligible impact on the practical world. Second, although the controversies over the use of brain or circulatory tests for death first came to medical and public attention in the context of declaring the death of organ transplant donors, they highlight essential biophilosophical concepts that exist independently of utilitarian transplantation considerations.

A Biophilosophical Analysis of Death

Numerous scholars have analyzed the definition and criterion of death over the past several decades. Thirty years ago, my Dartmouth colleagues and I contributed to this debate by offering a rigorous biophilosophical analytical method, proceeding from the conceptual to the tangible and measurable (Bernat et al., 1981), that since has been accepted by most other scholars, even including many of those who disagreed with our proposed definition or criterion of death. For example, Alan Shewmon, a scholar who rejects every brain criterion of death in favor of the circulatory criterion, recently described our analytic method as "virtually universally accepted" (Shewmon, 2010). A sequential, systematic analytic method provides a valuable tool because it proceeds in a logical order and permits one to pinpoint areas of scholarly disagreement and clarify the reasons for it.

Our four-stage sequential analytic method consists of paradigm, definition, criterion, and tests (Bernat, 2002). The paradigm is a set of conditions and assumptions that frame the argument by identifying its nature, clarifying the class of phenomena to which it belongs, and demarcating its conceptual boundaries (Bernat, 2002). Accepting the paradigm, like accepting a set of ground rules for a game, is a prerequisite for further discussion. There is no possibility of achieving scholarly consensus on the definition and criterion of death if there first cannot be consensus on the paradigm conditions because scholars will be discussing different classes of phenomena. Identifying the definition of death is the philosophical task of making explicit the meaning implicit in our ordinary use of the common and nontechnical term *death* that we all use correctly. Identifying the criterion of death is the philosophical and medical task of determining that measurable general condition that shows that the definition has been fulfilled by being both necessary and sufficient for death. Devising tests of death is the medical-scientific task whose goal is to demonstrate that the criterion of death has been fulfilled with no false-positive and minimal false-negative determinations.

Not all scholars endorse our sequential analytic method. Winston Chiong (2005) rejects beginning an analytic process with a definition of death because he claims that my colleagues and I rely on the misguided philosophical approach to determining a definition by trying to divine the essence of death. Chiong cited Wittgenstein's argument that some common terms, such as *games*, cannot have uniform definitions that are based on the possession of an essential meaning shared by all members of the set because all members of the set in question do not share an essential characteristic. Rather than communally sharing an essential characteristic, members of the set are related to each other in various other ways. Chiong claims that *death* is such a word. He argues that searching for the essence of the meaning of the word *death* from which to establish its definition is futile because there are no conditions that are both necessary and sufficient for death. He further observed that defining death is an unnecessary step to sustain a coherent argument supporting the whole-brain criterion of death. He concluded that our paradigm-definition-criterion-test sequential analytic method therefore should be rejected.

My philosopher colleague, Bernard Gert, refuted Chiong's criticism (Gert, 2006). Gert argued that Chiong misunderstood the correct meaning of a definition by accepting the discredited essentialist concept of a definition. The effort to choose a definition of death is not to make explicit the implicit essence of the concept of death but rather to make explicit the meaning implicit in our consensual and ordinary use of the nontechnical word *death*. Gert further pointed out that, given this proper intent of definition, Chiong, perhaps unknowingly, also relied on a definition of death—though one more diffuse than ours—in his defense of the whole-brain criterion of death. Therefore, Chiong's argument rejecting definition constituted an invalid criticism of our paradigm-definition-criterion-test method of analysis that requires starting with what is ordinarily meant by the term *death* before choosing its criterion.

In an essay on the semiotics of language describing death, Alan and Elisabeth Shewmon showed how each language has evolved unique words to describe death, and how these words themselves categorically limit our ability to state a definition of death that is acceptable among different cultures (Shewmon & Shewmon, 2004). The Shewmons asserted that death resists a uniform definition because it is an "ur-phenomenon [that is] conceptually fundamental in its class; no more basic concepts exist to which it can be reduced. It can only be intuited from our experience of it." Other biophilosophers have reached a similar conclusion about the futility of defining the phenomenon of human conscious awareness. Yet, these claims, while valid, do not preclude identifying the meaning of ordinary words like *death* that we all use correctly.

The Paradigm of Death

The paradigm of death has seven elements:

1. The word *death* is a common, nontechnical word that we all use correctly to refer to the cessation of the life of a human being or another higher-vertebrate species. The philosophical task of defining death seeks not to redefine it by contriving a new meaning, but rather to determine and make explicit the implicit meaning of death underlying our consensual usage of the word that has become ambiguous as a result of technological advances. Scholars should neither redefine death from its ordinary meaning to achieve an ideologically desired end nor overanalyze it to such a metaphysical level of abstraction that it is rendered devoid of its ordinary meaning.
2. Death is fundamentally a biological phenomenon. Because life is fundamentally a biological phenomenon, its cessation also must be. This condition does not denigrate the value of cultural and religious practices surrounding death and dying, nor does it deny societies the authority to establish laws regulating the determination and time of death. Because death is an immutable biological fact and is not a social contrivance, the paradigm concerns only the ontology of death and not its normative aspects.[1]
3. We restrict analysis to the death of higher-vertebrate species for which death is univocal: we mean the same concept of death when we say our cousin died as we do when we say our dog died. Simpler organisms and parts of organisms, such as cells or organs, also can die but our task purview is the death of the higher organism.
4. The term *death* can be applied directly and categorically only to organisms. All living organisms must die, and only living organisms can die. When we say "a person died," we are referring to the death of the formerly living human organism that embodied the person, not to a human organism that remains alive but ceases to have the attributes of a person. Personhood is a psychosocial, religious, moral, and legal construct that may be lost in some cases of severe brain damage but cannot die, except metaphorically.
5. A higher-vertebrate organism can reside in only one of two states, alive or dead. No organism can be in both states or in neither. However, we currently lack the technical ability always to accurately identify an organism's state and, at times, may know it only in retrospect. Alive and dead are mutually exclusive (nonoverlapping) and jointly exhaustive (no other) biological states.
6. Death is best regarded as an event and not a process. If there are only two exclusive and non-overlapping underlying states of an organism, the transition from one state to the other, at least in theory, must be sudden, discontinuous, and instantaneous, because of the absence of an intervening state. For technical reasons, the event of death may be determinable with confidence only in retrospect. As my colleagues and I noted, death is best conceptualized not as a process but as the event separating the true biological processes of dying and bodily disintegration (Bernat et al., 1981).
7. Death is irreversible. If the event of death were reversible, it would not be death, but rather incipient dying, that was interrupted and reversed.

Challenges to the Paradigm of Death

Several scholars have disagreed with elements of the paradigm. The most serious disagreement is over whether there can be a uniform concept of death for a human being or whether there must be two types of death: death of a human organism and death of a person. Jeff McMahan (1995, 2002) holds that because human beings are our persons and not simply our organisms, what counts most in a concept of death is the death of the person. He advocates having separate, dual accounts of death for persons and for human organisms, and acknowledges that this dichotomy represents a form of mind–body dualism. John Lizza (1999) reached the same conclusion using a similar argument.

McMahan and Lizza reached their dualistic conclusions because they offer a more expansive concept of person than merely one of a human organism endowed with certain attributes, such as the concept of person and personhood that Gert, Culver, and I endorse. McMahan and Lizza's idea of a person differs from ours because it incorporates a soul or at least an infused spiritual element that exists separately but in parallel with the bodily organism. This account of personhood therefore requires a dual account of death.[2]

Lee and George (2008) and Shewmon (2010) have further developed the concept that views a person as having both animal and mental components ("body-self dualism"), and assert that the mental component cannot be produced merely from the animal component. Shewmon (2010) further elucidated this concept: "reflective self-awareness, universal concept formation, abstract reasoning, and free will all have properties that transcend spatiality and cannot in principle emerge from a complex electrochemical network. They therefore derive from an immaterial principle, but nevertheless, one profoundly oriented to operate in and through a body." These scholars therefore deny the "reductive" claim accepted by most cognitive neuroscientists that the mind is solely the product of the brain.

Gert, Culver, and I require for our paradigm that human beings are only our human organisms, that self-awareness and other human behaviors are solely emergent functions of the brain that do not derive from an immaterial principle, and therefore human death is the death of the human organism. This approach is consistent with three other elements of the paradigm: (1) death is fundamentally a biological phenomenon; (2) only organisms can die; and (3) the univocal usage of the word *death* requires that it mean the same thing for humans as for other higher animals such as dogs unimbued with souls. We regard personhood as a set of psychosocial, legal, moral, and religious attributes of human beings that arguably may be lost by severe brain injury or illness but cannot die except metaphorically. In his monograph, Eric Olson (1997) more rigorously and expansively defends the position that human beings are our organisms.

Robert Veatch (1999) takes the libertarian view that because death is a socially and culturally defined phenomenon, each individual should be permitted to decide the criteria that physicians use to determine his or her own death. My understanding of his claim (clarified by discussions with him) is that it is only the determination of death that is relativistic and culturally defined, and not the underlying concept of death. It is therefore plausible to make Veatch's claim without rejecting the paradigm condition that death is fundamentally a biological phenomenon.

Linda Emanuel (1995) exemplifies a scholar who relies too heavily on metaphysics with her claim "there is no state of death . . . to say 'she is dead' is meaningless because 'she' is not compatible with 'dead.'" Emanuel's depth of metaphysical abstraction of the concept cannot identify a definition or criterion of death because it offers nothing to clarify the common usage of the term *death*. And as an experienced physician, she obviously does not truly believe that there is no state of death.

Halevy and Brody (1993) claim that defining death is impossible because an organism can reside in a transitional state between life and death that has features of both states but is congruent with neither state. Using the mathematical model of fuzzy logic, they postulate that whereas no organism can fully belong to both the sets of living and dead organisms, because the sets represent mutually exclusive states, some organisms can reside in a transitional state in which they have some features of each state but do not fully belong to either the set of living or dead organisms.

Our argument against this position emphasizes the distinction between the precise life-state of an organism and of our ability to accurately determine that state. Simply because, as a consequence of technical limitations, we may not be able to determine conclusively at all times whether a given organism is alive or dead does not mean that it must reside in a transitional state between alive and dead. The paradigm provides that all organisms are either dead or alive, but because of technical limitations, we may be able to make the accurate determination of its life-state only in retrospect. Future technological advances will improve the accuracy of this determination.

In their mathematical analysis of state discontinuities, Alan and Elisabeth Shewmon (2004) settled the longstanding debate over whether death is best understood as an event or as a process. The Shewmons showed that death must be an event because of the suddenness and discontinuity of the transition from the states of alive to dead, given the absence of an intervening state. They agreed that we may not always be able to identify the precise time of the event, and we may be able to identify it only in retrospect because of technical limitations. Everyone agrees that the biological phenomena of dying before death and of bodily disintegration after death are processes. Most scholars, including the Shewmons, now agree with us that death is best viewed as the event separating the process of dying from the process of bodily disintegration (Bernat et al., 1981).

The Definition of Death

A prerequisite for analyzing the definition of death is understanding the nature of an organism and, especially, the concept of the organism as a whole. The concept of the "organism as a whole" emphasizes the distinction between the life-state of the organism and the life-state of its component parts. A definition of death must address the level of the life-state of the organism, not of its component parts.

An organism comprises hierarchically arrayed interdependent units or subsystems that have evolved over many millions of years. Although each unit or subsystem is alive, none alone constitutes an organism. Living cells comprise living tissues that in turn comprise living organs that in turn comprise living organ systems. The organism's cells, tissues, organs, and organ systems are organized in functional groups displaying hierarchies of functions. The interrelationships of the many hierarchies of functional units create an integrated, coordinated, unified whole. That whole is the organism itself, the highest and most complex life form that is alive as a result of the functioning of its living component subsystems.

Functioning components of an organism create unique phenomena known as emergent functions. An emergent function is a function of a whole entity that is neither present within nor reducible to any of its component parts (Mahner & Bunge, 1997). Such a function is called "emergent" because, given the normal coordinated presence of bodily components in an operational unit, the new function emerges spontaneously. Thus, tissues have emergent functions beyond those of its component cells, and organs have emergent functions beyond those of its component tissues. Each emergent function is a more complex behavior than those of its component subunits. Given our current scientific understanding and mathematical modeling, emergent functions cannot be predicted or easily understood solely by studying the component subunits, their interrelationships, and their functions (Clayton & Kauffman, 2006). The most inscrutable example of an emergent function is that of human conscious awareness, an exquisite but ineffable phenomenon that emerges spontaneously from the integrated functioning of multiple distributed parallel hierarchical networks of brain neurons (Koch, 2004).

The life of the cellular, tissue, or organ components, while often necessary for the life of the organism, is not equivalent to the life of the organism. Because the life of its component parts is not equivalent to the life of an organism, an organism can die despite some of its component parts remaining alive as a consequence of technological support. The key to understanding the definition of death is the separation of the life of an organism from the life of its component parts.

The most accurate definition of death in our technological age is the irreversible cessation of functioning of the organism as a whole. The concept of "organism as a whole" was proposed by the early-twentieth-century biologist, Jacques Loeb, in a classic monograph of that name (Loeb, 1916). The "organism as a whole" refers not to the whole organism (the sum of its component parts) but to the emergent functions of the organism that are the consequence of the normal operation of but greater than the mere sum of its component parts. Intrinsic to the concept of "organism as a whole" is that the interrelatedness of the component parts provides emergent functions that create the coherent unity of the organism. To explore this concept further, it is necessary first to clarify a few fundamental facts about the biological nature of living organisms.

For many years, scientists and philosophers have attempted the daunting task of identifying the criteria of life. For example, the biologist, Jacques Monod, elucidated the characteristics that separate living from nonliving entities: (1) teleonomy, the correspondence between structure and function that suggests purpose; (2) autonomous morphogenesis or self-reproduction of form; and (3) reproductive invariance, the phenomenon in which the source of information expressed in the structure of a biological form results entirely and only from a structurally identical form

(Monod, 1971). Other scientists have created similar lists (Crick, 1981; Margulis & Sagan, 1995). All scholars acknowledge that it is easier to describe the functions of life than to define life, and that even exhaustive lists of the characteristics of life inevitably create ambiguities and exceptions (such as the classification of viruses or prions).

The specific criteria of life forms and higher organisms were recently analyzed by Raphael Bonelli and colleagues (Bonelli et al., 2009). They observed that all life forms have a delimited unity that is characterized by four criteria: (1) dynamics, or signs of life, such as metabolism, regeneration, growth, and propagation; (2) integration, the requirement that the life process derives from the mutual interaction of its component parts; (3) coordination, the requirement that the interaction of the component parts is maintained within a certain order; and (4) immanency, the requirement that the preceding characteristics originate from and are intrinsic to the life form. These are characteristics of all life forms, including the component parts of organisms.

Bonelli and colleagues then identifed four criteria that make a life form an integrated, unified, and whole organism: (1) completion, the requirement that an organism is not a component part of another living entity but is itself an intrinsically independent and completed whole; (2) indivisibility, the condition of intrinsic unity that no organism can be divided into more than one living organism; and, if such a division occurs and the organism survives, the completed organism must reside in one of the divided parts; (3) self-reference or auto-finality, the characteristic that the observable life processes and functions of the component parts serve the self-preservation of the whole, even at the expense of the survival of its parts, because the health and survival of the living whole is the primary end in itself; and (4) identity, the circumstance that, despite incremental changes in form and the loss or gain of certain component parts (that even could eventually result in the exchange of all component atoms), the living being remains one and the same throughout life (Bonelli et al., 2009).

Bonelli and colleagues concluded that the death of an organism is the loss of these four characteristics that render an organism no longer capable of functioning as a whole. They point out that in higher animal species, with the irreversible cessation of all functions of the entire brain ("brain death"), the organism has permanently lost the capacity to function as a whole and therefore is dead. The organism has lost immanency because its life processes no longer spring from itself but result from external intensive care support. The organism has lost auto-finality because whatever control over the component organ subsystem parts that remains now is directed at the level of the surviving parts and no longer at the whole. The organism has lost self-reference because the continued functioning of its parts no longer supports the function of the whole. The organism has lost completeness and indivisibility because its separate component parts and subsystems no longer belong to each other and no longer constitute a whole (Bonelli et al., 2009).

In our contemporary technological era in which skilled physicians with advanced technology can maintain the life of component parts of organisms outside or inside the body, the continued life of the organism versus the continued life of its component parts has become ambiguous. The essence of the death of a higher animal species is the irreversible cessation of the functioning of the organism as a whole. Once an organism has irreversibly lost its totality, completion, indivisibility, self-reference, and identity, it no longer functions as a whole and is dead.

A necessary but not sufficient feature of the organism as a whole is the integration and coordination of its component subsystems by a central control system. Julius Korein first championed this idea and provided an account using thermodynamics and entropy to argue that the brain is the critical system of the organism whose permanent loss of functioning equals death (Korein, 1978, 1997). Alan Shewmon later showed the inadequacy of relying solely on an integration-coordination rationale for "brain death" because certain control systems are integrated and coordinated by the spinal cord and by other structures outside the brain (Shewmon, 2001, 2004).

In their book, *Controversies in the Determination of Death*, the President's Council on Bioethics (2009) accepted Shewmon's critique and offered an alternative rationale to the integration-control concept. They supported the coherence and validity of "brain death" but argued that irreversible cessation of all brain functions was death not because of the organism's loss of integration but because it caused "the inability of the organism to conduct its self-preserving work" (President's Council 2009). In a critique, Shewmon refuted the President's Council's new rationale for a neurological standard of death by arguing that it suffered the same conceptual flaws as the integration rationale they replaced (Shewmon, 2009). But these criticisms are of the criterion of death, not of the definition of death as the irreversible cessation of the organism as a whole—one that the President's Council and Shewmon both accept.

The Criterion of Death

The criterion of death is the measurable general condition, suitable for inclusion in a death statute that shows that the definition has been fulfilled by being both necessary and sufficient for death. In published analyses of death, four principal choices for a criterion of death have been proposed, and each has been accepted by a group of scholars: the whole-brain, higher-brain, brainstem, and circulatory formulations. The first three are variants of the "brain death" concept, whereas the circulatory formulation rejects "brain death" and holds that a person is not dead until systemic circulation ceases irreversibly. An overwhelming majority of medical associations and jurisdictions have accepted the practice of "brain death," and accept the whole-brain criterion of death that my Dartmouth colleagues and I also accept. The brainstem formulation prevails in the UK, yet the tests for "brainstem death" in the UK and for "brain death" elsewhere are nearly identical (Pallis, 1995). No society or jurisdiction uses the higher-brain formulation. I have analyzed the shortcomings of the higher-brain formulation that have led to its total disregard by physicians and policy makers (Bernat, 1992, 1998).

The whole-brain criterion is necessary for death because the operations of the functions of the organism as a whole are distributed throughout the brain. The brainstem contains centers of respiration, circulation, and the reticular system necessary for wakefulness that is a prerequisite for conscious awareness. The diencephalon contains centers for neuroendocrine and autonomic control and homeostasis, integration of sensory input and motor output, and conscious awareness. The cerebral hemispheres are necessary for conscious awareness.

The irreversible cessation of brain functions serves as a criterion of death because it is a necessary and sufficient condition for the cessation of the organism as a whole. A brain-dead patient whose visceral organ functions are maintained only as a consequence of technological support has lost the functions of the organism as a whole and is only a living component part of a dead organism, analogous in type though not extent to a technologically supported isolated living organ or limb. The irreversible loss of the functions of the brain responsible for the emergent functions of the organism as a whole indicates that the brain-dead patient is a mechanically supported, living component part of a human organism who has already died.

Alan Shewmon (2001, 2004) and his followers reject any type of brain criterion of death and argue that the human organism is not dead until its systemic circulation stops irreversibly. They regard the brain as only one bodily organ that has no greater significance in a concept of death than any other organ. They regard a "brain dead" patient as severely disabled but one who remains alive on life-support technology. Shewmon agrees with the definition of death as the cessation of the organism as a whole but argues that the criterion fulfilling that definition is the cessation of systemic circulation. Our position is that the cessation of systemic circulation is a sufficient criterion of death, because the brain is always destroyed in this circumstance, but it is unnecessary because the brain can be destroyed in circumstances in which circulation to organs other than the brain can be maintained (Bernat et al., 1981).

In Shewmon's most recent re-analysis of death (2010), he now distinguishes two stages of death: (1) "passing away," which occurs at the moment of the permanent cessation of the organism as a whole, and which marks the human organism's relational and civil end; and (2) "deanimation," which occurs at the moment of irreversible cessation of the organism as a whole, and which marks the ontological end of the human organism. Noteworthy in this analysis is his acceptance of the definition of death as the cessation of the organism as a whole and his emphasis on the importance of the distinction between the *permanent* and *irreversible* cessation of organ functions in an analysis of death.

I agree with Shewmon that the distinction between *permanent* and *irreversible* cessation of function is critical in an analysis of death.[3] I have argued that a permanent cessation of function is one that *will not* return because it will neither return spontaneously nor be restored through resuscitative technology, whereas an irreversible cessation of function is one that *cannot* return using current technology (Bernat, 2006a, 2010). Although some death statutes stipulate the irreversible cessation of organ function, medical practices always have required only their permanent cessation. Society has authorized physicians to declare death at the moment of permanent cessation without requiring or proving the cessation of organ function to be irreversible because it allows death to be determined at the stage of "passing away" in Shewmon's terminology. The only case in which the difference between using a permanent or an irreversible standard in death determination becomes consequential is that of organ donation after circulatory death (DCD). A United States–Canadian expert panel recently provided guidelines for death determination in organ donors after circulatory death at the point of permanent cessation of circulatory and respiratory functions which has been accepted in all DCD protocols (Bernat et al., 2010).

An asymmetry in using permanent or irreversible cessation of functions arises when physicians determine death with brain tests or circulatory–respiratory tests. This asymmetry results from the timing of death determinations in the two circumstances. Tests showing absent brain functions are almost always performed in retrospect to show that death has occurred. They require showing that an irreversible cessation of clinical brain functions has occurred. Tests showing absent circulatory and respiratory functions more often are performed in prospect once these functions have been observed to cease. Therefore, it is sufficient for physicians declaring death to show only the permanent cessation of circulatory and respiratory functions, whereas they show the irreversible cessation of brain functions (Bernat, 2010).

Conclusion

There remain numerous areas of scholarly disagreement on the definition and criterion of death. Is it possible that these disagreements can be resolved in the future given the fact that they have persisted for the past four decades? The bad news is that the only means of achieving consensus is for scholars to accept the paradigm conditions for a death analysis as I have enumerated them. Yet, this requirement, too, remains a source of longstanding heated controversy. In the absence of future agreement on the paradigm conditions (which appears unlikely), it will not be possible for scholars to achieve consensus on the definition and criterion of death.

The good news is that it probably does not matter whether scholarly consensus can be achieved if societies can establish publicly and professionally acceptable guidelines for physicians to determine death in clinical and transplantation circumstances. Currently, physicians practice under a set of accepted medical guidelines and laws that endorse the whole-brain criterion of death. This issue has been well settled at the public-policy level leading to the enactment of uniform death statutes and a successful program of organ transplantation (Bernat, 2006b). Practicing physicians remain unaware of the scholarly contention within the academy over the definition and criterion of death because it simply has had no impact on the practical level of bedside death determination. Despite the scholarly controversies, there is no pressing need to change current medical practices and legal standards on death determination, and an expert commission studying this issue recently recommended no changes to public policy (President's Council, 2009).

On this practical level, Chiong is correct that society can accept and successfully implement the whole-brain criterion of death without first agreeing on a definition of death. But on a conceptual level, it would be far more satisfying if we could clarify and agree on the meaning of the word *death* that we all use correctly, and thereby justify the societal and professional acceptance of the whole-brain criterion of death.

Notes

1 Space does not permit an analysis of views of defining death in terms of personal identity, morality, or prudential value. For a discussion of these aspects of the definition of death, see DeGrazia (2007).

2 A more in-depth analysis of personhood is beyond the scope of this article. For such an analysis, see John Lizza's anthology of articles discussing different approaches to personhood, particularly as the concept applies to the definition of human death (Lizza, 2009).

3 See my further analysis of the definitions of *permanent* and *irreversible* cessation of organ functions as they pertain to death (Bernat, 2006a, 2010).

References

Ad Hoc Committee (1968). A definition of irreversible coma: Report of the ad hoc committee of the Harvard Medical School to examine the definition of brain death. *Journal of the American Medical Association, 205*, 337–340.

Bernat, J. L. (1992). How much of the brain must die in brain death? *Journal of Clinical Ethics, 3*, 21–26.

Bernat, J. L. (1998). A defense of the whole-brain concept of death. *Hastings Center Report, 28*(2), 14–23.

Bernat, J. L. (2002). The biophilosophical basis of whole-brain death. *Social Philosophy & Policy, 19*(2), 324–342.

Bernat, J. L. (2006a). Are organ donors after cardiac death really dead? *Journal of Clinical Ethics, 17*, 122–132.

Bernat, J. L. (2006b). The whole-brain concept of death remains optimum public policy, *Journal of Law, Medicine & Ethics, 34*, 35–43.

Bernat, J. L. (2010). How the distinction between "irreversible" and "permanent" illuminates circulatory–respiratory death determination. *Journal of Medicine and Philosophy, 35*(3), 242–255.

Bernat, J. L., Capron, A., Bleck, T., Blosser, S., Bratton, S . . . White, D. (2010). The circulatory–respiratory determination of death in organ donation. *Critical Care Medicine, 38*, 972–979.

Bernat, J. L., Culver, C. M., & Gert, B. (1981). On the definition and criterion of death. *Annals of Internal Medicine, 94*, 389–394.

Bonelli, R. M., Prat, E. H., Bonelli, J. (2009). Philosophical considerations on brain death and the concept of the organism as a whole. *Psychiatria Danubina, 21*, 3–8.

Chiong, W. (2005). Brain death without definitions. *Hastings Center Report, 35*(6), 20–30.

Clayton, P., & Kauffman, S. (2006). On emergence, agency, and organization. *Biology and Philosophy, 21*, 501–521.

Crick, F. (1981). *Life itself: Its origin and nature.* New York: Simon & Schuster.

DeGrazia, D. (2007). The definition of death. *Stanford encyclopedia of philosophy.* Retrieved from: http://plato.stanford.edu/entries/death-definition/

Emanuel, L. (1995). Re-examining death: The asymptotic model and a bounded zone definition. *Hastings Center Report, 25*(4), 27–35.

Fost, N. (1999). The unimportance of death. In S. Youngner, R. Arnold, & R. Schapiro (Eds.), *The definition of death: Contemporary controversies* (pp. 160–178). Baltimore, MD: Johns Hopkins University Press.

Gert, B. (2006). Matters of "life" and "death." *Hastings Center Report, 36*(3), 4.

Gervais, K. (1986). *Redefining death.* New Haven, CT: Yale University Press.

Halevy, A., & Brody, B. (1993). Brain death: Reconciling definitions, criteria, and tests. *Annals of Internal Medicine, 119*, 519–525.

Jonsen, A. (2008). *A short history of medical ethics.* Oxford: Oxford University Press.

Koch, C. (2004). *The quest for consciousness: A neurobiological approach.* Englewood, CO: Roberts & Company Publishers.

Korein, J. (1978). The problem of brain death: Development and history. *Annals of the New York Academy of Sciences, 315*, 19–38.

Korein, J. (1997). Ontogenesis of the brain in the human organism: Definitions of life and death of the human being and person. *Advances in Bioethics, 2*, 1–74.

Lee, P., & George, R. (2008). *Body-self dualism in contemporary ethics and politics.* Cambridge: Cambridge University Press.

Lizza, J. (1999). Defining death for persons and human organisms. *Theoretical Medicine and Bioethics, 20*, 439–453.

Lizza, J. (Ed.). (2009). *Defining the beginning and end of life: Readings on personal identity and bioethics.* Baltimore, MD: Johns Hopkins University Press.

Loeb, J. (1916). *The organism as a whole.* New York: G. P. Putnam's Sons.

Mahner, M., & Bunge, M. (1997). *Foundations of biophilosophy.* Berlin: Springer-Verlag.

Margulis, L., & Sagan, D. (1995). *What is life?* New York: Simon & Schuster.

McMahan, J. (1995). The metaphysics of brain death. *Bioethics, 9*, 91–126.

McMahan, J. (2002). *The ethics of killing: Problems at the margins of life.* Oxford: Oxford University Press.

Monod, J. (1971). *Chance and necessity: An essay on the natural philosophy of modern biology.* New York: Alfred A. Knopf.

Olson, E. (1997). *The human animal: Personal identity without psychology*. Oxford: Oxford University Press.

Pallis, C. (1995). *ABC of brainstem death*. London: British Medical Journal Publishers.

President's Commission for the Study of Ethical Problems in Medicine and Biomedical and Behavioral Research. (1981). *Defining death: Medical, legal and ethical Issues in the determination of death*. Washington, DC: US Government Printing Office.

President's Council on Bioethics. (2009). *Controversies in the determination of death: A white paper by the President's Council on Bioethics*. Washington, DC: President's Council on Bioethics.

Shewmon, D. A. (2001). The brain and somatic integration: Insights into the standard biological rationale for equating "brain death" with death. *Journal of Medicine and Philosophy, 26*, 457–478.

Shewmon, D. A. (2004). The "critical organ" for the organism as a whole: lessons from the lowly spinal cord. *Advances in Experimental Medicine and Biology, 550*, 23–42.

Shewmon, D. A. (2009). Brain death: Can it be resuscitated? *Hastings Center Report, 39*(2), 18–24.

Shewmon, D. A. (2010). Constructing the death elephant: a synthetic paradigm shift for the definition, criteria, and tests for death. *Journal of Medicine and Philosophy, 35*, 256–298.

Shewmon, D. A., & Shewmon, E. S. (2004). The semiotics of death and its medical implication. In C. Machado & D. A. Shewmon (Eds.), *Brain death and disorders of consciousness* (pp. 89–114). New York: Kluwer Academic Publishers.

Task Force on Death and Dying of the Institute of Society, Ethics, and the Life Sciences. (1972). Refinements in the criteria for the determination of death: An appraisal. *Journal of the American Medical Association, 221*, 48–53.

Veatch, R. M. (1993). The impending collapse of the whole-brain definition of death. *Hastings Center Report, 23*(4), 18–24.

Veatch, R. M. (1999). The conscience clause: How much individual choice in defining death can our society tolerate? In S. Youngner, R. Arnold, & R. Schapiro (Eds.), *The definition of death: Contemporary controversies* (pp. 137–160). Baltimore, MD: Johns Hopkins University Press.

Chapter Twenty Four

There Cannot Be Agreement as to What Constitutes Human Death

Against Definitions, Necessary and Sufficient Conditions, and Determinate Boundaries

Winston Chiong

In a series of influential articles, James Bernat, Bernard Gert, and Charles Culver have articulated and defended the *whole-brain criterion* of death, according to which a human being dies when his or her whole brain irreversibly ceases to function. On this framework, such debates should begin with a *definition* that captures the shared and implicit understanding that we associate with the word *death*, and on the basis of this definition should arrive at a *criterion* that gives necessary and sufficient conditions for death in human beings. While some authors accept this theoretical framework but reject the whole-brain criterion of death, I reject the framework itself. I actually consider the whole-brain criterion of death to be acceptable, if understood more modestly. First, I reject the claim that we should start by attempting to define, or *analyze*, the ordinary meaning of the word *death*. Second, I do not believe that there is a unique set of necessary and sufficient conditions, shared by all dead people, in virtue of which they are all dead. Finally, I reject the idea that it is always a determinate matter of fact whether someone is alive or dead—instead, some cases may represent a borderline area in no rational or scientific considerations dictate that we categorize someone as either living or dead.

Introduction

In a series of influential articles, James Bernat, Bernard Gert, and Charles Culver have articulated and defended the *whole-brain criterion* of death, according to which a human being dies when his or her whole brain irreversibly ceases to function. In the course of their arguments, these authors have advanced a theoretical framework for debates about death that has become widely accepted, even by authors who do not accept the whole-brain criterion. On this framework, such debates should begin with a *definition* that captures the shared and implicit understanding that we associate with the word *death*, and on the basis of this definition should arrive at a *criterion* that gives necessary and sufficient conditions for death in human beings. (Roughly speaking, these necessary and sufficient conditions tell us what unique feature or set of features all dead people have in common, in virtue of which they are all dead.) Bernat also claims that it is always a determinate matter of fact whether or not someone does or does not satisfy this criterion; while

Contemporary Debates in Bioethics, First Edition. Edited by Arthur L. Caplan and Robert Arp.

he acknowledges that in some cases we may be unable to determine (due to scientific or technical limitations) whether someone is alive or dead, he maintains that there are no true borderline cases in between life and death.

My objections to this view are somewhat complicated; while some authors accept this theoretical framework but reject the whole-brain criterion of death, I reject the framework itself. (I actually consider the whole-brain criterion of death to be acceptable, if understood more modestly.) First, I reject the claim that we should start by attempting to define, or *analyze*, the ordinary meaning of the word *death*. Second, I do not believe that there is a unique set of necessary and sufficient conditions, shared by all dead people, in virtue of which they are all dead. Finally, I reject the idea that it is always a determinate matter of fact whether someone is alive or dead—instead, some cases may represent a borderline area in no rational or scientific considerations dictate that we categorize someone as either living or dead.

Before articulating my objections to Bernat and his colleagues, I wish to highlight an important area of agreement. While the word *death* can be used in a variety of nonbiological and metaphorical ways (as when we speak of "dead languages," or even when it is said of a patient with advanced dementia that the *person* has died, even though their body continues to live), Bernat and I both accept that the sense of death relevant here is the biological death of a human organism. This sort of death is not *in principle* different from the deaths of other organisms, although the details of death in different species will vary with differences in their physiology. (For some reason, Bernat limits his discussion to the death of higher vertebrates, but it seems clear to me that we use the word *death* with the same biological meaning when we talk about the deaths of other organisms such as octopuses, or beetles, or trees.)

As one last point of introduction, I wish to say that many of my arguments are not novel. Many of my claims depend on some classic arguments about the nature of language by Ludwig Wittgenstein (1958), and a second set of influential arguments made by Saul Kripke (1972) and Hilary Putnam (1973). In applying these arguments to human biology, I have relied heavily on the work of Richard Boyd (1999). For fuller theoretical discussion of these points, I refer the reader to the original sources.

Three Examples of Death

Consider three different legal declarations of death—all quite different, though all in accordance with existing law and accepted medical practice in the United States. In the first case, a man with advanced-stage cancer dies, not unexpectedly, in his sleep at home. In the morning, his caregiver finds his body cold and unresponsive, and a physician is called to the bedside. She palpates his wrist and neck and finds no evidence of a pulse; taking her stethoscope from her bag, she listens to his chest for a heartbeat or breath sounds but hears none. The physician concludes that the man's heart has irreversibly stopped beating and that he has irreversibly stopped breathing, and she pronounces the man dead.

Let us note two details about this case. First, the physician makes no formal assessment of the man's brain function (beyond the fact that he has stopped breathing), basing her declaration on the fact that his heart and lungs have stopped working. Second, while the *legal* time of death is when the physician makes her determination, Bernat and I would both agree that his *actual* death is a biological event independent of the physician's judgment, and likely occurred long before the physician arrived.

In the second case, a woman falls to the ground and is brought to the emergency department in a coma. Because she cannot breathe safely on her own, a breathing tube is placed in her mouth and down her throat, and is attached to a mechanical ventilator that forces air into her lungs at set intervals. Her physicians determine that she has suffered a hemorrhagic stroke: a blood vessel in her brain has burst open and a large blood clot has collected inside her brain, compressing the surrounding brain tissue. Over a few days, though her other internal organs (including her heart) continue to function normally, her brain swells, and she becomes unresponsive even to painful stimulation. Two neurologists perform a detailed neurological examination according to hospital protocol and find no evidence of brain function; for a brief period, the ventilator is stopped, and the patient makes no attempt to breathe on her own. These physicians conclude that her brain has irreversibly stopped functioning, and pronounce the woman dead.

In the first case, the physician determines that the patient has died without making any formal assessment of the patient's brain function, basing her determination on the fact that his heart and lungs have stopped functioning. In the second case, the physicians determine that the patient has died on the basis of a detailed examination of the patient's brain function, even though her heart continues to beat, and her lungs continue to exchange gases (with the aid of mechanical ventilation). These two cases illustrate that, in the United States and in many other countries, physicians may determine that a patient has died on the basis of two quite different criteria. In the first case, the physician determines that the man has died on the basis of the traditional *circulatory–respiratory* (or *cardiopulmonary*) *criterion*; while in the second case, the physicians determine that the woman has died on the basis of the modern *whole-brain criterion* of death. At first glance, this discrepancy in practice should strike us as puzzling. As I have noted, on the framework advanced by Bernat and his colleagues, there should be some feature or set of features that is common to all dead people; and therefore, we should expect careful physicians to evaluate the same physiological functions, particularly given the importance of the task determining whether someone has died. We may then be tempted to ask: is it the irreversible loss of function of the heart and lungs, or of the brain, that *actually* makes a person dead?

A common way of reconciling these two cases is to say that the *whole-brain criterion* of death is actually the correct one, and that the *circulatory–respiratory criterion* is merely acceptable as a rough approximation in certain cases (President's Commission, 1981; Bernat et al., 1982). After all, the cells that make up the brain are exquisitely dependent on the supply of oxygen and nutrients from the bloodstream, so that after the heart stops circulating blood, the brain will suffer irreversible injury in a matter of minutes. When the physician in our first example arrives at the patient's home and finds that his heart and lungs have stopped functioning, she might simply presume that his brain has irreversibly stopped functioning as well; and so we might think that a detailed neurological examination in his home would be an unnecessary formality. Thus, someone might claim that the whole-brain criterion is the precise account of death, which must be followed in complicated cases in high-technology settings like a hospital intensive-care unit, while the circulatory–respiratory criterion may be a reliable enough indicator of death to be used in simple and low-technology cases like an expected death at home.

However, this explanation does not account for a third case of *donation after cardiac death*, which has become an increasingly common practice over the last decade (Bernat et al., 2006). Consider a man with amyotrophic lateral sclerosis (ALS, also known as Lou Gehrig's disease), a disease that causes progressive paralysis due to the loss of neurons that control muscle movements, while in most cases sparing other parts of the brain and spinal cord. In this case, the disease has progressed to the point that the man cannot breathe on his own, depending on a mechanical ventilator that forces air into his lungs through a tube attached to his trachea; he is also unable to move without a motorized wheelchair, and depends on a feeding tube because he is unable to chew or swallow. Knowing that his condition will continue to deteriorate, and judging that his quality of life with these interventions is unacceptably poor, he instructs his doctors to stop the ventilator and allow him to die. After the ventilator is stopped, the lack of oxygen and accumulation of carbon dioxide will cause his heart to stop beating in about half an hour.

However, because his other organs are still in good condition, he wants to be an organ donor, which he regards as his last opportunity to help others. Unfortunately, if his ventilator is stopped in the usual way at home, the prolonged loss of blood flow to his internal organs will result in irreversible damage, and these organs will be unusable for transplantation. These organs can only be used if taken out of his body very quickly after his heart stops beating. To honor his request, his physicians initiate a complicated protocol: he is brought to an operating room while on the ventilator, still alive, and put under anesthesia. The ventilator is stopped, and after half an hour his heart stops beating—the physicians do not attempt to restart his heart because he has refused resuscitation in advance. After waiting for a prespecified interval of 5 min, his physicians determine that his heart has permanently stopped beating,[1] and pronounce him dead on the basis of the permanent loss of circulation and breathing. After he is pronounced dead, his organs can be used for transplantation, and are quickly removed from his body.

In this case, we cannot claim that the circulatory–respiratory criterion is merely used as a low-technology approximation of the whole-brain criterion of death; this death takes place in one of the most technologically sophisticated settings in modern medicine. The physicians do not perform a detailed neurological examination to document the loss of brain function, in part because this examination is time-consuming, and any delay would result in further injury to his organs. However, we cannot simply presume that his whole brain is irreversibly injured, as we know that many people retain some primitive brain functions (such as the gag reflex) for several minutes after their hearts stop beating. If we really believe that the whole-brain criterion is the precise account of when someone has died, then we should regard the application of the circulatory–respiratory criterion in this case as a sham, as it leaves open the possibility that some brain functions persist, and therefore that (according to the whole-brain criterion) the patient is still alive.

In this chapter, however, I will propose a different way of understanding this heterogeneity in our practices of determining death. On this view, there is no unique feature or set of features common to all dead organisms in virtue of which they are dead rather than alive. Instead, we should understand living and dead organisms in terms of an interrelated cluster of features, which may be present or absent in different cases. In some cases, a subset of these features will be sufficient for a particular organism to be dead; whereas, in other cases, a different subset of these features may be sufficient.

Definitions, Criteria, and Biological Kinds

Bernat and his colleagues have proposed that a theoretical investigation of life and death should begin with a *definition* that "[makes] explicit the indispensable characteristics of death that comprise our implicit, consensually agreed-upon concept of death," and then should proceed to a *criterion* "that satisfies the definition by being both necessary and sufficient for death" (Bernat, 2002). This model of rigorous theorizing owes much to the philosophical tradition of *conceptual analysis*, developed by Gottlob Frege, Bertrand Russell, and G. E. Moore in the early twentieth century. As a trivial example, consider a theorist who wants to know how to determine whether or not someone is a bachelor. According to this model, this theorist should start by analyzing the English word *bachelor*. By examining the implicit, shared understanding of ordinary English speakers, the theorist would arrive at a definition of the word *bachelor* as "an unmarried adult male person." If correct, this definition provides us with a unique set of four conditions that are both necessary and sufficient for being a bachelor: that is, for something to be a bachelor it must satisfy these four conditions, and anything that does satisfy these four conditions is a bachelor.

Such an analysis does more than just indicate whether or not something is a bachelor. Metaphysically, this analysis tells us *what it is* to be a bachelor—that is, what features all bachelors have in common in virtue of which they are bachelors, and thus gives an account of the truth conditions of the claim that something is a bachelor. And semantically, the implicit mental contents associated with the word *bachelor* explain how the word secures reference—which is to say that ordinary English speakers, when they use the word *bachelor*, succeed in referring to the set of all bachelors because they implicitly associate this word with a definition that provides necessary and sufficient conditions for bachelorhood. By contrast, if someone does not understand that a bachelor is an unmarried adult male person, then we would judge that this person does not have a sufficient conceptual grasp of the term *bachelor* to make any meaningful statements, whether true or false, about bachelors.

While this model is intuitively appealing for terms like *bachelor*, it breaks down when we consider terms that refer to *natural kinds*. These involve categories that occur in nature and independently of human interests, such as *gold* or *tigers*, and are contrasted with *nominal kinds* such as *chair* or *bachelor* that answer specifically to human interests. One important feature of natural kinds is that they have an underlying nature, about which the speakers of a given language may be unaware or misinformed; therefore, simply analyzing the implicit understandings that people associate with a term may not tell us much at all about what it takes to belong to the relevant natural kind. For instance, there is a necessary and sufficient condition for something to be gold, which is having atomic number 79. However, in contrast with the term *bachelor*, ordinary speakers do not need to know this in order to use the word "gold" in making and understanding meaningful claims about gold. In fact, they do not need to share the same conception of gold—one person might have only a vague concept of gold as that yellowish metal that is typically used in jewelry, while another simply conceives of it as the valuable stuff guarded in Fort Knox. The situation is even worse when we consider ordinary English speakers before the advent of modern chemistry, when *no one* knew that the necessary and sufficient condition for being gold was having atomic number 79. In contrast with terms like *bachelor*, we cannot discover indispensable characteristics of natural kinds by attempting to analyze implicit, consensually agreed-upon concepts that speakers associate with them—instead, such discovery is a matter for empirical, rather than merely conceptual, investigation (Kripke, 1972).

Then, consider the next step in Bernat's model, which is to seek out a criterion that gives necessary and sufficient conditions for death. In the case of some natural kinds like *gold*, necessary and sufficient conditions for membership in the kind do exist, even if they are not discoverable by conceptual analysis. However, kinds like *living organism* and *dead organism* (or, perhaps, *dead higher vertebrate*) are biological natural kinds; and it has long been recognized in the philosophy of biology that biological kinds typically do not have such necessary and sufficient conditions (Hull, 1978). To illustrate: is there any feature, or any set of features, that all tigers have in common and that all nontigers lack?

We might start, as an exercise, by attempting the sort of definition advocated by Bernat and his colleagues, analyzing the implicit and shared understandings that ordinary English speakers associate with the term *tiger*. For simplicity's sake, in this discussion I will leave out the fact that this ordinary concept includes that tigers are cats, or that they are animals, since *cat* and *animal* are themselves natural kind terms that present similar difficulties—so we might start by saying that our shared implicit understanding of tigers includes that they are large, predatory, four-legged, have black and orange stripes, and live in Africa and Asia. But in contrast with the four conditions we identified for the term *bachelor*, none of these features is a necessary condition for being a tiger. That is: something cannot be a bachelor if it is not unmarried, or not male, or not an adult, or not a person. However, we can easily imagine mutant or damaged tigers that are not large, or not predatory (perhaps after brain damage), or not four-legged (perhaps after injury), or do not have black and orange stripes, or do not live in Africa or Asia. Furthermore, these conditions together are not sufficient for being a tiger: we might imagine a mutant lion with black and orange stripes that satisfies all of these conditions, in which case we would say that "while that animal might have the features that we implicitly associate with tigers, it is not *really* a tiger." By contrast, at least if our analysis of bachelorhood is correct, there is no unmarried male adult person of whom we would say, "while that man might have the features that we implicitly associate with bachelors, he is not *really* a bachelor" (see Kripke, 1972).

Setting aside our implicit and shared understandings associated with the term *tiger*, might we turn to scientific investigation to find the necessary and sufficient conditions for being a tiger? (After all, we did discover a necessary and sufficient condition for being gold, even if this was not as a result of analyzing our shared understandings about gold.) The most promising approach might be an appeal to genetics; however, it is clear that there is no "tiger gene" that all tigers have in common, in virtue of which they are all tigers. For any candidate gene, we might imagine a mutant tiger with a missing or variant version of the gene that yet remains a tiger, or we might imagine a mutant lion that has the candidate gene yet remains a lion. And when we broaden our view to encompass the entire genome, there is of course no sequence of base-pairs that all tigers have in common that makes them all tigers. Each individual organism's genome is unique, not only from the novel reassortment of parental genes, but also from the 100 or so spontaneous genetic mutations that arise in each individual (Xue et al., 2009).

The broader point here is that natural kinds in biology, unlike natural kinds in physics or chemistry, encompass populations that exhibit tremendous genetic and phenotypic diversity. Each individual begins life with a unique genome and matures under a unique set of environmental influences, which can interact in unpredictable ways. For this reason, scientific statements about biological kinds are typically true only in general, or true only for typical cases. As an example, when we say that gold atoms have 79 protons, this statement is exceptionless. However, when we say that human beings have 46 chromosomes, this is true only in general—people with Down's syndrome have 47 chromosomes and are unquestionably human, while people with Turner's syndrome have 45. Such variation illustrates why biological natural kinds typically do not have necessary and sufficient conditions for membership. Therefore, not only does *tiger* lack an analytic definition as required by Bernat's model (because examining the implicit, shared understandings associated with this word does not reveal any indispensable characteristics of tigerhood), but also there are no criteria for being a tiger in Bernat's sense, as there is no unique set of features that is both necessary and sufficient for being a tiger (Boyd, 1999).

As a final point, recall that Bernat claims that it is always a determinate matter of fact whether or not something is alive or dead. However, biological natural kinds typically admit of borderline cases, in which it is unclear whether or not something belongs to the relevant kind. One example of this indeterminacy concerns speciation. According to evolutionary theory, at some point in the distant past the species *tiger* evolved from some earlier species of large cats. If we had complete information about the entire lineage stretching back in time, in most cases we would be able to say determinately whether a given organism was a tiger, or whether it belonged to this ancestral species. However, given that speciation is a gradual process, it is implausible to think that there is any bright line that demarcates these species—for instance, that there was some particular generation of cats that were determinately all tigers, but whose parents were determinately all members of the ancestral species. Instead, it makes most sense to think that some of the organisms occupied a borderline state between the two species, such that no rational or scientific considerations dictate whether we should classify them as tigers or as members of the earlier species (Boyd, 1999).

Life and Death as Biological Natural Kinds

I hope to have demonstrated that, at least for an important group of terms like *tiger*, the theoretical model of definitions and criteria proposed by Bernat and his colleagues simply will not work, for three specific reasons. First, our use of the term may not be governed by any shared and implicit understanding that gives indispensable characteristics for its successful application. Second, there are no necessary and sufficient conditions for belonging to the relevant kind. And third, there are borderline cases in which it is unclear whether or not something belongs to the relevant kind. However, I have admitted that Bernat's model might work for another group of terms like *bachelor*. What remains at issue between us, then, is whether the terms *life* and *death* are more like the term *tiger*, or more like the term *bachelor*.

Let us begin by considering whether we can find a definition of life or death that captures the indispensable characteristics that comprise our implicit, consensually agreed-upon understanding of life and death. In the case of terms like *bachelor*, it appears that in order to use this word in mutual conversation, we must all agree on the definition of *bachelor* as "an unmarried male adult person." As an illustration, imagine meeting someone like Humpty Dumpty in *Through the Looking Glass*, who insists on defining *bachelor* not as "an unmarried male person" but instead as "a nice knock-down argument." It would be pointless to have a conversation with Humpty Dumpty about bachelors; for instance, you might ask him whether bachelors have a higher average salary than married men, and he might respond by saying that in all bachelors the conclusions follow logically from the premises. In an important sense, the two of you would *not even be disagreeing*, because although you are using the same words you are actually talking about entirely different things. So, we might observe that for terms like *bachelor*, a shared definition of the term is a precondition for genuine disagreement about bachelors.

Bernat claims that *death* also has an analytic definition, which is "the permanent cessation of the critical functions of the organism as a whole" (Bernat, 2002). Does this definition provide us with indispensable characteristics of death that comprise an implicit, consensually agreed-upon concept of death possessed by all English speakers, in the same way that our definition of *bachelor* does? One initial ground for doubt is simply that terms like "critical function" and "organism as a whole," as used by Bernat, have such precise technical meanings that it is implausible to think that ordinary speakers have them in mind, or have consensually agreed upon them, when they use the word *death*. Furthermore, I suspect that if we were to ask people to explicitly state their implicit concept of death, we would find more variation than consensus. For instance, many people would define *death* as "the departure of the immaterial soul from the physical body," while adherents of Chinese medicine might define *death* as "the transformation of *Qi* from a condensed to a dispersed form."

The problem here is not just that people disagree. The real problem for Bernat's model is that it seems to make genuine disagreement impossible—if these people do not share the same definition of *death*, then we cannot even be sure that we are talking about the same thing, just like in our example of Humpty Dumpty's use of the term *bachelor*. I think the solution here is to give up the claim that *life* and *death* have semantics like the term *bachelor*, and thus Bernat's claim that we should be able to discover characteristics of life and death by examining the shared, implicit understandings that ordinary English speakers have about life and death. Instead, the terms *life* and *death* operate like *gold*, *tigers*, and other natural kind terms, which people can use without implicitly sharing any definition that gives indispensable characteristics of death, or gold, or of tigers. For instance, two people can argue about whether the indispensable characteristic of gold is having atomic number 79 or atomic number 80, without us having the Humpty-Dumptyish worry that only one is talking about gold, and the other is actually talking about mercury, because gold is a natural kind that both can identify using its accidental features, such as being the yellow metal typically used in jewelry (Putnam, 1973). Similarly, two people can argue about whether the indispensable characteristic of death is the permanent cessation of the critical functions of the organism of the whole, or is the dispersal of *Qi*, because death has an underlying nature (the details of which might really be unknown to both of them) and can be identified for conversational purposes in virtue of accidental features—such as through our own personal experiences of death among our family members and friends.

Thus, contrary to Bernat and his colleagues' model, there is no analytic definition of death that makes explicit the indispensable characteristics of death by analyzing our implicit and shared concept of death. In addition, contrary to Bernat's claims, there is no unique set of features that is both necessary and sufficient for death; and life and death (like the natural kind *tiger*) admit of borderline cases in which no rational or scientific considerations dictate whether we should classify something as living or dead. In an earlier paper (Chiong, 2005), I have argued for both of these claims by considering our intuitive responses to a number of real and imagined cases.

To see the gist of this argument, we might start by taking a step back and asking: why have theorists' efforts to provide necessary and sufficient conditions for death proven so unsatisfying? In the case of the whole-brain criterion favored by Bernat, he claims that *only* the functions of the whole brain are relevant to determining whether someone is alive or dead, and that other bodily functions are irrelevant. Consider an unusual case of whole-brain death, one of many real-life cases presented by Alan Shewmon (1998): a pregnant woman suffers a devastating brain injury and is placed on life support including mechanical ventilation. Unfortunately, her brain injury is irreversible, and all of her (measurable) brain functions are lost; however, her body is maintained on life support for several weeks until her fetus is mature enough to be delivered by cesarean section. To my mind, the ability of a brain-dead body to gestate a fetus successfully to viability (although with intensive medical support) is truly remarkable. While I disagree with Shewmon's claim that this ability clearly shows that the woman still remains alive, I do believe that this ability is relevant in considering whether or not she is alive. However, because of his position that *only* the functions of the whole brain are relevant to the question of whether a person has died, Bernat must insist that this ability has no bearing at all in determining whether she is alive or dead.

On the other hand, consider the traditional circulatory–respiratory criterion favored by Shewmon. According to this criterion, the irreversible cessation of blood flow and gas exchange are necessary and sufficient for death; and thus, according to this view the functions of the brain are irrelevant to the question of whether a person has died. Consider then a different case: a man suffers a penetrating chest wound that stops his heart and paralyzes his diaphragm, rendering him unable to circulate blood or to breathe. In such a case, consciousness might be retained for roughly 20 s before he lapses into unconsciousness from the lack of blood flow to his brain. Let us set aside the argumentative question of whether the circulatory–respiratory criterion can be modified in some way to account for this delay, and focus on the question: is the fact that the man retains consciousness during this period relevant to determining whether he is alive (though dying) or already dead? In this case, a defender of the circulatory–respiratory criterion must insist that consciousness, in itself, has no bearing at all in such a determination.

In both cases, the attempt to provide strict necessary and sufficient conditions for death has left us with impoverished accounts of life and death that force us to ignore important features of individual cases. Furthermore, since the theoretical model of definitions and criteria is based upon a faulty conception of how language works, there is no reason for us to abide by these restrictions. Following Richard Boyd's interpretation of Wittgenstein (Wittgenstein, 1958; Boyd, 1999), I have proposed a *cluster account* of life and death that does not attempt to state necessary and sufficient conditions for life and death, but instead recognizes a variety of features that may be relevant to the determination that an individual organism is alive or dead (Chiong, 2005). These features include, but are not limited to:

1. Consciousness.
2. What might be called, at the risk of circularity, spontaneous vital functions. These may vary from organism to organism (the functions that are vital for plants are very different from those that are vital for animals), but by *vital* I mean in general those functions that are necessary for the persistence of the other functions of the organism. By *spontaneous* I mean that these functions are regulated and maintained by activities that are internal rather than external to the organism.
3. Behavior; that is, functional responsiveness to environmental stimuli, regardless of the presence of consciousness.
4. Integrated and coordinated functioning of multiple subsystems—a certain degree of organizational complexity and coherence.
5. The ability to resist decay and putrefaction.
6. The capacity to reproduce.
7. The capacity to grow via the assimilation of nutrients.

Note that this list of features is not like the list of features that define bachelorhood. A bachelor must possess all of those features, and therefore something cannot be a bachelor if it is not unmarried, or not male, or not an adult, or not a person. However, a living organism does not need to possess all of these features to be alive. For example, prepubertal children and postmenopausal women do not have the capacity to reproduce, yet this fact does not make them any less alive than anyone else. Meanwhile, having this feature in the absence of others does not guarantee that something is alive—prions can replicate themselves but are not living organisms. Still, whether or not something has this capacity, perhaps in concert with other features on this list (as in the case of brain-dead pregnant bodies) is certainly relevant to the question of whether or not something is a living organism.

In most cases of life and death, these features tend to be either present together or absent together, so determining whether or not something is alive or dead is straightforward. In other cases, one or two of these features might be missing (as in the case of postmenopausal women and reproduction), but the presence of the other features makes it obvious that something is still a living organism; or alternatively, one or two of the features might be present (as in the functionally responsive behavior of a Roomba vacuum cleaner), but the absence of the other features makes it obvious that something is not a living organism. In between, however, there will be extremely difficult cases, that lack many central features of living organisms yet retain others. In such borderline cases (and I believe that the brain-dead pregnant woman is one of them), we could know all of the relevant physiological facts and still be unable to determine whether someone is alive or dead.

This leaves us with the practical problem of what to do in these borderline, indeterminate cases. One solution, which we commonly apply in other cases of indeterminacy, is to adopt an artificially defined boundary for legal and social purposes, even when we know as a fact that the underlying phenomenon is continuous. This is like adopting an artificial cutoff for adulthood at 18 years, even though we know that maturation is a gradual process that takes place over many years. While the whole-brain criterion represents one acceptable boundary, there are other cutoffs that we could choose to adopt in certain circumstances or for special purposes. To return, for instance, to the example of the ALS patient who wishes to donate his organs, our understanding of brain physiology suggests that the capacity for consciousness would be irreversibly lost after half an hour without breathing and 5 min without a heartbeat, although some more primitive brain functions may be retained. Given that, in addition, his heart has stopped beating, and he has stopped breathing, this case in my view would represent at most a borderline case between life and death, rather than a clear case of a still-living organism. It would then be reasonable to adopt a boundary that treats such people as dead, even if some primitive brain functions (such as the gag reflex) are still present.

Note

1 For the purposes of my discussion, I will pass over a second problem with this case, which is that while circulation in this patient may have ceased permanently (in that the heart will not restart), it may not be the case that circulation has ceased irreversibly (i.e., that the heart could not be restarted by CPR or defibrillation). For discussion, see Bernat (2006), Truog and Cochrane (2006), and Marquis (2010).

References

Bernat, J. L. (2002). The biophilosophical basis of whole-brain death. *Social philosophy & policy, 19*(2), 324–342.

Bernat, J. L. (2006). Are donors after cardiac death really dead? *Journal of Clinical Ethics, 17*(6), 122–132.

Bernat, J. L., Culver, C. M., & Gert, B. (1982). Defining death in theory and practice. *Hastings Center Report, 12*(1), 5–9.

Bernat, J. L., D'Alessandro, A. M., Port, F. K., Bleck, T. P., Heard, S. O., Medina, J., ... Delmonico, F. L. (2006). Report of a national conference on donation after cardiac death. *American Journal of Transplantation, 6*(2), 281–291.

Boyd, R. (1999). Homeostasis, species, and higher taxa. In R. A. Wilson (Ed.), *Species: New interdisciplinary essays* (pp. 141–185). Cambridge, MA: MIT Press.

Chiong, W. (2005). Brain death without definitions. *Hastings Center Report, 35*(6), 20–30.

Hull, D. (1978). A matter of individuality. *Philosophy of Science, 45*, 335–360.

Kripke, S. (1972). *Naming and necessity*. Cambridge, MA: Harvard University Press.

Marquis, D. (2010). Are DCD donors dead? *Hastings Center Report, 40*(3), 24–31.

President's Commission for the Study of Ethical Problems in Medicine and Biomedical and Behavioral Research. (1981). *Defining death: Medical, legal and ethical issues in the determination of death*. Washington, DC: US Government Printing Office.

Putnam, H. (1973). Meaning and reference. *Journal of Philosophy, 70*(19), 699–711.

Shewmon, D. A. (1998). Chronic "brain death": meta-analysis and conceptual consequences. *Neurology, 51*(6), 1538–1545.

Truog, R. D., & Cochrane, T. I. (2006) The truth about "donation after cardiac death." *Journal of Clinical Ethics, 17*(6), 133–136.

Wittgenstein, L. (1958). *Philosophical investigations* (G. E. M. Anscombe, Trans.). New York: Macmillan.

Xue, Y., Wang, Q., Long, Q., Ng, B. L., Swerdlow, H., Burton, J., ... Tyler-Smith, C. (2009). Human Y chromosome base-substitution mutation rate measured by direct sequencing in a deep-rooting pedigree. *Current Biology 19*(17), 1453–1457.

Reply to Chiong

James L. Bernat

In his rejection of the analysis of death that my Dartmouth colleagues and I advocate, Winston Chiong argues that it is impossible to define the word *death* or to identify a set of necessary and sufficient conditions that are shared by all dead people, by virtue of which they are dead, and that it is not always a determinate matter of fact whether someone is alive or dead. He concludes that, despite these conditions, it remains possible for society, as he does, to accept the whole-brain criterion of death.

My colleagues and I assert that *death* is a common and nontechnical word, and that in our analysis, defining death requires making explicit the meaning that is implicit in the way everyone consensually uses the word. In my 2002 article that Chiong cites in which I advocated first striving to identify the essence of death (Bernat, 2002), I failed to make this point clearly, but my colleague, Bernard Gert, clarified it his 2006 letter (Gert, 2006) critiquing Chiong's (2005) article. Chiong did not address whether Gert's clarification of this point and critique of Chiong's claim that definitions were unnecessary—that I explain in this here—changed his analysis or opinion.

I agree with Chiong that although defining death as "the cessation of functioning of the organism as a whole" may represent an accurate biophilosophical conceptualization of death, it is not what most people mean when they say "death." Most people conceptualize the easy cases in which death is a unitary phenomenon in which all vital systems have ceased functioning more or less simultaneously. The tough cases introduced by technology include those with mechanical support of organ subsystems and those requiring physicians to determine death in a very timely manner, such as for organ donor after a circulatory determination of death. It is for these tough cases that a rigorous biophilosophical analysis is necessary.

Despite his rejection of our definitional prerequisite, Chiong supports the whole-brain criterion of death. Yet, he does not address the question raised by brain-death opponents of why a "brain-dead" human being is dead. He did address this question in his 2005 article (Chiong, 2005), but it is also relevant to his current critique. The essence of that justification lies in the distinction between the survival of living components of the organism and the continued life of the organism itself. This distinction is based on the concept of the functioning of the organism as a whole. Although I continue to hold that the organism as a whole concept forms the nucleus of understanding the death of the human organism, I concede that it has inherent vagueness.

In place of a definition-criterion-tests framework, Chiong proposes a "cluster account" of life and death that replaces the necessary and sufficient conditions for life or death with a list of features relevant to the determination that an organism is alive or dead. While

Contemporary Debates in Bioethics, First Edition. Edited by Arthur L. Caplan and Robert Arp.

acknowledging the complexity of the subject and not disputing his proposed list of features, I find this account to be even more vague in its capacity to provide specific criteria that physicians can use to determine life or death in the tough cases.

At the most fundamental level, most scholars who have analyzed death accept the logic that a conceptual account of death must precede the task of devising procedures for the bedside determination of death. Following this orderly sequence requires a definition, however broadly or narrowly it is conceived and formulated. Because Chiong's analysis also requires a concept of death, my colleagues and I hold that it, too, falls within the broad domain of a definition.

References

Bernat, J. L. (2002). The biophilosophical basis of whole-brain death, *Social Philosophy & Policy*, *19*(2), 324–342.

Chiong, W. (2005). Brain death without definitions. *Hastings Center Report*, *35*(6), 20–30.

Gert, B. (2006). Matters of "life" and "death." *Hastings Center Report*, *36*(3), 4.

Reply to Bernat

Winston Chiong

It gives me great pleasure to participate in this discussion with Jim Bernat—who, I wish to note, is the person who first encouraged me to think critically about brain death several years ago. While I have highlighted points of disagreement between us in my chapter (and will continue to do so in these remarks), there are many other matters about which we agree. As he notes, we both accept the whole-brain criterion of death; we also believe that death should be understood as a biological event, and we both maintain (in my case, with some ambivalence) that the determination that someone has died should precede procurement of vital organs for transplantation in situations like donation after cardiac death. One way, then, to interpret my view is as an attempt to find a firmer foundation and a deeper theoretical understanding for commitments that we both share.

Bernat refers to a letter in response to my 2005 paper (Chiong, 2005) by his Dartmouth colleague, Bernard Gert (2006). Here, I would like to expand upon the brief remarks I made in my reply to Gert's letter (Chiong, 2006). As I have argued, there is an important difference between terms like *bachelor*, in which we can determine necessary and sufficient conditions for a term's application by analyzing the implicit mental contents that speakers associate with it; and terms like *tiger* (and, I argue, *living organism* and *dead organism*), whose referents have an underlying nature that may be unknown to ordinary speakers. In my reply to Gert, I took an example from Gert et al. (1997, p. 253; also 2006, p. 285), in which Gert and his colleagues claim that "whales ceased to be fish when a new classification scheme was adopted." This suggests that in pre-Linnaean times, it was scientifically correct to claim that whales are fish, and this claim is now false only because it violates our linguistic conventions. I think this is wrong. On my view, it was a *mistake* to have ever thought that whales were fish, and it was a scientific *discovery* (rather than merely a linguistic agreement) that, despite their outward appearances and our previous assumptions, whales are actually mammals. Or to put it more bluntly: when I tell my son that "whales are not fish," I am not teaching him English, I am teaching biology. (In contrast, when I tell him that "bachelors are not married," I am merely teaching him how to use the English word *bachelor*.)

Where do Gert and his colleagues go wrong? I think their rough idea is that, in earlier times, there was a linguistic agreement to use the word *fish* just to mean something like "an aquatic creature with bones, fins and a tail," which included not only the animals that we now call fish, but also dolphins and whales; and that people later *decided* to adopt a more useful classificatory scheme on which *fish* is now specified in phylogenetic terms. On grounds originally presented by Kripke and Putnam, I think this is the wrong picture. Instead, the word *fish* has always referred to a natural kind whose members have some underlying

Contemporary Debates in Bioethics, First Edition. Edited by Arthur L. Caplan and Robert Arp.

nature, the details of which were unknown to pre-Linnaean speakers; and it was a scientific discovery that, despite appearances, whales do not partake in these underlying features and therefore are not (and never truly were) fish. An interesting wrinkle of this account is that pre-Linnaean English speakers could use the word *fish* without *even being able to tell* fish apart from some things (like whales) that were not fish. (Just as English speakers in an earlier period might have used the word *gold* without being able to distinguish gold and iron pyrite.)

For a term like *bachelor*, the meaning is settled by what the community of English speakers thinks it is; whereas, in the case of terms for natural kinds (like *fish* or *gold* or *tiger*), the community of speakers can make mistakes about the proper application of the term, which are then revisable in light of later evidence. Despite Bernat and Gert's effort to frame their view about the definition of death more modestly, I still find an ambiguity between these two possibilities in their view. On one hand, Bernat writes that "defining death requires making explicit the meaning that is implicit in the way everyone consensually uses the word." This suggests that, in formulating our definition, our standard for its correctness is whether it matches the implicit consensus of the community of speakers. But on the other hand, he writes that his definition of death (as "the cessation of functioning of the organism as a whole") "is not what most people mean when they say *death*"—in part because people do not conceptualize the difficult cases. If our definition is justified by appealing to how the community of speakers uses the word, and most members of this community have never thought about (and would probably be quite puzzled about) how to apply the word in difficult cases, then it seems like a stretch to expect such a definition to yield verdicts (indeed, fully determinate verdicts) about complicated cases like an ALS patient whose ventilator is stopped, or a brain-dead pregnant woman who is being intensively supported long enough to deliver her fetus.

Bernat and Gert both suggest that in my own account, I also rely upon a definition of death; such that, despite my rejection of their analytic framework, I am (perhaps unwittingly) relying upon it in framing my own view. There is a weaker sense of "definition" upon which I do rely—Putnam (1973) calls this an "operational definition" that helps us to focus on the object of our inquiry, even if it does not reveal the underlying nature of the object. This is like starting out by saying that gold is the yellow metal typically used in jewelry, which establishes an object of inquiry that scientific investigation might later reveal to have atomic number 79. But such operational definitions do not have the features required by Bernat and Gert's model: they may appeal to merely accidental rather than indispensable characteristics of the object; they do not commit us to finding necessary and sufficient conditions for the term's application; and there is no guarantee that it is always a determinate matter whether the term applies.

Thus, as Bernat notes, in my account I also depend on the notion of a living organism. But in my account, this is only because *living organism* and *dead organism* (as opposed, say, to *living cell* and *dead cell*) are the natural kinds relevant to the question of whether or not someone has died—so this is a matter of "defining terms" at the outset just to be clear about the object of our inquiry. By contrast, Bernat's model requires that the very concept of a living organism (which we all share) can itself provide necessary and sufficient conditions for life and death with enough specificity to establish that, for instance, a ventilated woman with no brain function gestating a viable fetus is determinately dead. Since my view commits me to no such claim, my view is not an application of their model; instead, I have argued that we cannot expect to arrive at determinate verdicts about previously unimagined cases by examining our shared implicit associations with death, or the way that people use terms like *life* and *death*.

References

Chiong, W. (2005). Brain death without definitions. *Hastings Center Report, 35*(6), 20–30.

Chiong, W. (2006). Matters of "life" and "death" [author reply]. *Hastings Center Report, 36*(3), 5–6.

Gert, B. (2006). Matters of "life" and "death." *Hastings Center Report, 36*(3), 4.

Gert, B., Culver, C. M., & Clouser, K. D. (1997). *Bioethics: A return to fundamentals*. Oxford: Oxford University Press.

Gert, B., Culver, C. M., & Clouser, K. D. (2006). *Bioethics: A systematic approach*. Oxford: Oxford University Press.

Putnam, H. (1973). Meaning and reference. *Journal of Philosophy, 70*(19), 699–711.

Part 13

Is There Ever a Circumstance in Which a Doctor May Withhold Information?

Introduction

"Many Doctors in Survey Admit Lying to Patients" reads the headline article in the Health section of *The Seattle Times* on February 8, 2012 (Neergaard, 2012). The subtitle to the article continues, "More than half of doctors surveyed admitted describing someone's prognosis in a way they knew was too rosy." The head researcher of the 2009 survey of 1800 physicians around the US, Dr Lisa Iezzoni, noted, "I don't think that physicians set out to be dishonest," but speculates (common sensibly) that not revealing the whole truth, or possibly downplaying grim findings, is a way for a doctor to give the patient hope (Iezzoni et al., 2012). Doctors are people with emotions and shortcomings, too, and it is easy for us to imagine that it would be incredibly difficult for Dr Smith to be brutally honest about the prognosis concerning 35-year-old Jane's stage IV adenocarcinoma of the lung in his office with Jane's husband, Jack, there holding her hand, the both of them sobbing while Jack's mother is watching the three grandkids out in the waiting room.

When one inspects data gathered from surveys of doctors over the years (and probably, anecdotally, if you just asked any doctor), one sees that almost all doctors agree that they *should always* tell the truth about a patient's diagnosis and prognosis, revealing any and all known facts, hypotheses, and informed speculations, even if they admit to not living up to this imperative (Holland et al., 1987; Miyaji, 1993; Quirt et al., 1997; Hingorani et al., 1999; Iezzoni et al., 2012; the papers in Surbone et al., 2013). Yet, as is the case oftentimes in applied ethics and real-life cases, what *should be* done and what *actually is* done do not match up with one another. A priori—in classrooms, on paper in articles and books, and in hospital cafeteria conversations—it is easy to lay out the shoulds and should-nots; but a posteriori—in the moment, situation, circumstance, or experience itself—those imperatives are not always abided by.

Contemporary Debates in Bioethics, First Edition. Edited by Arthur L. Caplan and Robert Arp.

It is not an exaggeration to claim that Immanuel Kant's (1724–1804) deontological moral theory—with its emphasis upon abiding by rational principles that have been erected and articulated based upon consistency, autonomy, respect for persons, and blind justice—as well as John Stuart Mill's (1806–1873) utilitarian moral theory—with its emphasis upon bringing about the most nonharmful (and hence, pleasurable) and beneficial consequences to a person (or sentient being) affected by an action—have acted as the basis for practical moral decision-making of every stripe, since the theories were formulated in the eighteenth and nineteenth centuries (Kant, 1785/1998; Mill, 1861/2001; O'Neill, 1990; Korsgaard, 1996; Baron, 1999; Hooker, 2000). It is from Kant that the modern basis for "Thou shalt not lie, *no matter what*" and "One should *always* tell the truth, *as a matter of duty and principle*" have been formulated, while it is from Millian-inspired rule utilitarians that we derive the general rule that one ought to tell the truth, based upon the fact that lying regularly brings about detrimental consequences in almost every situation (Lewis, 1972; Shaw, 1999). Starting in the middle of the twentieth century, a third perspective based in Aristotle's (384–322 BCE) virtue theory has become influential in moral decision-making and a viable contender with the theories of Kant and Mill (Aristotle, 1962; MacIntyre, 1981; Statman, 1997). From the virtue ethics perspective, where the actor performing the action is significant, one should not lie because not only will lying make one into a liar, but also it contributes to an unhealthy, imbalanced, vicious personality.

Kant's moral theory sets him apart as the foremost proponent of a secular *deontology* (Kant, 1775–1789/1963, 1785/1998, 1797a/1996a, 1797b/1996b). The term is a combination of two Greek words: *deontos*, which means, "duty," and *logos*, which means "the logic of" or "the study of." Kant argues that whether an act is moral or immoral depends wholly on one's *duty* to act according to a moral principle concerning that action. Duties, for Kant, are not a matter of considering the consequences of an action; they are a matter of pure rationality.

Kant articulates his duty-based theory in three forms—referred to as formulations of the *categorical imperative*—two of which we will mention here. The first can be paraphrased as follows: Whenever you act, make sure that your action is something that can be universalized without contradiction. In other words, ask yourself the question: "What if everyone did what I'm about to do?" and if it undermines or negates what you want to do, then it is immoral, and you should not do it. For example, say you wanted to borrow money from someone knowing that you will not pay it back. Now, think what would happen logically—not the empirical, but *logical* consequences—if all people *universally* did this: the very idea of "borrowing" would completely go away, since no one would ever trust another person to borrow because Person A would know that s/he would never get the money back from Person B. And, you yourself, then, could never borrow any money with *or without* the intent of paying back. So, you would be contradicting or undermining your own action, which is irrational and unreasonable to do; hence, it is immoral.

When you universalize in this Kantian way, so too: (1) Suicide is immoral because it contradicts self-preservation of one's life, and if everyone committed suicide there would be no life to kill, including your own; (2) giving discounts to friends at your place of business is immoral because it contradicts fair prices for all, effectively negating any possibility of giving discounts in the first place; (3) lying is immoral because it contradicts truth-telling, and when you lie, you depend upon the very idea of truth-telling so that people will believe your lies. It is a rationally based—and absolutist—moral theory through and through, and any kind of "performative contradiction" like those mentioned above is immoral. Kant is able to use this universalizability method to show that truth-telling *really is* rational and, hence, moral, while lying *really is* irrational and, hence, immoral.

We can paraphrase Kant's second formulation of his rational principle this way: Whenever you act, always treat yourself and others as an end in themselves, and never *merely* as a means to an end. In other words, do not ever use yourself or another person instrumentally *merely* to achieve some other goal, no matter the consequences. The basis for this has to do with the fact that humans are conscious, rational, precious, sacred beings having an *intrinsic* value (as ends) and not an *instrumental* value (as a means to an end) like some object, tool, thing, or instrument. From this perspective, morally right decisions are those decisions where a person is treated as an end, and morally wrong decisions are those where someone is treated as a mere instrument or means to an end. Kant thought that always telling the truth is not only universalizable but also a way to respect the intrinsic value of the self and others. Whereas when one lies or even hides part of the truth from someone, s/he disrespects that person who is always deserving of the truth. "By a lie a man throws away and, as it were, annihilates his dignity as a man," claimed Kant in his *Metaphysics of Morals* (1797b/1996b).

One final point about Kant: Kant argues that if a person's motivation or reason for a supposed moral act is anything other than dutifully acting from respect for morality—whether it be the good consequences that result from an action, benefits to self or others, your own desires or inclinations, or *even love itself*—then the act cannot rightly be considered moral. In fact, Kant says that Jesus' command in the Christian Scriptures to "love your enemies" is a clear case of dutifully acting in accordance with a moral principle and *not* acting according to your own inclination/desire, which is to hate your enemy. This does not mean that actions motivated by emotions, inclinations, circumstances, and consequences *are not* morally good, only that we *could never tell* whether you are acting morally when you act according to those motivations.

In contrast to Kant's duty-based, absolutist approach to morality, which does not consider the empirical consequences of an act, Millian-inspired utilitarians argue that morality depends *wholly* on the consequences of an action. Whereas a Kantian would say, "It is the principle of the matter, and I am not concerned with the consequences to me or anyone else," a utilitarian would say something like, "I am concerned only with the consequences of the act to me and all affected, and I do not care about principles if they are going to bring about bad consequences." The way in which the utilitarian determines the good consequences to all affected in a situation is through a pro vs. con kind of calculus, or adding up all of the gains/pleasures/goods/benefits on one side and comparing them with all of the losses/pains/bads/deficits on the other side. The moral decision, then, is the one where the most gains will result. Also, since everyone is considered completely equal in terms of their worth, it appears to be a fair way to determine actions. We can think of the decision-making process of a utilitarian like a cost–benefit analysis used in many complex business and institutional decisions and, indeed, considering "what's best for the company" or "what's good for the organization" are commonly heard, and accepted, kinds of claims (O'Neill, 2008).

Given the emphasis upon bringing about good consequences, utilitarians argue that the *end* of bringing about good consequences can, at times, justify the *means* of doing something like lying in order to bring the good about. A Kantian has an obligation not to lie, since lying would use an intrinsically valuable person as if they were merely extrinsically valuable—that is, valuable for the liar's end. But a utilitarian—specifically, a *rule* utilitarian—may also have a moral obligation not to lie, since lying often leads to more interpersonal conflict than it resolves, or sets up an atmosphere of distrust. Therefore, telling the truth seems to bring about good consequences, more often than not, so we should tell the truth as a general rule. But again, a utilitarian will endorse, and indeed actually promote, lying, if the lie is necessary to bring about the most benefit for the majority in a particular situation or set of circumstances.

Opposed to both Kantian-based and consequence-based moral theories—which try to establish what people should *do* and then assess whether they have actually done so—there are character-based moral theories, such as Aristotle's virtue ethics, which evaluate the value of a person's *character* and then assess which actions best contribute to a certain kind of character. The central idea of virtue ethics is that character and behavior are mutually forming. Having a certain type of character will determine how you act, and how you act over time will determine what kind of character you have. If someone has a virtuous character, then they will often do what is best. Similarly, if someone does what is best over time, her/his character will develop in such a way that s/he will be more likely to do what is best in the future. After all, we want to perform duty-bound, right actions according to rational principles (Kantian-based) that have good consequences (utilitarian-based), but we also want to be *virtuous people* performing right actions that have good consequences. Though you may be able to convince a demon to do the right thing (according to some principled duty) or to bring about good consequences (according to some utilitarian calculus), the agent is still a demon. Thus, virtue ethics can act as a kind of complement to the Kantian and utilitarian positions, rounding out our moral lives.

Our characters result from forming certain good habits starting in childhood and acquiring practical wisdom in maturity. *Virtue* is a good habit whereby one fosters a kind of *balance* in one's character, promoting "not too much" and "not too little" of some character trait, but "just the right amount," so that our actions and reactions reflect a healthy, harmonious, functional, appropriate character. Virtues are the traits that fall within the mean, or average, of the extremes of too much (the vice of excess) and too little (the vice of deficiency). Virtue ethicists identify a general list of virtues, including courage, prudence, generosity, integrity, affability, respect, and honesty, to name just a few.

The virtuous person has cultivated the kind of character whereby s/he knows how to act and react in the right way, at the right time, in the right manner, and for the right reasons in each and every moral dilemma encountered. However, the way in which one cultivates a virtuous character is through choosing actions that are conducive to building that virtuous character. So, for example, if one wants to cultivate the virtue of honesty so that one can actually be an honest person, then one needs to *act* honestly time and time again so that the virtue can "sink in" to the person's character. The more Johnny actually tells the truth when asked whether he has done something wrong, the more Johnny cultivates the virtue of honesty. The more Suzy lies when asked whether she has done something wrong, the more she cultivates the vice of dishonesty. So, whereas the Kantian would say that one has a duty-bound, rational reason to tell the truth in principle, and the utilitarian would say that one should tell the truth generally to facilitate good—or, at least, nonharmful—consequences, the virtue ethicist would say that one should tell the truth for the sake of one's psychological well-being, as well as for the well-being and social harmony of the community.

The 2001 American Medical Association's "Principles of Medical Ethics" (AMA, 2001) includes a reference to honesty (so does the 1980 version) that sounds as if it was written by a virtue ethicist: "II. A physician shall uphold the standards of professionalism, be honest in all professional interactions, and strive to report physicians deficient in character or competence, or engaging in fraud or deception, to appropriate entities."

There is a now commonly understood and morally intuitive difference between the following:

1. lying to someone with the intention to deceive so that the one lying may gain profit, pleasure, or advantage—or to avoid hassles, pain, or disadvantage—as a result of the lie and deception;
2. withholding the truth (not revealing any or all known facts, hypotheses, and informed speculations) from someone so that the one withholding the truth may gain profit, pleasure, or advantage—or to avoid hassles, pain, or disadvantage—as a result of the withholding;
3. lying to someone to avoid a perceived negative, detrimental, or painful physical or psychological consequence—or to promote a perceived positive, healthy, or pleasurable consequence—for the person to whom one is lying;
4. withholding the truth (not revealing any or all known facts, hypotheses, and informed speculations) from someone to avoid a perceived negative, detrimental, or painful physical or psychological consequence—or to promote a perceived positive, healthy, or pleasurable consequence—for the person to whom one is withholding the truth.

There is nearly universal agreement that (1) is immoral for a variety of obvious reasons—Kantian-based, utilitarian-based, and virtue ethics-based ones—but most people see (1) as wholly impractical, too, since society would likely collapse altogether if everyone lied in this way, or if there were not a serious punishment for doing so. Also, it is arguable that there is a kind of moral scale that goes from (1) being most morally offensive to (4) being least morally offensive. (4) occurs all of the time, for example, when a boss decides before a worker's review that she will highlight the worker's strengths, and not mention any of his weaknesses, during the actual review because she knows that positive reinforcement works for him. Teachers use this kind of "accentuate only the positive" technique all of the time in their classrooms with students and even during parent–teacher conferences with the parents themselves. Or, a witness to a horribly gruesome motorcycle accident has the opportunity to sit down with the accident victim's mother several months later to chat about the accident so as to bring some closure to the mother, and the witness makes it a point to leave out many of the gruesome details when the mother asks, "Could you please tell me what happened to my boy and what you saw that day of the accident?"

(3) occurs all of the time, too, in situations where parents, teachers, or other adults try to shelter children from emotional scare or psychological damage. For example, at Cokeville Elementary School in Cokeville, WY on May 16, 1986, a husband-and-wife team held 150 students and teachers hostage with a bomb in a classroom. Not wanting to scare her students during the ordeal, the first-grade teacher told them, "the nice people are helping us with a fire drill." The bomb actually went off several hours later, killing only the husband and wife (WG, 2012).

A clear example of (1) occurred in North Wales in 2006 when a nine-month-old girl was brought into Wrexham Maelor Hospital and was diagnosed by a junior doctor with viral tonsillitis. In the examination room, the girl's parents asked the junior doctor for a second opinion from the senior doctor overseeing the junior doctor's cases. The junior doctor left the room for 45 min, then came back in to tell the girl's parents that, "his 'boss' agreed with his diagnosis" of viral tonsillitis. In actuality, the junior doctor had not consulted the senior doctor at all and had lied, in a straightforwardly deceptive way, to the parents. The parents and their baby girl left the hospital, but later returned to the emergency room where the girl was diagnosed with pneumococcal meningitis and treated. Although doctors were able to save the girl's life, she suffered brain damage and went blind and deaf, and has chronic lung disease and several other complications resulting from the meningitis. The case went to Mold County Court in Wales in 2012 and was settled with the girl's parents receiving £1 million (DP, 2012; Narain, 2012) from the hospital.

As was expected, the parents of the little girl, various members of the community in North Wales where the family lived, other doctors, and numerous bioethicists have been outraged by the junior doctor's lie, and called for his license to practice medicine to be revoked, at the very least. From the Kantian perspective, it is clear that what the doctor did was immoral in telling the lie and violating a foundational rational principle as well as disrespecting the parents, while from the utilitarian perspective, telling the lie was immoral because it prevented the possibility of more testing to determine the real cause of the girl's illness, sooner rather than later, which may have helped prevent the resulting brain damage or other complications. And from the virtue ethics perspective, the doctor was not only a liar—or taking vicious steps toward becoming a liar—but also being downright irresponsible, another vicious trait according to virtue ethicists.

Lying in the sense of (3) above, however, usually does not illicit the same kind of moral outrage and, from a certain utilitarian perspective, might even be the morally obliged thing to do. Consider the following fictitious, but certainly possible, case: Mary is a clinically depressed 70-year-old woman who has been in and out of treatment centers three times in her life, twice for suicide attempts. She is a divorcee who has been married twice, and she reveals in therapy sessions that both of her ex-husbands claimed she was "overly pessimistic and irrational." A major regret she has often voiced throughout her life is the fact that she was never able to have children, and indeed, she voiced this regret in therapy sessions following both of her suicide attempts at the treatment centers. For the past 10 years, Mary has used a general surgeon named Dr Jones to remove cysts in her breast and on her thyroid gland, and he is aware of Mary's saturnine and surly disposition, as well as her suicide attempts. Mary goes to Dr Jones for surgery to repair an inguinal hernia, and he discovers that she has an undescended testicle, indicating that she has XY Androgen Insensitivity Syndrome (AIS), a syndrome whereby one phenotypically/outwardly appears to be female, but genetically is male. The undescended testicle poses no health risks to Mary, and it appears as if he is the only doctor to be aware of Mary's AIS. Knowing Mary's fragile personality and psychological history—and thinking to himself that she might actually succeed in committing suicide this time—Dr Jones decides not to reveal the discovery of the undescended testicle and the AIS to Mary. He also thinks to himself, "The poor old woman is nearing the end of her life—better to not have this weigh on her." Dr Jones's not revealing this information is an example of (4) above.

However, consider what happens next. Mary had seen a show on TV that featured people with AIS not too long before her hernia surgery and, after hearing of the experiences of the people on the show and reflecting upon her own experiences as a child growing up, was excessively preoccupied about the possibility that she may also have AIS. So, in his office during a follow-up session to her hernia surgery, she asks Dr Jones point blank, "Dr Jones, I watched this show about people with AIS, and I was wondering if you thought that I might have AIS too? I'm scared I might have it. What do you think?" Again, considering Mary's age, fears, and fragile disposition, Dr Jones replies, "No Mary. I don't think you have AIS, and I wouldn't worry about it anymore." Now, Dr Jones has clearly lied in the sense of (3) above; however, many people—including certain utilitarians—would argue that he did the morally correct thing here.

Still, with the Mary case, we are left with the nagging moral sense that Dr Jones should not have withheld any information from Mary, and certainly should not have lied to her when she asked her question about AIS, and we feel this nag probably for the reasons given by Kant: (1) we should not withhold truth from another human out of respect for that human's autonomy and worth as an end in and of her/himself; (2) and we simply just should not lie, ever, as a matter of moral principle.

The first author in this section, Tom Beauchamp, wrote a book with the theologian and philosopher, James Childress, *Principles of Biomedical Ethics* (Beauchamp & Childress, 1979/2009) that expresses four principles that have been influential in bioethical decision-making over the years. Two of these principles, autonomy and justice, have a Kantian basis; the other two, nonmaleficence and beneficence, have more of a utilitarian basis. In his chapter here, Beauchamp discusses the principles of autonomy, noting that "this principle invites—indeed, many think, *demands*—painstakingly honest disclosures by physicians with no withholding of information that is material to a patient's decision." He also discusses beneficence and its implications, claiming that, "by virtue of their role in healthcare, physicians are riveted on providing medical benefits. Almost everything else is a secondary consideration."

In line with what we have hinted at in this introduction already concerning Kantian deontology and Millian utilitarianism, Beauchamp makes the point that these two principles often conflict with one another and "as contexts change (e.g., as a patient becomes increasingly frightened or agitated), the weights of the two competing moral demands of respect for autonomy and beneficence will vary, and no decision rule is available to determine that one obligation outweighs the other. The question in medical practice typically is whether a patient will benefit maximally by not being given some upsetting or otherwise harm-causing information." Thus, with respect to truth telling, Beauchamp argues that "careful management of medical information—including limited disclosure, staged disclosure, and even non-disclosure—is justified in various circumstances."

He gives three cases where it is morally appropriate to withhold information in the sense of (4) above, as well as lie in the sense of (3) above: the first case deals with withholding information from a patient until a second test can be performed to determine if the patient has cancer, or not; the second deals with not revealing the "whole package of bad news" to someone who has been diagnosed with liver cancer; the third deals with a physician mentioned in the story *Schindler's List* who injects cyanide into four immobile patients at a hospital—unbeknownst to them or anyone else—so that they may be saved from the Nazi SS guards, who will undoubtedly take them away, likely torturing them or using them for human experiments. In the end, for special circumstances where the principle of beneficence is appropriate to utilize, Beauchamp endorses a staged disclosure of information for physicians whereby they reveal information little by little to their patients during the course of treatment.

"The most fundamental moral argument against therapeutic deception is the Kantian imperative to respect persons insofar as they are *rational* and *autonomous* agents." So claims Jason Eberl, the second author in this section. "Failure to disclose all relevant information to a rational, autonomous patient is to *infantilize* her," maintains Eberl, "to treat her as being somehow less of a rational, autonomous agent." Further than this, imagine if you found out that your doctor knew some piece of information relevant to your own body, and decided not to disclose that to you. Any patient in that situation would feel angry, frustrated, and especially mistrustful of that doctor.

Importantly, Eberl points out that full disclosure on the part of the doctor leads to full trust on the part of the patient, and he quotes from the Council on Ethical and Judicial Affairs of the American Medical Association: "In practice, medical information should never be permanently withheld from the patient because doing so represents a clear violation of patients' trust." Eberl also points out that full disclosure helps the patient to participate actively in her/his own healthcare. When a patient has *all* of the relevant information—positive or negative—s/he can assist the doctor in addressing her/his own needs, even possibly giving the doctor some insight into a proposed treatment plan.

Eberl does acknowledge, however, that nondisclosure "should be reserved only for extreme cases in which a patient is not substantially autonomous, or lacks the intrinsic capacity to rationally receive and incorporate such information into a deliberative, cooperative process of working with the physician to devise and execute a proper treatment strategy." In this sense, then, his position seems aligned with the example of the fictitious divorcee we mentioned earlier, Mary, who lacks the "intrinsic capacity to rationally receive" her news about the AIS. In his reply to Beauchamp, Eberl characterizes the difference between his position and Beauchamp's: "The primary difference between us is that Beauchamp authorizes a physician to engage—under certain restricted circumstances—in *complete nondisclosure*; whereas I do not believe a physician's role of beneficent guardian of her patients' best interests ever justifies such wholesale withholding of information that is materially relevant to a patient's decision at hand." Both Eberl and Beauchamp probably would agree with the following from Dr James Drane (2012): "Harm may be rare, but still it must be guarded against. The doctor who tells a dreadful truth must do so at a certain time, and in a certain way. The communication of truth always involves a clinical judgment. Truth telling in every clinical context must be sensitive and take into consideration the patient's personality and clinical history. Generally speaking, however, in case of doubt it is better to tell a patient the truth."

References

AMA (American Medical Association). (2001). AMA principles of medical ethics. Retrieved from: http://www.cirp.org/library/statements/ama/

Aristotle. (1962). *Nicomachean ethics* (M. Oswald, Trans.). Upper Saddle River, NJ: Prentice-Hall.

Baron, M. (1999). *Kantian ethics almost without apology*. Ithaca, NY: Cornell University Press.

Beauchamp, T., & Childress, J. (1979/2009). *Principles of biomedical ethics*. Oxford: Oxford University Press.

DP (Daily Post). (2012). North Wales couple 'wasted six years fighting' over daughter's brain damage. *DailyPost.co.uk*, April 27. Retrieved from: http://www.dailypost.co.uk/news/north-wales-news/2012/04/27/north-wales-couple-wasted-six-years-fighting-over-daughter-s-brain-damage-55578-30849563/

Drane, J. (2012). Honesty in medicine: Should doctors tell the truth? *Centro Interdisciplinario de Estudios en Bioetica*. Retrieved from: http://www.uchile.cl/portal/investigacion/centro-interdisciplinario-de-estudios-en-bioetica/publicaciones/76983/honesty-in-medicine-should-doctors-tell-the-truth

Hingorani, M., Wong, T., & Vafidis, G. (1999). Patients' and doctors attitudes to amount of information given after unintended injury during treatment: Cross sectional, questionnaire survey. *British Medical Journal, 318*, 640.

Holland, J., Holland, J. C., Geary, N., Marchini, A., & Tross, S. (1987). Psychosocial issues: An international survey of physician attitudes and practice in regard to revealing the diagnosis of cancer. *Informa Healthcare, 5*, 151–154.

Hooker, B. (2000). *Ideal code, real world: A rule-consequentialist theory of morality*. Oxford: Oxford University Press.

Iezzoni, L., Rao, S., DesRoches, C., Vogeli, C., & Campbell, E. (2012). Survey shows that at least some physicians are not always open or honest with patients. *Health Affairs, 31*, 383–391.

Kant, I. (1775–1789/1963). *Lectures on ethics* (L. Infield, Trans.). Indianapolis, IN: Hackett Publishing.

Kant, I. (1785/1998). *Groundwork of the metaphysics of morals* (M. Gregor, Trans.). (Section I: Transition from common rational to philosophic moral cognition). Cambridge: Cambridge University Press.

Kant, I. (1797a/1996a). *Practical philosophy* (M. Gregor, Trans.). Cambridge: Cambridge University Press.

Kant, I. (1797b/1996b). *The metaphysics of morals* (M. Gregor, Trans.). Cambridge: Cambridge University Press.

Korsgaard, C. (1996). *Creating the kingdom of ends*. Cambridge: Cambridge University Press.

Lewis, D. (1972). Utilitarianism and truthfulness. *Australasian Journal of Philosophy, 50*, 17–19.

MacIntyre, A. (1981). *After virtue*. Notre Dame, IN: Notre Dame Press.

Mill, J. S. (1861/2001). *Utilitarianism*. Indianapolis, IN: Hackett Publishing Company.

Miyaji, N. (1993). The power of compassion: Truth-telling among American doctors in the care of dying patients. *Social Science & Medicine, 36*, 249–264.

Narain, J. (2012). 'Lying doctor failed to spot meningitis' that wrecked a girl's life: Now she is set for a seven-figure sum. *MailOnLine*, April 27. Retrieved from: http://www.dailymail.co.uk/health/article-2135543/Lying-doctor-failed-spot-meningitis-wrecked-girls-life-Now-set-seven-figure-sum.html

Neergaard, L. (2012). Many doctors in survey admit to lying to patients. *The Seattle Times*, February 8. Retrieved from: http://seattletimes.com/html/health/2017459899_medicalfibs09.html

O'Neill, O. (1990). *Constructions of reason: Explorations of Kant's practical philosophy*. Cambridge: Cambridge University Press.

O'Neill, O. (2008). Kant and utilitarianism contrasted. In J. Arthur & S. Scalet (Eds.), *Morality and moral controversies: Readings in moral, social and political philosophy* (pp. 40–45). New York: Pearson.

Quirt, C., Mackillop, W., Ginsburg, A., Sheldon, L., Brundage, M., Dixon, P., & Ginsburg, L. (1997). Do doctors know when their patients don't? A survey of doctor–patient communication in lung cancer. *Lung Cancer, 18*, 1–27.

Shaw, W. (1999). *Contemporary ethics: Taking account of utilitarianism*. Cambridge, MA: Blackwell Publishers.

Statman, D. (Ed.). (1997). *Virtue ethics*. Edinburgh: Edinburgh University Press.

Surbone, A., Zwitter, M. Rajer, M., & Stiefel, R. (Eds.). (2013). *New challenges in communication with cancer patients*. London: Springer.

WG (Wyoming Government State Parks & Cultural Resources) (2012). Survivor is my name. Retrieved from: http://wyospcr.state.wy.us/MultiMedia/Display.aspx?ID=86&icon=1

Chapter Twenty Five

There Are Circumstances in Which a Doctor May Withhold Information

Tom L. Beauchamp

Are there conditions under which patients should not be given full information by their physicians about their medical circumstances? Legal and moral doctrines of informed consent have led many physicians, lawyers, and writers in bioethics to the belief that patients have both a right to full disclosure and a right to consent. At least since the Nuremberg trials, which exposed abusive medical experimentation without any form of truth-telling or consent, bioethics has placed disclosure by physicians and voluntary consent by patients and research subjects at the forefront of its concerns. However, there is much more to the legitimate and appropriate management of information in medical practice than the doctrine of informed consent suggests. I will argue that healthcare professionals have an obligation to manage information in a way that sometimes withholds information and at other times stages disclosures over time.

Introduction

Although information disclosure and truth-telling are the subjects under investigation, many topics in bioethics fall roughly under the scope of the title of this chapter. They include medical confidentiality, informed consent, informed refusal, placebo treatment, randomized clinical trials, genetic counseling, and the duty to warn third parties. In each of these areas, questions have arisen about whether withholding information to patients is justified and, if so, under which conditions. For example, in randomized clinical trials, which are generally regarded as the gold standard of accurate data gathering in clinical research, patients commonly do not know whether they are receiving an investigational drug of interest or rather are receiving no treatment at all. It has been very sensibly argued that it is ethically acceptable, and highly desirable in some situations, to randomize patients without their express knowledge and consent in trials comparing widely used, approved interventions that pose no additional risk (Truog et al., 1999). However, these problems of research ethics do not raise quite the same questions about withholding information as those that arise in clinical ethics. I will confine attention almost entirely to clinical ethics.

Historical Background of the Problem

Prior to the early 1970s, there was no strong commitment in medicine to physician truth-telling. Nor was there any basis in medical codes of ethics to indicate that patients have a right to diagnostic information or

Contemporary Debates in Bioethics, First Edition. Edited by Arthur L. Caplan and Robert Arp.

to make a decision about treatment recommendations. This is not to say that no physicians were committed to truthfulness in disclosures to patients and research subjects. Many were so committed, but patients' rights to be told the truth were rarely discussed and had never been acknowledged in formal codes. The prevailing Hippocratic tradition had for over 2000 years neglected almost all problems of truthfulness, privacy, patients' rights, and the like. An excellent example of how this tradition was distilled into a systematic medical ethics is found in Thomas Percival's (1803) *Medical Ethics; or a Code of Institutes and Precepts, Adapted to the Professional Conduct of Physicians and Surgeons*. Percival's work was the pattern for the American Medical Association's (AMA) first code of ethics in 1847 (Pellegrino & Thomasma, 1993; Jonsen, 1998).

The *Principles of Medical Ethics* of the AMA (1847) from its origins made no mention of an obligation or virtue of veracity. The strongest case by a physician for truth-telling prior to the twentieth century that I have been able to locate is the following thesis of nineteenth-century physician, Worthington Hooker: "There are cases in which [withholding information] should be done. All that I claim is this—that in withholding the truth no deception should be practised, and that if sacrifice of the truth be the necessary price for obtaining the object, no such sacrifice should be made" (Hooker, 1849, p. 380; also Smith, 1946). Hooker offers a simple, but profoundly important, thesis: Withholding can be permissible in medical practice, and sometimes should be done, but only if it does not involve deception, lying, sacrifice of the truth, and the like. Hooker puts his finger on the primary problem before us, but is his position defensible?

In the mid-1970s, a different climate began to develop in medicine. There arose—primarily through developments in law and ethics—an interest in general moral principles that would allow for impartial judgments in medicine, ones that took into consideration both the autonomy interests and the welfare interests of patients and research subjects (Beauchamp & Faden, 1986, chs. 3–6). A goal of various writers from roughly 1975 to the present has been to develop a set of principles or rules that would alter healthcare's traditional, near-exclusive preoccupation with obligations to medically benefit patients, while not addressing interests that patients have in receiving information and making their own decisions. The idea was to shift medical ethics in the direction of better serving the autonomy of patients and improving informational exchanges.

The result of several decades of writings on the subject has been to shift medical ethics in the direction of increased disclosure and far less withholding of information. Many changes were imposed on medicine through nonmedical forms of authority, most notably judges in courts and government bodies or officials in regulatory agencies. In particular, rules of obtaining informed consent have gone from being nonexistent to being canonical in medical practice. In fact, a study done in the mid-1960s, conducted by a lawyer–surgeon team (Hershey & Bushkoff, 1969), showed that consent forms were not yet a ubiquitous feature, even of the practice of surgery—let alone elsewhere in medicine. However, the pendulum may now have swung too far in the direction of seeing the landscape of physician responsibility in terms of patients' rights to information. Especially dangerous is the model of a one-time delivery of all relevant information, by contrast to a staged delivery of information over time. I will argue that the proper view is one in which different interests are balanced, which entails that sometimes a physician is morally justified in withholding information. Careful management of medical information—including limited disclosure, staged disclosure, and even nondisclosure—is justified in various circumstances I will discuss.

A Framework of Principles for Biomedical Ethics

I begin with a framework of principles that I developed with my colleague, James Childress, as a general, principled-based approach to deliberating on such questions of bioethics (Beauchamp & Childress, 1979/2009). This framework helps establish why problems of withholding information are problems of moral principle that do not have obvious answers based on a firm general rule of truth-telling or right to information.

The moral principles in our framework are grouped under four general categories: (1) *respect for autonomy*, a principle requiring respect for the decision-making capacities of autonomous persons, (2) *nonmaleficence*, a principle requiring not causing harm to others), (3) *beneficence*, a group of principles requiring that we prevent harm, provide benefits, and balance benefits against risks and costs, and (4) *justice*, a group of principles requiring fair and appropriate distribution of benefits, risks, and costs. For the purposes of this chapter, the two most important principles are respect for autonomy and beneficence. Although the other principles are important moral considerations, we need here discuss only these two principles and the ways they come into conflict with each other:

- *Respect for autonomy*. Personal autonomy refers to personal self-governance: personal rule of the self by adequate understanding while remaining free from controlling interferences by others and from personal limitations that prevent choice. "Autonomy" means freedom from external constraint and the presence of critical mental capacities such as understanding, intending, and voluntary decision-making capacity (Beauchamp, 2005; Kukla, 2005). The *principle* of respect for autonomy requires that there be respectful treatment when disclosing information and requires that someone in a health-professional role be able to help patients make genuinely autonomous decisions. This principle invites—indeed, many think, *demands*—painstakingly honest disclosures by physicians with no withholding of information that is material to a patient's decision.
- *Beneficence*. The second principle, beneficence, presents a moral obligation to act for the benefit of others. Traditional notions of the physician's obligations were uniformly expressed in terms of both beneficence and nonmaleficence, as the following much-quoted Hippocratic statement indicates: "As to disease, make a habit of two things—*to help, or at least to do no harm*" (Jones, 1923). Still today, no demand of medical ethics is more important in taking care of patients: The welfare of patients is medicine's context and purpose. Many basic duties in medicine, nursing, public health, and research are expressed in terms of a positive obligation to come to the assistance of those in need of treatment or in danger of injury. By virtue of their role in healthcare, physicians are riveted on providing medical benefits. Almost everything else is a secondary consideration.

Controversial moral problems about use of these principles arise when we must interpret their weight and significance in particular contexts and determine precise limits on their application. Several controversies involve questions about the conditions under which a person's right to autonomous choice demands a disclosure by a physician that would either harm the patient or harm someone connected to the patient—such as a family partner or a partner who might be harmed either by a disclosure or by a failure to disclose information.

The most important aspect of this problem is that, as contexts change (e.g., as a patient becomes increasingly frightened or agitated), the weights of the two competing moral demands of respect for autonomy and beneficence will vary, and no decision rule is available to determine that one obligation outweighs the other. The question in medical practice typically is whether a patient will benefit maximally by not being given some upsetting or otherwise harm-causing information. No one in moral theory has been able to formulate a hierarchical-ordering rule that requires that respect for the autonomy of patients (and full disclosure of information) always overrides the physician's obligations to make a good medical judgment so as to protect patients from harm-causing conditions. I believe this goal is impossible to achieve, which means, for present purposes, that there are no general theoretical considerations to show that physicians must never withhold information. Everything depends, I will argue, on the weight, in the circumstance, of a medical benefit and the importance of an item of information for the patient.

Problems of Autonomy Limitation: The Harm Principle and Medical Paternalism

Problems about whether physicians can withhold information from their patients seem to come down to one major problem in moral theory: Can we justifiably limit the autonomous choices and actions of patients for reasons of medical paternalism? However, paternalism is not the only justifying reason that might be offered for nondisclosure. For example, a physician might withhold information in order to protect another person, such as a family member or sexual partner, from harm. These problems of paternalism and protection of others are both instances of what I will call *autonomy-limiting principles.* These principles provide the philosophical structure of justification for withholding information that I will use hereafter, especially paternalism.

The Nature of Autonomy-Limiting Principles

The history of this problem is traceable to John Stuart Mill's (1849/1977) attack on various principles that restrict liberty in his classic *On Liberty*. Mill argues that an individual's liberty rights are justifiably overridden when that person's choices conflict with other rights or moral principles, such as those protecting health and welfare. For example, we require people by law to do many things they wish not to do, such as paying taxes; and we require them to not do many things they might wish to do, such as driving an automobile at high speeds on city streets. We have good reasons for restricting their actions in these ways. Joel Feinberg (1986, vol. 4, p. 9), following Mill's model, called the principles that have been put forward to constrain our freedom of action "liberty-limiting principles" and "coercion-legitimizing principles," but I prefer the designation "autonomy-limiting principles" and will use it here.

The two principles we need in order to address physician-withholding of information are these:

1. *The harm principle*: A person's autonomy is justifiably restricted to prevent harm to others caused by that person's actions.
2. *The principle of paternalism*: A person's autonomy is justifiably restricted to prevent harm to one's self caused by one's own actions, irrespective of whether any harm is caused to others.

Mill (1849/1977) defended the first principle and rejected the second. He delivered the following blistering attack on paternalism: "The only purpose for which power can be rightfully exercised over any member of a civilized community, against his will, is to prevent harm to others. His own good, either physical or moral, is not a sufficient warrant" (p. 223). The first principle would permit a physician to withhold information from a patient in order to prevent harm from occurring to a third party. However, no form of paternalism—including withholding information for the patient's own good—can ever be justified, in Mill's view.

A serious philosophical problem for Mill is that his utilitarian moral theory is threatened by it. His utilitarian theory does not support absolute restrictions of the sort his critique of paternalism strongly suggests. Mill's formulations of utilitarianism require that actors consider the various interests of all parties affected by an action in order to bring about the best state of affairs. A philosophy grounded in the importance of balancing different welfare interests of all affected parties is ill-suited to the rejection of medical paternalism, which itself demands such a balancing of different welfare interests for individual patients. I will use such a balancing account (though not a utilitarian one) to argue both that Mill's apparent rejection of withholding information in clinical encounters is unwarranted by his own philosophy and that such balancing is sometimes justifiably present when physicians paternalistically customize disclosures to patients. My thesis is that balancing different autonomy and welfare interests is basic to moral deliberation in medical practice and that there are circumstances in which a physician may withhold information—though, of course, there are also circumstances in which a physician may not withhold information. The right decision depends on the weight of the moral considerations of beneficence and autonomy at work in particular circumstances.

The Harm Principle and Its Import for Withholding Information from Patients

I start with Mill's harm principle, which is accepted by virtually everyone in both theoretical and practical ethics. It is part of ordinary morality that we can justifiably use coercive power to limit certain types of actions, against the will of the actors, to prevent them from causing harm to other parties. This principle retains its strength in relevant cases of withholding of information from patients.

In a famous case known as *Tarasoff v. Regents of University of California* (TvR, 1976) a patient confided to his psychologist that he intended to kill a third party. Psychotherapeutic practice has long honored strict rules of confidentiality, which require that information divulged in psychotherapy by a patient to the therapist may not be shared with other individuals without the patient's prior consent. This rule descends from the Hippocratic Oath, in which the physician vows, "Whatever, in connection with my professional practice ... I see or hear, in the life of men, which ought not to be spoken of abroad, I will not divulge, as reckoning that all such should be kept secret." This rule is based on the need for the patient to trust the therapist and is an expression of respect for the privacy of patients. Another widely, though not universally, accepted rule is that a physician or other health professional is morally obligated to take reasonable steps to prevent or warn of major harm to another individual or group (a third party, in my language here) if the therapist is situated to do so and can do so without significant personal risk. Maintaining confidentiality sometimes come into direct conflict with this second rule: Taking steps to warn a third party, based on confidentially disclosed information, infringes the rule of confidentiality.

The psychologist in *Tarasoff* faced the choice of either preserving the confidentiality of information disclosed by the patient or warning a young woman that her life is in danger because of plans the patient has. The psychologist decided to inform the police of the threat (so that the police could protect the woman) and did not tell the patient that confidentiality would be infringed or that it had been infringed. A legal judgment later reached is this case held that a threat of serious bodily injury to a third party justified the infringement in this case and did not compel disclosure of that fact to the patient. The judges reached the reasonable conclusion that the endangered person's interests have more moral weight than the interests of the patient or the loss of confidentiality. Concealment of the notification to police was warranted by the seriousness of the threat. This balancing of interests is entirely correct, in my view, though it does not solve all moral problems.

One issue is whether the psychologist had an obligation to disclose to his patient both that he had broken confidentiality and that he would not be able to continue treating the patient. This information is, beyond a reasonable doubt, a matter of material interest to the patient. The traditional moral premise in confidentiality provisions is that, in the absence of an explicit disclosure to the patient that confidentiality does *not* (or hereafter will not) hold, the patient is always entitled to assume that it does hold. Mill's harm principle again is a relevant consideration assessing the role of this traditional rule. In the case before us, disclosure would create a situation of a high risk of personal injury for the psychologist because his life would be in danger as a consequence of the disclosure. At each step of the decision chain, a health professional must balance risks and benefits. As the risks and benefits go up or down in such cases of withholding information and infringing confidentiality, a health professional should adjust his or her thinking about whether it is acceptable to breach confidentialilty—and whether to hide such a breach from the patient.

With this case behind us, I now shift to the more important principle of paternalism, where we will get the same result of justified withholding, though for different reasons.

The Principle of Paternalism and Its Import for Withholding Information from Patients

Whether there are valid paternalistic justifications for withholding information from patients now becomes the main issue. Paternalism is the intentional overriding or limitation of one person's autonomous choices or actions by another person or institution, where the latter justifies the action (here a physician's withholding information) by appeal to the goal of providing a benefit or of preventing or mitigating harm to the person whose choices or actions are limited or overridden. This definition is value-neutral because it does not presume whether paternalism is or is not justified. The term "paternalism" therefore has neither a negative nor a positive valence. The definition assumes that there is an act of beneficence analogous to parental beneficence, but it does not assume that the beneficent act is justified, obligatory, or unjustified (Dworkin, 1992; Arneson, 1980; Archard, 1990).

Examples of paternalism in medicine in this strong sense include court orders for blood transfusions when patients have refused them, involuntary commitment to institutions for treatment, intervention to stop rational suicides, resuscitating patients who have asked not to be resuscitated, and, of course, withholding medical information that is relevant to patients' decision-making. The motivation is the beneficent promotion of physical or psychological health and welfare of those whose autonomous choice is limited or overridden.

No one seriously doubts that the harm principle is a justified liberty-limiting principle, but there has been deep concern since Mill about the justifiability of a principle of paternalism. The debate in the literature is nuanced, but the crux of the account I will offer of justified paternalistic actions is that risks and benefits for a patient should be placed on a scale with the patient's autonomy interests (in information), and then the interests should be balanced: As a patient's interests in autonomy increase (i.e., as the information becomes more important) and the benefits for that person decrease (e.g., withholding provides only a minor medical benefit), the justification of paternalistic action becomes increasingly less plausible; conversely, as benefits for a person increase and autonomy interests decrease, the justification of paternalistic action becomes increasingly more plausible. Accordingly, a physician who prevents only minor harms or provides only minor benefits while withholding information will lack plausible justification for an intervention. However, actions that prevent major harms or provide major benefits, while only trivially disrespecting autonomy (by withholding pieces of relatively insignificant information), will often be justified paternalistic actions.

The moral thesis is that as risk to a patient's welfare increases, and as the information disclosure is less important, the likelihood of a justified paternalistic intervention correspondingly increases. For example, if a dying patient who will live for a month or less is in an extreme form of pain but refuses pain medication on grounds that he might become addicted to it, it is plausibly justified for a physician to initiate an undetectable pain-control medication without informing the patient of the intervention. I will now further explore this thesis about justified withholding of information by examining three situations in which justified paternalistic actions involving withholding occur. The first two are common in medicine and, I believe, are justified practices, but the third is a most unusual situation that illustrates how extreme emergencies can justify paternalistic withholding of information that would not be justified in ordinary circumstances.

1. *Withholding Information Prior to a Second Diagnostic Procedure*. Here is a relatively simple starting case: A physician obtains the results of a lumbar myelogram (a picture of the spinal region made from X-rays and a contrast material) following examination of a patient. The procedure yields inconclusive results and must be repeated, but it also strongly suggests a serious pathology. When the patient asks what the physician has learned, the physician withholds the potentially negative information about a possible pathology because he appreciates that the patient would be distressed and agitated by the information, which could turn out to be inaccurate. The physician is confident that the patient will consent to another myelogram. The physician is committed to being completely truthful with the patient in the future about the results of the second procedure and about needed procedures (Beauchamp & Childress, 1979/2009).

This physician's act of nondisclosure is a warranted paternalistic withholding of information. The physician's reasoning is that disclosure of a suspicion of a serious pathology would provide no medical benefit or useful information to the patient, and therefore the patient's autonomy interests in knowing about a possible pathology are extremely low. The physician balances this need for information against the risks of confusion and stress that will be present until the results of the second procedure are available. It is completely within the bounds of good medical practice and good medical ethics for the physician to make this paternalistic judgment. The withholding prevents what could be an agonizing period of time for the patient while awaiting the results of the second procedure, and there is only a minor disrespecting of autonomy.

2. *Caring for Patients Who Have Received Bad News.* Some patients with whom physicians interact are fearful and stressed after having been told the basics of some bad news about their medical condition, for example, that a test indicates they have liver cancer. They have not yet been told the whole package of bad news—e.g., they may have been told almost nothing about how much pain they will suffer, the costs and complications of treatment, how long they have to live, the side effects of the available medical treatments, the specialists they will have to see (or have the option of seeing), the full course of future procedures, and the like. These patients have not lost the capacity for autonomous judgment. Indeed, many have an excellent understanding of their situation and want to exercise the best judgment they can about how to proceed. Nonetheless, these patients are fragile, fearful, subject to being upset, and even devastated by additional bad news beyond that already received.

In this situation, the primary concern of doctors and nurses should not at the outset be the disclosure of all available relevant information. Some information can be delayed and then spread over a period of time, and some of it may justifiably never be mentioned. The physician's fundamental obligation at the beginning of the process of disclosure is to calm down and reassure this patient, while engaging sympathetically with the patient's feelings and conveying the presence of a caring, knowledgeable medical authority (cf. Quill & Townsend, 1991). The physician's emotional investment in the patient's feelings should be joined with a detached evaluation of what the patient's medical and informational needs are. Cases in which risk of harm and burden will be substantially increased if all pertinent information is disclosed call for a skilled management of each item of information. The question almost always is how much information can justifiably be withheld to provide the best form of care for the patient. For some period of time, and perhaps throughout the course of the entire episode of care, the physician's obligations of taking care may take moral precedence over obligations to disclose information.

Each such encounter a therapist has with a patient calls for a response that is inadequately captured by sweeping and inflexible rules of truth-telling (Carse, 1998). Behavior that in the context of one delicate patient is a caring response and a balancing of an appropriate level of information will not be so for another patient. There are no precise rules about how to care for such patients. In clinical judgments, considerations of compassion, objective assessment, caring responsiveness, reassurance, management of information, and the like all have a role. In these common situations in medicine, it is a wooden premise that there morally cannot be a withholding of information that will be hurtful to patients and of no practical consequence. For example, it would be morally contemptible to tell a patient who has just been diagnosed with cancer of the tongue that she will never again sing in her church choir and will encounter profound difficulty in being understood when speaking. What she should be told is that she will need speech therapy that will help her to regain some lost capacities of speech. It is obligatory in such a case to withhold hurtful information while giving hope where that hope may have some basis. There is no other appropriate form of care for the patient. It would not be fitting for a caring physician in these cases to act on a rule of never withholding devastating information such as that the patient might eventually lose their ability to speak.

3. *Patients in Extraordinary Circumstances.* I have thus far been dealing with more or less common encounters in medicine. Now, I turn to an extraordinary circumstance in which the issue arises whether even highly relevant information may be justifiably withheld. In *Schindler's List*, a chronicle of life under the Nazi SS in the Jewish ghetto in Cracow, Poland, Thomas Keneally (1983) describes a physician faced with an inescapable moral dilemma: In the next few minutes either inject cyanide into four immobile patients or abandon them to the SS, who were at that moment emptying the ghetto and had already demonstrated that they would brutally torture and kill their captives, including hospitalized patients. This physician "suffered painfully from a set of ethics as intimate to him as the organs of his own body" (pp. 176–180). Here is a person of high moral character who, in unprecedented circumstances, seeks to find the morally right action. Ultimately, with

uncertainty and reluctance, the physician elected euthanasia without telling the four doomed patients of the decision—an act universally denounced by the abstract general rules in codes of professional medical ethics. Even if one thinks that the physician's act of withholding information that the injection would cause death was wrong and blameworthy—a judgment I reject—no blame or demerit can be directed at the physician's motives or character. Having already risked death, by choosing to remain at his patients' beds in the hospital rather than take a prepared escape route, the physician is a moral hero who understandably does not disclose the decision to use lethal means to terminate the lives of the patients.

I have argued in this section that various paternalistic withholdings of information are justified, even though other similar actions are unjustified. In medical ethics, it should be left an open question whether, in particular cases, reasonably minor withholdings of information are justified in light of the critical needs of the patients—and in extraordinary cases whether more than minor items of information may justifiably be withheld. It will serve moral reflection well if we do not follow Mill in his absolute banishment of all forms of paternalism.

Clinical Judgment and Strategies of Information Disclosure

When clinical judgment is exercised to withhold information, which strategies are justified, and which arguments support use of these strategies?

One justified strategy is staged disclosure of information, which involves withholding information for periods of time during an episode of care. Staged disclosure over time can be the most desirable strategy in the bad-news situations involving fragile patients previously discussed. This approach will not, of course, be justified in all circumstances. There is some threat to trust between clinicians and patients, but not such a threat (at least in many cases) that staged disclosure is rendered impermissible. To the contrary, my arguments and case analyses above suggest that this strategy should be part of the balancing act and in some cases will be morally the best way to manage some fragile patients. Staged disclosure using carefully selected language is apparent in the following case from rehabilitation medicine first put forward by Joel Stein (1990):

> For close to a month, a physician in a stroke rehabilitation unit carefully managed information in his interactions with a patient who had suffered a stroke and who asked during a first session how long it would take for his arm to improve. From the beginning the doctor knew that the patient was unlikely to recover significant use of his arm, and he offered caveats and uncertainty that did not fully match what he believed or felt. He stressed the limitations of prognostication, the unpredictability of recovery, and the need to give the brain a chance to heal. The patient received these answers well at the time, apparently preferring the physician's "ambiguous statements about the future to the alternative judgment of the permanent paralysis he fears." This indefinite, but caring and supportive, exchange continued, with the physician praising the patient's progress in walking and performing daily activities, despite residual weakness. After two weeks, the patient was enthusiastic about his progress and asked, "How about my arm?" The physician responded, "The arm may not recover as much as the leg." Although this statement confirmed his fears, the patient focused on his overall progress. He had a strong hope that the physician might be mistaken, since he had repeatedly stressed his inability to prognosticate accurately. (pp. 305–306)

This physician had learned that his patients generally have a strong hope for a return to their previous capabilities, so much so that a straight dose of bad news, unless carefully staged, tends to overpower any good news about the possibilities of rehabilitation. He was entirely convinced, based on years of clinical experience, that patients need to learn many of the facts about their situation slowly during the course of their adjustment to a rehabilitation hospital. They need from the start to have a strong infusion of hope, and they need time to settle into certain facts about their disabilities. This physician is right to regard staged disclosures as an appropriate form of medical care of patients.

Although moral, legal, and professional norms generally call for honest and thorough provision of information about diagnoses, therapeutic options, and treatment recommendations, physicians have not been expected to follow this same script in discussing *prognoses*. Physicians are particularly cautious in discussing prognoses. They prefer to instill hope in patients. This strategy is justified, and not merely on the basis of paternalistic beneficence. It is part of the good medical care of patients to give hope and to combat hopelessness and dejection.

In some cases, usually owing to fears patients have, full disclosure from the outset can leave patients with a misleading picture of the possibilities for good therapeutic outcomes. Much information in medicine needs to be framed so that patients are not misled or given to misimpressions. Some patients have difficulty in *accepting* as true the information medical professionals have given them—even if they *comprehend* the information. For example, patients sometimes have false beliefs that they bring to the context of the discussion. Seriously ill patients who have been adequately informed of their circumstance and asked to make a treatment decision refuse a recommended treatment because they have a false belief that they are not truly sick. Some patients continue for weeks believing that what they have been told is false.

After a half century now of dealing with difficulties of obtaining informed consents in medicine and research, physicians are very aware of how tangled and difficult lines of communication and decision-making can be in medicine. They appreciate what law and morals require in the way of honest disclosures and understanding by patients—as well as the dangers of underdisclosure, but they also know that there are many ways to respect the autonomy of patients. What we should ask of physicians is an educated and caring sensitivity to the patient's informational and therapeutic needs while also carefully managing the quantity and quality of information disclosed and the pace of the disclosure. Attending to a particular patient's need for information is complicated, and that fact is not going to change.

References

AMA (American Medical Association). (1847). *Proceedings of the National Medical Conventions, held in New York, May 1846, and in Philadelphia, May 1847*. Philadelphia: T. K. & P. G. Collins, Printers.

Archard, D. (1990). Paternalism defined. *Analysis, 50*, 36–42.

Arneson, R. (1980). Mill versus paternalism. *Ethics, 90*, 470–489.

Beauchamp, T. L. (2005). Who deserves autonomy and whose autonomy deserves respect? In J. Taylor (Ed.), *Personal autonomy: New essays in personal autonomy and its role in contemporary moral philosophy* (pp. 310–329). Cambridge: Cambridge University Press.

Beauchamp, T. L., & Childress, J. (1979/2009). *Principles of biomedical ethics*. Oxford: Oxford University Press.

Beauchamp, T. L., & Faden, R. (1986). *A history and theory of informed consent*. Oxford: Oxford University Press.

Carse, A. (1998). Impartial principle and moral context: Securing a place for the particular in ethical theory. *Journal of Medicine and Philosophy, 23*, 153–169.

Dworkin, G., (1992). Paternalism. In L. Becker (Ed.), *Encyclopedia of ethics* (pp. 939–942). New York: Garland Publishing.

Feinberg, J. (1986). *The moral limits of the criminal law*. Oxford: Oxford University Press.

Hershey, N., & Bushkoff, S. (1969). *Informed consent study: The surgeon's responsibility for disclosure to patients*. Pittsburgh, PA: Aspen Systems Corporation.

Hooker, W. (1849). *Physician and patient, or a practical view of the mutual duties, relations and interests of the medical profession and the community*. New York: Baker and Scribner.

Jones, W. (Ed.). (1923). *Hippocrates: Epidemics 1.11*. Cambridge, MA: Harvard University Press.

Jonsen, A. (1998). *The birth of bioethics*. Oxford: Oxford University Press.

Keneally, T. (1983). *Schindler's list*. New York: Penguin Books.

Kukla, R. (2005). Conscientious autonomy: Displacing decisions in health care. *Hastings Center Report, 25*, 34–44.

Mill, J. S. (1849/1977). *On liberty*. Toronto: University of Toronto Press.

Pellegrino, E., & Thomasma, D. (1993). *The virtues in medical practice*. Oxford: Oxford University Press.

Percival, T. (1803). *Medical ethics, or a code of institutes and precepts, adapted to the professional conduct of physicians and surgeons*. Manchester: S. Russell.

Quill, T., & Townsend, P. (1991). Bad news: Delivery, dialogue, and dilemmas. *Archives of Internal Medicine, 151*, 463–464.

Smith, H. (1946). Therapeutic privilege to withhold specific diagnosis from patient sick with serious or fatal illness. *Tennessee Law Review, 19*, 340–351.

Stein, J. (2000). A fragile commodity. *Journal of the American Medical Association, 283*, 305–306.

Truog, R., Robinson, W., Randolph, A., & Morris, A. (1999). Is informed consent always necessary for randomized, controlled trials? *The New England Journal of Medicine, 11*, 804–806.

TvR (*Tarasoff v. Regents of the University of California*) (1976). 7 Cal. 3d 425, 551 P.2d 334, 131 Cal. Rptr. 14 (Cal. 1976).

Chapter Twenty Six

There Are No Circumstances in Which a Doctor May Withhold Information

Jason T. Eberl

May a physician withhold certain information from a patient that may be harmful? This question is examined from four theoretical foundations: utilitarian, libertarian, Kantian, and Aristotelian. I conclude that the imperative to promote patients' capacity to render voluntary and informed decisions should lead physicians to work cooperatively with their patients to design and implement a treatment plan that would best serve each patient's healthcare goals. While concerns regarding psychologically or emotionally vulnerable patients' capacity to receive and process distressing information may support temporary nondisclosure or "staged" disclosure, a complete withholding of information that would be materially relevant to patients' exercise of their autonomy is never justified.

Introduction

Two patients are under the care of a physician, who has diagnosed both of them with an incurable form of cancer. The first is a stoic, self-made individual who demands that the doctor "give it to him straight." The other is emotionally unstable and prone to bouts of depression, and has even contemplated suicide in the past over romantic break-ups and job losses. Knowing the respective personalities of her two patients, the physician decides to approach each patient differently. To the first, she says quite directly, "I'm afraid you have an incurable form of cancer with a prognosis of less than nine months' survival." The patient thanks the physician for her candor and leaves to start putting his affairs in order. To the second patient, she hedges a bit, "Your test results indicate some sort of growth. It may be malignant, but we need to study the results further before confirming a diagnosis." She takes this approach so as to warm the patient up to the idea that he might have cancer. In later visits, she plans to reveal to him first that he does have cancer, and then later reveal that his cancer is incurable. She hopes that, by taking this "staged" approach to revealing the grim diagnosis, the patient will be able to adjust to the news and not sink into a potentially suicidal state of depression.

This case represents just one of many ways in which physicians may elect to withhold certain information from their patients, at least temporarily. In some cases, though, a physician may intend *never* to reveal the undisclosed information. Consider a case involving a medical error: a patient's blood is drawn for a cholesterol screening, but the vial is mislabeled, and the sample is accidentally tested for HIV without the patient's consent. If the results of the test are positive,

Contemporary Debates in Bioethics, First Edition. Edited by Arthur L. Caplan and Robert Arp.

is the physician ethically obligated to reveal both the mistake and the patient's HIV+ status to him? Perhaps so, especially given the public health concern at stake. But what if the test results are negative? Must the physician reveal to the patient that his blood was accidentally screened for HIV if there is no health benefit to doing so; nor is there any cost in concealing the mistake?

This essay will focus on the first type of case described, in which a physician elects to withhold, either temporarily or permanently, certain information from a patient for arguably *beneficent* reasons. That is, the physician is not being self-serving, to herself or her institution, by not revealing this information. Rather, the goal is purely to promote what the physician believes to be in the patient's best interest by withholding information that may be *harmful* to him. This practice of informational guardianship is known as the "therapeutic privilege." This discussion will thus also be limited to *clinical* interactions and not explicitly discuss withholding information from research subjects, which raises distinct ethical issues and elicits different reasons used to justify or nullify the moral permissibility of nondisclosure.

History and Definition of Therapeutic Privilege

"The longer I practice medicine the more I am convinced that every physician should cultivate lying as a fine art." This statement by Joseph Collins (1927) reflects not just his personal opinion, but a general attitude of his day, in which physicians felt perfectly justified in adopting a *paternalistic* attitude toward their patients and acting appropriately, including not only withholding information judged to be potentially harmful, but even lying outright. A generation later, Donald Oken (1961) conducted a survey of physicians in which nearly 90% reported withholding a diagnosis of cancer from their patients. Less than two decades later, though, a similar survey revealed a reversal of attitude: 97% of physicians surveyed indicated a preference for informing patients of their cancer diagnosis (Novack et al., 1979). From a legal perspective, US courts have upheld the permissibility of physicians to withhold certain types of information from patients, primarily related to the disclosure of particular risks associated with a therapeutic intervention: "The [therapeutic privilege] exception obtains [if] risk-disclosure poses such a threat of detriment to the patient as to become unfeasible or contraindicated from a medical point of view. It is recognized that patients occasionally become so ill or emotionally distraught on disclosure as to foreclose a rational decision, or complicate or hinder the treatment, or perhaps even pose psychological damage to the patient" (*Canterbury v. Spence*, 464 F.2d 772 (D.C. Cir, 1972) at 789; quoted in Faden & Beauchamp, 1986, p. 37).

A few clarifications are in order here. First, the modern concept of therapeutic privilege does not directly justify *lying* to a patient, as Collins (1927) recommends; but rather involves nondisclosure of certain information, which is at least a form of deception that may be morally equivalent to lying. Second, cases in which therapeutic privilege is invoked are distinct from cases in which disclosure is simply infeasible—e.g., emergency situations or patients who lack the capacity to give voluntary informed consent. Third, therapeutic privilege is aimed directly at the *patient's* good, not that of the physician, healthcare institution, or third parties. Therapeutic privilege thus stands at the crossroads of three ethical principles that impact the physician–patient relationship: respect for autonomy, which requires that a patient give *informed consent* to any therapeutic or research-related intervention; beneficence, i.e., promoting a patient's well-being; and nonmaleficence, i.e., not causing undue harm to a patient (Beauchamp & Childress, 2009).

Although withholding of information is not the same, ontologically speaking, as an act of lying, it may nevertheless count as a form of deception that is morally on a par with lying. While there has been considerable debate on this point (Jackson, 1991, 1993; Bakhurst, 1992; Benn, 2001), I will follow Daniel Sokol (2006), who concludes his analysis of this debate by defining deception as follows: "Deception is a communicative act intended to induce or maintain what the agent believes to be a false belief in the target when (1) the target's expectation of truthfulness is reasonable and (2) the agent is successful in producing the intended deceptive outcome" (p. 462). By "communicative act," Sokol refers to not only speech acts, but also nonverbal behavior and even silence that may be "content-full" in certain contexts. Concealment of relevant information may thus also meet the criteria for being deceptive. Hence, the question at hand is whether a physician may be justified in being *deceptive* in certain circumstances, regardless of what particular actions or nonactions—lying, nondisclosure, etc.—may be employed.

Ethical Frameworks for Analysis

There are myriad ethical approaches that may be adopted—depending on one's overall moral worldview—in order to analyze the permissibility of therapeutic deception (as I will refer to it from here on). Three theoretical foundations have been predominant in the literature representing both sides of this debate: utilitarian, libertarian, and Kantian. I will also elucidate a fourth perspective: Aristotelian.

Utilitarianism, as a *consequentialist* theory, takes as the starting-point for moral evaluation the results of a particular action—or of following a rule upon which particular actions are based—and whether the net value of such results is overall beneficial or harmful to all affected parties. There is thus no intrinsic rightness or wrongness to any given action or rule; rather, different circumstances will yield different moral judgments depending upon whether the action, or rule upon which the action is based, leads to greater net benefit or harm than the available alternatives. Thus, it may be the case that therapeutic deception would be the right course of action in certain types of circumstances, while being unjustified in others; or it could be the case that therapeutic deception is never justifiable if there are no circumstances in which it would lead to greater net benefit than being honest and providing full disclosure of all material information.

Libertarianism, as premised upon the John Stuart Mill's classic essay, "On Liberty" (Mill, 1859/2006), holds each individual person, of mature faculties, to be sovereign over their own mind and body. Most pertinent to the issue at hand is Mill's assertion that each person "is the proper guardian of his own health, whether bodily, or mental and spiritual" (p. 623). This principle grounds the moral obligation to respect an individual patient's exercise of freedom in choosing to elect or refuse a particular treatment or to participate in research: "if the physician denies the patient liberty, the physician is in effect denying the patient free will, which is essential to being human" (Pirakitikulr & Bursztajn, 2006, p. 307). In order to rationally exercise one's freedom in this regard, all relevant information should be disclosed. On the other hand, an individual may wish to be free *from* information (Vandeveer, 1980, p. 204). Perhaps the patient fears how he may react upon hearing news of a terminal illness, or knows himself well enough to foresee that, if every possible risk of a surgical intervention were explained to him, he may not have the courage to go through with it, or simply wants to go through life blissfully unaware of his impending death.

A Kantian evaluation of this question appeals to the moral imperative to respect persons as ends in themselves (Kant, 1998), which includes, most fundamentally, respecting a person as an *autonomous* agent who, as in Mill's libertarian theory, is sovereign over her own self and her own moral acts. Thus, one of the guiding principles of biomedical ethics is to respect a patient's autonomy (O'Neill, 2002). Such respect involves both a *negative* obligation not to restrict a patient's exercise of autonomously chosen actions and a *positive* obligation to support autonomous decision-making by, among other things, disclosing all relevant information that may impact the patient's deliberation (Beauchamp & Childress, 2009, p. 104). It may be the case, though, that disclosure of certain types of information to certain types of patients—even if they are rational and autonomous on the whole—or an "overload" of disclosed information may *inhibit* rather than promote rational deliberation and autonomous choice (Epstein et al., 2010).

An Aristotelian approach emphasizes the moral imperative to seek the *flourishing* of oneself and others as living, sentient, social, and *rational* animals. This last quality, which Aristotle identifies as human beings' unique "species-defining" characteristic—at least among other members of the animal kingdom—grounds certain specific obligations to provide for the cultivation of various intellectual virtues of both speculative and practical reasoning (Aristotle, 1999; MacIntyre, 2001). Martha Nussbaum (2011) has developed a contemporary version of Aristotelianism termed the "capabilities approach," in which the overarching goal of moral activity is to foster the development of fundamental human capabilities—e.g., to exercise rational autonomy—so that individuals may pursue their particular vision of "the good life." As with Kantianism, this ethical standpoint may also lead to divergent conclusions regarding therapeutic deception: while providing all pertinent information for a patient to exercise their capacity for rational autonomous choice would seem to be warranted in all cases, there may yet be cases in which a patient's irrational fear or confusion—prompted by too great an influx of certain types of distressing information—may lessen their capacity to render a rationally deliberated, autonomously chosen decision regarding treatment.

Numerous reasons have been utilized to support the moral permissibility of therapeutic deception under certain circumstances within the clinical context, premised upon one or more of the theories described above. In the following sections, I will describe and critique each of these rationales, and then elucidate arguments against the validity of therapeutic deception.

Reasons Supporting Therapeutic Deception

The most popular and arguably powerful reason not to disclose certain types of information to some patients is to *prevent harm* insofar as such information, if disclosed, would cause the patient anxiety, destroy their hope, retard or erase a therapeutic outcome, or lead them to commit suicide (Beauchamp & Childress, 2009, p. 290). In some instances, such information may even be irrelevant to determining prognosis or to the patient's choosing among available treatment options (Epstein et al., 2010). Faden and Beauchamp (1980) conducted a survey focused on how disclosed information affects patients' decision-making process and found that only 12% of patients cited the disclosed information as the "most important factor" in determining their consent decision (p. 319).

If it is presumed that information should be disclosed unless there is a clear indication that it may cause great harm, establishing practical criteria by which a physician may accurately judge whether such a "clear indication" is present is no easy task, and there may be implicit paternalistic presumptions at play. For example, in a case of nondisclosure of a terminal illness to prevent a patient from falling into a suicidal depression, Allen Buchanan (1978) notes three relevant facts that are often overlooked in evaluating the physician's justification: (1) the physician is employing an "unqualified *psychiatric* generalization"; (2) it is doubtful that even psychiatric specialists may render reliable generalizations about which types of patients may be prone to suicidal depression based on such news; and (3) the physician is assuming that suicide cannot be a rationally chosen course of action for a terminally ill patient (p. 379). In short, a physician, even a psychiatrist, is not competent to render an accurate and value-neutral prognosis concerning how a patient will or ought to react upon learning that they are terminally ill.

Another argument appeals to the impracticability of disclosing the *whole truth* to patients (Lipkin, 2008). In fact, attempting to provide every minute detail—including, for example, the improbable side-effects of a medication or incidental findings of a diagnostic test—exhausts precious time in the clinical encounter and may distract a patient from more relevant information that should play a more determinative role in their ultimate decision regarding treatment (Epstein et al., 2010). This requires the formulation of "a standard of *substantial* completeness" in the disclosure of information that is material to a patient's decision-making regarding a particular treatment (Beauchamp & Childress, 2009, p. 292). Devising and following such a standard is not problematic, since it recognizes that not every single detailed bit of information will be relevant to a patient's decision-making. As Cullen and Klein (2008) note, "All a patient requires is an understanding adequate to appreciate the nature and seriousness of his illness and the potential benefits and risks of the available therapies. A diabetic need not know the stages of oxidative phosphorylation to grasp the importance of insulin and role of diet in maintaining her health" (p. 159).

Furthermore, adhering to such a standard does not empower physicians to withhold information that would be material to the patient's capacity to render an informed decision, which is what is ultimately of moral import. Emphasizing the *material relevance* of the disclosed information allows for some degree of professional judgment on the part of physicians to potentially withhold, for example, negligible risks associated with a particular treatment in cases where the physician has good reason to suspect that the patient may formulate an irrationally overblown perception of such risks. Even in such cases, though, the appropriate course of action may be not nondisclosure of such risks, but rather a modified or staged disclosure in which the physician first informs the patient that no medical intervention is without risk, then ascertains the extent to which the patient wants to be informed of all possible risks—this "contractual" approach to disclosure strategy will be discussed below—and finally presents desired information in a clear and easily understandable form (Palmboom et al., 2007, p. 70).

A related concern regards a patient's capacity to *understand* the disclosed information (Beauchamp & Childress, 2009, p. 292). If the disclosed information may confuse the patient or even lead to the formulation of a false belief, then it may be better to disguise that particular datum. Buchanan (1978) counters that this line of reasoning "relies upon dubious and extremely broad psychological generalizations," and notes that the ethical obligation of informed consent requires that physicians "make a reasonable effort to be understood" (p. 386). Robert Higgs (2009) accuses medical professionals who justify nondisclosure based on this rationale of being either arrogant or lazy and elaborates upon physicians' fundamental duty in this regard: "Any skilled person who is at the interface with the public must be able to explain what they are up to. Those who cannot must learn how to do so. Medicine is a good deal less complex than many activities. As science advances, things may appear to become more complicated, but professionals have a duty all the time to bring their public up to date. To dress up simple ideas or uncertainties as mysteries is the mark of the charlatan" (p. 522).

Finally, some patients may *not want* to know the truth about their condition and either they *explicitly* state their wishes thus, or family members make clear that the patient would be better off without knowing such information (Beauchamp & Childress, 2009, pp. 292–293). Cullen and Klein (2008) argue that it does not violate a patient's autonomy not to disclose information in such a case; rather, a patient's explicit desire to remain ignorant "is as much an expression of autonomy as is the wish to be informed" (p. 157). This conclusion follows, though, only if respecting a patient's explicit autonomous choices is the only or indisputably paramount moral obligation on the part of physicians. As Beauchamp and Childress (2009) make clear, the ethical obligation to respect a patient's autonomy is but one of at least four fundamental prima facie moral duties in the biomedical context.

In fact, it may be the case that a patient's desire to have certain information withheld may impair his capacity to give autonomous consent to a therapeutic intervention to such an extent as to constitute an *unreasonable* desire on his part, such that acceding to this desire will ultimately fail to positively *promote* the patient's exercise of his autonomy. For example, it would be eminently unreasonable for a patient to consent to a procedure that carries a significant risk of causing debilitation or death without being aware of such risk; if knowledge of the risk ultimately leads the patient not to consent to the procedure, this would seem to be a reasonable choice on his part due to the danger involved if the procedure itself is not required as a life-saving intervention. If the patient explicitly states that he does not want to be told of the attendant risks of the procedure out of fear that he will not then consent to it, we must ask whether it is more reasonable for the patient to render a final treatment decision based upon such fear-driven ignorance or upon a reasonable fear of the disclosed risks.

Furthermore, as Pirakitikulr and Bursztajn (2006) note, there are various practical difficulties, such as eliciting patients' "preferences for information regarding scenarios that are difficult to imagine" (p. 308). Such epistemic hurdles may become full-on roadblocks to a patient's capacity to exercise rational deliberation in determining the direction of their autonomous will.

While the first rationale supporting the moral permissibility of withholding certain types of information from certain types of patients is best understood as balancing the prima facie duties of beneficence and nonmaleficence against that of respecting patient autonomy, the other cited reasons converge in a general concern regarding how best to facilitate patients' exercise of autonomy by not distracting them with distressing but largely irrelevant information, "overloading" them with minutiae and technical details that may cloud their understanding, or contradicting their desire not to be burdened with such information.

These latter concerns, however, may be alleviated to some extent by taking care with respect to *how* information is disclosed to patients:

> What these cases do, surely, is argue, not for no telling, but for better telling, for sensitivity and care in determining how much the patient wants to know, explaining carefully in ways the patient can understand, and providing full support and "aftercare" as in other treatments. (Higgs, 2006, p. 615; cf. Higgs, 2009, p. 526; Weiss, 2002, pp. 98–100)

It is certainly reasonable for physicians not to disclose information that clearly would not be at all material to a patient's informed decision-making—e.g., the technical minutiae describing how the physician arrived at her diagnosis of the patient's condition. Also, certain types of *quantitative* information may not need to be disclosed if it does not impede the patient's overall understanding of his diagnosis, prognosis, and attendant risks or potential benefits of possible therapeutic interventions (Schwartz, 2011). Finally, there may be an ethical obligation not to reveal specific types of information about which the patient has explicitly expressed a desire not to know, provided that the physician is confident that ignorance of such information would not skew the patient's decision-making process to a clearly unreasonable conclusion that would go against the patient's other known or reasonably presumed desires—e.g., not to accept a significant risk of death by consenting to a nonlife-saving intervention.

Reasons Against Therapeutic Deception

The most fundamental moral argument against therapeutic deception is the Kantian imperative to respect persons insofar as they are *rational* and *autonomous* agents. While this principle allows for exceptions in cases of patients who are not substantially autonomous or capable of giving voluntary consent, it supports a duty to honesty—including full disclosure of all information that may be material to a patient's decision-making—in all other cases. Failure to disclose all relevant information to a rational, autonomous patient is to *infantilize* her, to treat her as being somehow less of a rational, autonomous agent as the physician electing to withhold said information: "to mislead patients is to deny them due respect; it implies they are incapable of understanding, accepting, and controlling their situation. Lying or deception is therefore an abuse of power that infringes the patient's right to self-determination and self-knowledge. It is, in short, an affront to the patient's dignity and autonomy. Moreover, the practice of deceiving patients contributes to the cult of expertise surrounding the medical profession, and to a view of doctors not as providing a service, but as guardians of a special wisdom, which they may determine when, and to whom, to divulge" (Bakhurst, 1992, p. 65).

Physicians who withhold relevant information from their patients may be guilty not only of deception, but also of *discrimination* in treating patients in a way that physicians themselves would not want to be treated—a double-standard revealed by various surveys (Higgs, 2006, p. 614). This harkens back to another Kantian moral imperative—viz. the principle of *universalizability*: "act only in accordance with that maxim through which you can at the same time will that it become a universal law" (Kant, 1998, p. 31). Insofar as a physician could not will that the moral universe be such that information relevant to his healthcare could be paternalistically withheld from him, he cannot exempt himself from following the contrary rule that requires disclosure.

In the days of yesteryear, when Collins (1927) recommended that physicians ought to be as well practiced in the art of deception as they are in any practical medical skill, patients were generally of the opinion that physicians did possess a "special wisdom" and were often more than happy to buy into the "cult of expertise." Times have changed, however, and while some patients may submit to this bygone perception, public sentiment is often cynical with respect to the healthcare profession—perhaps more directed at private insurers than at physicians themselves. Nevertheless, any diminishment in *trust* between a patient and her physician, or between the public and the medical profession in general, can only be detrimental to effective caregiving (Bostick et al., 2006). As Higgs (2006) puts it succinctly, "If truth is the first casualty, trust must be second" (p. 611).

Even if a physician's trustworthiness is not negated wholesale by the discovery of undisclosed information, the *suspicion* on the patient's part that she is not being told all pertinent information could lead to undesirable consequences, such as confusion, false beliefs, exaggerated weighting of the suspected withheld information, and misinterpretation of other information that is disclosed (Grill & Hansson, 2005, pp. 650–651). And while advocates of therapeutic deception are concerned that increased confusion and anxiety may result from disclosure in certain cases, Faden and Beauchamp's (1980) study revealed "no evidence that disclosure resulted in excessive or incapacitating confusion or anxiety" (p. 325). Granted, this study is limited in scope—focusing solely on consent for nonsurgical contraceptive techniques—but the authors cite at least one other study that showed similar results for kidney donors (p. 328).

What is arguably most vital in the clinical encounter is the formation of an evermore *open relationship* between physician and patient (Higgs, 2009, p. 528) that underwrites *meaningful discourse*, leading to a "therapeutic alliance" that can help patients "bear pain without the compounding bitterness, helplessness, and hopelessness that accompany aloneness" (Pirakitikulr & Bursztajn, 2006, p. 308). Suspicion or outright lack of trust will only serve to either precipitate or exacerbate a patient's negative perception of her vulnerable and lonely state, whereas a patient's *participation* in her own healthcare management, facilitated by having all relevant information at her disposal, can be *empowering* and itself a form of healing.

The concept of a therapeutic alliance coheres well with Nussbaum's "capabilities approach" insofar as the goal of full disclosure of all relevant information is to facilitate the patient's ability to cooperate with her physician—and the larger healthcare team—to devise desirable and effective treatment strategies in line not only with the patient's basic interest in survival and good health, but also with any pertinent religious or moral values she may have that would be factored into her decision-making. One of the fundamental capabilities Nussbaum identifies as essential to living a flourishing human life is *freedom of choice*, which includes the capacity to engage in *rational deliberation* about the various options from which one may choose. Assuming a patient is substantially autonomous, then respecting her personal dignity requires the facilitation of her capacities for rational deliberation and freedom of choice, which in turn demands that all material information be disclosed. In this way, patients are "capacitated" to be not merely *passive* recipients of healthcare administered by others—even if such others are competent and caring medical professionals—but rather to be *agents* who take personal responsibility for their healthcare and are invested in the treatment plan because they cooperated, through their *informed* autonomous consent given at the end of a process of rational deliberation, with the design and implementation of said plan. While the rational deliberative process may indeed be thrown askew by information that is not "well received" by the patient, if we assume that the patient is substantially autonomous and capable of understanding the disclosed information, then the physician's duty is to find a way of disclosing the information in such a way as to ensure—to the extent possible—the patient's calm and rational reception of it. Nondisclosure, however, should be reserved only for extreme cases in which a patient is not substantially autonomous, or lacks the intrinsic capacity to rationally receive and incorporate such information into a deliberative, cooperative process of working with the physician to devise and execute a proper treatment strategy.

AMA Policy

The Council on Ethical and Judicial Affairs (CEJA) of the American Medical Association has affirmed the following:

> In practice, medical information should never be permanently withheld from the patient because doing so represents a clear violation of patients' trust. However, physicians' obligations of beneficence may allow (or compel) them to postpone the full disclosure of information to patients whose capacity to make competent medical decisions may be compromised, or when disclosure is other medically contraindicated. Delayed

> disclosure, however, is not justified when physicians merely intend to prevent a patient's refusal of medically necessary treatments, or to instill hope for the future. (Bostick et al., 2006, p. 303)

This judgment does not rule out all cases of nondisclosure. For example, Raanan Gillon (1993) refers to the case of thyrotoxicosis, in which a potentially fatal complication known as "thyroid crisis" or "thyroid storm" may be precipitated by worry, anxiety, or anger. Therapeutic deception was thus often utilized to prevent such a complication. While this case is obsolete insofar as the specific cause of patient anxiety—the necessity of thyroidectomy—is no longer necessary to treat this condition, it remains a justifiable case of nondisclosure based upon "medical contraindication" due to the fact that there is a clearly identifiable health risk to the patient that is *directly related* to the anxiety that could reasonably be expected to be caused, though maybe not in all patients, by disclosing specific diagnostic or prognostic information. This is a quite different case, however, from a more nebulous, general concern about a patient's psychological or emotional well-being based upon the disclosure of distressing information. But even in the well-defined "medically contraindicated" case, at some point, the relevant information must be disclosed: a patient could not have a thyroidectomy performed without having previously consented to the procedure: hence the CEJA's judgment that only *temporary* nondisclosure could ever be ethically justifiable.

Another potential avenue for justifying nondisclosure are cases in which a physician "contracts" with the patient not to reveal certain types of information the patient would rather not know. The CEJA concludes:

> Withholding medical information from patients without their knowledge or consent is ethically unacceptable. Physicians should encourage patients to specify their preferences regarding communication of their medical information, preferably before the information becomes available. Moreover, physicians should honor patient requests not to be informed of certain medical information or to convey the information to a designated proxy, provided these requests appear to genuinely represent the patient's own wishes. (Bostick et al., 2006, p. 305)

Buchanan (1978) raises a couple of significant issues with proposal. First, insofar as a patient may not be able to specify precisely which type(s) of medical information he would like to have withheld, but rather authorizes the physician not to disclose any "harmful" information, it becomes incumbent upon the physician to judge which type(s) of information may be harmful for this particular patient to hear, which goes outside the physician's training and purview. Second, since any agreement between a physician and her patient will be subject to limitations—allowing, for example, the patient to terminate his relationship with the physician if he believes her to be violating the terms of the agreement by not disclosing information the patient did not authorize her to withhold—the patient needs to be in an epistemic position to determine whether such limitations are being observed (pp. 383–385). Edmund Howe (2006) further contends that, particularly in cases where the patient's diagnosis is already known by the physician, it becomes very difficult to inquire about what information the patient would prefer to know or not know without risking harm to or destruction of the patient's trust in the physician. Finally, as noted above, there may be an epistemic gap that bears upon a patient's ability to state an explicit preference for information related to future scenarios that are hard for him to imagine (Pirakitikulr & Bursztajn, 2006).

A different cooperative framework between physician and patient, instead of focusing on a nondisclosure contract, would be "to invite active participation by patients or subjects in the context of an informational exchange.... Professionals would do well to end their traditional preoccupation with disclosure and instead ask questions, elicit the concerns and interests of the patient or subject, and establish a climate that encourages the patient or subject to ask questions" (Faden & Beauchamp, 1986, p. 307). While this approach may still lead to some degree of nondisclosure based on a patient's expressed desire not to receive certain types of information or the withheld information not being materially relevant to the patient's decision-making, near-maximal disclosure will remain the standard of practice premised upon the greatest degree of respect for a patient's autonomy and the actualization of his capacity to render voluntary and informed consent to a jointly devised treatment plan.

Conclusion

I have argued that the standard reasons given to support withholding materially relevant medical information from patients fail to justify even the most well-intended beneficent nondisclosures on the part of physicians. Furthermore, respect for patients' autonomy and the moral imperative to promote patients' capacity to render voluntary and informed decisions should lead physicians to work *cooperatively* with their patients to jointly design and implement a treatment plan, including any necessary follow-up care, which would best serve each patient's healthcare goals. While concerns regarding psychologically or emotionally vulnerable patients' capacity to receive and process distressing information are legitimate, such concerns function best by directing physicians to consider carefully *how* such information is conveyed, not *whether* it is conveyed. This conclusion would support temporary nondisclosure or "staged" disclosure in certain, restricted cases, but would never justify a complete withholding of information that would be materially relevant to patients' exercise of their autonomy either with respect to electing a treatment option or to making other life-decisions based upon the diagnosis or prognosis of their condition.

References

Aristotle (1999). *Nicomachean ethics* (T. Irwin, Trans.), 2nd ed. Indianapolis, IN: Hackett.

Bakhurst, D. (1992). On lying and deceiving. *Journal of Medical Ethics, 19*, 63–66.

Beauchamp, T. L., & Childress, J. F. (2009). *Principles of biomedical ethics*, 6th ed. New York: Oxford University Press.

Benn, P. (2001). Medicine, lies and deceptions. *Journal of Medical Ethics, 27*, 130–134.

Bostick, N. A., Sade, R., McMahon, J. W., & Benjamin, R. (2006). Report of the American Medical Association Council on Ethical and Judicial Affairs: Withholding information from patients: Rethinking the propriety of "therapeutic privilege." *Journal of Clinical Ethics, 17*, 302–306.

Buchanan, A. (1978). Medical paternalism. *Philosophy and Public Affairs*, 7, 370–390.

Collins, J. (1927). Should doctors tell the truth? *Harper's Monthly Magazine, 155*, 320–326.

Cullen, S., & Klein, M. (2008). Respect for patients, physicians, and the truth. In R. Munson (Ed.), *Intervention and reflection: Basic issues in medical ethics*, 8th ed. Belmont, CA: Thomson-Wadsworth.

Epstein, R. M., Korones, D. N., & Quill, T. E. (2010). Withholding information from patients—When less is more. *New England Journal of Medicine, 362*, 380–381.

Faden, R. R., & Beauchamp, T. L. (1980). Decision-making and informed consent: A study of the impact of disclosed information. *Social Indicators Research*, 7, 313–336.

Faden, R. R., & Beauchamp, T. L. (1986). *A history and theory of informed consent*. New York: Oxford University Press.

Gillon, R. (1993). Is there an important moral distinction for medical ethics between lying and other forms of deception? *Journal of Medical Ethics, 19*, 131–132.

Grill, K., & Hansson, S. O. (2005). Epistemic paternalism in public health. *Journal of Medical Ethics, 31*, 648–653.

Higgs, R. (2006). On telling patients the truth. In H. Kuhse & P. Singer (Eds.), *Bioethics: An anthology*, 2nd ed. Malden, MA: Blackwell.

Higgs, R. (2009). Truth-telling. In H. Kuhse & P. Singer (Eds.), *A companion to bioethics*, 2nd ed. Malden, MA: Blackwell.

Howe, E. G. (2006). Comment on the CEJA guidelines: Treating patients who deny reality. *Journal of Clinical Ethics, 17*, 317–322.

Jackson, J. (1991). Telling the truth. *Journal of Medical Ethics, 17*, 5–9.

Jackson, J. (1993). On the morality of deception—does method matter? A reply to David Bakhurst. *Journal of Medical Ethics, 19*, 183–187.

Kant, I. (1998) *Groundwork of the metaphysics of morals* (M. Gregor, Trans.). New York: Cambridge University Press.

Lipkin, M. (2008). On telling patients the truth. In R. Munson (Ed.), *Intervention and reflection: Basic issues in medical ethics*, 8th ed. Belmont, CA: Thomson-Wadsworth.

MacIntyre, A. (2001). *Dependent rational animals: Why human beings need the virtues*. Chicago, IL: Open Court.

Mill, J. S. (2006). On liberty. In H. Kuhse & P. Singer (Eds.), *Bioethics: An anthology*, 2nd ed. Malden, MA: Blackwell.

Novack, D. H., Plumer, R., Smith, R. L., Ochitill, H., Morrow, G. R., & Bennett, J. M. (1979). Changes in physicians' attitudes toward telling the cancer patient. *Journal of the American Medical Association, 241*, 897–900.

Nussbaum, M. (2011). *Creating capabilities: The human development approach*. Cambridge, MA: Harvard University Press.

Oken, D. (1961). What to tell cancer patients: A study of medical attitudes. *Journal of the American Medical Association, 175*, 1120–1128.

O'Neill, O. (2002). *Autonomy and trust in bioethics*. New York: Cambridge University Press.

Palmboom, G. G., Willems, D. L., Janssen, N. B. A. T., & de Haes, J. C. J. M. (2007). Doctor's views on disclosing or withholding information on low risks of complication. *Journal of Medical Ethics*, *33*, 67–70.

Pirakitikulr, D., & Bursztajn, H. J. (2006). The Grand Inquisitor's choice: Comment on the CEJA report on withholding information from patients. *Journal of Clinical Ethics*, *17*, 307–311.

Schwartz, P. H. (2011). Questioning the quantitative imperative: Decision aids, prevention, and the ethics of disclosure. *Hastings Center Report*, *41*, 30–39.

Sokol, D. K. (2006). Dissecting "deception." *Cambridge Quarterly of Healthcare Ethics*, *15*, 457–464.

Vandeveer, D. (1980). The contractual argument for withholding medical information. *Philosophy and Public Affairs*, *9*, 198–205.

Weiss, G. G. (2002). Patients' rights: Who should know what? *Medical Economics*, *79*, 97–104.

Reply to Eberl

Tom L. Beauchamp

The title of Jason Eberl's compelling chapter is "There Are No Circumstances in Which a Doctor May Withhold Information." I will call this claim *the bold thesis*. Consistent with the argument in my chapter, I will now argue that the bold thesis either (1) is not defensible without such heavy qualification that it loses its boldness or (2) rests on an unsustainable absolutist moral principle, though Eberl's representations are not absolutist.

At times, it seems that Eberl himself does not accept the bold thesis, only a weakened version of it. For example, he writes that in some cases in which "the physician has good reason to suspect that the patient may formulate an irrationally overblown perception of . . . risks . . . the appropriate course of action may be not nondisclosure of such risks, but rather a modified or staged disclosure in which the physician first informs the patient that no medical intervention is without risk, then ascertains the extent to which the patient wants to be informed of all possible risks." This claim might seem consistent with the bold thesis, because the goal is either to disclose the bulk of the relevant information or to phase it in over time. However, modified and staged disclosure are both circumstances in which *withholding of information occurs*—and therefore the boldest form of the bold thesis has been relinquished. That is, if staged disclosure is used, withholding is part of the physician's larger plan. I argued earlier that plans of initial nondisclosure together with staged disclosure are often justified, but to a defender of the bold thesis, such withholding should be unacceptable. The scope of its acceptabililty to Eberl is unclear to me.

Eberl also raises a question about what should happen in a circumstance in which a patient has autonomously requested that information not be disclosed (in effect, a waiver of the right to give an informed consent):

> Cullen and Klein (2008) argue that it does not violate a patient's autonomy not to disclose information in such a case; rather, a patient's explicit desire to remain ignorant "is as much an expression of autonomy as is the wish to be informed" (p. 157). This conclusion follows, though, only if respecting a patient's explicit autonomous choices is the only or indisputably paramount moral obligation on the part of physicians. As Beauchamp and Childress (2009) make clear, the ethical obligation to respect a patient's autonomy is but one of at least four fundamental prima facie moral duties in the biomedical context.

This line of argument presents several problems that threaten the bold thesis, including weakened versions of it such as Eberl's. I agree that "autonomy is but one" of the prima facie principles or duties that may play a justificatory role in any given context. As I argued in my chapter, depending on the precise context, the moral demands of respect for autonomy and beneficence will have different weights, and no a

Contemporary Debates in Bioethics, First Edition. Edited by Arthur L. Caplan and Robert Arp.

priori decision rule is available to determine that one outweighs the other. Any one of these principles may morally override any other principle in a given situation, and therefore beneficent treatment of patients may override the demands of respect for autonomy.

This position undercuts both the bold thesis and Eberl's version of it. The framework of prima facie principles is directly linked to the balancing position I defended previously on valid disclosure and nondisclosure. Allowing a plural body of prima facie principles to govern the discussion of physician withholding of information is the backbone my position, and Eberl seems to come close to the acceptance of this view here. His acknowledgment of several valid prima facie principles rightly recognizes that autonomy may not be the paramount and overriding consideration, depending on the specific case, which strongly implies a balancing position that contradicts the bold thesis. However, his position in the chapter overall seems to require that respect for autonomy (or at least a principle not allowing withholding of information) be an absolute principle, irrespective of balancing considerations. Neither of these two positions is the one he seems to defend, but I do not see how he can escape one or the other. If he is to stick with the bold thesis, I do not see how it in particular can be defended without either turning respect for autonomy into an absolute principle or hierarchically ranking autonomy above all other considerations in the context of physician disclosure.

In the above quoted passage, Eberl says, "This conclusion [namely, 'it does not violate a patient's autonomy not to disclose information in such a case' of waiver of information] follows, though, only if respecting a patient's explicit autonomous choices is the only or indisputably paramount moral obligation on the part of physicians." This argument seems to have a revealing gap. The conclusion actually *does follow* without any need for an "only if" condition; that is, it is correct to say that there is no violation of the principle of respect autonomy (or, better, of a patient's rights of autonomy) even in the absence of the mentioned qualification about a paramount moral obligation. What *does not follow*, and what Eberl may have in mind, is that this nonviolation of the patient's rights of autonomy does not by itself (without further argument) justify the action of withholding information or mean that it is the right action to perform. Even if no violation would occur by nondisclosure, there still might be a good reason to disclose rather than to withhold. Nonviolation of autonomy when a person's autonomous wishes have been expressed is not always a morally sufficient basis to justify the requested withholding of information (independent of all features of the case and all relevant principles). Perhaps, under the circumstances, the physician should make disclosures that the patient has requested not be made. In every such case, we need a justification of either the claim that withholding is acceptable or the claim that withholding is unacceptable.

Suppose the patient's reason for wanting to remain ignorant of relevant information is that he fears that, in the face of certain kinds of negative information, he will fall into despair and will not follow a prescribed medical regimen. (This patient is like someone on a diet who does not want to learn his weight during the course of the diet for fear that he will despair from lack of progress and give up on the diet.) In this medical scenario, the physician may justifiably reach the conclusion that *the paramount obligation is to withhold, a decision that is justified by appeal to both respect for autonomy and medical beneficence* (that is, by appeal to the patient's waiver of the right to information together with the achievement of a medical good for the patient). Eberl's argument has no resources to assert that the physician is unjustified in withholding information in such a case. If the reasons given by the physician (drawn from two prima facie duties) jointly provide a sufficient justification, then the bold thesis cannot be correct. Once one acknowledges that principles other than respect for autonomy can, in some cases, have sufficient weight to override the weight of that principle or to join with it to justify withholding, the case for the bold thesis has been lost.

Eberl appeals at one point to a passage in Roger Higgs for support of his position, as follows:

> What these cases do, surely, is argue, not for no telling, but for better telling, for sensitivity and care in determining how much the patient wants to know, explaining carefully in ways the patient can understand, and providing full support and "aftercare" as in other treatments.

Higgs' observation seems to beg the question. Some cases argue for better telling, but others argue for no telling, staged telling, or limited telling. It is inaccurate to say that these cases "argue not for no telling" and only for "better telling." Some of the cases argue strongly not for better telling, but for no telling. Higgs's statement seems an absolutist evasion of the issues.

Eberl, too, is threatened by this problem, which may explain why, in a later section, he maintains that,

> The most fundamental moral argument against therapeutic deception is the Kantian imperative to respect persons insofar as they are *rational* and *autonomous* agents. . . . Failure to disclose all relevant information to a rational, autonomous patient is to *infantilize* her, to treat her as being somehow less of a rational, autonomous agent as the physician electing to withhold said information.

This Kantian imperative is an absolutist principle of just the sort that I have maintained is essential to defense of the bold thesis. In general, I think there is no good defense of this Kantian position, but I will not argue here for this claim. I only note, again, that I do not see that Eberl has a defense of the kind of principle needed to sustain the Kantian imperative or the bold thesis.

Reply to Beauchamp

Jason T. Eberl

Given the moral complexity of many issues in biomedical ethics, particularly those that arise within the clinical encounter, it is not surprising that Professor Beauchamp and I find ourselves to have many points of agreement. There remain some significant points of disagreement, though, in which a difference in how each of us weighs the value of respecting patients' autonomy against other competing goods becomes evident.

Beauchamp and I agree first and foremost on the general moral value of truthfulness. The fact that one of us may allow for a physician to withhold information in cases where the other one would not does not in any way betray a cavalier attitude towards the truth or the prima facie obligation to disclose relevant information to patients so that they may make an informed decision regarding their course of treatment. We also agree that the obligation to respect a patient's autonomy, either through disclosure or by any other means, is neither an *absolute* moral duty nor one that necessarily trumps all other moral considerations in a given case. Because of the correlative prima facie duties of beneficence and nonmaleficence that must be balanced with the duty to respect and facilitate autonomous decision-making, it is apparent that the utilization of "staged disclosure," in which a patient is not given every bit of potentially devastating news all at once—particularly when there is still a reasonable degree of epistemic uncertainty, e.g., awaiting a second round of confirmatory test results—"is only a minor disrespecting of autonomy" that is consistent with a physician's caring attitude towards her patient. Along the same lines, we concur that information must be properly framed to avoid giving patients a false impression or otherwise mislead them to a hasty or erroneous conclusion. Care must especially be taken with respect to *prognoses* in which the degree of epistemic uncertainty is typically higher than in the case of *diagnostic* information.

Where Beauchamp and I disagree concerns the normative weight we assign to respecting a patient's autonomy against other competing moral obligations. The primary difference between us is that Beauchamp authorizes a physician to engage—under certain restricted circumstances—in *complete nondisclosure*, whereas I do not believe a physician's role of beneficent guardian of her patients' best interests ever justifies such wholesale withholding of information that is materially relevant to a patient's decision at hand. Of course, what counts as "materially relevant" information will be subject to the physician's judgment; but the possibility of employing some sort of standard, either in the form of explicit guidelines or by appeal to what a "reasonable person" would need to know in order to render an adequately informed decision, lessens the risk that a physician may fail to disclose pertinent information. Beauchamp's sliding-scale strategy, on the other hand, in which the justification

Contemporary Debates in Bioethics, First Edition. Edited by Arthur L. Caplan and Robert Arp.

for nondisclosure is proportionally related to the net value of the patient's autonomy interests combined with the benefits that would accrue to the patient if the information is withheld, strikes me as less amenable to standardization in clinical practice. As a result, justification of nondisclosure will rely more on an individual physician's subjective judgment, and there is a significant potential for physicians to misjudge the relative strength of the patient's autonomy interests balanced against the benefits of nondisclosure.

In addition to this fundamental point of divergence between our views, there are problematic features with Beauchamp's analyses of three particular cases he raises. In the first case, Beauchamp contends:

> if a dying patient who will live for a month or less is in an extreme form of pain but refuses pain medication on the grounds that he might become addicted to it, it is plausibly justified of a physician to initiate an undetectable pain-control medication without informing the patient of the intervention.

One option Beauchamp does not consider is *reasoning* with the patient to help him to understand that the danger of becoming addicted to the pain medication given his projected life-expectancy—I am presuming that the patient is already aware of his prognosis—is virtually nonexistent or would not constitute a harm to the patient, since he will require pain-control medication for the remainder of his life. Of course, this is not at all how the conversation with the patient should be *framed*, but rather should be delivered in such as manner as to demonstrate compassion while also attempting to be effectively persuasive. The point is that, even by Beauchamp's own standards, he seems to move too quickly to justifying the clandestine administration of an explicitly refused medication. If the patient were steadfast in his refusal of the medication, then the physician may need to explore—with the assistance of a psychiatric consult—whether there are any other unspoken motivations for the patient's refusal and address those. In the end, though, after having exhausted every persuasive avenue and assuming the patient is not otherwise delusional or incompetent to make a rational, autonomous decision, the physician is obligated to accede to the patient's continued refusal of pain-control medication.

In another case he describes, Beauchamp asserts that "it would be morally contemptible to tell a patient who has just been diagnosed with cancer of the tongue that she will never again sing in her church choir and will encounter profound difficulty in being understood when speaking." To a certain extent, I agree with Beauchamp's exhortation insofar as the withheld information is *prognostic* in nature, and thereby subject to some degree of epistemic uncertainty; such information need not be *volunteered* to the patient, especially considering that it is not relevant to any treatment decision she may need to make. But what if the patient directly asks how this cancer will affect her ability to sing in the church choir? It is one thing not to volunteer information; it is another not to respond honestly to a patient's direct inquiry. Given that a negative response is likely true, even if subject to some degree of uncertainty, the physician ought to answer the patient, explaining the degree of probability involved and obviously framing the response in the most compassionate way possible. With respect to the patient's projected inability to be understood by others, honest disclosure is more imperative insofar as she may need to prepare, for example, by procuring a telecommunications device that would facilitate her ability to communicate in case the recommended speech therapy is not sufficiently effective. While I disagree with Beauchamp concerning whether such hurtful information may be permanently withheld, I concur with him that the physician should also provide for "hope where that hope may have some basis."

In the final, and most challenging, case he presents, Beauchamp considers patients in extraordinary circumstances: specifically, the euthanization of four hospitalized patients instead of allowing them to be tortured and killed by Nazi soldiers. Let us assume for the sake of discussion that the act of euthanasia itself, in these circumstances, is morally permissible. The relevant question then is whether the four patients were *conscious* of their circumstances. If they were not conscious, then I would concur with Beauchamp's ethical appraisal of the situation. If, however, the patients were conscious and thus able to give consent, then the physician ought to have asked each patient if they would prefer to be euthanized or left in the hands of the Nazis—although the physician had only a few minutes at his disposal, this would have been a feasible course of action, given the small number of patients. While we may reasonably assume that most, if not all, of the patients would have chosen to be euthanized anyway, one or more of them may have considered accepting euthanasia as tantamount to suicide and thus would have preferred to allow the soldiers to bear the moral weight of their deaths, or perhaps would have preferred to endure suffering at the hands of the Nazis for the sake of some spiritual purpose that is meaningful to them.

Neither Beauchamp nor I adopt an extreme, absolutist view that would require a physician either to disclose every bit of information to patients, no matter how distressing or potentially irrelevant to their decision-making, or to treat the truth in a cavalier manner as the pendulum swung back to an outdated paternalistic model of "doctor knows best." The downside of not adopting an absolutist view, though, is that competing moral goods and obligations must be weighed against each other, and this is where space is created for disagreement among well-intentioned parties. While conclusions may differ among bioethicists with respect to *applying* general ethical principles, such as respect for autonomy, beneficence, nonmaleficence, and justice, to specific types of cases, the inherent validity of the principles themselves should nevertheless be apparent in this discussion.

Part 14

Should In Vitro Fertilization Be an Option for a Woman?

Introduction

The Latin in vitro literally means "in glass," and the first attempts at animal in vitro fertilization (IVF) occurred utilizing glass Petri dishes. IVF is a process whereby a sperm fertilizes an egg outside of the body in some fluid medium, and then is placed back into the uterus of the female to allow for natural pregnancy and birth of offspring. Gregory Goodwin Pincus (1936) utilized IVF to produce "test-tube rabbits" at Harvard in 1934, having fertilized rabbit eggs with rabbit sperm in test tubes. Since then, mice, rats, cats, dogs, horses, cows, hamsters, guinea pigs, and numerous other animal offspring have been safely produced through IVF (Brackett, 2001). Born on July 25, 1978, Louise Brown is famous for being the first "test-tube baby"—it was a Petri dish, actually—and she was born as a result of what is known as *natural-cycle IVF*, which was developed by Robert G. Edwards, who won the Nobel Prize in Physiology or Medicine in 2010 (Walsh, 2008; Wade, 2010). In natural-cycle IVF, eggs are collected from a woman's fallopian tubes or uterus after ovulation during her natural menstrual cycle without the use of any drugs. *Ovarian hyperstimulation*, the most common method for obtaining eggs today, is a process whereby a woman is given protein hormones to facilitate the production of a larger-than-normal number of eggs before they are collected. There are other IVF methods and procedures (see the papers in Nagy et al., 2012).

IVF has been used to produce more than 5 million babies worldwide since 1978, the obvious reason for its use being that a woman has found it difficult to become pregnant (Mail, 2012). The Catholic Church holds the position that human reproduction should occur only within the context of sexual intercourse, given that intercourse is a natural behavior meant solely for the purposes of procreation and intimacy between husband and wife in a marriage (HV, 1968). Thus, the Church (CCC, 1994) is somewhat of a lone beacon in opposing IVF:

> Techniques involving only the married couple (homologous artificial insemination and fertilization) are perhaps less reprehensible, yet remain morally unacceptable. They dissociate the sexual act from the procreative act.

Contemporary Debates in Bioethics, First Edition. Edited by Arthur L. Caplan and Robert Arp.

> The act which brings the child into existence is no longer an act by which two persons give themselves to one another, but one that "entrusts the life and identity of the embryo into the power of doctors and biologists and establishes the domination of technology over the origin and destiny of the human person. Such a relationship of domination is in itself contrary to the dignity and equality that must be common to parents and children." (¶ 2377)

Instead of IVF, the Church (CCC, 1994) recommends that, "spouses who still suffer from infertility after exhausting legitimate medical procedures should unite themselves with the Lord's Cross, the source of all spiritual fecundity. They can give expression to their generosity by adopting abandoned children or performing demanding services for others" (¶ 2379).

Another reason the Church opposes IVF has to do with the fact that, in the process, zygotes and early-stage embryos are created and, if not used, often times discarded or utilized in medical research. The official Church position is that human life begins at the moment of conception, and that this life is as dignified, valued, and deserving of protection as any other human life, no matter what stage of human development (zygote, embryo, fetus, infant, child, young adult, adult, elderly adult). Given this inherent value, a human zygote or embryo should never be harmed, for any reason whatsoever (John Paul II, 2001; DHC, 2004; NCBC, 2009; O'Brien, 2011). Fr. Tad Pacholczyk (2006) of the National Catholic Bioethics Center sums it up: "in a gesture that reduces young humans to commodities or manipulable products . . . embryonic humans should not be generated in laboratory glassware where they can be prodded, invaded, and violated." One could argue for the same conclusion on secular grounds pertaining to inherent value, too (Kant, 1775–1789/1963,1785/1998, 1797a/1996a, 1797b/1996b; Dworkin, 1993; Lachmann, 2001; Novak, 2001; cf. Manninen, 2008).

It is important to note that Advanced Cell Technologies was awarded a patent from the United States Patent and Trademark Office for what is referred to as *single-blastomere* technology (US Patent # 7893315), a method that "uses a one-cell biopsy approach similar to pre-implantation genetic diagnosis (PGD), which is sometimes used in the in vitro fertilization (IVF) process and does not appear to interfere with the embryo's developmental potential. The stem cells generated using this approach are apparently healthy and completely normal, and differentiate into all the cell types of the human body, including insulin-producing cells, blood cells, beating heart cells, cartilage, and other cell types of therapeutic importance" (ACT, 2010, 2011; Lang, 2011). What is significant about this technology is that the embryos are *not* destroyed as a result of the stem cells being harvested from them (Klimanskaya et al., 2006, 2007), in which case, there need not be any moral outrage associated with the killing of human embryos. Still, one may argue that, along the lines of Fr. Pacholczyk's thinking, single-blastomere technology is nonetheless immoral—one reason being that any kind of human manipulation of nature or natural processes whatsoever is immoral.

There are many who would argue that the kind of value and inherent rights that the Catholic Church affords to human beings at any stage of development *whatsoever* is incorrect. Consider the fact that we make classifications by distinguishing things on the basis of both their form (or shape) and their function (or purposive activity). When it comes to human-made things, this way of classifying is easy to understand. The knife in one's kitchen is of a different form and has a different function from that of the computer keyboard on which one types emails. The knife has a blade and a handle, and is used for cutting; the keyboard is rectangular, has keys, and is used for word processing. With living things, we still can do a decent job of classifying things as being distinct from one another, even when it comes to classifying the developmental stages of one kind of living thing. For example, the form and function of a butterfly egg are distinct from that of the larva (caterpillar), which is distinct from the pupa (chrysalis), and adult butterfly. One can easily see that each of these stages represents a different form and function of a specific entity; yet, all of these entities make up the various stages of a butterfly's life. Similarly, we can see that there is an obvious developmental distinction between a human zygote, a human embryo, a human fetus, an infant, a toddler, a teenager, and a middle-aged, fully coherent individual; researchers in physical and psychological human development document and explain these differences quite thoroughly (Kail & Cavanaugh, 2010; Sadler, 2011; Newman & Newman, 2012). Equating potentiality with actuality in terms of moral standing—an acorn with a tree seems to be quite a moral stretch.

The issue of using and possibly discarding human zygotes and embryos in IVF is paralleled in the abortion debate where the definition of personhood—as well as *who* or *what* counts as a person—is often front and center. Catholics and many Evangelical Protestants want to either (1) equate personhood with humanity or being human at any stage in the human's development or (2) afford the exact same rights and privileges to human beings, no matter what their stage of human development, or particular mental or physical state (e.g., mentally handicapped, mentally ill, or demented individuals, or individuals in a persistent vegetative state; EV, 1995). Contrary to the Catholic position, in 1971 Judith Jarvis Thomson claimed in the last line of her famous article, "A Defense of Abortion," that a "very early abortion is surely not the killing of a person" (Thomson, 1971), while in her important article, "On the Moral and Legal Status of Abortion," Mary Ann Warren (1973) lays out criteria for personhood—viz., consciousness, reasoning, self-motivated activity, the capacity to communicate, and self-awareness—noting that "a fetus, even a fully developed one, is considerably less person-like than is the average mature mammal, indeed the average fish" (p. 48; also see English, 1973; Warren, 1997). If zygotes, embryos, and even fetuses are not persons, then they do not have full moral rights and privileges, and we perhaps need not think that we have done anything immoral when we abort them, do experiments resulting in their destruction, or discard them after IVF.

The first author in this section, Laura Purdy, thinks that arguments where the fertilized egg is equated with persons "having full human rights, are unpersuasive." Further than this, she points out that the Catholic position has problems. First, given the standard pluralistic society—and a pluralistic world—she intimates that it is difficult not only to prove the existence of one god, but also to prove that the Catholic God's moral pronouncements are the correct ones. Second, the Catholic position commits what is known as the *naturalistic fallacy*, which, in this case, is the fallacy of concluding to what ought to be the case from premises having to do with what is in fact the case. Catholics think that because it is the case that intercourse leads to procreation, then therefore (1) human genitalia ought to be reserved for intercourse only and (2) couples ought to engage in intercourse only with the intention of procreation. Of course, these conclusions need not necessarily follow, since it can be argued that human genitalia should be used for other sexual purposes at times, and couples should—again, at times—engage in intercourse without having to procreate. Third, according to Purdy, Catholics argue "in a circle by claiming to read into nature what is in fact only the reflection of their previously chosen values." She then goes on to point out the fact that Catholics think that nature is inherently valuable, whereas it is we who imbue nature with value.

Purdy also addresses the typical Catholic claim that in many IVF procedures—especially *ovarian hyperstimulation*, where a larger-than-normal number of eggs and then embryos using them are produced—there are extra eggs that are discarded or used in research (if they are not donated to someone else) and this discarding is wholly immoral, given the sanctity of human life at any stage of development. In response to this, she notes, "More relevant to the objection that IVF 'wastes' extra embryos not transferred to women's uteruses, most embryos created by sexual activity are ejected from women's bodies early in the process of development," the obvious point being that the end result of attempts at fertilization are the same with IVF or straightforward natural processes.

Purdy focuses most of her chapter on the morality surrounding the various risks and possible harms associated with IVF. For example, ovarian hyperstimulation can cause *ovarian hyperstimulation syndrome*, which can cause death. There is also the possibility of infection in the embryo-transfer process of IVF, and injury, bleeding, or infections are always real considerations in the egg-retrieval process (see Complications of Treatment section of Gardner et al., 2008). Further, although more studies need to be performed, there is a correlation that has been made between IVF and certain cancers in women, specifically ovarian cancer (see the research in van Leeuwen et al., 2012). Purdy responds to these and other objections throughout her chapter, pointing out that women need to obtain more information about the risks of IVF before jumping into the procedure, as well as consider all realistic options surrounding infertility. "The reality is that we, as a society, allow people to choose treatments that can harm, even for goals some judge frivolous or sick, like cosmetic surgery or sex change procedures," claims Purdy. "Still more importantly, mainstream disease treatments can also maim or kill, sometimes with little promise of benefit, as in last-ditch cancer procedures. Allowing access to IVF—under the kinds of conditions argued for here—is required for consistency with these other practices and policies."

"The characterizing of surplus or in other ways deficient embryos as 'spares'—and the consignment of such embryos to fates such as long-term or permanent cryopreservation, scientific research, or simple discarding," notes the second author in this section, Christopher Tollefsen, "all these are well-known parts of the IVF industry." This claim comes on the heels of Tollefsen pointing out that children are "the fulfillment, or fruition of that marital love" between a man and a woman having an obvious inherent sacredness and value that can be contrasted with the evil character from the *Harry Potter* series, Voldemort's, command to his henchman, Wormtail, to "kill the spare" human being. Tollefsen is trying to get us to see that human life should not be considered a spare, or a superfluous, unnecessary thing—or collateral in commodity and commerce—as it can be in the IVF process that entails drugs, medical procedures, research, and, of course, money paid for all of this (Spar, 2006).

Echoing the Catholic moral position, Tollefsen argues that human zygotes and embryos have the *capacity* for rationality, consciousness, and other person-like attributes in a state of *potentiality*, meaning that, if left to develop, the human zygote would eventually become an older human who would be able to *actually exercise* rationality, consciousness, and other person-like behaviors stemming from the fact of being a human. This seems commonsensible enough: barring severe mental disabilities, it is not as if human zygotes develop into lizards, dogs, monkeys, great apes, or any other biological kind of thing lacking in personhood! In the same way that acorns are actually potentially full-blown oak trees, kittens are actually potentially full-blown cats, and other living things are actually potentially what they are, no matter what stage of life they are in. Given that human zygotes and embryos *actually already* have a capacity/potential for personhood, "fairness," claims Tollefsen, "requires that one treat all human beings with the same fundamental forms of moral respect."

The main crux of Tollefsen's argument against IVF goes something like this: Given that in the IVF process embryos are often thought of as spares as well as useful only insofar as at least one of them succeeds in the pregnancy, they have mere instrumental, useful worth to the parents or mother trying to conceive a "child of *one's own*" (his italics). "This language suggests, though it does not prove, that *all* the embryos which are created are viewed as products—at least at the time of their creation—and have a kind of conditional status hovering over them: if they are not good enough, they will be discarded." And then, according to Tollefsen, this conditional status "would further suggest two related moral deficiencies in IVF: first, that the parents involved love their children, at least at their origins, only conditionally, and second, that they treat their children as things, something incompatible with respectful treatment of persons." Even if later in life, once the zygote becomes the child, and the child is treated with worth, dignity, and inherent value, Tollefsen argues that it was still immoral to have devalued this human being in the early stages of life, analogous to the way that Huck Finn—in the Mark Twain book, *Adventures of Huckleberry Finn*—was wrong to have devalued "Nigger Jim" when he first met him, even though later Huck respects Jim and apologizes to him for his initial disrespect.

In his response to Purdy, Tollefsen mentions that treating "a person as a mere means only is, as Kant recognized, always wrong." Kant's second formulation of his categorical imperative—which has been used as a basis for moral decision-making since it was first formulated near the end of the eighteenth century—goes something like this: Whenever you act, always treat yourself and others as an end in themselves, and never *merely* as a means to an end. In other words, do not ever use yourself or another person instrumentally *merely* to achieve some other goal, no matter the consequences. The basis for this has to do with the fact that humans are conscious, rational, precious, sacred beings having an *intrinsic* value (as ends) and not an *instrumental* value (as a means to an end) like some object, tool, thing, or instrument. From this perspective, morally right decisions are those decisions where a person is treated as an end, and morally wrong decisions are those where someone is treated as a mere instrument or means to an end (Kant, 1775–1789/1963, 1785/1998, 1797a/1996a, 1797b/1996b). If there is a way to make Kant's argument work for human embryos that are *actually*, *already*, *potentially* conscious, rational beings (cf. Oduncu, 2003; Manninen, 2008), then Tollefsen can use this deontological secular position to bolster a Catholic religious-based position.

References

ACT (Advanced Cell Technologies). (2010). Advanced Cell Technology receives FDA clearance for the first clinical trial using embryonic stem cells to treat macular degeneration. Retrieved from: http://www.advancedcell.com/news-and-media/press-releases/advanced-cell-technology-receives-fda-clearance-for-the-first-clinical-trial-using-embryonic-stem-cel/index.asp

ACT (Advanced Cell Technologies). (2011). ACT secures patent to generate embryonic stem cells without embryo destruction. Retrieved from: http://www.advancedcell.com/news-and-media/press-releases/act-secures-patent-to-generate-embryonic-stem-cells-without-embryo-destruction/index.asp

Brackett, B. (2001). Advances in animal in vitro fertilization. In D. P. Wolf & M. Zelinski-Wooten (Eds.), *Contemporary endocrinology: Assisted fertilization and nuclear transfer in mammals* (pp. 21–51). London: Springer.

CCC (*The Catechism of the Catholic Church*). (1994). Chicago: Liguori Publications and Libreria Editrice Vaticana.

DHC (Document of the Holy See on Human Cloning). (2004). Retrieved from: http://www.vatican.va/roman_curia/secretariat_state/2004/documents/rc_seg-st_20040927_cloning_en.html

Dworkin, R. (1993). *Life's dominion: An argument about abortion, euthanasia and individual freedom*. New York: Alfred A. Knopf.

English, J. (1973). Abortion and the concept of a person. *Canadian Journal of Philosophy*, *5*(2), 233–243.

EV (*Evangelium Vitae*). (1995). Retrieved from: http://www.vatican.va/edocs/ENG0141/_INDEX.HTM

Gardner, D., Weissman, A., Howles, C., & Shoham, Z. (Eds.). (2008). *Textbook of assisted reproductive technologies: Laboratory and clinical perspectives*. London: Informa.

HV (*Humanae Vitae*). (1968). Retrieved from: http://www.vatican.va/holy_father/paul_vi/encyclicals/documents/hf_p-vi_enc_25071968_humanae-vitae_lt.html

John Paul II. (2001). Pope's address to President Bush at Castel Gandolfo, Italy, July 23, 2001. Retrieved from: http://www.americancatholic.org/news/stemcell/pope_to_bush.asp

Kail, R., & Cavanaugh, J. (2010). *Human development: A lifespan view*. Belmont, CA: Wadsworth.

Kant, I. (1775–1789/1963). *Lectures on ethics* (L. Infield, Trans.). Indianapolis, IN: Hackett Publishing.

Kant, I. (1785/1998). *Groundwork of the metaphysics of morals* (M. Gregor, Trans.). (Section I: Transition from common rational to philosophic moral cognition). Cambridge: Cambridge University Press.

Kant, I. (1797a/1996a). *Practical philosophy* (M. Gregor, Trans.). Cambridge: Cambridge University Press.

Kant, I. (1797b/1996b). *The metaphysics of morals* (M. Gregor, Trans.). Cambridge: Cambridge University Press.

Klimanskaya, I., Chung, Y., Becker, S., Lu, S-J., & Lanza, R. (2006). Human embryonic stem cell lines derived from single blastomeres. *Nature*, *444*, 481–485.

Klimanskaya, I., Chung, Y., Becker, S., Lu, S-J., & Lanza, R. (2007). Derivation of human embryonic stem cells from single blastomeres. *Nature Protocols*, *2*, 1963–1972.

Lachmann, P. (2001). Stem cell research—why is it regarded as a threat? An investigation of the economic and ethical arguments made against research with human embryonic stem cells. *European Molecular Biology Organization (EMBO) Reports*, *2*(3), 165–168.

Lang, M. (2011). ACT awarded patent for stem cell generation technique. *Mass High Tech*, February 25. Retrieved from: http://www.masshightech.com/stories/2011/02/21/daily53-ACT-awarded-patent-for-stem-cell-generation-technique.html

Mail (*MailOnline*). (2012). Number of IVF babies passes 5 m worldwide with demand for techniques still rising. *MailOnline*, July 1. Retrieved from: http://www.dailymail.co.uk/health/article-2167509/Number-IVF-babies-passes-5m-worldwide-demand-techniques-rising.html#ixzz28Sug4zKs

Manninen, B. (2008). Are human embryos Kantian persons? Kantian considerations in favor of embryonic stem cell research. *Philosophy, Ethics, and Humanities in Medicine*, *3*(4). Retrieved from: http://www.peh-med.com/content/3/1/4

Nagy, Z., Varghese, A., & Agarwal, A. (Eds.). (2012). *Practical manual of in vitro fertilization: Advanced methods and novel devices*. London: Springer.

NCBC (National Catholic Bioethics Center). (2009). *A Catholic guide to ethical clinical research*. Philadelphia: National Catholic Bioethics Center.

Newman, B., & Newman, R. (2012). *Development through life: A psychosocial approach*. Belmont, CA: Wadsworth.

Novak, M. (2001). The stem cell side: Be alert to the beginnings of evil. In M. Ruse & C. Pynes (Eds.), *The stem cell controversy: Debating the issues* (pp. 111–116). Amherst, NY: Prometheus Books.

O'Brien, N. (2011). Science, religion not in conflict, US bishops say in stem-cell document. *AmericanCatholic.Org*.

Retrieved from: http://www.americancatholic.org/News/StemCell/stemcelldocument.asp

Oduncu, F. (2003). Stem cell research in Germany: Ethics of healing vs. human dignity. *Medical Health Care and Philosophy*, *6*, 11–12.

Pacholczyk, T. (2006). Guilt-free pluripotent stem cells? National Catholic Bioethics Center. Retrieved from: http://www.ncbcenter.org/Page.aspx?pid=287

Pincus, G. (1936). *The eggs of mammals*. New York: Macmillan.

Sadler, T. (2011). *Langman's medical embryology*. Hagerstown, MD: Lippincott, Williams & Wilkins.

Spar, B. (2006). *The baby business: How money, science, and politics drive the commerce of conception*. Boston: Harvard Business School Press.

Thomson, J. J. (1971). A defense of abortion. *Philosophy and Public Affairs*, *1*, 47–66.

van Leeuwen, F., Mooij, T., & Burger, C. (2012). Reply: In vitro fertilization and ovarian malignancies: Potential implications for the individual patient and for the community. *Human Reproduction*, *27*, 2879.

Wade, N. (2010). Pioneer in in vitro fertilization wins Nobel Prize. *The New York Times*, October 4. Retrieved from: http://www.nytimes.com/2010/10/05/health/research/05nobel.html?pagewanted=all

Walsh, F. (2008). 30th birthday for first IVF baby. *BBC News*, July 14. Retrieved from: http://news.bbc.co.uk/2/hi/health/7505635.stm

Warren, M. A. (1973). On the moral and legal status of abortion. *The Monist*, *57*, 43–61.

Warren, M. A. (1997). *Moral status: Obligations to persons and other living things*. Oxford: Oxford University Press.

Chapter Twenty Seven

In Vitro Fertilization Should Be an Option for a Woman

Laura Purdy

In this chapter, I argue that in vitro fertilization (IVF) should, under tightly regulated conditions, be available to women. The most urgent (and doable) steps are to ensure that women are better informed about the risks and benefits of IVF, and to promote professional guidelines to minimize instances of multiple pregnancy. In addition, we need a comprehensive policy focusing on the prevention of infertility and alternative approaches to it. These changes would be promoted most successfully by converting the treatment of infertility to a nonprofit activity. And, some of the impetus for IVF could be reduced by attending to the social, rather than genetic value of childrearing, as well as countering pronatalism and sexism. There are numerous moral concerns about IVF. Nevertheless, on balance, there is a better case for ensuring that it remains available to women than for legally prohibiting it. The worries involve both IVF itself, and the other technologies for which it is a steppingstone. However, the latter need to be evaluated on their own merits, so the major focus here should be IVF itself. Some objections, such as those advanced by proponents of the view that fertilized eggs have full human rights, are unpersuasive. However, there are still problems aplenty, involving mainly the treatments' risks for women and children, known and unknown. The problems are exacerbated by the social and political context within which IVF care is delivered. Some are so fundamental that there is little reason to think that they can be remedied, but concerted action could mitigate others sufficiently so that it would be inconsistent to ban IVF but not other treatments vulnerable to similar criticisms.

Introduction

When word of Nadya Suleman's octuplets got out in January 2009, there was an uproar. Suleman—immediately christened "Octomom"—was already the mother of six young children, and had just produced (via IVF) eight more. Suleman also looked completely unprepared to care well for the resulting brood, as she was single, unemployed, and dependent financially on government assistance; she lived with her parents in a small house, and three of her older children had health problems (Rosenthal, 2010).

Although much of the furor no doubt arose from the fact that the public might ultimately be responsible for astronomical hospital bills for the eight preemies—estimated at between $1.5 and $3 million (Petok, 2008), this situation raised plenty of other legitimate worries. First and foremost, such "supertwin" pregnancies are extremely risky for fetuses and the children they become, as well as for the pregnant woman. In addition, although media glorification of earlier octuplet births had failed to emphasize the impossibility of anybody meeting the physical and emotional needs of so many same-aged children, the presence

Contemporary Debates in Bioethics, First Edition. Edited by Arthur L. Caplan and Robert Arp.

of the six older children in this case apparently did the trick (Purdy, 2007). Given these issues, the question was inescapable: should women have unrestricted access to technologies like in vitro fertilization that can be used in such an irresponsible way?

Lurking in the background were other doubts about the technologies, controversial ever since Louise Brown's birth in 1978 brought advances in what soon became known as new or artificial reproductive technologies to the public's attention.

The worries were diverse and came from many quarters. The focus at the time was—and to some extent still is, despite its now widespread deployment—IVF. IVF is at the heart of efforts to combat infertility.

What precisely is IVF? Conception usually takes place in women's fallopian tubes. When they are blocked or damaged, conception cannot occur. IVF circumvents this problem by manually extracting women's eggs, fertilizing them in a Petri dish, and then returning them to the uterus. This basic form of IVF permits women to gestate their "own" genetically related children.

IVF (or its components) are also essential for additional technologies that seek goals some consider even more controversial. For example, male infertility can sometimes be overcome by intracytoplasmic sperm injection (ICSI). Other refinements include freezing gametes and embryos, and "assisted hatching" to increase the number of viable embryos. IVF is also required to obtain donor eggs for reproduction and research. In addition, IVF facilitates preimplantation genetic diagnosis, which enables couples to prevent the birth of individuals with genetic traits causing diseases like Huntington's Disease, to do sex selection, and to choose embryos with compatible traits to donate materials to older siblings with devastating diseases, becoming so-called "savior siblings." IVF is also required for gestational contract pregnancy, where the gestating woman nurtures a fetus grown from the egg of another. Also, women over 40 turn out to have a higher probability of a successful pregnancy using donor eggs with IVF. Components of IVF are also the gateway for such brave-new-world possibilities as reproductive cloning, human embryo stem-cell research, genetic engineering required to produce so-called "designer babies," and research on artificial gametes. It also facilitates genetically related reproduction by singles and homosexuals without sexual intercourse.

IVF's morality is thus central for the morality of each of its "progeny." Thus, for instance, evaluating ICSI requires both that IVF be permissible and that ICSI itself pass moral muster. So, we need to consider such questions as whether the apparent risks of infertility or other abnormalities in sons born of ICSI constitute a moral barrier to it (Purdy, 2008).

Does this state of affairs risk a slippery slope for IVF, such that although IVF itself may be morally permissible, it necessarily leads to morally impermissible activities? There is vigorous debate about all these technologies, and a persuasive case against any of them may yet be made. However, the fact of the slippery slope would still remain to be established.

Why might access to IVF be morally desirable? The reason is that most people appear to have an extremely strong preference for genetically related children. Many women also want to gestate their children, if possible. People will go to very considerable lengths to satisfy the desire for these things, as the rapid development of reproductive technologies demonstrates—despite the judgment by some philosophers (like Michael Bayles) that wanting genetically related children is irrational (Bayles, 1984). But it is not clear that any such alleged irrationality is the morally salient issue: what matters is whether individuals undertake disproportionate risks in pursuing their goals. If so, it would be good if people were less attached to them. The moral baseline, though, should be that, other things being equal, it is good for desires to be satisfied.

Critiques of IVF

Let us now consider moral objections to IVF. There is a huge range of arguments against IVF, and it would take books to address them all. The task is still further complicated by the necessity for distinguishing between arguments that it is immoral and the conclusion that it should be legally prohibited. Here, only the most important concerns will therefore be addressed.

I will concentrate primarily on consequentialist worries about IVF to see whether there are grounds for arguing that it is immoral or that it should be banned. Understanding these concerns requires a somewhat more detailed examination of IVF procedures and outcomes.

IVF is most successful when many eggs can be fertilized, and the best transplanted into the uterus. However, encouraging many eggs to ripen simultaneously requires women to take powerful fertility drugs. Their ripe eggs are then gathered by inserting a long needle into the vagina. After fertilization, the healthiest looking eggs are then placed in the uterus with a rigid catheter. Those remaining are either frozen for possible later use or discarded.

These procedures involve risk. Fertility drugs can cause a variety of problems, most notably ovarian hyperstimulation syndrome, which can sometimes cause death (Purdy, 2008). Bleeding, infection, or injury to blood vessels and viscera may be caused by the egg-retrieval process, and embryo transfer may expose women to infection.

Moreover, there is still little solid information about possible long-term risk (either for women or for children), despite the fact that there is reason to fear that taking powerful hormones might lead to various kinds of cancers (Ehrenfeld, 2006).

IVF pregnancies are more risky for women because of their higher-than-average risk of spontaneous abortion and bleeding. Most dangerous is ectopic pregnancy, where the embryo implants in a woman's fallopian tube, threatening to kill her when the growing fetus causes it to burst (Purdy, 2008).

IVF treatments are also problematic because of the broader social and political context. IVF success rates vary tremendously, depending on the woman's situation and the effectiveness of the particular clinic. In the best case, close to 50% come away with a baby, but many still do not, despite multiple cycles. Until very recently, there was little solid information about the probable benefit of such persistence. Clinics that treat infertility are very profitable (Spar, 2006). Each cycle now costs about $12,400 (Chang, 2010), and the more cycles performed, the more money is made. In the absence of good information about the value of additional cycles, the conflict of interest inherent in the fee-for-service structure creates a bias toward treatment such that it is difficult to know when to say "enough." This problem is exacerbated by the weak regulation of infertility clinics that makes accurate information about their success rates hard to come by (Donchin, 2011). But undertaking multiple cycles adds to the discomfort and risk women undertake.

Last, and not least, what about risks specific to children? IVF has hugely increased the incidence of multiple pregnancies (MPs), primarily as a result of decisions to transfer many embryos at a time. However, the more fetuses women carry, the greater the risks to themselves and to the fetuses (Purdy, 2007). By some measures, even twins fare worse than singletons, let alone higher-order pregnancies (Purdy, 2006). Women carrying MPs are at additional risk for anemia, preterm labor, hypertension, thrombophlebitis, preterm delivery, and hemorrhage (Mahowald, 2006). The children are still more at risk. They may suffer from a variety of problems in the uterus, and some or all of the fetuses may die there. Those who survive to birth will likely be very premature, a cause of major health problems. A significant percentage of such premature, low-birth-rate babies have such severe problems (such as low intelligence, major vision problems, or cerebral palsy) that they must be in special-education programs (Mahowald, 2006; Purdy, 2007).

Recall Nadya Suleman's story mentioned above. In fact, she was remarkably lucky in that all of her babies survived and do not appear to have any major health problems. An earlier mother of octuplets, Nkem Chukwu, lost one soon after the birth in 1998; none weighed even two pounds. All spent months in the hospital, and four of them were critically ill; one spent 6 months there. Luckily, they appear to be doing well now. But that is not the norm. Many families with supertwins are struggling with the harsh reality of one or more children with serious problems. For example, all the Aymond quintuplets have serious health problems. One is blind, four of them are in speech therapy, three are in occupational therapy, and three are in physical therapy (Purdy, 2007). These common, harsh realities tend to be obscured by the feel-good reporting common in the media.

Why do women accept MP? Some, like Suleman, may believe that their embryos have a right to life, and so it is wrong to freeze or discard them. Others may do so in the belief that it will increase the probability that their pregnancy will result in the baby they seek.

As we will see below, there is reason to think that most MPs can be prevented. However, it also turns out that even singletons born of IVF have a somewhat higher probability of birth defects, and the long-term risks are currently unknown. Louise Brown, the first IVF baby, born in 1978, is currently healthy, and has had a child the usual way. But with IVF becoming common only recently, it is too early to be fully reassured that the children born of it face no additional late-developing risks.

Given all this, the major moral issue is whether those undertaking IVF are in a position to make fully informed and autonomous decisions, both about their own health and about that of any resulting children.

The literature on informed consent is not particularly reassuring, either in general or with respect to reproductive treatments (Houmard & Seifer, 1999; Stewart et al., 2001; Corrigan, 2003). The difficulty in conveying even straightforward information to healthy individuals—let alone more complicated issues for those under stress—is well established. Some studies show that even among highly qualified practitioners, fewer than half discussed the possibility that treatment might contribute to higher rates of ovarian cancer, and among those, most had started doing so only shortly before the study (Houmard & Seifer, 1999). And only some had changed their practice patterns to reflect that worry, for example, by limiting the number of treatment cycles they offer women (Houmard & Seifer, 1999). Another chilling study reinforced the fact that women are woefully uninformed about IVF and are thus unprepared to protect their own interests, despite their strong desire to participate in treatment decisions. They seriously overestimated the probability of a live birth, and were unaware that there might be long-term risks, such as ovarian cancer, resulting from the procedures. What they did know, they mostly learned on their own. They underestimated how difficult it is to detect or treat such cancers, and most thought their doctors could suggest ways to reduce the risk (Stewart et al., 2001). These facts are still more disturbing, given that women may undertake IVF not because they themselves are infertile, but to offer their mates a genetically related child (Lorber, 1989).

Examining the broader context of reproductive medicine both suggests further worries and points the way toward reducing some of these risks.

On the one hand, the existence of IVF may be leading women to sign up for infertility treatment when there might be better alternatives. Thus, for instance, in a different world—less sexist, pronatalist, less focused on genetic relationships—many infertile women might be quite content to remain childless, or adopt instead. Adoption is not necessarily the panacea some believe, but it could well make sense in some cases.

This world would also have created other, more desirable alternatives. Critics of Western medicine, especially US medicine, have long noted its bias toward aggressive, invasive, high-tech solutions (Payer, 1996). A rational approach to infertility would have focused on its causes, aiming at prevention. Thus, it would have pursued the evidence that pollution can cause it (Mann, 2010); the problematic chemicals are ubiquitous (phthalates, BPA, perfluorinated compounds in nonstick cookware, triclosan, and mercury). Also, there are intriguing hints that such factors as stress, smoking, diet, or obesity might play a role in infertility. Last and not least, the need to establish careers during the most fertile years leads many professional women to delay childbearing until their less fertile years. Social conditions, including poverty, create still further barriers to fertility in developing countries (Donchin, 2010). But there is no coordinated approach to problems, starting with prevention. Whether or when a particular issue is taken up, and by what branch of medicine, is often a matter of chance; medicalizing infertility simply buttresses society's piecemeal and backwards approach to the issue.

Still more broadly, reproductive medicine, taken as a whole, reflects and reinforces pervasive and harmful social values. Sexism, pronatalism, and the paramount value placed on genetic relationships lead girls to assume that *of course* they will have children and that no life is complete without them (Hollingworth, 1974; Meyers, 2001). Such socialization might have been essential for species survival when high death rates were a threat, but that is no longer our chief problem, and even if it were, it is hardly clear that women have a moral obligation to remedy it (Overall, 2012).

Given this less-than-optimal state of affairs, should women therefore be denied access to IVF? No. Unfortunately, ethics and policy often need to devise ways to cope with bad situations that might have been prevented. Closing off dangerous options may in some cases be the solution. But IVF does offer important benefits for some who would make good parents and who are infertile or incapable of reproducing because of their social situation. Thus, the best solution would be to promote a multi-pronged advance along the paths already indicated.

Addressing Consequentialist Concerns

So, an obvious first step is making research on the causes of infertility a top priority, along with studying possible low-risk alternatives to IVF like improving diet, weight loss, and stress reduction, with practitioners recommending such approaches to patients before moving on to IVF. More broadly, society as a whole clearly needs to focus more on both individual practices aimed at better overall health, and the more comprehensive social changes need to encourage and facilitate such practices. Needless to say, this is a tall order, given the entrenched interests, such as agribusiness, that benefit from the status quo. Nonetheless, even piecemeal approaches can benefit individuals.

Second, more stringent regulation of IVF and reproductive medicine itself is clearly necessary—also a politically daunting prospect. At a minimum, much more transparency about procedures, risks, and success rates as measured by the number of live births per cycle is required. Equally important, procedures themselves must be more tightly controlled to reflect current best practices. For example, new research suggests that there is little benefit for most women after two or three cycles (Chang, 2010). That should become the firm standard of care.

A related, and equally politically sensitive issue, is tackling incentives for high-tech treatment built into the current profit-oriented, fee-for-service system (Cohen, 2001). Unfortunately, the most effective way to make progress here would be to convert for-profit clinics into nonprofit organizations. That would mitigate the more aggressive (and profitable) approaches, such as offering women experimental protocols in the guise of established treatments, waiting instead for the results of rigorous studies of the risks and benefits of innovations. And that would also reduce the temptation to skimp on unprofitable but essential elements of excellent care, like aiding patients to make good decisions and careful follow-up. Ideally, most or all healthcare should be delivered by nonprofit providers, for these and related reasons. It is hard to picture this happening in the US anytime soon, despite well-documented drawbacks of the current system (Kuttner, 1996; Elliott, 2010). But even in the absence of such thoroughgoing reform, other changes discussed here could go a substantial way toward achieving the goals of nonprofit infertility care.

The foregoing proposals would go quite far toward protecting children and women from IVF risks. But one more big change is required: reducing or eliminating MP, especially higher-order MP. Fortunately, so-called "single embryo transfer" (SET) is turning out to be as effective for some groups of women as implanting multiple embryos. Embryos are grown for an extra two days, making it easier to judge which are most likely to flourish, and raising the probability of implantation. SET is already common in Europe—in Sweden, for instance, some 70% of IVF is done using SET. Pregnancy rates for younger women are about as good, but have far less risk (Petok, 2008). Freezing other good embryos for later attempts is also as successful as transferring two embryos (Milingos & Bhattacharya, 2009). Given the dangers of MP, SET should be considered the norm.

What about the conscience rights of those who think letting embryos die is murder? It would be morally reasonable to offer them the choice between fertilizing fewer eggs, or agreeing to freezing or embryo adoption. It is one thing to respect people's basic moral convictions; it is quite another to let them set all the terms on which that is done.

Even if MP can be drastically reduced, as we have seen, IVF still clearly poses some risk to children, given the somewhat higher probability of birth defects, although their extent is unclear because of poor follow-up. This lack of information, particularly about possible long-term risk of serious late-onset problems, is especially troubling (Kennedy, 2005; Kolata, 2009). Louise Brown was born only in 1978, and even if she and all subsequent IVF children were being systematically studied (which they are not), that would not be enough time to reveal all the potential dangers.

Is a moratorium on these grounds warranted? There are some grounds for thinking that would be a good idea but also some reasons for resisting it.

Oddly, those who seek IVF are apparently unworried about such potential risks. For example, as Gina Kolata comments, in her *New York Times* article on the possible dangers of IVF, patients rarely ask about them, and those who do—despite information in consent forms—are never dissuaded from going forward by the answers. According to Richard G. Rawlins of the Rush Centers for Advanced Reproductive Care in Chicago, few physicians appear to be worried about the IVF procedures, either (Kolata, 2009). Needless to say, good ethics cannot be inferred from what people think, but such facts are nonetheless a measure of people's priorities.

More importantly, there is a good deal of disagreement about whether we are morally required to prevent the birth of individuals at risk for disease or disability. Some, most notably certain leading disability-rights activists, believe that it is discriminatory, insulting, and immoral (Parens & Asch, 2000). Although their focus is on genetic services, it seems to me that the same arguments should be applied to other relevant contexts like this one. Another group of thinkers—mostly liberal philosophers—see no moral urgency here, either, as they believe that as long as the people we create are not so miserable that they wish they were dead, there is no moral objection to going forward (Parfit, 1984).

Although there is reason to think that the arguments for these positions are weak, their existence shows that a ban would be more controversial than one might think (Purdy, 2001; McBrayer, 2008). In addition, even if the moral case against IVF on these grounds were stronger, it would not follow that the treatment should be made illegal. It is one thing to try to educate or persuade about a given activity; quite another to bring the power of the state to bear on it.

The key justification for such state action is to prevent serious harm. But applying this principle requires well-founded criteria for line drawing. MP poses such serious risks to children that it would be justifiable to prohibit the transfer of more than two embryos. However, there is no such clear evidence of highly probable risk of serious harm from IVF itself.

Even, more crucially, society's concern about potential harm to children is highly selective at best. The US, for instance, tolerates known and serious harms such as lack of access to healthcare, nutritious food, and nonviolent, nontoxic environments. In the absence of such basic measures to prevent harm, how can it be justifiable to single out a service like IVF in the name of child protection? This point has not prevented women from being jailed for allegedly putting their fetuses at risk, but does that not seem rather out of line, considering the social ambivalence (at best) about other sources of risk to fetuses? Banning IVF now would be another step toward holding women, but not society in general, accountable.

Might the remaining risks to women from IVF procedures (especially the fertility drugs now in use) justify limiting access to IVF? Eliminating MP would drastically reduce—but not eradicate—risk, as would the other measures already discussed. Clearly, it means so much to some women who see IVF as their only hope for the child they seek, despite possible risks to themselves, that one might reasonably conclude that the choice should be theirs.

This is not to say that no treatments should ever be taken off the market because of their risks. Some are so risky, with so little counterbalancing benefit, that no well-informed individual would choose them. But that does not appear to be the case here.

Moreover, the reality is that we, as a society, allow people to choose treatments that can harm, even for goals some judge frivolous or sick, like cosmetic surgery or sex-change procedures (Elliott, 2003). Still more importantly, mainstream disease treatments can also maim or kill, sometimes with little promise of benefit, as in last-ditch cancer procedures. Allowing access to IVF—under the kinds of conditions argued for here—is required for consistency with these other practices and policies. (Notice here that the focus here is on the paradigm case of egg retrieval for women's own use; donation raises additional issues (Dickenson, 2001).

Feminists have rightly pointed out that having more choices is not always liberating or beneficial (Sherwin, 1992; Nelson, 1995). Problematic procedures can become difficult-to-refuse standards of care, especially for the relatively vulnerable. This is a genuine problem, but prohibitions are also problematic. First, which procedures get prohibited, and who gets to choose them? Abortion? Contraception? IVF?

Prohibitions also have a way of creating black markets, which may endanger women still more. Second, these days, many prohibitions would be relatively futile, as reproductive tourism—seeking IVF in other, less highly regulated countries—would in any case provide access for the relatively well off (Donchin, 2010). Such "escape hatches" should not always militate against legislation, but the inequities created by them must be taken into account where prohibitions are contemplated.

Last, we need to consider whether the scarcity of healthcare resources might not create a case against access to IVF. But in the US (and, in a more limited way, in most other countries that have large publically funded programs), healthcare providers generally make available services people want and will pay for. The results can hardly be said to optimize human welfare, as providers turn to specialties like cosmetic surgery instead of primary-care medicine, and drug companies focus on the most profitable, not the most needed, drugs. But under these circumstances, it would be inconsistent to ban IVF services on this ground. Where attempts are made to allocate resources to maximize benefit, this conclusion calls for further scrutiny. Interestingly, then, the province of Ontario has chosen to provide some access to IVF, even if only for women with blocked fallopian tubes, and for no more than three cycles.

It follows from all this that if at least three of the remedies suggested here are implemented (meaningful regulation aimed at facilitating more effective informed consent procedures, establishing no more than two or three cycles as the norm, and eradicating MP), IVF would be morally and politically permissible in the US. Researching and implementing preventive measures to reduce infertility, and mitigating the cultural pressures that promote the desire for genetically related children would reduce the negative impact of infertility as well.

It would be naïve to underestimate the difficulty of these measures. But perhaps the Suleman case will turn out to be something of a watershed. In 2009, her IVF specialist, Dr Michael Kamrava, lost his membership of the American Society for Reproductive Medicine. In October, 2010, the state of California began negligence hearings that could lead to his license being suspended or revoked. He is alleged to have transferred 12 embryos to Suleman, and to have failed to refer her for a mental-health evaluation, despite the fact that she already had babies of 17 and four months at the time, when the standard of care for women of Suleman's age is, in any case, to transfer no more than two embryos (Patsner, 2009). He is also accused of negligence, having gone forward with IVF for another patient who should have been referred for a cancer screening, and who later turned out to have stage 3 disease (Mohajer, 2010).

No IVF!

However, some would reject even this quite limited access to IVF, based on what they view as far more fundamental moral objections. The most sweeping objection to IVF (and other reproductive technologies) comes from the Roman Catholic Church, which holds that it is wrong to separate sex and reproduction. The inseparability thesis prohibits sex that is not open to reproduction but also reproduction without sex (Cohen, 1969). That thesis rests on natural law (NL) theory. NL holds that God embedded moral values in the natural world, and that reason provides us with a means for reading those values from it; secular NL sees values inherent in nature itself.

Neither version of NL is compelling. The first depends on the existence of a monotheistic, all-powerful God; the second fails to explain how values could be embedded in nature. Neither explains how to evaluate disagreement among proponents of NL. Even if, for the sake of argument, we accept these premises, NL commits either the naturalistic fallacy or begs key questions.

The naturalistic fallacy is committed when it is argued that the way things are is the way they ought to be. As David Hume noted, this happens when the premises of an argument contain only references to how things are, yet the conclusion advances a claim about how they ought to be. No sound argument can advance claims in the conclusion that are not already implicit in the premises (Hume, 1739).

Proponents of NL also beg questions, arguing in a circle by claiming to read into nature what is in fact only the reflection of their previously chosen values. For example, traditional NL theorists believe that nature teaches us that human life is always valuable, despite the fact that the natural world supports no such inference. Without human "interference" in the form of public-health measures and modern medicine, death rates from disease have been enormously high. Human violence continues to exact an enormous toll as well, although that issue raises the interesting question whether "human nature" is really part of "nature" (Pierce, 1970). More relevant to the objection that IVF "wastes" extra embryos not transferred to women's uteruses, most embryos created by sexual activity are ejected from women's bodies early in the process of development (Gilbert, 2008). How is this compatible with the NL principle that embryos are inherently valuable? In fact, the more we learn about biology, the clearer it becomes that some influential ethical views, like this one, are based on inaccurate information (Rachels, 2003, ch. 4; Gilbert, 2008).

Aside from the Vatican rejection of reproduction without sex, there are other religiously based objections to IVF. Among them are the moral status of ensouled embryos, concern about playing God, and the belief that suffering is intrinsically valuable (Evans, 2010). What legal standing might these views have? In the US, the First Amendment generally entitles individuals to follow their religious principles in such personal matters, but that same Amendment prohibits making these principles applicable to all without compelling independent grounds. Any other approach violates the First Amendment rights of those with competing religious or philosophical convictions. Thus, for instance, some conservative religions that discourage contraception diverge from Roman Catholicism by declaring IVF to be permissible. Their underlying value is pronatalism, the view that childbearing is a top moral priority, and it trumps the Vatican's inseparability principle (Joyce, 2009). It follows that none of these should ground IVF regulation.

Conclusion

Let us now return to the Suleman case that initially pressed the question whether women should have access to IVF. Should Suleman's actions be condoned? Of course not: what she (and her physician) did was irresponsible. But it is important to be clear about where the problem lies. The problem precisely was her insistence (and her physician's acquiescence) that all her embryos be transferred, when she already had several very young children. The changes suggested here, together with existing guidelines, would have prevented that outcome.

What if a woman used IVF to get pregnant 14 times? These proposals would leave this decision in her hands, and it is not clear that we would want to change that, no matter how unwise one might think such a course. First, she could do it without IVF, either the usual way or by using artificial insemination by donor. Second, despite the morally reasonable idea that people should not have children unless they can support them decently, we should think twice about enshrining this principle into law. What does "decently" mean? And what about the many Americans who cannot offer their children nutritious food, safe housing, or high-quality medical care and education? Should they refrain from childbearing altogether? What about their existing children? For the most part, focusing on this state of affairs ignores the politics of inequality that has led to it, and it would surely be better to remedy that before we empower government to interfere in decisions about whether to have children. Would that change prevent a few, like Suleman, from having children they cannot support? Of course not, but it would make ensuring their offsprings' welfare far more manageable.

So: IVF? In a better world, there would be considerably less need or interest in it, and less risk, too. We should be working toward that better world. In the meantime, we must formulate ethics and policy for this world, ones that will both meet our needs now and help lead us toward that better one.

References

Bayles, M. (1984). *Reproductive ethics*. Engelwood Cliffs, NJ: Prentice-Hall.

Chang, A. (2010). More not always better with in vitro fertilization. *Salon*, February 10. Retrieved from: http://www.salon.com/wires/allwires/2010/10/27/D9J45L6G2_us_med_fertility_success/index.html

Cohen, C. (1969). Sex, birth control, and human life. *Ethics*, *79*, 251–263.

Cohen, C. (2001). Unmanaged care: The need to regulate new reproductive technologies in the United States. *Bioethics*, *11*, 348–365.

Corrigan, O. (2003). Empty ethics: The problem with informed consent. *Sociology of Health & Illness*, *25*, 768–798.

Dickenson, D. (2001). Property and women's alienation from their own reproductive labour, *Bioethics*, *15*, 205–217.

Donchin, A. (2010). Reproductive tourism and the quest for global gender justice. *Bioethics*, *24*, 323–332.

Donchin, A. (2011). In whose interest? Policy and politics in assisted reproduction. *Bioethics*, *25*, 92–101.

Ehrenfeld, P. (2006). Bioethics and women's rights. Blog. Retrieved from: http://www.iheu.org/node/1911

Elliott, C. (2003). *Better than well: American medicine meets the American dream*. New York: W. W. Norton & Company.

Elliott, C. (2010). *White coat, black hat: Adventures on the dark side of medicine*. Boston: Beacon Press.

Evans, J. H. (2010). *Contested reproduction: Genetic technologies, religion, and public debate*. Chicago: University of Chicago Press.

Gilbert, S. F. (2008). When "personhood" begins in the embryo: Avoiding a syllabus of errors. *Birth Defects Research (Part C)*, *84*, 164–173.

Hollingworth, L. S. (1916). Social devices for impelling women to bear and rear children. *American Journal of Sociology*, *22*, 19–29.

Houmard B. S., & Seifer, D. (1999). Infertility treatment and informed consent: Current practices of reproductive endocrinologists. *Obstetrics & Gynecology*, *93*, 252–257.

Hume, D. (1739). *A treatise of human nature*. London: John Noon.

Joyce, K. (2009). *Quiverfull: Inside the Christian patriarchy movement*. Boston: Beacon Press.

Kennedy, R. (2005). Risks and complications of assisted conception. British Fertility Society Factsheet. Retrieved from: http://www.britishfertilitysociety.org.uk/public/factsheets/conceptionrisks.html

Kolata, G. (2009). Picture emerging on genetic risks of IVF. *New York Times*, February 16. Retrieved from: http://www.nytimes.com/2009/02/17/health/17ivf.html?Pagewanted=all

Kuttner, R. (1996). *Everything for sale: The virtues and limits of markets*. Chicago: University of Chicago Press.

Lorber, J. (1989). Choice, gift, or patriarchal bargain? Women's consent to *In Vitro* fertilization in male infertility. *Hypatia*, *4*, 23–36.

Mahowald, M. (2006). *Bioethics and women: Across the life span*. Oxford: Oxford University Press.

Mann, D. (2010). Household chemicals linked to early puberty, infertility. *WebMD Health News*, November 18. Retrieved from: http://www.webmd.com/infertility-and-reproduction/news/20101118/household-chemicals-linked-early-puberty-infertility

Meyers, D. T. (2001). The rush to motherhood: Pronatalist discourse and women's autonomy. *Signs*, *26*, 735–773.

McBrayer, J. (2008). Rights, indirect harms and the non-identity problem. *Bioethics*, *22*(6), 299–306.

Milingos D., & Bhattacharya, S. (2009). Single embryo transplant. *Obstetrics, Gynaecology & Reproductive Medicine*, *19*, 229–231.

Mohajer, S. (2010). Licensing hearing wraps up for Octomom's fertility doctor, decision in coming months. Retrieved from: http://www.themonitor.com/articles/kamrava-43678-suleman-health.html

Nelson, H.L. (1995). Dethroning choice: Analogy, personhood, and the new reproductive technologies. *Journal of Law, Medicine & Ethics*, *23*, 129–135.

Overall, C. (2012). *Why have children? The ethical debate*. Cambridge, MA: MIT Press.

Parens, E., & Asch, A. (Eds.). (2000). *Prenatal testing and disability rights*. Washington, DC: Georgetown University Press.

Parfit, D. (1984). *Reasons and persons*. Oxford: Clarendon Press.

Patsner, B. (2009). The octuplets: A medical mistake needing more regulation? *Health Law Perspectives*. Retrieved from: www.law.uh.edu/healthlaw/perspectives/homepage.asp

Payer, L. (1996). *Medicine and culture*. New York: Holt Paperbacks.

Petok, W. D. (2008). Single embryo transplant: Why not put all your eggs in one basket? *American Fertility Association*. Retrieved from: http://www.theafa.org/library/article/single_embryo_transfer_why_not_put_all_your_eggs_in_one_basket/

Pierce, C. (1970). Natural law language and women. *Eros and Epistemology*, *17*, 3.

Purdy, L. (2001). Review of *Prenatal testing and disability Rights*, Erik Parens and Adrienne Asch, (Eds.). *Social Theory and Practice*, *27*, 681–687.

Purdy, L. (2006). Women's reproductive autonomy: Medicalization and beyond. *Journal of Medical Ethics*, *32*, 287–291.

Purdy, L. (2007). Could there be a right not to be born an octuplet? In S. Brennan & R. Noggle (Eds.), *Taking responsibility for children* (pp. 157–168). Waterloo, ON: Wilfrid Laurier Press.

Purdy, L. (2008). The bioethics of assisted reproduction. *Encyclopedia of Life Sciences*. Wiley Online. Retrieved from: http://onlinelibrary.wiley.com/doi/10.1002/9780470015902.a0003479.pub2/references

Rachels, J. (2003). *The elements of moral philosophy*. New York: McGraw-Hill.

Rosenthal, M. (2010). A preventive ethics approach to IVF in the age of octuplets. *Fertility and Sterility*, *93*, 339–340.

Sherwin, S. (1992). *No longer patient: Feminist ethics & health care*. Philadelphia: Temple University Press.

Spar, B. (2006). *The baby business: How money, science, and politics drive the commerce of conception*. Boston: Harvard Business School Press.

Stewart, D., Rosen, B., Irvine, J., Ritvo, R., Shapiro, R. ... Deber, R. (2001). The disconnect: Infertility patients' information and the role they wish to play in decision making. *Medscape General Medicine*, *3*, 1154–1168.

Chapter Twenty Eight

In Vitro Fertilization Should Not Be an Option for a Woman

Christopher Tollefsen

In this chapter, I argue that in vitro fertilization (IVF) is an inapt way for bringing children into the world. In Section I, I discuss the desire to have children, framing this desire in the context of marital love. In Section II, I raise some embryo-centered considerations against IVF. These considerations do not themselves rise to the level of principled objections to the procedure itself, but only to the way it is currently practiced in the US. Nevertheless, these considerations point us in the direction of a more principled argument. In Sections III and IV, I make that principled argument against IVF on the grounds that in this procedure, parents seek not to beget but to produce persons, an act I argue is always wrong. Later sections address further moral, political, and practical concerns.

I

In this chapter, I have the unenviable task of arguing that a procedure, which seems to most reasonable persons both morally unproblematic and to provide a very significant benefit, is in fact morally *impermissible*, and should not, at least morally, and perhaps politically, be an option for women. Such a position can seem cold and heartless, and inadequately sensitive to the tragedy of infertility, and unfulfilled desire for children. It is therefore especially important to begin this chapter with an acknowledgment of the nature and significance of the desire for children, and the pain and sorrow that ensue when that desire cannot be satisfied.

As regards the first, the desire for children, many reasons are given by philosophers explaining why this desire has such a hold on us: children are thought by Aristotle, for example, to ensure a form of immortality; desire for children is thus an extension of the desire for one's own continued existence. Similarly, children and their lives are sometimes thought of as a clean slate on which parents extend their own personal narratives, writing into their children's lives their own life plans and projects, which their child(ren) will fulfill.

Because it will be important to my argument later, I will describe a different view of the desire for children, one which begins with an account of marital love: in marriage, couples join in a commitment to a complete sharing of lives at all levels of their existence. Sexual union in marriage is a completion of that commitment at the physical level: a husband and wife become one flesh, one bodily organism, through their bodies working together to perform, or attempting to perform, a biological function that each on his or her

Contemporary Debates in Bioethics, First Edition. Edited by Arthur L. Caplan and Robert Arp.

own is incapable of performing: reproduction. Success in reproduction, then, is a further completion of that initial commitment, which now becomes bodied forth in the life of a new person, whom we could describe as the fulfillment, or fruition, of that marital love (Gergis et al., 2010).

Infertility is a deep pain and tragedy for this reason especially: in the paradigm case, parents bring forth new life out of, and as an expression and realization of, their love for one another. Their love is no less real, when biological children are not forthcoming (and indeed, I believe that adopted children, in the paradigm case, are also truly children of their parents *through* their parents' mutual love for one another; see Tollefsen, 2010); yet it can seem, for it really is the case, that an important way in which all love operates is missing: for all love seeks to bring forth something new, and romantic love seeks to bring forth something new, bodily, organic, and personal.

As the possibility of adoption suggests, love's fecundity may be adaptive when its more usual possibilities for creation are blocked, and no doubt infertile couples can body forth their love for one another into the world around them by projects of socially significant service. But our capacity to bring forth *new persons* out of our love is such a deep and even metaphysically significant feature of ourselves, and so central to the meaning of romantic love, that damage to that capacity cannot but be felt as a constant and tragic reminder of the brokenness of our world.

Nevertheless, I do not believe that all possible responses to that tragedy are equally morally permissible, and in this chapter, I will argue that IVF, in particular, is an inapt way for children to be brought into the world. The inaptness will be brought out in part precisely by contrast with the way in which sexual union is *apt* for the *begetting of persons*. In Sections III and IV of this chapter, I will make a principled argument against IVF on the grounds that, in this procedure, parents seek not to beget, but to produce persons, an act I will argue is always wrong. But in Part II of this chapter, I discuss some other important considerations, which do not themselves rise to the level of a principled argument against IVF, but which are very significant, and which point us, ultimately, in the direction of those principled arguments.

II

I was struck, in my initial (and, with my children, subsequent!) reading of J. K. Rowling's *Harry Potter* series, by a scene in *Harry Potter and the Goblet of Fire*. Harry has just arrived at a graveyard for a crucial battle with Voldemort, but he is accompanied, unexpectedly, by Cedric Diggory. Lord Voldemort issues the following directive to his minion, Wormtail: "Kill the spare."

The breathtaking lack of concern for the person that is Cedric is characteristic of Voldemort: what is in his way, and not to his purposes, is to be destroyed without qualm. It is difficult to imagine taking such an attitude towards our fellow human beings, and almost impossible to imagine taking it towards our own children. Yet, the consigning of "spare" embryos to fates such as long-term or permanent cryopreservation, scientific research, or simple discarding is a well-known part of the IVF industry.

These aspects of IVF would not, of course, be morally problematic (or at least not in the same way) were the early embryos in question *not* human beings, or *not* human persons. Philosophers and others have advocated both positions, both to justify the termination of embryonic human lives after IVF, and as part of a more comprehensive justification for both embryonic stem-cell research, and abortion. But I believe that both claims are in error.

As regards the first, that human zygotes and human embryos are early-stage human beings, members of the same biological species to which you, the readers, and I, the author, of this chapter, belong seems to me to be well-established scientific fact. In standard textbooks of developmental biology, we find passages such as the following, uttered as part of received scientific wisdom:

> *Human development begins at fertilization* when a male gamete or sperm (spermatozoon) unites with a female gamete or oocyte (ovum) to produce a single cell—a zygote. This highly specialized, totipotent cell marked the beginning of each of us as a unique individual. The zygote, just visible to the unaided eye as a tiny speck, contains chromosomes and genes (units of genetic information) that are derived from the mother and father. The unicellular zygote divides many times and

> becomes progressively transformed into a multicellular human being through cell division, migration, growth, and differentiation. (Moore & Persaud, 2003, p. 16)

If this claim is correct, then the destruction of leftover, and of many deficient, embryos from IVF procedures is the destruction of human beings. There is good reason to think that this is seriously morally wrong (George & Tollefsen, 2008).

Some philosophers deny this claim, on the grounds that a being, such as the embryo, which is not currently capable of rational thought or self-consciousness, is not a *person*. Such a claim denies that all human beings are worthy of fundamental moral respect, and holds instead that only a subset of human beings is so worthy, the subset that is capable of rational activity.

Yet "capable of" and "capacity" are ambiguous terms. No being goes from an inability to think to an ability to think, without changing what it fundamentally is, unless it *already* has a capacity—we could call it a radical capacity to indicate that it is there from the beginning—to develop itself to the point of being able to manifest thought. The capacity to think is not instilled in a being from without, but is the realization of a radical capacity already present in the being of that sort; and if the capacity is not present, as it is not in cats and dogs, no amount of development will ever bring that being to the state of rationality.

Human zygotes and embryos thus *do* have a capacity for rationality (and consciousness, self-consciousness, and various other personal attributes); the question is then whether it is the status of possessing those capacities in radical form, or the achievement of having developed those capacities, that qualifies a being for full moral status. I believe this question is a fundamentally moral question: it is the question of whether to treat all beings of the same kind as us—human beings—in the same fundamental ways that we would wish to be treated—or whether it is permissible to introduce radical differences of treatment—killing some, protecting others—on the basis of nonessential differences. Fairness, I believe, requires that one treat all human beings with the same fundamental forms of moral respect. But because persons just are those beings to whom fundamental moral respect is owed, a consequence of this argument (rather than, strictly speaking, a premise of it) is that all human beings are persons.

Because the IVF industry, especially in the United States, is highly unregulated, and contains inducements to the creation of surplus embryos, and few restrictions on the disposal of such embryos, the IVF industry as a whole is characterized by wide impermissible destruction of human beings, a moral wrong, albeit in service of the rectification of the natural tragedy of infertility. For this reason alone, at a minimum, the practice of IVF should be radically rethought, and no couple should cooperate with the project of producing more embryos than they plan to implant right away (for, if the embryo is a human person, it is surely disrespectful to "store" that person in cryopreservation until such time as one might later want to "use" or implant him or her).

Still, as I noted earlier, this argument cannot be considered an "in principle" argument against IVF. Such an argument would show that there was something morally problematic or wrong about IVF as such; but the argument thus far has shown only that there is something (systematically, in the US at least) wrong with the *practice* of IVF. Since that practice could be reformed, the argument does not address the permissibility of a practice of IVF in which only the embryos to be implanted were created, and which involved no "spares," to be destroyed or otherwise.

III

Despite the conditional nature of the argument in the previous section, I believe it contains the germ of an idea that is crucial to understanding the morality of IVF, and of some other forms of assisted reproduction, such as reproductive cloning. I will first, in this section, set out the argument in a brief and, I hope, somewhat intuitive way, and will then argue in Section IV at greater length.

Consider again Lord Voldemort's words, "Kill the spare," and consider what we identified as the chilling insensitivity to the humanity, the personhood, of Diggory. For something to be a spare is for it to be a mere thing, to be kept if useful or needed, but to be discarded otherwise. What is "spare" is a mere object, subordinated to the will of him or her who possesses, or has power over it.

Now, the fact that embryos left over from an IVF regimen can be called "spares," and discarded if not needed, certainly tells us something about how *those* embryos are thought of. But the fact that the language of "spares," and of embryo "grading," and of "selective reduction" and even, perhaps of "*wanting* a child of *one's own*" are parts of the practice of IVF generally might be indicative of a further fact: that this objectifying attitude is *intrinsic* to the IVF procedure itself. This language suggests, though it does not prove, that *all* the embryos that are created are viewed as products—at least at the time of their creation—and have a kind of conditional status hovering over them: if they are not good enough, they will be discarded. And this would further suggest two related moral deficiencies in IVF: first, that the parents involved love their children, at least at their origins, only conditionally, and second, that they treat their children as things, something incompatible with respectful treatment of persons.

There is an obvious objection to the first of these claims, namely, that parents of IVF children clearly love them just as much as other parents love their children. But two points should be made in response. First, this claim is clearly false at the outset for at least those parents who create extra embryos and then choose which embryos to implant. *Those* parents' future love is conditional on both the grading and the selection, not just with respect to those embryos which in fact are eventually discarded, but with regard to all those that might be; and this might strike us as morally disturbing. Second, a morally problematic attitude towards, and treatment of, another human being at one stage of life does not make impossible, and can be quite compatible with, an improved attitude towards, and treatment of, that same person at another time. Huck Finn began his journey with Jim convinced that Jim was a "nigger," a nonperson; yet his attitude became sufficiently reformed through acquaintance with Jim that he eventually recognized the imperative to "humble himself" before Jim and apologize for his mistreatment of him. But Huck's eventual respect for Jim did not negate the moral wrongs of his initial mistreatment.

Intuitively, then, one might be led to wonder whether there is something intrinsic to IVF that inclines agents towards, or even necessarily involves, those agents treating their children as objects, even if only for some time, and in ways that can later be overcome. It is to this question that I now turn.

IV

In this section, I argue that to engage in IVF is to attempt to make a child, or at least to do something morally similar, in problematic ways, to making a child. I show further why this "making" attitude or approach is disrespectful of the child, and discuss what I take to be a complementary argument that takes the notion of "benefit" as its key concept. I then show in Section V how sexual reproduction in the context of married love is not disrespectful in the ways identified by the making and benefiting arguments, and is, on the contrary, a uniquely respectful way to bring children into the world. In Section VI, I raise some political questions about IVF; and in Section VII, I then very briefly discuss the morality of adoption, and of embryo adoption.

Why should we think that IVF is similar in relevant ways to the production of something? To answer, we first need to look at other contexts in which production is (typically permissibly) pursued.

Consider the inventor of something: Smith wants a better way of keeping time than observance of the sun, and he has recently been experimenting with gears and other devices. Thinking about the goal he wishes to pursue, that of accurate time keeping, and the materials at his disposal, he attempts to put the materials into such a shape as will enable him to be successful in accomplishing what he desires. Three points are worth noticing about what Smith does here, and his attitudes towards what he does.

First, Smith takes his engagement with the materials to be something he does in service to what he himself needs or wants, or, perhaps, in service of someone else's needs or wants. His activity is governed by a good that he seeks, and that good determines how he will engage the materials at hand, and also governs what will be considered a success in that engagement. Smith's activity is not for the sake of the material product itself, even when, as in the creation of a work of art, Smith (or others) will later take pleasure in the work of art itself; for even then, the work exists for the benefit of Smith and those others who will take (valuable) pleasure in it.

Second, Smith aspires for his labor with the materials to be *sufficient* for the eventual orientation of those materials towards his end. That is, Smith hopes to have a kind of mastery over the materials, eliminating as much as possible of luck or chance, and bringing the materials as much as possible under his control, so that those materials will, in their new configuration, do for him what he wants them to. Of course, sometimes Smith will work with others in the production of an artifact, and when he does so, he will not have the kind of control over those with whom he cooperates as he hopes to have over the materials; but collectively, all the agents working together will aspire to bring as complete a form of mastery over their materials as they can.

Third, and following from the first two points, when Smith's control fails—when the material has been too refractory, or his skill inadequate, or his plans flawed, and his materials are inadequate for his purposes, then, in principle, the product is, just so far forth, something to be discarded as a failure. Of course, what is a failure in one respect might be seen as a success in another, and thus kept, or it could be kept for sentimental reasons, or because nothing better is on the horizon. But disposability and replaceability are features of our treatment of what is made, for, as the first point noted, what is made is made as subject to our desires, and, as the second point noted, we aspire to subject our materials to our skills. When the materials are not so subjected, or our skills are deficient, and the product does not serve our needs, then the product is acceptable *only* insofar as there is no *more* successful product available to us.

Now, this description seems to characterize in various ways the creation of embryonic human beings through IVF. First, as in the production of artifacts, IVF begins with a problem that needs to be solved (infertility) or a desire that is otherwise going to go unmet (for a child), and takes that desire and problem as a sufficient reason for engaging in whatever process is suggested, with a view to solving the problem and satisfying the desire. As some have pointed out, in fact, there is really no *other* reason why one would want to engage in IVF—it has no meaning or value of its own, but has significance only as a solution.

Second, IVF involves an attempt to bring a kind of mastery—scientific, rather than, say, culinary or artistic—to a set of materials, in this case, the gametic materials of sperm and ovum. These materials must be treated in certain ways in order to be more serviceable—sperm must be artificially capacitated in order to allow them to penetrate the ovum's glycoprotein sheath, and oocytes must often be procured in greater number than usual by hyperstimulating the woman's ovaries; and then the technician attempts to exert as precise and exacting a form of control as possible over the materials to improve, to whatever degree possible, the chances of success. Researchers continue to hone these techniques, occasionally coming up with new breakthroughs, such as intracytoplasmic sperm injection (ICSI), by which a single sperm is inserted into the oocyte. And IVF clinics boast, through advertisements, of their relative success rates (an IVF researcher once told me, "I get women pregnant when their husbands can't").

Third, as we have discussed, failed, deficient, or even simply unwanted efforts at creating embryonic human beings are regularly discarded, artificially preserved, or made subject to lethal experimentation. Nor is this discarding limited to the pre-implantation stage of the embryo. IVF is subject to an unusually high degree of multiple births, not, primarily, because multiple embryos are implanted, but because IVF embryos appear to have a higher-than-usual rate of twinning. But, in cases in which there are *too many* embryos in a woman's womb, selective reduction—a form of targeted abortion—may be undergone to eliminate some of the extra embryos, which will, in at least some cases, be perfectly healthy and "normal."

So, there is a plausible case for the claim that parents involved in IVF (as well as any doctors and lab technicians that might be involved) are attempting to *make a child*. By why should this be thought problematic? And is it not the case that "making a child" is precisely what parents who deliberately procreate sexually are also doing? Does not the argument prove too much?

I will postpone the challenge about sexual procreation until the next section, and here discuss only the wrong of making a child, and, correspondingly, the wrong of treating a child as a product, as something to be made.

As has been clear, in making a product, the maker takes an attitude of supremacy over that product, an attitude that is related to the supremacy that he or she attempts to exert over the materials. Because the product is brought into existence because of some desires or problem of the artificer, the product's creation is subject to the will of the artificer at its origins; and because the product is so subject, it is further subordinate to the artificer's judgments regarding success or failure. But all such attitudes and judgments are inconsistent with treatment of embryonic human beings as our *equals*, that is, as equal to the artificer, and to all other human beings, in their personhood. To be treated as a product is to be treated as a thing, and things are, by their nature, nonpersonal. To treat a person as a thing is therefore implicitly to deny and act against the personhood of the person, in a way akin to the treatment of slaves, who were bought and sold as property. Moreover, this would appear to be true even if, in actual fact, the producers of the child break with the production paradigm at some point. So, parents who do *not* treat the resulting embryos as "gradeable" or disposable, because, for example, they recognize them as human persons, are thereby breaking from a pattern of subordination and instrumentalization of the embryonic human being, but this does not change the fact that they have *already* treated the child as a product to be made prior to this point.

There is likely to be some push-back against the notion that the parents of an IVF child thereby treat the child as subordinate to their desires, needs, or goals. Here is where the complementary argument can be helpful. The philosopher, Joseph Spoerl, has argued that, because the child-to-be does not exist prior to his or her creation in IVF, IVF therefore cannot be seen as of benefit to that child, for it does not bring the child from a worse to a better state—there simply was no child in a "worse" state prior to the IVF procedure (Spoerl, 2000). Claims of benefit to a person, in other words, can only be made of already-existing persons and are inapplicable to the situation in which a person begins to be.

If it is impossible to benefit the child who is being created in IVF, however, it is necessary to ask who *is* being benefited, for all action plausibly seeks to realize some good or benefit (else why would one act in the first place?). If not the child, then the most plausible answer is the parents: the child is being brought into being as a benefit to the parents (here we see an analogue to my first claim about making, above); the child is brought into being because the parents feel unfulfilled, or desire someone to love, and so on. But if all the benefit in creating the child is for the sake of the parents, then the child is being made, and hence being treated, as something whose existence is, at least in the choice to create, for the sake of another, namely the parents. And this is tantamount to saying that the child is being treated *merely* as a means to someone else's ends, a violation of the Kantian Categorical Imperative that one treat humanity, whether in one's own person or another, always as an end, and never merely as a means.

Now, surely, the second objection that I raised above comes back with a vengeance: if it is wrong to make a child or, more broadly, to bring a child into being for one's own ends (it being impossible to do so for the benefit of the child), then does this not also mean that sexual reproduction between spouses, many of whom engage in intercourse with a view to the possibility of a child, is equally wrong? In the next section, I address this difficulty.

V

Do parents who procreate sexually make a child? I will take for my paradigm case parents who are in the sort of loving marital relationship I described in Section I, parents who make a mutual commitment to a complete sharing of lives with one another, a sharing to be realized not just spiritually, say, but also physically, in the action of marital intercourse. Is what such a couple does, when their marital union is fruitful, and they bring forth new human life, a *production* of that child? And is their intercourse, when, say, it is planned to maximize their chances of conception, an attempt to make a child?

In most cases, I argue, the answer is negative. Consider for example, the lack of parallel to an attempted mastery of materials to serve one's ends. In the paradigm case, a loving couple engages in sexual intercourse to express and realize their love for one another. But this is something that they *do*;

they engage in an action that does not go out into some external material, as in the production of something but rather remains, in a sense, immanent in their persons. The distinction, which goes back to Aristotle, between acting and making seems very apt here. So far forth, then, there is a lack of parallel between the couple's actions and those of the IVF parents.

But do not loving couples often engage in intercourse precisely because they know that "the time is right," i.e., because they wish to have children and know that having intercourse today will likely be successful in bringing children about? Not quite: in the paradigm case, I suggest, it is reasonable for the couple to *hope* that their loving union will be fruitful; but it is wildly unrealistic for a couple to think that in engaging in sexual union, even at a most conducive time, they are thereby engaged in the production of their child; for the coming into being of that child is well out of their hands, once they have engaged in intercourse. "Making love" is quite unlike making a cake, and is very inaptly described as "making a baby," even though that is sometimes how we colloquially speak. A reasonable couple welcomes the possibility of a child coming to be as the fullest completion of their bodily union, but does not aspire to create that child.

Nevertheless, moral errors are possible here. Historically it has not been unknown for a man to take a wife in marriage, and then have sexual relations with her, precisely for the sake of bringing about an heir, to the family estate, or perhaps the throne. And perhaps this attitude of sexual intercourse precisely for the sake of a child is, and has been, taken by the woman who "wants a child" from this man; and perhaps the attitude could be taken by both parents. In any such case, there appears to be not just the deficient attitude towards the child described earlier in the discussion of IVF, but also a deficient attitude of one or both members of the couple towards the other, as their action with each other becomes better described as action *on* the other. Engaging in sexual relations precisely with a view to having a baby seems far from the paradigm case of marital love expressed and realized in sex.

If so, then while sexual intercourse between a couple *could* be engaged in with the same set of instrumentalizing attitudes characteristic of IVF, it *need* not be. Moreover, from a slightly different perspective, we can see precisely why being the fruit of marital intercourse is an especially apt way for a human being to come into existence, for such a human being comes to be as the fruit of the love of two human beings for one another, and as a result of the willingness of those loving beings to allow their physical realization of their love its greatest possible fulfillment. This seems to be a notably appropriate origin for a being of the profoundly special sort that human beings are.

VI

I have argued that IVF should not *morally* be an option for women; and that politically, *at least* considerable overhaul of the assisted reproduction industry is called for. Before turning at the end to the question of adoption and embryo adoption, it is worth addressing the political question of IVF as such; however, my treatment will be far from exhaustive, and indeed, rather tentative.

The political state exists, I believe, in large part for the protection of human persons from threats to their existence and well-being that they would otherwise be insufficient adequately to address themselves. The obligation of the state to step in on behalf of persons within its borders grows insofar as the threat to such persons is serious—particularly if the threat imperils their lives or bodily persons, and perhaps their property; and insofar as the threat can be addressed without disproportionate disruptions to the good of the individuals protected or the rest of the citizens of the state. So, minor threats to persons are often not significant enough to justify state intervention, and even more serious threats can be such that it is prudent for the state to take a hands-off approach if rectification of the situation would involve, for example, significant breaches of privacy.

Judged by these standards, to repeat, the case for radical overhaul of the assisted reproduction industry is very strong: currently, many hundreds of thousands of "spare" human embryos exist in cryopreservation, and many such embryos have been destroyed or used in experiments. The mandate of the state to protect persons requires that it intervene to stop such abuses. But the case is less clear if we are considering the possibility of a strongly regulated industry, one that does not create or destroy surplus embryos. Such circumstances exist, for example, in certain European countries. I have argued that even in these cases, the practice of IVF is disrespectful of the children conceived, and that would-be parents should not, accordingly, opt for this practice. The forms of disrespect present in IVF no doubt have some other negative consequences too, possibly leading to an increasingly instrumental view of the value of human life more broadly. Yet in the hypothetical situation under consideration, human embryos would not be destroyed or otherwise subjected to the indignities of cryopreservation and medical experimentation. It seems to me that the case for further intervention here is not as strong.

Nevertheless, I believe that the state should avoid in any way promoting IVF; and I believe that the state *could* reasonably decide to ban the procedure in an effort to witness the respect owed to human beings, including the respect owed at the origins of human life. But whether it is obligatory for the state to do so, in a deeply pluralistic culture, is difficult for me to say.

VII

One thing that I believe the state most definitely should do is to promote to a significant degree the practice of adoption by married couples, both by couples without and by couples with children. Adoption can be, as I suggested in Section I, one way for the love of a married couple to go forth into the world in a creative capacity, for in adoption, as I see it, the couple act through their love in such a way that something new comes into being: a child previously without a family becomes part of a family; having been without parents, he or she becomes the child—the son or daughter—of this particular couple. In this respect, the existence of the child as a son or daughter is, as it were, morally and even metaphysically parallel, and not less than, the sonship or daughtership of a child conceived as the fruit of marital love in sexual intercourse.

Seeing that this is the case—that the child becomes the son or daughter of the couple precisely through their marital love—is essential to correcting a potential misunderstanding about adoption. The error of IVF begins, arguably, with seeing infertility as a problem for which a solution is needed; the couple then turn to technology to generate the solution in the form of a child. Similarly, adoption too can be seen as a "solution" to the "problem" of infertility—it is just another *means*, perhaps less morally problematic in some ways—to address the frustrated desire on the part of the couple.

But frustrated desire is not the starting-point of love; nor should frustrated desire be conflated with the pain and sorrow that are possible as a result of infertility. That pain and sorrow can be not the result of frustrated desire—a loss of what one could *get*—but recognition of the loss of one possible, and tremendously valuable, way for one's love to *give*; for love, as I noted earlier, finds its expression in the bringing forth into the world of what is good. In Section I, I referred to the possibility of adoption as one way for love's orientation towards fecundity to adapt to its circumstances; but this is a very different thing than thinking of adoption as a way of fixing something that has gone wrong.

Thus, adoption is a very appropriate response to the tragedy of infertility, and so, I want to close by suggesting, is the more limited case of embryo adoption. In embryo adoption, a couple recognizes the need of a child, here at the embryonic stages of his or her life, for a family, for parents, and they undertake the action of adoption at a much earlier stage in the child's life than usual by transferring the unimplanted embryo into the woman's womb. Some moralists who are, as I obviously am, pessimistic about the morality of IVF are similarly dubious of the permissibility of embryo adoption, perhaps because they see the situation as that of the woman being made pregnant by someone other than her husband. But from the perspective just sketched, in embryo adoption a child becomes, through the love of *both* parents, the son or daughter of that couple. For couples whose love seeks to bring forth something new, whether they are biologically fertile or not, embryo adoption and more conventional forms of adoption go right in ways that embryo production through IVF does not.

References

George, R., & Tollefsen, C. (2008). *Embryo: A defense of human life*. New York: Doubleday.

Gergis, S., George, R., & Anderson, R. (2010). What is marriage? *Harvard Journal of Law and Public Policy, 34*, 245–287.

Moore, K., & Persaud, T. (2003). *The developing human*. New York: W. B. Saunders.

Spoerl, J. (2000). Making law on making babies: Ethics, public policy, and reproductive technology. *American Journal of Jurisprudence, 93*, 93–115.

Tollefsen, C. (2010). Divine, human, and embryo adoption: Some criticisms of *Dignitas personae*. *National Catholic Bioethics Quarterly, 10*, 75–85.

Reply to Tollefsen

Laura Purdy

Christopher Tollefsen concludes that, morally, IVF should not be an option for women. He also argues that the state should ban IVF procedures that produce embryos that will not be immediately implanted, and that it might not be unreasonable to ban IVF altogether.

Tollefsen's thoughtful argument for these conclusions owes much to natural-law thinking, and relies on a variety of additional premises and more recent expansions of that general tradition. Particularly crucial is the claim that embryos are human persons who should be treated with the same respect as any others. His position also owes a good deal to Leon Kass's concerns about nonsexual child production.

The argument proceeds roughly as follows. Tollefsen sees marriage as a commitment to completely sharing lives, and having children as the physical expression of that commitment at the physical level. Adoption, but not IVF, counts as fulfilling this commitment.

Why? In part, because IVF, as currently practiced in the US, creates many "surplus" embryos. Because embryos are human persons, they are seriously wronged by being frozen, destroyed, or used in research. This state of affairs could be remedied by ensuring that all embryos are implanted. But banning the creation of excess embryos would still not address the "instrumentalizing" attitudes towards embryos Tollefsen regards as intrinsic to IVF.

Tollefsen sees embryo creation as just another form of "production." "Production" necessarily aims at one's own satisfaction (or that of others), uses science and technology to achieve the desired product, and leads to discarding output regarded as unsuccessful. Thus, embryo creation necessarily leads parents—at least at the outset—to love their embryos only conditionally, and to treat their children as things, rather than as persons. This position is bolstered by the claim that children are not benefited by being brought to life via IVF: they did not exist before that, and so one cannot judge that they are better off now than they were before. Worse still, it follows that such children are created for their parents' sake, and thus are treated as mere means, anathema for any Kantian system of morality. Politically, it follows from all this that because the state has a serious obligation to protect humans' lives and welfare, at the very least it should ban the production of surplus embryos.

Any position based on this many assumptions and arguments could be vulnerable at many points, and space here is very limited. So, I will simply flag a few such vulnerable points, leaving a more comprehensive critique for another day.

One is the view that embryos have full moral status. Tollefsen relies on embryos' species membership, as well as what he argues is their capacity—albeit unrealized at this stage—for reason and self-consciousness.

Contemporary Debates in Bioethics, First Edition. Edited by Arthur L. Caplan and Robert Arp.

But one might wonder whether this position is speciesist, and whether potentiality is not being mistaken for capacity. In addition, to the extent that this is a position based in natural law, one might also wonder whether nature's rough treatment of embryos—ejecting up to 80% of them from women's uteruses before their time—signals anything about their intrinsic value.

Another is the claim that doing IVF necessarily has more in common with the production of tools and other goods than with making babies via sexual intercourse. I am simply unconvinced that the actions and intentions that count most here imply that embryos must necessarily be seen as products in the narrow sense alleged. If adoption is morally acceptable, despite the fact that the new family member was not created by loving sexual activity on the part of the couple, why not IVF, if the couple is focused on creating a child to love for its own sake? In any case, their attitudes and assumptions should be a matter for empirical research, not a priori argumentation. And, the work of researchers like Golombok showing that IVF families are doing well should trump such speculation.

The conclusion that IVF children are being used as mere means by their parents is equally unconvincing. For starters, it seems to prove too much, since, in its present form, it applies equally to children created the usual way. Tollefsen denies this objection, maintaining that sex—even if consciously aiming at conception—more centrally aims at expressing the couple's love. Thus, it is something they do, not just a means to having a child. After all, there are no guarantees that a given act of sex will in fact lead to conception.

But it is hardly clear why the fact that we have limited control over conception should be thought to make such a difference in the moral assessment of the act. Moreover, although it is wonderful when sex does express a couple's love, the reality is that most human sex surely fails to meet this exacting standard. One might thus wonder whether it makes sense to uphold it as the only morally acceptable sex, condemning the rest as morally deficient. Surely it would be better to keep our eye more directly on the ball, focusing on any resulting children's welfare—regardless of how they were brought to life—not to mention the satisfaction of the participants' aims (pleasure, bonding, children).

No liberal society would prevent those who see the world through something like Tollefsen's lens from creating their families accordingly. However, if his recommendations about IVF were to be implemented politically, those who do not share it would not be given similar latitude. Requiring all embryos to be implanted would probably increase the incidence of dangerous multiple pregnancies. A full ban would deprive many who would make excellent, loving parents of the opportunity to have children. Pluralistic societies must surely, other things being equal, offer their members the liberty to choose among competing philosophical ideals about sexual and reproductive morality. Of course, I have argued for fairly stringent limits on IVF myself, but those limits are intended to prevent immediate and objective harm. In my view, Tollefsen has not persuasively shown that IVF necessarily involves such harm.

Reply to Purdy

Christopher Tollefsen

I am impressed by Laura Purdy's honest assessment of IVF's flaws and failings. She rightly notes a number of ways in which IVF is bad for women, and bad for children; I agree with her that these failings are given insufficient attention, especially at the level of public policy. Moreover, I believe she points to an important cultural difficulty surrounding issues of infertility: our lack of imagination, in the face of the promises of science, in dealing with the difficulties of infertility. This lack of imagination encourages reliance on scientific fixes, while failing to attend sufficiently to the causes of the problem, some of which seem environmental or lifestyle related, or to alternative solutions, such as adoption or a childlessness lived in service to others.

Purdy and I disagree about some matters of principle, however, three of which I will simply mention here; a full accounting of the differences and a full engagement between the competing views and arguments are well beyond the scope of this brief comment.

The first concerns the desire for children. Purdy recognizes that this desire is something that has to be taken seriously by political philosophy, but she does not say much about it beyond simply specifying it as a very strong desire. Other things being equal, she writes, "it is morally good for desires to be satisfied."

I give a somewhat different account of the desire for children, as grounded in the marital commitment to the couple's complete sharing of lives; desire for children is a natural outgrowth of the desire that the one-flesh union that consummates that sharing of lives be fruitful. But this account has already narrowed the subject from the very broad "desire to have children" to something much more normatively focused: not all desires for children have equal moral standing on my normativized view, but only those that emerge from the marital union. I think these differences in our starting-points give rise to many interesting and important issues that should be explored in future work.

Second, Purdy and I disagree about the moral status of the embryonic human being. She writes that "the more we learn about biology," the clearer it is that my claims about the inherent worth of the embryo are "based on inaccurate information." Purdy cites at this point an essay by the very respected developmental biologist, Scott F. Gilbert, who has accused those who hold my view of subscribing to a "Syllabus of Errors" (Gilbert, 2008). However, as I have pointed out elsewhere, Gilbert's own *biological* work supports, in my opinion, the claim that the early embryo is fully a human being (Tollefsen, 2010); while the view that all human beings are inherently valuable is a claim of *ethics*, not biology. For Gilbert to lend his scientific authority to claims about "personhood" or "inherent value" is for him to abuse that authority.

Purdy herself points to the high rate of embryo loss as evidence that human life is not inherently valuable,

Contemporary Debates in Bioethics, First Edition. Edited by Arthur L. Caplan and Robert Arp.

but I see no sound inference here: high infant mortality rates historically, and continuing in some parts of the world today, give no evidence that the lives of infants are of less-than-inherent value. Similar inferential restraint should be the norm where embryo loss is concerned.

Third, Purdy and I disagree about both the nature and value of so-called "natural law" theory and reasoning. Purdy suggests that such reasoning infers values from nature, or from straightforwardly theological premises. But I agree that inferring values from facts is an instance of the "naturalistic fallacy," and that such a procedure is hugely faulty. I do make claims about values in my essay, of course: I hold, for example, that the union of shared lives characteristic of marriage is a good; and that the life of human persons is a good. I believe such claims are, at their deepest levels of meaning, not factual claims at all, but practical claims, orienting persons towards protection and promotion of such goods. Other goods too are picked out by such practical propositions: knowledge is a good to be pursued, as is friendship, as is personal integrity, for example. But human beings do not *infer* that these are goods to be pursued; they *recognize* that such goods offer genuine opportunities for betterment, for flourishing, and assent, at least in their practical lives, to the propositions in question.

It is then a crucial question whether some particular contemplated option for action really is such as only to promote and pursue goods, or whether it might not also, in some or all cases, be such as to damage or destroy such goods. The choice to end suffering by killing might promote the good of friendship, in some cases, but only by the intentional destruction of the good of human life. My natural-law approach thus rules out such a choice, though again, with no illicit inference from fact to value.

Moreover, my natural-law account holds that persons ought to exist in a form of community with other persons that recognizes and treats those persons *as* persons—as beings that can be fulfilled by human goods, and accordingly, as beings whose value must never be made instrumental or subordinate to our own. Thus, treating a person as a mere means only is, as Kant recognized, always wrong.

Thus, if my overall account of the wrong of IVF is misguided, it is not, I think, because of the naturalistic fallacy, but because I have wrongly understood marriage and human life to be basic human goods; or because I have wrongly analyzed the action of IVF as one of *making* a human being; or because I have wrongly identified the making of a human being as involving a wrongful treatment of a human person as a mere thing. All these claims are controversial, of course, and I have hardly done more than to suggest their plausibility; but I do believe they are true, and indeed, when fully defended, convincing.

References

Gilbert, S. F. (2008). When "personhood" begins in the embryo: Avoiding a syllabus of errors. *Birth Defects Research (Part C)*, *84*, 164–173.

Tollefsen, C. (2010). Incarnate reason and the embryo: A response to Dabrock. *Christian Bioethics*, *16*, 177–186.

Part 15
Are International Clinical Trials Exploitative?

Introduction

According to the US National Institutes of Health's (NIH) organization, ClinicalTrials.gov, a *clinical trial* (also known as an *interventional study*), is a "clinical study in which human participants are assigned to receive one or more interventions (or no intervention)—namely, drugs, medical devices, procedures, vaccines, and other products that are either investigational or already available—so that researchers can evaluate the effects of the interventions on biomedical or health-related outcomes" (CT, 2012). Beside the information that can be found at ClinicalTrials.gov, The NIH's Eunice Kennedy Shriver National Institute of Child Health & Human Development provides a simple and clear description of the clinical trial process in its "Steps Involved in Clinical Research Efforts" on its website at: http://www.nichd.nih.gov/health/clinical research/steps.cfm.

Exploitation refers to the act of using someone else to one's own advantage, gain, or pleasure with the one being exploited standing to be disadvantaged or harmed. Also, usually—though not always or necessarily—the one being exploited does not realize that the exploitation is occurring. This strikes many as straightforwardly immoral, with the further idea that in the exploitation, people are objectified—treated as mere instruments, tools, or objects—adding to the immorality (Wertheimer, 1999, 2008). During the Holocaust, in concentration camps such as Auschwitz, non-Nazis were exploited and objectified by Nazis for slave labor and experiments, and to create anatomical samples. Many of those who did not meet these fates—such as the elderly, the mentally handicapped, and the feeble—were killed using cyanide gas produced from Zyklon B pellets; then their hair was cut from their corpses for usage as industrial-spun felt and yarn, and their gold fillings were pulled from their teeth with pliers and melted down into gold bars (Lifton, 2000, p. 149; TNP, 2012). This is exploitation and objectification at its most egregious, and these activities horrify, stupefy, sicken, and anger us.

During and after the Nuremberg trials (1945–1946), where numerous Nazis were tried for a variety of atrocious crimes, the Nuremberg Code was devised and codified in response to the systematic abuse of human subjects in research. The Code includes basic biomedical principles related to clinical trials such as absence of coercion in recruiting subjects, the necessity of informed consent, nonmaleficence toward participants

Contemporary Debates in Bioethics, First Edition. Edited by Arthur L. Caplan and Robert Arp.

in experiments, and the correct formulation of a scientific protocol (Caplan, 1992; Emanuel et al., 2003, part II; Weindling, 2004; Schmidt & Frewer, 2007; Emanuel et al., 2011; NIH, 2011a, 2011b).

Human exploitation in the name of medicine and other sciences has occurred numerous times throughout human history (Moreno, 2000; Dresser, 2001; Goliszek, 2003; Guerrini, 2003; Hawkins & Emanuel, 2008; Millum & Emanuel, 2012). For example, the world learned in 1972 that, for 40 years, an experiment monitoring the effects of syphilis upon poor, rural, and illiterate African-American men—who, having been lied to by researchers, *thought* they were being treated for the disease but in fact were not—had been conducted by the US Public Health Service and Centers for Disease Control and Prevention. The Tuskegee Syphilis Experiment—so named because Tuskegee Institute was a willing participant—began as an observational study in 1932 with 600 African-American men, 399 with syphilis and 201 without the disease. In 1972, when the study became known through whistle-blowing in the media, 74 of the 600 men were still alive. Concerning the original 399 men with syphilis, 28 died of syphilis, and 100 died of syphilis-related complications, while 40 of their wives were infected with syphilis, and 19 of their children were born with syphilis (Jones, 1992; Reverby, 2009). What makes this experiment all the more insidious is the fact that, by 1945, penicillin was being mass-produced in the US to treat diseases like syphilis; the infected men in the experiment easily could have been treated after 1945, and many lives would have been saved as well as much pain and suffering avoided (Katz & Warren, 2011).

But the discovery of penicillin, unfortunately, led to further human exploitation. In 2011, a report titled, *Ethically Impossible: STD Research in Guatemala from 1946 to 1948*, was published by the US Presidential Commission for the Study of Bioethical Issues (USP, 2011). From 1946 to 1948, with the approval of the Guatemalan government, US medical officials infected some 5500 Guatemalan prisoners, mental patients, soldiers, and others with syphilis—without their consent—in order to study the effects of penicillin on the disease. At least 83 people died over the course of the experiments (DN, 2011). They were conducted during the time the Nuremburg trials were being prosecuted.

In response to the Tuskegee Syphilis Experiment as well as increased public awareness of other unethical experiments conducted in the US and in other countries (Beecher, 1966), in 1974 the National Research Act (Pub. L. 93–348) of the US established the National Commission for the Protection of Human Subjects of Biomedical and Behavioral Research (1974–1978), and in 1979 the Commission issued a landmark document for biomedicine or clinical research called, "The Belmont Report: Ethical Principles and Guidelines for the Protection of Human Subjects of Research." It was named "The Belmont Report" for the Smithsonian Institution's Belmont Conference Center (Elkridge, MD) where the Commission met in February of 1976 when first drafting the report (Childress et al., 2005; NIH, 2011b). The Belmont Report affirmed all of the basic bioethical principles found in the Nuremberg Code, as well as articulated other principles, including the principle of justice whereby "equals ought to be treated equally" (Emanuel et al., 2003, 2011).

If you thought that exploitation and objectification like that found in the Tuskegee and Guatemala experiments were a thing of the distant past, think again. In 1996, a meningitis epidemic in northern Nigeria killed upwards of 15,000 people, despite many having taken the anti-meningitis drug, ceftriaxone. During that time, the American drug company, Pfizer, sent a team to the city of Kano, Nigeria to test its new antibiotic, trovafloxacin (Trovan), on 100 children who already were severely ill with meningitis. At the Kano Infectious Disease Hospital, they monitored 200 children total, 100 who were given Trovan, and 100 who were given a deliberately lowered dose of ceftriaxone. Of the 100 children given trovafloxacin, five died, while six more who were given ceftriaxone died. There was the lack of proper consent from the families of the 200 children involved. Parents claimed that they did not realize their children were receiving an experimental treatment (Stephens, 2000; Wise, 2001; Macklin, 2004, pp. 99–101).

Many also questioned whether an epidemic is the appropriate time to perform a study, while meningitis specialist, Dr George McCracken, noted of the study: "I just wouldn't do a study that way myself. I know they (Pfizer's team) wanted to get the data. They wanted to go fast. They wanted to move ahead. I'm not sure they made a smart decision" (quoted in Stephens, 2000). The faster a company can recruit people to participate in a clinical trial, the faster the study can be completed; and the lower the cost of experimenting, the quicker drugs get approved and compete in the economic market. Pfizer spokesperson, Betsy Raymond, said of the study: "We had to move quickly. You would not be able to find those numbers of children with spinal meningitis in the US" (quoted in Stephens, 2000).

Even with informed consent and other kinds of mechanisms in place for revealing all of the potential risks involved in a clinical trial, many would argue that it is still possible to exploit and objectify a "willing" participant. It is not usually healthy, wealthy, educated folks who volunteer, or are recruited, for trials in the developing world—it is usually poor, uninsured, uneducated people whose choices truly are limited by their life's circumstances (Angell, 1997; Snibbe & Markus, 2005; Hughes, 2012; Snyder, 2012). And it is arguable that drug companies and researchers know this and are willing to utilize and perhaps exploit them. As Susan Perry (2010) has noted: "Clinical trials can still exploit study subjects, only the exploitation has taken a different form. Medical researchers may no longer be going out and intentionally making people sick, as they did in the Guatemala study (and in the infamous Tuskegee syphilis study), but they still can—and do—recruit vulnerable people (the uninsured, the poor) and often fail to give them adequate treatment while the subjects are in the trial."

Another issue raising concern about exploitation is that studies oftentimes are not for the benefit of the participants. Rather, the purpose can be to gather data and information that may eventually help others in more advantaged circumstances. "Sick people can't think of themselves as research subjects. They don't want to feel like they're being used as guinea pigs. They want to feel like patients," according to bioethicist and human-rights lawyer, George Annas; but the cold reality is that "they're not. They're guinea pigs" (Grady, 1999).

In the history of Western philosophy, we can point to two significant philosophical positions that act as the justification for why we should not exploit or objectify human beings: Kantian deontology and Millian utilitarianism/consequentialism.

Followers of Immanuel Kant (1724–1804) and his deontological moral philosophy ground moral decision-making in the fact that persons are conscious, rational beings, capable of their own free and informed decisions. In this sense, a person is a kind of sanctified being who not only has an innate worth and dignity that ought to be respected, but also must always be treated as an end in her/himself and never used as a means to some end. In other words, because they are conscious, rational beings, persons are precious in having an *intrinsic* value (as ends) and not an *instrumental* value (as a means to an end) like some object, tool, thing, or instrument (Kant, 1775–1789/1963, 1785/1998, 1797a/1996a, 1797b/1996b). From this perspective, morally right decisions are those decisions where a person is treated as an end, and morally wrong decisions are those where someone is treated as a mere instrument or means to an end (Hill, 1991; Korsgaard, 1996).

So, it would be immoral to use a person A as a means to further some end, goal, or purpose of another person B, since, by doing so, person A is reduced to the status of a mere object or thing to be used for person B's own purposes (O'Neill, 1990, 2008; Baron, 1999). For example, say some psychopath has a big bomb and will not blow up a city of 250,000 people on the one condition that his old eighth-grade teacher—whom the psychopath despises because he feels that the teacher is solely responsible for ruining his life—is brought out onto the steps of city hall and executed. A Kantian of this stripe would say that it would be immoral to execute the eighth-grade teacher, even if doing so meant saving the city folk, because the teacher would be used as an object to fulfill the needs of the psychopath as well as save the city (Dworkin, 1981; MacKinnon, 1988).

Followers of John Stuart Mill's (1806–1873) moral philosophy argue that an action is morally good insofar as its consequences promote the most benefit, pay-off, or pleasure for the most persons affected by the decision (Mill, 1861/2001; Singer, 1979; Scheffler, 1982, 1988; Scarre, 1996). This view has been termed *utilitarian* because of the apparent usefulness to be found in generating such a huge amount of satisfaction for the group of persons. In opposition to the Kantian view that persons never should be used as means to some end (however, see Garry, 1993; Madigan, 1998; Schwarzenbach, 1998), the utilitarian position may be used—though not necessarily—to justify the treating of persons as means to the greater good of achieving benefit for the majority. If the greater consequence of saving a group of 250,000 people from some evil-doer requires killing one, two, or even 100 people in the process, then, according to some utilitarians, this could be morally correct.

If consequences are the key to determining whether objectification is morally wrong, then we can see that treating persons as objects *as a general rule*—maybe not in isolated cases—has negative ramifications and, hence, is morally unacceptable. Think of all of the instances of slavery throughout human history where one group of persons has been subjugated by another group, and all of the negative consequences of such horrible situations. Or, think of all of the instances of totalitarian regimes, like Stalin's Soviet Union, Hitler's Third Reich, or Gaddafi's Libya, where persons were tortured, tormented, displaced from their homes, manipulated, and murdered all for the greater "good" of some state or ideology. Further, consider the consequences to our communities of treating women or men solely as sex objects, the way in which is done in pornography or advertising. Such objectification has been linked to violence against women, date rape, eating disorders, and a general disrespect for the sanctity of intimate relationships (Friedman, 1993; Barry, 1995; Dwyer, 1995; Andrew, 2001; Tessman, 2001; cf. Brake, 2003). Hence, on utilitarian grounds, one can argue that these forms of objectification are immoral and should be condemned *as a general rule*.

Consider again the example of the psychopath and his desire to have his eighth-grade teacher killed, or else he will blow up the city. If we gave into every psychopath's desire to kill his eighth-grade teacher, and people knew that there was a real possibility that they might be next to be used in situations like this or similar ones, then we would probably facilitate a community of paranoid, dysfunctional, and unstable individuals who are always "on the look out" so as not to get used or exploited. Such an environment is bad for the majority, so we would not want to facilitate it. Thus, because objectification of this sort would have negative consequences in our social interactions, it is immoral.

"Are poor people in developing countries being exploited in research for the benefit of patients in the developed world where subject recruitment to a randomized trial would be difficult?" This is a central question posed in a 2012 article by Amitav Banerjee and Clark Baker titled, "Ethical Concerns of the Study" (Banerjee & Baker, 2012). The first author in this section, Jamie Watson, thinks that it is likely that poor people in developing countries are being exploited. First, after considering various necessary and sufficient conditions for exploitation, Watson puts forward a definition: "An act by a morally competent person or group of persons, *A*, is wrongfully exploitative if and only if that act employs the behavior of a moral subject, *B*, in successfully obtaining *A*'s ends under circumstances in which *B* stands an unreasonable risk of losing something of fundamental value to *B*." Among other activities, "cases of coercion or deception are paradigm cases" of exploitation, according to Watson, "including fraud, slavery, armed robbery, lying for personal gain, and Ponzi schemes."

In the first paragraph of this introduction, it was noted that exploitation often goes hand in hand with a lack of awareness on the part of the person(s) being exploited. Beside the knowledge of health risks afforded to participants in a clinical trial—for example, direct effects and/or side effects of a drug—one of the reasons that informed consent is so vital in clincial trials is to minimize the possibility of researchers treating the participants like guinea pigs. "If a subject is not in a position to genuinely consent, either by lack of physical or mental capacity, or because complete information is withheld or biased, then in offering her admittance to the study, researchers are situating her such that she cannot reasonably refuse to participate, and thereby wrongfully exploiting her," claims Watson; and not only does he point to instances where researchers seem to have skirted consent altogether, but also he gives a couple of examples of studies where information was misunderstood by the participants. Given the nature of international trials, coupled with the fact that medical jargon is tough enough to understand in one's native language, it makes sense that important information would be "lost in translation" in communication from, for example, researcher X from Australia who speaks English to clinical trial participant Y from Nigeria who speaks Yoruba. Especially since we are usually talking about high-risk situations with international clinical trials, it is morally important to be extra attentive to communication issues.

Watson also mentions that researchers will often use a utilitarian, cost–benefit/pain–pleasure calculus in their moral considerations as to whether to run a study in a particular area of the world, or not, which seems sensible enough. Still, Watson warns: "Researchers can make informed judgments about treatments and outcomes, but subjects know their values. Therefore, presumably, researchers and test subjects must communicate in an atmosphere of mutual respect. Thus, any utilitarian calculation that does not take subjects' personal value assessments into consideration is likely to place those subjects at risk in ways they could not genuinely consent to accept and, therefore, is more likely to exploit them for what researchers take to be the *greater good*." Again, communication between researcher and participant is key here.

The second author in this section, Richard Arneson, urges that, "where informed consent really is beyond reach, because subjects cannot comprehend the contract that is being offered, nothing inherently precludes proxy consent from working effectively to safeguard the interests of these subjects." As a common example from clinical trials performed in third-world kinds of areas, Arneson notes: "the political system with its checks and balances operating in [a] village, or the virtue and wisdom of the chieftain, may well bring it about that she acts effectively as a trustee, and that this is manifest to the agents of the company conducting the research, so the study can be done without wrongfully exploiting participants."

Interestingly enough, Arneson hints that the picture of the huge, heartless drug corporation using, demeaning, and disrespecting the poor, helpless townspeople in the exploitative clinical trial is simplistic and stereotypical. Further than this, there are other regulators and checks at work to help minimize exploitation: "Customers of the medical firm can threaten to boycott its products if it engages in sleazy deals that take milk from the mouths of hungry babes in third-world countries. International ethical guidelines can be promulgated and enforced by treaty or international regulatory bodies or aggressive jawboning by nongovernmental organizations such as Doctors Without Borders. Media campaigns in host countries can target abusers of the weak and vulnerable. Governments in poor countries can establish regulations that offset the undeniable bargaining advantages of powerful corporations."

Arneson claims that his position is "resolutely" what is known as an *act-consequentialist* perspective. Whereas a rule consequentialist (or rule utilitarian) devises prima facie general laws/rules/principles based upon what brings about the greatest good/benefit/pleasure for the most people affected by a decision (the principle of utility, POU), an act consequentialist does not have general principles established already, but instead applies the POU on a case-by-case basis. In other words, for the act consequentialist, the POU is applied directly to particular actions under particular circumstances; for the rule consequentialist, the POU is used to establish the selection of a set of rules, which are then used to determine what to do in particular situations.

Thus, in polar opposition to Kantian deontology with its a priori set of principles that already place restrictions on actions *before* experiences, events, or circumstances in the real world even occur, Arneson maintains from his resolutely act consequentialist perspective that "any remotely credible view about deontological rules will have to allow that when the consequences of abiding by the rule are sufficiently bad, the rules should give way. So, for example, when it comes to exploitation, if the overall long-term consequences of what in a narrow view looks to be Tom's unfairly taking advantage of Randy are good enough, the presumption that what Tom is doing is morally wrong is overturned." The idea is something like this: if you are being exploited by someone, and eventually you benefit from the exploitation, then there is nothing morally problematic with this situation; yet, a Kantian morality would focus on the "unfairly taking advantage" part of the situation and condemn the exploitation before it even occurs, thus denying you the consequential benefit which is a good that ought to be pursued.

Further than this, Arneson maintains in his reply to Watson: "If I am duped or tricked into accepting a transaction that generously benefits me, and does not yield disproportionate benefit to other participants, I am not exploited." So, Arneson takes *ostensibly* immoral activities—"unfairly taking advantage" and "duping" and "tricking"—and shows how such activities can be made wholly moral from an act-consequentialist/

utilitarian perspective. In other words, who cares if you are being exploited, used, objectified, lied to, and the like, by some researcher, doctor, drug company, or whoever, as long as you—as well as the exploiters—stand to benefit in the end?

Near the end of his reply to Watson, Arneson leaves us with the following, which we can ponder with respect to bioethical decisions, or *any* applied ethical decision, really: "The moral rules we should accept, as rational agents, are the rules that in given circumstances would help us come closer in our conduct to the conduct that would bring about best outcomes (better lives for people, fairly distributed)."

References

Andrew, B. (2001). Angels, rubbish collectors, and pursuers of erotic joy: The image of ethical women. In P. DesAutels & J. Waugh (Eds.), *Feminists doing ethics* (pp. 119–134). Lanham, MD: Rowman and Littlefield.

Angell, M. (1997). Editorial: The ethics of clinical research in the Third World. *The New England Journal of Medicine, 337*, 847.

Banerjee, A., & Baker, C. (2012). Ethical concerns of the study. *WebmedCentral: Bioethics, 3*, 9–15.

Baron, M. (1999). *Kantian ethics almost without apology*. Ithaca, NY: Cornell University Press.

Barry, K. (1995). *The prostitution of sexuality*. New York: New York University Press.

Beecher, H. (1966). Ethics and clinical research. *New England Journal of Medicine, 274*, 1354–1360.

Brake, E. (2003). Sexual objectification and Kantian ethics. *Proceedings and Addresses of the American Philosophical Association, 76*, 120–131.

Caplan, A. (Ed.). (1992). *When medicine went mad: Bioethics and the Holocaust*. Totowa, NJ: Humana Press.

Childress, J., Meslin, E., & Shapiro, H. (Eds.). (2005). *Belmont revisited: Ethical principles for research with human subjects*. Washington, DC: Georgetown University Press.

CT (ClinicalTrials.gov). (2012). Glossary of common site terms. Retrieved from: http://clinical trials.gov/ct2/about-studies/glossary#interventional-study

DN (Democracy Now). (2011). As grim details emerge, Guatemalan victims seek justice for US medical experiments in 1940s. *Democracy Now*, August 31. Retrieved from: http://www.democracynow.org/2011/8/31/as_grim_details_emerge_guatemalan_victims

Dresser, R. (2001). *When science offers salvation: Patient advocacy and research ethics*. Oxford: Oxford University Press.

Dworkin, A. (1981). *Pornography: Men possessing women*. New York: Perigee Press.

Dwyer, S. (1995). *The problems of pornography*. Belmont, CA: Wadsworth.

Emanuel, E., Crouch, R., Arras, J., Moreno, J., & Grady, C. (Eds.). (2003). *Ethical and regulatory aspects of clinical research: Readings and commentary*. Baltimore, MD: Johns Hopkins University Press.

Emanuel, E., Grady, C., Crouch, R., Lie, R., Miller, F., Wendler, D. (Eds.). (2011). *The Oxford textbook of clinical research ethics*. Oxford: Oxford University Press.

Friedman, M. (1993). *What are friends for? Feminist perspectives on personal relationships and moral theory*. Ithaca, NY: Cornell University Press.

Garry, A. (1993). Pornography and respect for women. In J. Arthur (Ed.), *Morality and moral controversies: Readings in moral, social and political philosophy* (pp. 395–421). Upper Saddle River, NJ: Prentice-Hall.

Goliszek, A. (2003). *In the name of science: A history of secret programs, medical research, and human experimentation*. New York: St. Martin's Press.

Grady, D. (1999). Patient or guinea pig: Dilemma of clinical trials. *The New York Times*, January 5. Retrieved from: http://www.nytimes.com/1999/01/05/science/patient-or-guinea-pig-dilemma-of-clinical-trials.html?pagewanted=all&src=pm

Guerrini, A. (2003). *Experimenting with humans and animals: From Galen to animal rights*. Baltimore, MD: The Johns Hopkins University Press.

Hawkins J., & Emanuel, E. (Eds.). (2008). *Exploitation and developing countries: The ethics of clinical research*. Princeton, NJ: Princeton University Press.

Hill, T. (1991). *Autonomy and self respect*. New York: Cambridge University Press.

Hughes, R. (2012). Individual risk and community benefit in international research. *Journal of Medical Ethics, 38*, 626–629.

Jones, J. (1992). *Bad blood: The Tuskegee syphilis experiment*. New York: The Free Press.

Kant, I. (1775–1789/1963). *Lectures on ethics* (L. Infield, Trans.). Indianapolis, IN: Hackett Publishing.

Kant, I. (1785/1998). *Groundwork of the metaphysics of morals* (M. Gregor, Trans.). (Section I: Transition from common rational to philosophic moral cognition). Cambridge: Cambridge University Press.

Kant, I. (1797a/1996a). *Practical philosophy* (M. Gregor, Trans.). Cambridge: Cambridge University Press.

Kant, I. (1797b/1996b). *The metaphysics of morals* (M. Gregor, Trans.). Cambridge: Cambridge University Press.

Katz, R., & Warren, R. (Eds.). (2011). *The search for the legacy of the USPHS syphilis study at Tuskegee*. Lanham, MD: Lexington Books.

Korsgaard, C. (1996). *The sources of normativity*. New York: Cambridge University Press.

Lifton, R. (2000). *The Nazi doctors: Medical killing and the psychology of genocide*. New York: Basic Books.

MacKinnon, C. (1988). *Feminism unmodified: Discourses on life and law*. Cambridge, MA: Harvard University Press.

Macklin, R. (2004). *Double standards in medical research in developing countries*. Cambridge: Cambridge University Press.

Madigan, T. (1998). The discarded lemon: Kant, prostitution and respect for persons. *Philosophy Now*, *21*, 14–16.

Mill, J. S. (1861/2001). *Utilitarianism*. Indianapolis, IN: Hackett Publishing Company.

Millum, J., & Emanuel, E. (Eds.). (2012). *Global justice and bioethics*. Oxford: Oxford University Press.

Moreno, J. (2000). *Undue risk: Secret state experiments on humans*. London: Routledge.

NIH (National Institutes of Health). (2011a). *Trials of war criminals before the Nuremberg military tribunals under control council law no. 10, vol. 2*, pp. 181–182. Washington, DC: US Government Printing Office, 1949. Retrieved from: http://ohsr.od.nih.gov/guide lines/nuremberg.html

NIH (National Institutes of Health). (2011b). The Belmont report: Ethical principles and guidelines for the protection of human subjects of research, April 18, 1979. Retrieved from: http://ohsr.od.nih.gov/guidelines/belmont.html.Perry, S. (2010). *MinnPost*, October 14. Retrieved from: http://www.minnpost.com/second-opinion/2010/10/too-many-clinical-trials-still-exploit-poor-and-other-vulnerable-people-says-

O'Neill, O. (1990). *Constructions of reason: Explorations of Kant's practical philosophy*. Cambridge: Cambridge University Press.

O'Neill, O. (2008). Kant and utilitarianism contrasted. In J. Arthur & S. Scalet (Eds.), *Morality and moral controversies: Readings in moral, social and political philosophy* (pp. 40–45). New York: Pearson.

Perry, S. (2010). *MinnPost*, October 14. Retrieved from: http://www.minnpost.com/second-opinion/2010/10/too-many-clinical-trials-still-exploit-poor-and-other-vulnerable-people-says-

Reverby, S. (2009). *Examining Tuskegee: The infamous syphilis study and its legacy*. Chapel Hill: The University of North Carolina Press.

Scarre, G. (1996). *Utilitarianism*. London: Routledge.

Scheffler, S. (1982). *The rejection of consequentialism*. Oxford: Clarendon Press.

Scheffler, S. (Ed.). (1988). *Consequentialism and its critics*. Oxford: Oxford University Press.

Schmidt, U., Frewer, A. (Eds.). (2007). *History and theory of human experimentation: The Declaration of Helsinki and modern medical ethics*. New York: Franz Steiner.

Schwarzenbach, S. (1998). On owning the body. In J. Elias, V. Bullough, V. Elias, & G. Brewer (Eds.), *Prostitution: On whores, hustlers, and johns* (pp. 345–351). Amherst, NY: Prometheus Books, 1998.

Singer, P. (1979). *Practical ethics*. Cambridge: Cambridge University Press.

Snibbe, A., & Markus, H. (2005). You can't always get what you want: Educational attainment, agency, and choice. *Journal of Personality and Social Psychology*, *88*, 703–720.

Snyder, J. (2012). Exploitations and their complications: The necessity of identifying the multiple forms of exploitation in pharmaceutical trials. *Bioethics*, *26*, 251–258.

Stephens, J. (2000). Where profits and lives hang in the balance: Finding an abundance of subjects and lack of oversight abroad, big drug companies test offshore to speed products to market. *The Washington Post*, December 17. Retrieved from: http://www.washingtonpost.com/wp-dyn/content/story/2008/10/01/ST2008100 101390.html

Tessman, L. (2001). Critical virtue ethics: Understanding oppression as morally damaging. In P. DesAutels & J. Waugh (Eds.), *Feminists doing ethics* (pp. 79–99). Lanham, MD: Rowman and Littlefield.

TNP (The Nizkor Project). (2012). The trial of German major war criminals: Sitting at Nuremberg, Germany 29th July to 8th August 1946. Retrieved from: http://www.nizkor.org/hweb/imt/tgmwc/tgmwc-20/tgmwc-20-195-08.shtml

USP (US Presidential Commission for the Study of Bioethical Issues). (2011). *Ethically impossible: STD research in Guatemala from 1946 to 1948*. Retrieved from: http://bio ethics.gov/cms/sites/default/files/Ethically-Impossible_PCSBI.pdf

Weindling, P. (2004). *Nazi medicine and the Nuremberg trials: from medical war crimes to informed consent*. New York: Palgrave Macmillan.

Wertheimer, A. (1999). *Exploitation*. Princeton, NJ: Princeton University Press.

Wertheimer, A. (2008). Exploitation. *The Stanford Encyclopedia of Philosophy*. Retrieved from: http://plato.stanford.edu/entries/exploitation/

Wise, J. (2001). Pfizer accused of testing new drug without ethical approval. *British Medical Journal*, *322*, 194.

Chapter Twenty Nine

Clinical Trials Are Inherently Exploitative

The Likelihood That They Are Is High

Jamie Carlin Watson

I will offer a set of conditions minimally necessary and sufficient for wrongful exploitation and argue that, while international clinical trials are not inherently wrongfully exploitative, problems with informed consent, the prevalence of misapplied moral theories among researchers, and the weakness of human moral motivation make it likely that any particular international clinical trial is wrongfully exploitative.

Introduction

The term *exploitation* is often used in politically charged contexts to incite public outrage against some behavior that the inciter finds offensive (e.g., Walker, 2011). Some argue that college athletics programs exploit their athletes, since players' compensation (college tuition) is far outstripped by the schools' proceeds (e.g., Associated Press, 2007; Taylor, 2010). Similarly, some argue that surrogate motherhood should be legally prohibited because such a contract would inevitably be exploitative. The difficulty, of course, is that very few writers explain what they mean by *exploitation*, which makes it difficult to justify such claims. And until recently, moral philosophers have expended little ink to identify precisely what constitutes an exploitative act. Whether any of the above cases is actually exploitative and, if so, whether these instances of exploitation are morally impermissible depend on the plausibility of the account of exploitation invoked. Thus, to evaluate whether international clinical trials are wrongfully exploitative, we will need a plausible account of wrongful exploitation.

As with many philosophical concepts, I take it that the most efficient method of discovering or constructing an adequate account of exploitation involves testing hypothesized necessary and sufficient conditions against rational intuitions about counterexamples. Nevertheless, a review of the current literature reveals that there is widespread disagreement over the necessary and sufficient conditions for wrongful exploitation. Some regard wrongful exploitation as a primarily economic term, referring to a particular type of relationship between workers and rulers in a society. Others argue that it requires some sort of harm, or rights violation, or coercion. Some have even rejected the idea that there is a single set of necessary and sufficient conditions and that some types of

Contemporary Debates in Bioethics, First Edition. Edited by Arthur L. Caplan and Robert Arp.

wrongful exploitation may be incommensurable with others. For instance, Alan Wertheimer (1999, 2008) suggests that wrongful exploitation may be analyzed along a number of mutually exclusive dimensions, for instance, exploitation that is consensual or nonconsensual, volitional or nonvolitional, or identified by outcome or process.

Unfortunately, there is not space here to swim these waters deeply. Rather than address these disagreements directly, I will begin with Mikhail Valdman's (2009) important recent analysis of wrongful exploitation, and I will highlight what I take to be its strengths and deficiencies. In response to these deficiencies, I will offer what I take to be a set of minimally necessary and sufficient conditions for wrongful exploitation that capture the intuitions that Valdman's and others have attempted to isolate, while providing a framework for adapting to various dimensions of an action, such as those noted by Wertheimer. The result suggests a way of unifying our intuitions about wrongful exploitation and provides a standard against which to evaluate whether international clinical trials are wrongfully exploitative. In the second half of this chapter, I offer three lines of evidence to show that it is *highly likely* that any particular international clinical trial meets the conditions for wrongful exploitation.

Exploitation and Valdman's Position

Traditional Western usage of *exploitation* suggests, at the very least, *the use of one person by another for the latter's benefit*. And it seems intuitive that, in its broadest sense, exploitation need not imply moral impermissibility. For instance, hiring employees, directing volunteers, and building houses all fall within the scope of colloquial phrases such as "exploiting resources" and "exploiting advantages" without implying, even prima facie, negative moral implications. As such, these are not the instances of exploitation with which we are primarily concerned. We want to know what constitutes *morally impermissible*, or *wrongful*, exploitation.

An analysis of wrongful exploitation cited widely in the biomedical literature comes from Alan Wertheimer (1999): *A* exploits *B* when *B* receives an unfair level of benefits as a result of *B*'s interactions with *A* (Emanuel et al., 2000, 2004; AAAS Policy Forum, 2002). This analysis has two conditions: (1) *A* interacts with *B*, and (2) an unfair level of benefit to one party is a result of this interaction. Though this analysis is fairly clear and captures some of our intuitions about wrongful exploitation, it is somewhat unfortunate that it is cited so widely; Wertheimer uses this analysis only as a starting-point for a more rigorous discussion of exploitation, and to see why, we need only consider an example.

Consider that most cases of buyer's remorse meet both conditions. If *B* purchases object *X* from *A* and, subsequently, *B* decides that *X* is not really worth the amount that he paid, *B* now perceives that *A* has received an unfair level of benefit from the transaction. There are at least two problems here: one with the temporal relationship between the transaction and the feeling of unfairness, and one of determining what counts as "unfair." Presumably, irrespective of temporal considerations, if a transaction is voluntary, both parties value what they receive more than what they are giving up—I am willing to sell my iPod to you for $100 because I value your $100 more than my iPod, and vice versa (and this explains why both parties can say, "Thank you."). But few would regard buyer's remorse as an instance of exploitation, wrongful or otherwise. This case suggests that this account lacks the sophistication we need to adequately identify instances of wrongful exploitation.

An alternative starting-point is Mikhail Valdman's (2009), "A Theory of Wrongful Exploitation." Valdman asks us to consider what he calls the *Antidote Case*: "Person *B* is bitten by a rare poisonous snake while hiking in a remote forest. His death is imminent. Fortunately, another hiker, *A*, happens by and offers to sell *B* the antidote. . . . Though it retails for $10, *A* insists that he will accept no less than $20,000. Since *B* would rather lose his money than his life, he accepts *A*'s offer (p. 3)." According to Valdman, not only is this a case where, "*A* wrongly exploited *B*," but, "Indeed, this is about as clear a case of wrongful exploitation as I can imagine. If some theory suggested otherwise, I would take that as evidence against it" (p. 3). Valdman argues that *A*'s offer is wrongfully exploitative because *A* "extracts excessive benefits from someone who cannot, or cannot reasonably, refuse one's offer" (p. 9).

His analysis includes three conditions that, combined with a circumstance in which *A* uses *B*'s behavior for his own gain, are sufficient for *wrongful* exploitation: (1) *B*'s urgent need; (2) *A*'s monopoly power; and (3) *A*'s excessive benefit. Thus, the Antidote Case is wrongfully exploitative because *A* uses *B*'s behavior for his own gain in conditions where (1) the antidote is something that *B urgently needs*, (2) *A* holds *monopoly power* over the antidote, such that *B* is not in a position to "reasonably refuse" any offer *A* makes, and (3) *A* exacts *excessive benefit* from *B* in charging him $20,000 rather than the market rate of $10.

While I ultimately agree with Valdman that this is an instance of wrongful exploitation, I am skeptical of his analysis. I take it, first, that condition (1) is irrelevant. Unless you are a certain type of consequentialist (à la Peter Singer and Peter Unger), *need* alone, even *urgent need*, does not establish a moral obligation that someone meet that need. And even if a refusal to meet some types of need is immoral, it is not clear that such a refusal meets conditions sufficient for wrongful *exploitation*. We can see this clearly with a slight modification of the case, in which *A*, who still has the antidote in his possession, thinks it likely that he will need the antidote soon, either for himself or for a member of his family. If he thinks the likelihood high enough, he might reasonably decide to refuse to give or sell the antidote to *B*. In this case, *A* refuses to sell or give *B* what *B* urgently needs, and *A* holds monopoly power over *B*, and yet it would be inappropriate to say that *A exploits B*. And Valdman agrees that "an obligation not to wrongly exploit is different from an obligation to rescue" (p. 12). Therefore, by "urgent need," he must mean something other than *desperate* or *vital* need. And, in fact, *B*'s need seems relevant only insofar as *B*'s *death* is an *unreasonable* option *for B* in the contract offered by *A*, so that *B* cannot reasonably refuse any offer. But this points us away from need and toward condition (ii).

Condition (ii) is more intuitive but, I think, misdirected except as it relates to *B*'s ability to reasonably refuse. Hold fixed *B*'s urgent need, but consider a modification in which another hiker, also with the antidote, approaches, learns of the situation, and offers to sell hers to *B* for only $15,000. This removes *A*'s monopoly on the antidote. And, if one additional antidote-seller is not enough, increase the number as much as you like until you are confident that there is no longer a "monopoly" on the antidote. Presumably, none of these competitors would sell it for $10, given its worth *to B* at that particular moment. And yet something about this bidding war strikes us as "unfair" to *B*. Therefore, *that* someone holds monopoly power does not add any force to a case of putative exploitation. More plausibly, the worry about *A*'s offer stems from the fact that *B* cannot reasonably refuse *A*'s—or any number of other vendors'—offer. I will return to the ability to reasonably refuse below.

Further, Valdman's condition (iii)—that *A* extracts excessive benefit from *B*—seems unnecessary because it depends on the implausible assumption that there are objective normative standards of exchange value by which to evaluate the permissibility of transactions. In this case, Valdman assumes there is some *objective* truth about what the antidote is *worth* independently of any consideration of *B*'s interests (cf. Snyder, 2008, 2012). But value transactions (e.g., monetary exchanges, barter exchanges, companionship, love, etc.) are not conducted according to *objective* standards of value; they are conducted according to *subjective*, consumer standards of value. The fact that most people are not *willing to pay* more than $10 for the antidote does not mean it is not *worth* vastly more *to B* in these circumstances. We can imagine some piece of sci-fi memorabilia that is not worth a dollar to most people, but for which some eager fan is willing to pay a large sum. In that case, we would not say the seller has exploited the fan. (Valdman seems to agree with this point, as indicated by an example he offers of a stamp collector willing to pay an exorbitant rate for a stamp in advance of its official release.) The seller has no *obligation to sell* the item at all, much less for some "objectively" determined normative value. Similarly, if *B* has no money whatsoever, even $10 is "excessive," since it is physically impossible for him to pay it. Thus, whether the demanded price is "excessive" can only be determined by the consumer. Absent other considerations, *A* is merely acting prudently. Therefore, contra Valdman, it is implausible that a theory of wrongful exploitation depends on a case's meeting such a condition. Incidentally, Valdman argues that, without condition (3), the Antidote Case is no longer exploitative. In a modification of the Antidote Case where *A* offers *B* the antidote for $10, Valdman writes,

"… surely *A* did not wrongly exploit *B*. Indeed, here it seems that *A* didn't even wrong *B*" (p. 12).

So, if the Antidote Case really is wrongfully exploitative, but none of Valdman's conditions are independently or jointly sufficient for wrongful exploitation, what accounts for the wrongness of *A*'s offer to *B*? It is now time to consider the previous suggestion that it is *B*'s inability to reasonably refuse *A*'s offer. As with "excessive benefit," saying precisely what is "reasonable" is tricky; all sorts of conditions may undermine our abilities to reasonably refuse a contract without broaching wrongful exploitation. A car salesman may be able to take far greater advantage of me than my father. But I have not been wrongfully exploited when I have bought cars; I have simply lacked the requisite virtue of fortitude for pursuing my interests. Nevertheless, there seem to be some unambiguous cases in which it would not be my fault that I could not enter appropriately into a contract, particularly cases where I would stand an *unreasonable risk of losing something of fundamental value.* Recall that, if *B* is destitute, *A*'s charging *B* $10 for the antidote is as inappropriate as *A*'s demand of $20,000. We may note, similarly, that $20,000 would not seem inappropriate or excessive if *B* were extremely wealthy. Therefore, what seems relevant to wrongful exploitation is not *A*'s excessive benefit, or *A*'s monopoly over the antidote, or *B*'s mere need, or any combination of the three, but *B*'s *risk of excessive loss*, as determined by *B*'s subjective assessment of his values.

Thus, Valdman's intuitions about "urgent need" and "monopoly power" can be captured more plausibly by a condition that a responsible agent cannot reasonably reject a contract, where the inability to reasonably reject means that the agent perceives that he stands an unreasonable risk of losing something he considers fundamentally valuable (e.g., his life, the lives of his family, his religious commitments, his financial stability, etc.). In the Antidote Case, if *B* is like many of us in that he is not very wealthy, *B* stands a 100% chance of losing something he considers of fundamental value: if he refuses the offer, he will lose his life; if he accepts the offer, he will lose his financial stability. Since it is likely that *B* perceives either choice as an unreasonable risk, any contract that *A* enters with *B*, apart from brute charity (which may be wrongfully exploitative for other reasons), is wrongfully exploitative.

This subjective condition allows responsible agents to enter into employment contracts as firemen or soldiers without the spectre of wrongful exploitation. Similarly, in cases where a corporation opens a plant in a rural third-world country, workers are wrongfully exploited only if they accept an agreement that, *to them*, constitutes an unreasonable risk of losing something of fundamental value (life or health in return for insufficient financial return).

So far, I have attempted to show that intuitions that the Antidote Case is wrongfully exploitative are not supported by considerations stemming from the particular amount *A* is charging *B* (there is no objective standard of value), *A*'s monopoly over the antidote (we would think it exploitative even if *A* were not the only vendor), or *A*'s obligation to rescue *B* from death (even if refusing is immoral, it is not obviously exploitative). What *does* seem relevant is that *B* is in *a position in which he cannot reasonably refuse* any offer *A* is willing to make. *B*'s life is on the line, so it may be that the stakes are too high for him to enter competently into an exchange of value (money for life) with *A*, irrespective of who else is selling, and regardless of any particular price. If this is right, *B* lacks the requisite capacity to enter into a morally binding contract with *A*. Thus, in order to avoid wrongful exploitation, it would seem that *A* is morally obligated either to withhold the antidote or to give *B* the antidote for free.

The ability to reasonably refuse an offer is closely related to the capacity to *consent* to a morally binding agreement. By "the capacity to consent," I mean that a subject, *S*, has both the autonomy and the rational ability to enter into a contractual relationship with another agent similarly situated. By "rational ability," I mean the ability to draw reliable inferences from information relevant to *S*'s decisions regarding the pursuit of her values. We restrict children and the severely mentally handicapped from driving and owning firearms on the grounds that they are not in a position to understand the moral implications of their decisions and are, therefore, not morally responsible for their actions. The ability to reasonably refuse a morally binding agreement entails the capacity to consent. Thus, if someone (a child, coma patient, etc.) lacks the ability to consent, she also lacks the ability to reasonably refuse an offer. This relationship is, however, asymmetric. Someone may lack the ability to reasonably refuse an offer, yet have the ability to consent more generally (e.g., a victim of fraud, Valdman's snakebite victim). All of this implies that not committing wrongful exploitation requires that *A* knows something of *B*'s values prior to offering a voluntary exchange.

Given these considerations, I propose the following analysis of what I will call a set of minimally necessary and sufficient conditions for wrongful exploitation, or Minimally Wrongful Exploitation (MWE): An act by a morally competent person or group of persons, *A*, is wrongfully exploitative if and only if that act employs the behavior of a moral subject, *B*, in successfully obtaining *A*'s ends under circumstances in which *B* stands an unreasonable risk of losing something of fundamental value to *B*.

I take it that wrongful exploitation occurs only in instances where *A successfully* obtains his ends at *B*'s unreasonable expense. Instances where other conditions are met but *A* is unsuccessful constitute *attempted* wrongful exploitation, which may have similar moral implications to actual wrongful exploitation. Further, an "unreasonable risk of losing something of fundamental value to *B*" is an epistemic condition (hereafter, URLV). To avoid wrongful exploitation, *A* must be justified in believing that *B* has the ability to reasonably refuse a morally binding contract, and *B* must agree. In the Antidote Case, for example, under the putatively normal circumstances in which *B* is not wealthy, *A* has independent reasons for believing that, if he were to charge $20,000 for the antidote, *B* stands a URLV. *A* would have these reasons irrespective of what *B* says under duress.

MWE implies that some acts are wrongfully exploitative, even when consistent with *B*'s ends, for instance, when some child performers are paid handsomely for exploitative performances. MWE rules out wrongful exploitation in cases where a subject is offered an opportunity that merely constitutes a risk of losing something *B* perceives to be of fundamental valuable, either for the sake of other values or out of a sense of self-sacrifice. Instances of this may include volunteering for charity organizations, or working as a police officer or emergency medical technician, where a subject is often called to aid strangers in dangerous circumstances.

To be sure, one or more of these conditions may need to be expanded to accommodate more complicated cases. Nevertheless, MWE accounts for most intuitive cases of wrongful exploitation. Cases of coercion or deception are paradigm cases, including fraud, slavery, armed robbery, lying for personal gain, and Ponzi schemes. It also includes, somewhat less intuitively, many violations of intellectual property law, including nonconsensual plagiarism. In addition, cases of factory "sweatshop" labor, an oft-decried example of putative exploitation, meet the conditions for MWE if the workers are enslaved or sexually abused, or have their wages withheld. Further, even in cases where these other conditions are not present, if factory workers perceive that they have *nothing of value* to offer in exchange for pursuing their interests other than *their labor in a particular factory*, such that their livelihoods depend on it and they cannot reasonably refuse the offer of a job, then the factory owners are wrongfully exploiting them. Similarly, surrogacy is wrongfully exploitative if and only if the surrogacy contract implies that one party stands a URLV.

The challenge, now, is to evaluate international clinical trials in light of MWE. In the next section, I will briefly review some of the motivations for conducting research in places other than researchers' home countries and the conditions under which research is conducted in them, and I will then show that these lead to a high likelihood of wrongfully exploitative behavior.

The Motivation for International Clinical Trials

In first-world countries, researchers seem to have access to an ample number of willing research participants. So, why conduct clinical trials in countries outside researchers' own, especially in developing, third-world countries? A survey of the literature reveals two primary reasons. First, some diseases for which researchers are seeking treatment affect people in higher concentrations in developing countries. For example, on the continent of Africa, approximately 22.9 million adults and children are infected with AIDS, compared to only 1.5 million in North America

(WHO, 2009). Similarly, in 2009 the incidence rate of tuberculosis in Zimbabwe was 742, and in the Asian country of Timor-Leste, the rate was calculated at 498. In stark contrast, in the same year in the US, the incidence rate of tuberculosis was only 4.1 (WHO, 2011). By conducting trials in areas with higher concentrations of affected people, research can be conducted more efficiently than is possible in researchers' home countries, which then decreases the amount of time it takes for a new discovery to be introduced into the market, thereby increasing the profits of the researching agencies and more quickly alleviating much suffering around the world.

A second motivation for international clinical trials is that government regulations in some countries are less restrictive than in researchers' home countries. For example, Lurie and Wolfe (1997, 2007) claim that researchers often choose test groups in undeveloped or developing countries precisely to avoid the restrictions of guidelines established to prevent immoral actions. Whether this is morally worrisome depends, of course, on whether these guidelines are appropriately aimed at the morality of actions or whether they are overly broad cautions. We know that policy makers are no better than anyone else at determining the moral permissibility of certain types of research, and we know that most regulations are too broad and too narrow to capture all the cases intended. In one case, for instance, a WHO guideline mandates that researchers from one country apply the same stringent standards to their research in a foreign country as they do in their own: "An external sponsoring organization and individual investigators should submit the research protocol for ethical and scientific review in the country of the sponsoring organization, and the ethical standards applied should be no less stringent than they would be for research carried out in that country" (WHO, 2002).

Yet, there are sometimes moral reasons for seeking countries with fewer restrictions than researchers' own. For instance, if regulations in researchers' home countries restrict research organizations from pursuing treatments that, to the best estimate of the researchers, present no foreseeable dangers to test subjects, and in some cases makes them better off, pursuing this research in countries without this restriction may be in the moral interests of all involved.

Nevertheless, when strong profit motives and esteemed faculty positions are on the line, researchers can be tempted to ignore moral considerations. We are all tempted to cut corners when we think it is in our long-term interests, and when medical researchers cut corners, wrongful exploitation is one likely result (recall the infamous Tuskegee Syphilis Study). Emanuel et al. (2004) write that, in developing countries, "the regulatory infrastructures and independent oversight processes that might minimize the risk of exploitation may be less well established, less supported financially, and less effective in developing countries." But is there any evidence that international clinical trials are *actually* wrongfully exploitative? In the next three sections, I offer evidence that it is highly likely that any particular international clinical trial—particularly those conducted in undeveloped or developing countries—is wrongfully exploitative. To be sure, I do not argue that international clinical trials are *inherently* wrongfully exploitative. There seems nothing inherent in the construction or implementation of a randomized experimental study that undermines a subject's autonomy or rationality in a way that meets MWE. If researchers are sensitive to linguistic, cultural, and moral boundaries when entering into a morally binding contract with a test subject, and subjects have a reasonable ability to refuse to participate, researchers are lowering the likelihood that anyone stands an unreasonable risk of losing something of fundamental value.

Problems with Obtaining Informed Consent in Developing Countries

Informed consent is a psychological state of a test subject, in which (1) she understands the nature and risks of the experiment in which she is being asked to participate, and (2) she agrees to participate. The process of obtaining informed consent typically involves a written or oral explanation of the experiment and its potential benefits and risks by a researcher to a patient who the researcher believes mentally competent to understand and assent to morally binding contracts. Obtaining genuine informed consent constitutes a necessary (though not sufficient) condition for determining whether a subject stands a URLV. If a subject is not in a position to genuinely consent, either by lack of physical or mental capacity, or because complete information is withheld or biased, then in offering her admittance to the study, researchers are situating her such that she cannot reasonably refuse to participate, and thereby wrongfully exploiting her. Note that "genuine consent" here is a matter not of being able to *volunteer* or *sign a consent form* but of having *the ability to assess the personal risk* involved in participating. There are at least three obstacles to obtaining genuinely informed consent in any particular international clinical trial.

Conceptual obstacles to genuine consent

Ruth Macklin (1999, pp. 86–108) highlights the fact that people will often confuse *informed consent* with the informed consent documentation itself. Macklin cites an example from a workshop she attended in the Philippines, where a doctor objected to informed consent on the grounds that, "... in the Philippines patients place great trust in their physicians. Doctors do not need to protect themselves against lawsuits by having patients sign a consent form." She then notes: "The Filipino physician misunderstood two things: first, the ethical basis for informed consent; and second, the difference between the process of informing and obtaining ... the piece of paper ..." If physicians and medical researchers are misinformed about the moral justification of informed consent, or are simply lazy in their consideration of their subjects, the likelihood rises that patients and test subjects will be placed in a position where they stand a URLV.

Cultural and institutional obstacles to genuine consent

Even in cases where a complex medical concept or procedure can be explained in a way sufficient for a subject's understanding, there may be cultural mores that inhibit an accurate assessment of procedure options, or reduce a subject to unreasonable treatment options. What counts as a significant likelihood of harm to a researcher from Great Britain may not sound so daunting to someone who lives under constant threat of poisonous snake bite, malaria, or gunfire from warring tribes. To someone from a culture that values large families, the threat of impotence may be more significant than the threat of prolonged illness. Out of ignorance or a concern for efficiency, researchers may ignore these considerations altogether (for further examples, see Bagenda & Musoke-Mudido, 1997).

In addition, knowing exactly which cultural features will help a test subject make an informed decision about whether to participate is difficult. Torbjörn Tännsjö (1994) explains how a subject's religious commitments can limit the treatment options to which he can reasonably consent: "The doctor should, for example, not force a blood transfusion upon a patient who for religious reasons refuses to accept it, even if it means that patient dies. But the latter is objectionable; it conforms to no reasonable rule of thumb in our medical practice. The doctor should not, if he can avoid it, put his religious patient in a situation where the patient needs a blood transfusion, if he knows the patient will reject it" (p. 528). A researcher must be aware of the patient's cultural background in order to take these sorts of commitments into consideration. And while this may be somewhat easier in countries relatively homogeneous with the researchers', it is certainly more difficult in cultures where a rich religious or social heritage determines much of what constitutes acceptable behavior.

In addition, in less politically stable countries like Mexico, Uganda, and Egypt, exaggerated perceptions of medical professionals and corrupt courts allow little opportunity for challenging medical and research practices. Patients are politically and culturally encouraged to feel at the mercy of the medical community. Macklin interviewed an Egyptian doctor, who explained that "in Egypt there is no process by which consent is obtained in clinical practice.... Patients who ask questions are viewed by doctors as 'impolite,' and in any case doctors do not like to answer questions posed by patients" (1996, p. 665). She also spoke with a Mexican colleague, who explained that Mexico does not officially recognize patients' rights, and that the Mexican people are much more tolerant of corruption in political and legal spheres (p. 666). These cultural tendencies clearly extend to medical research cases, where researchers are perceived as physicians offering a remedy for their suffering.

If a researcher is unaware of cultural distinctives that make some treatments an unreasonable option to a particular subject or if subjects implicitly trust anyone they perceive to be medical professionals, the likelihood of obtaining genuinely informed consent is low, and therefore, the likelihood of wrongful exploitation is high.

Urgency obstacles to genuine consent

The severity of a potential test subject's disease raises concerns about exploitation in all types of clinical trials. Sherlock (1986) and Cassell et al. (2001) argue that a subject's illness may diminish her ability to reason clearly about her medical decisions. But given MWE, simply facing a life-threatening disease may undermine her ability to reasonably refuse to participate in a clinical trial relevant to treating that disease.

Consider, again, Valdman's Antidote Case. The fact that *B*'s life is on the line places *B* in a position such that he cannot reasonably refuse any request *A* may make in return for the antidote. Many international clinical trials are designed to discover treatments for or preventions of life-threatening diseases, including HIV, AIDS, malaria, and tuberculosis. If any of these diseases constitute a threat to something of fundamental value, subjects may not be a position to reasonably refuse the risks offered by an experimental treatment. In being faced with the opportunity to participate in a clinical trial, a person may rightly perceive her options to be: (a) do not participate and die, or (b) participate and gamble on obtaining a better quality of life or dying. If a researcher understands this, she may be able to avoid placing a subject in a position where he stands a URLV. If not, the risk of meeting the conditions for MWE increases.

The Possibility of Misapplied Moral Theories

A second line of evidence showing that international clinical trials are wrongfully exploitative is the possibility that moral theories are misapplied in the context of nondomestic trials. While moral philosophy is more visible in the field of medical research than ever before, researchers in developed domestic contexts may comfortably rely on the regulations and guidelines of their country of origin to protect them from moral failure. Once out of these contexts, researchers are presented with the opportunity to question those regulations and to make independent, morally significant decisions. For researchers who have a grasp of sophisticated models of moral reasoning, this situation is less worrisome. But for those who are largely ignorant of moral philosophy, making such decisions can have devastating implications.

Take, for example, an attempt to apply consequentialism to the question of how to conduct a clinical trial. Consequentialism is the normative moral theory that the consequences of an action determine whether that act is permissible, impermissible, obligatory, or supererogatory. *Rule utilitarianism*—as opposed to *act utilitarianism*, according to which an act is morally obligatory if the consequences of that particular action increase the overall happiness of all involved—is, in its most general formulation, the consequentialist view that an act is morally obligatory if it is the result of a principle of reasoning that, in general, leads to greater overall happiness, where overall happiness is defined as the most pleasure for the largest number of people over the longest amount of time, and where pleasure includes both sensual pleasure and deep satisfaction. For instance, in the standard trolley dilemma, five people are stuck on one trolley track, and one person is stuck on a side track; you, as the conductor, face the mutually exclusive options of doing nothing and allowing the trolley to kill the five people and of changing the track so that the trolley kills only one person. According to standard accounts of rule utilitarianism, you have an obligation to change the track. Performing the action increases the happiness of the five and decreases the happiness of the one (plus yours for having to participate in such a horrifying event), thereby increasing overall happiness.

Now, in contrast to very general formulations of the theory, which are subject to damning counterexamples, sophisticated versions of rule utilitarianism often yield intuitively satisfying results. Sophisticated rule utilitarianism offers powerful explanations for our intuitions about the "rightness" of helping the poor and hungry, and for our desire that a certain minimum amount of healthcare is available to everyone. Some sophisticated utilitarians even argue that their theory entails decisions that are very similar, if not indistinguishable, from sophisticated deontological theories (Railton, 1988). But many who come away from basic courses in moral philosophy do not grasp the subtleties of sophisticated versions of moral theories. They often come away with very general views that sound more like Sunday School ethics than serious moral philosophy.

Unfortunately, however, on the basis of quite unsophisticated versions of utilitarianism, many medical researchers defend "paternalistic" policies in medical research, according to which "professionals have a superior knowledge of medicine; therefore, they and they alone are privileged, because of their long and specialized training, to decide what is in the best interest of patients and their families" (Thiroux & Krasemann, 2007, p. 342). Consider, for example, that Susan Dodds and Karen Jones (1989) argue that lawmakers are in a better position than a mother to decide what is in a mother's best interests: "Certainly, it would be *paternalistic* to interfere with a woman's choice to become a surrogate mother, but this does not mean that it must be *wrong* to do so" (p. 101, italics theirs). Similarly, Laura Purdy (1996, pp. 39–49) argues that doctors are better able to assess whether citizens have a right to reproduce than the potential parents: ".... it is morally wrong to reproduce when we know there is a high risk of transmitting a serious disease or defect. This thesis ... denies that people should be free to reproduce mindless of the consequences." In his case against allowing patients to sign "living wills," Christopher James Ryan (1996) cites evidence that: "Human beings are, I suggest, very poor at determining their attitudes to treatment for some hypothetical future terminal illness and very frequently grossly under-estimate their future desire to go on living" (p. 99).

In all of these cases, the underlying implication is clear: As an expert in medicine, I know how to calculate the risk of procedure *X* better than my patient/test subject, and regardless of any particular negative consequences to this particular patient/test subject, more people will be better off in the long run. And yet, it also seems clear how each of these claims could lead to clinical circumstances meeting MWE. Researchers restrict the options a test subject is permitted to choose from on the basis of unreflective utility calculations.

To be sure, a researcher's utility calculations may, in fact, be more accurate than a test subject's. But at least two factors challenge the plausibility of this claim for *any* clinical context. First, the difficulty already mentioned with cultural obstacles is relevant here. If a researcher does not know what a subject values, then regardless of how accurate her calculations on the information she has, she does not have all the relevant information. Carl Elliott (2003) describes a growing phenomenon of people who desire to have healthy limbs amputated. Although some anecdotal evidence suggests that this desire is not different from desires for cosmetic surgery or trans-gender operations, the medical community stigmatizes this desire as a disease, and seeks to ban it. Yet Elliott points out that the same reasons given for categorizing this desire as a "psycho-sexual disease" were also offered against gender modification, which is now largely viewed as elective surgery.

The question is: Who is in the *best* position to determine what is in a subject's best interests? Researchers can make informed judgments about treatments and outcomes, but subjects know their values. Therefore, presumably, researchers and test subjects must communicate in an atmosphere of mutual respect. Thus, any utilitarian calculation that does not take subjects' personal value assessments into consideration is likely to place those subjects at risk in ways they could not genuinely consent to accept and, therefore, is more likely to exploit them for what researchers take to be the *greater good*.

A second challenge to the idea that researchers are better suited to calculate the risks than test subjects is that there is no objective standard for calculating utility in complicated medical cases. This becomes clear when we look at cases where utilitarian calculations differ among professionals. For example, Torbjörn Tännsjö (1994) cites a clinical trial for which he was asked to be an ethical advisor. Researchers were attempting to determine whether a new drug, ddI, is as effective at postponing the time it takes for an HIV-positive patient to develop AIDS than the most effective drug at the time, zidovudine. At the outset, there was no reason to believe that ddI alone was more or less effective than zidovudine alone, there was some evidence available that the combination of the two was more effective than zidovudine alone, and there was also evidence that about one in 500 patients who took ddI died because it seems to cause a fatal form of pancreatitis. Subjects entering the new trial were assigned to one of three groups: the first third received zidovudine only, the second third received ddI only, and the third group alternated between the two drugs.

After calculating what researchers took to be the relevant considerations, Tännsjö concluded: "Given our assumptions, it turned out that, if a patient in the third category, who alternated between the two drugs, gained on average more than, roughly, one week of life without too serious symptoms of AIDS, it would be rational to volunteer" (p. 19). Unfortunately, however, not every consequentialist agreed with this conclusion. Some critics objected on the basis of a calculation principle used by insurance companies, which starts from a baseline assumption about which risks "just aren't worth taking" (p. 19):

> A company selling insurance does not sell if it means that, should the worse come to the worst (no matter how improbable this is), the company would go bankrupt. Only after such alternatives have been eliminated is the company prepared to maximize expected utility. By the same token, these doctors argued, we ought not to try a new drug, even if it offers good hope of prolonging (somewhat) the life of a patient if, at the same time, there is a not negligible probability that it will end at once. (pp. 19–20)

Which utility calculation is morally best? It is not the case that both conclusions avoid placing a test subject in a position where he stands a URLV, since they have vastly different implications, and it is possible that neither will. What is the solution? Presumably, a rejection of this sort of paternalistic model of decision-making. Even John Stuart Mill (1859/2002), the most outspoken proponent of utilitarianism, admits that such a calculus is implausible and argues that attempts to protect test subjects from themselves are wrongheaded. It would seem that this implication applies mutatis mutandis to all unsophisticated versions of plausible moral theories, especially those that include no obvious method for resolving conflicts among values. And if the number of researchers reasoning from these unsophisticated theories is nontrivial, then the likelihood that international clinical trials are wrongfully exploitative increases.

The Weakness of Human Moral Motivation and Interpretation

The final line of evidence is simply the weakness of human nature. All of us, from medical researchers to moral philosophers, are not always motivated to act morally. This is not to say we are *bad* people; it simply means that we tend to allow nonmoral motives to take priority over moral considerations. Consider a series of 16 drug trials in which researchers wanted to evaluate the effectiveness of new, less expensive treatments for reducing the transmission of HIV from mother to infants during labor, as compared with an accepted and effective but expensive treatment called the ACTG 076 intervention treatment (Lurie & Wolfe, 1997). The question arose as to how to test the effectiveness of these less expensive treatments: independently, against placebo groups, or in comparison with groups being treated with the known and effective ACTG 076 regimen.

Researchers, along with the NIH, CDC, and WHO, cite two reasons for preferring the placebo-controlled trials over the nonplacebo equivalency studies. First, they claim that "differences in the duration and route of administration of antiretroviral agents in the shorter regimens, as compared with the ACTG 076 regimen, justify the use of a placebo group" (p. 535). Second, they claim that placebo-controlled trials "require fewer subjects than equivalency studies and can therefore be completed more rapidly" (p. 536).

Note that both reasons are *efficiency* considerations: placebo-controlled trials allow researchers more accurate information about the shorter regimen treatments in less time. But efficiency considerations do not obviously outweigh moral considerations. In fact, if only the placebo-controlled trials are offered to potential test subjects, it would seem that these trials meet the conditions for MWE.

A thought experiment for determining whether this is, in fact, a case of wrongful exploitation is to imagine confronting potential test subjects with a choice between the placebo- and nonplacebo-controlled designs. If it is conceivable that one person could reasonably conclude that the overall potential benefits of the nonplacebo-controlled trial outweigh the overall potential benefits of the placebo-controlled trial, then in offering only one of the experimental designs, researchers are subjecting subjects to a URLV. Lurie and Wolfe (1997) discovered this to be the case in 15 of the 16 trials conducted in developing countries.

The Argument

With MWE and three lines of evidence highlighting the difficulties in developing countries of offering contracts to participate in medical research that present a reasonable opportunity for refusal, we can formulate the following argument:

1. MWE occurs when an act by a morally competent person or group of persons, *A*, employs the behavior of a moral subject, *B*, in successfully obtaining *A*'s ends under circumstances in which *B* stands an unreasonable risk of losing something of fundamental value to *B*.
2. Problems with informed consent, the prevalence of misapplied moral theories, and the weakness of human moral motivation make it highly likely that clinical researchers in developing countries employ test subjects' behavior in obtaining their ends under circumstances in which *B* stands an unreasonable risk of losing something of fundamental value.
3. Therefore, it is highly likely that any particular international clinical trial is wrongfully exploitative.

Conclusions

I have offered a set of minimally necessary and sufficient conditions for wrongful exploitation and argued that three considerations render it likely that any particular international trial is wrongfully exploitative. The burden is, therefore, on medical researchers conducting trials in developing countries to provide evidence that their experimental designs avoid meeting the conditions of MWE. How might we encourage this behavior? The most common response is to introduce more and stricter regulations. But as economists consistently warn, this is almost always an inefficient option; the costs of establishing such regulation are high; the regulation is, by necessity, restricted to its country of origin; and clever lawyers can always discover myriad loopholes. Instead, I suggest two more plausible options: more comprehensive moral education and freer economic markets.

To efficiently reduce wrongful exploitation, philosophers should encourage better moral education in secondary schools and more exposure to moral philosophy in college (the International Society for Ethics Across the Curriculum program is a good example of the latter). In addition to expanded moral education, philosophers should not shy away from emphasizing individual rights and personal responsibility among patients, medical professionals, and legal organizations in public and political arenas. Just as informed dialogue has moved us away from racism, sexism, and even animal cruelty, so it has the potential to reduce the likelihood of wrongful exploitation committed by medical researchers.

In addition, a renewed public emphasis on individual rights and personal responsibility will encourage fewer governmental regulations on exchanges of value among free people. Removing policies against the sale of insurance across state lines and restrictions on access to nondomestic pharmaceuticals will prevent collusion and increase competition among economically powerful entities, reduce costs, and increase access. These changes have the potential to reduce significantly the number of opportunities for wrongful exploitation. In addition, fewer restrictive policies will lead to clarity and simplicity in legal proceedings, making corruption easier to eliminate. No amount of well-intended coercion can stamp out immoral activity in any context. But freer markets and better access to fair legal reparations will reduce the number and severity of incidents, and, consequently, increase our confidence in the research results.

References

AAAS Policy Forum (2002). Fair benefits for research in developing countries. *Science, 298,* 2133–2134.

Associated Press. (2007). Buckeyes receiver says college athletes are exploited. *CBS Sports,* January 2. Retrieved from: http://www.cstv.com/sports/m-footbl/stories/010407aag.html

Bagenda, D., & Musoke-Mudido, P. (1997). A look at ethics and AIDS: We're trying to help our sickest people, not exploit them. *The Washington Post,* September 28. Retrieved from: http://www.ncbi.nlm.nih.gov/pubmed/11647249

Cassell, E., Leon, A., & Kaufman, S. (2001). Preliminary evidence of impaired thinking in sick patients. *Annals of Internal Medicine, 132,* 1120–1123.

Dodds, S., & Jones, K. (1989). A response to Purdy. *Bioethics, 3,* 35–39.

Elliott, C. (2003). *Better than well: American medicine meets the American dream.* New York: W. W. Norton & Company.

Emanuel, E., Wendler, D., & Grady, C. (2000). What makes clinical research ethical? *Journal of the American Medical Association, 283,* 2701–2711.

Emanuel, E., Wendler, D., Killen, J., & Grady, C. (2004). What makes clinical research in developing countries ethical? The benchmarks of ethical research. *The Journal of Infectious Diseases, 189,* 930–937.

Lurie, P., & Wolfe, S. (1997). Unethical trials of interventions to reduce perinatal transmission of the human immunodeficiency virus in developing countries. *New England Journal of Medicine, 337,* 853–856.

Lurie, P., & Wolfe, S. (2007). The developing world as the 'answer' to the dreams of pharmaceutical companies: The Surfaxin story. In J. Lavery, C. Grady, E. Wahl & Emmanuel, E. (Eds.), *Ethical issues in international biomedical research: A casebook* (pp. 159–170). Oxford: Oxford University Press.

Macklin, R. (1999). *Against relativism: Cultural diversity and the search for ethical universals in medicine.* Oxford: Oxford University Press.

Mill, J. S. (1859/2002). *On liberty.* New York: The Modern Library.

Purdy, L. (1996). *Reproducing persons: Issues in feminist bioethics.* Ithaca, NY: Cornell University Press.

Railton, P. (1988). Alienation, consequentialism, and the demands of morality. In S. Scheffler (Ed.), *Consequentialism and its critics* (pp. 93–133). Oxford: Oxford University Press.

Ryan, C. (1996). Betting your life: An argument against certain advance directives. *Journal of Medical Ethics, 22,* 95–99.

Sherlock, R. (1986). Reasonable men and sick human beings. *American Journal of Medicine, 80,* 2–4.

Snyder, J. (2008). Needs exploitation. *Ethical Theory and Moral Practice, 11,* 389–405.

Snyder, J. (2012). Exploitations and their complications: The necessity of identifying the multiple forms of exploitation in pharmaceutical trials. *Bioethics, 26,* 251–258.

Tännsjö, T. (1994). The morality of clinical research: A case study. *Journal of Medicine and Philosophy, 19,* 7–21.

Taylor, P. (2010). Indentured servants, college athletes are an exploited class. *The Pilot,* April 11. Retrieved from: http://www.thepilot.com/news/2010/apr/11/indentured-servants-college-athletes-are-an/

Thiroux, J., & Krasemann, K. (2007). *Ethics: Theory and practice.* Upper Saddle River, NJ: Prentice-Hall.

Valdman, M. (2009). A theory of wrongful exploitation. *Philosopher's Imprint, 9,* 1–14.

Walker, J. B. (2011). Religious exploitation should be called out. *The Washington Post,* February 22. Retrieved from: http://onfaith.washingtonpost.com/onfaith/panelists/j_brent_walker/2011/02/religious_exploitation_should_be_called_out.html

Wertheimer, A. (1999). *Exploitation.* Princeton, NJ: Princeton University Press.

Wertheimer, A. (2008). Exploitation. *The Stanford Encyclopedia of Philosophy.* Retrieved from: http://plato.stanford.edu/entries/exploitation/

WHO (World Health Organization). (2002). International ethical guidelines for biomedical research involving human subjects: Guideline 3. Retrieved from: http://www.fhi.org/training/fr/retc/pdf_files/cioms.pdf

WHO (World Health Organization). (2009). Global report 2009. Retrieved from: http://www.who.int/hiv/data/en/index.html

WHO (World Health Organization). (2011). Incidence of tuberculosis. Retrieved from: http://apps.who.int/ghodata/?vid=510

Chapter Thirty

International Clinical Trials Are Not Inherently Exploitative

Richard J. Arneson

The act consequentialist holds that one morally ought always to choose the act or policy of those available that would bring about the best outcome. In this chapter, I argue from an act-consequentialist standpoint that international clinical trials have no inherent tendency to be exploitative. They might be, but need not be. My account delivers a principled way of deciding whether fair labor standards or international regulations fixing standards of fairness for clinical trials in poor countries are morally acceptable or not.

Introduction

Corporations that sell prescription drugs for medical treatment have an interest in developing new products for sale. To be able to sell a patented medical prescription drug legally, the company must be able to adduce evidence of the safety and efficacy of the new drug for its proposed use. Scientific studies are needed.

There are reasons to carry out these studies in poor countries. If the incidence of the disease of interest to us is much greater in a poor country than in affluent countries, testing a remedy for that disease may be much easier in the poor country, simply because it is easier there to find a sufficient number of cases to treat with the remedy whose efficacy we are trying to determine. Another consideration is that the legal regulations governing clinical trials may be far more extensive and demanding in a rich country than in a poor country, so the cost of compliance with such regulations is much less in the latter setting.

Questions arise regarding the moral acceptability of excursions of profit-seeking companies into poor countries to conduct clinical trials. Here are two examples (one imaginary) to illustrate salient concerns:

1. Company Z has dispatched a team of medical doctors and staff to a remote rural region in the hinterlands of a poor country. By virtue of its elevation above sea level, the region happens to be an ideal site on which to carry out a clinical trial testing the efficacy of a drug the company is interested in marketing. The test will take a year to complete, and the terms on which the test will be conducted are, let us stipulate, generous and fair to volunteer participants in the study and to inhabitants of the region in which the study is to occur. The hitch is that cultural barriers preclude genuine informed consent on the part of each participant in the study. The villagers have had only slight contact with medical doctors, and the ideas of a doctor being an experimentalist rather than a clinician and of performing a double-blind controlled experiment as opposed to other types

Contemporary Debates in Bioethics, First Edition. Edited by Arthur L. Caplan and Robert Arp.

are simply alien to them. It is possible to induce potential participants to sign the informed consent papers, but genuine informed consent to the procedure being undertaken is not achievable. The medical team makes do by consulting with the village chieftain, who has a reputation for integrity and statesmanship, and who clearly understands the nature of the clinical trial being proposed and negotiates shrewdly on behalf of the experimental participants and the region as a whole. She agrees to the deal, and following her lead, others cooperate, but the fact remains that the experimental procedure is going forward without obtaining the informed consent of the experimental subjects.

2. In 2000, a private US drug company, Discovery Labs, proposed to conduct a double-blind, randomized, placebo-controlled trial testing its potential new treatment for respiratory distress syndrome (RDS) in 650 premature infants in Bolivia showing symptoms of RDS (see Hawkins & Emanuel, 2008, ch. 2). RDS is a common cause of fatality in premature infants worldwide. There are treatments involving administration of surfactin—a protein that helps weak infant lungs to function—that significantly reduce the risk of death from RDS. These treatments are commonly used in affluent countries but too expensive for general use in poor countries including Bolivia.

Discovery Labs calculated it was unclear that a test of Surfaxin versus the best currently approved surfactant treatment would yield a result that would clear the way to Food and Drug Administration (FDA) approval to market Surfaxin. However, a successful clinical trial showing that Surfaxin was an effective treatment by comparison with administration of a placebo would likely yield approval to market. Suppose Surfaxin is tested against the current approved surfactant medication in what is called an active-controlled trial. In a double-blind setting, some research surfactants are randomly assigned to get the standard treatment and some Surfaxin. If the test does not yield the result that Surfaxin is superior to the standard treatment, approval to market Surfaxin may be denied. If, instead, Surfaxin is tested against a placebo and proves efficacious in that test, the likelihood of gaining FDA approval, Discovery Labs judges, will be greater than if the active-control trial were run instead and yielded an ambiguous result. Notice that in conducting a placebo-controlled trial, the experimenters can be viewed as declining to rescue the sick infants who happen to be assigned the placebo treatment (because they could have been given the standard remedy in the active-controlled alternative trial). Such a study could not legally be performed in a developed country, where legal rules forbid placebo-controlled tests of drugs proposed for treatment of a disease condition for which there is already an established efficacious treatment.

Giving the placebo when the normal standard of clinical care requires administration of an approved treatment violates the ethical duty of the doctor to the patient involved in the trial. However, though surfactant treatments are approved for use in poor countries including Bolivia, they are far too expensive to be standardly used in treatment of premature infants except those born into wealthy families. So, in conducting a placebo-controlled trial in Bolivia, Discovery Labs would be administering a nontreatment (a placebo) to infants at risk of dying from RDS when there is a known efficacious treatment for the condition, albeit one that is not part of standard medical care in Bolivia and not one that any of these infants in the rural region would have received in the normal course of events if the clinical trial had not been conducted.

Each parent could regard enrolling her sick child in the placebo-controlled trial as gaining a lottery ticket that will pay off if the child gets the nonplacebo treatment and will leave him no worse off if he gets the placebo. (This statement needs to be qualified, because it is possible that the new treatment being tested is actually harmful. But an efficacy trial of this sort is preceded by safety trials that are supposed to eliminate this risk.)

In the event, the clinical trial had gone forward and had been successful, the drug Surfaxin approved for treatment for RDS would be too expensive to be affordable for any except a wealthy elite of Bolivian families. The benefits, if any, would accrue to Discovery Labs and perhaps to infants with RDS in wealthy nations. In these circumstances, was the Surfaxin trial as proposed exploitative in its dealings with Bolivian children enrolled in the study and their parents? Might terms be arranged that would render the proposed clinical trial fair and overall morally acceptable to conduct?

In these examples, the practices of the pharmaceutical corporation enterprises appear morally troubling. The practices are morally problematic at best and morally beyond the pale according to some plausible standards of ethical practice.

Are international clinical medical trials inherently exploitative or overwhelmingly likely to be so? Here are two arguments:

1. A distinguished scholar of law and medical ethics, George Annas, once observed, "I'd argue that you can't do studies ethically in a country where there is no basic healthcare. You can tell a person that this is research, but they hear they have a chance to get care or else refuse their only good chance at care. How can you put them in that position and then say they are giving informed consent?" (cited from Hawkins & Emanuel, 2008, p. 7). But one can voluntarily consent to an offer that one cannot reasonably refuse. I can voluntarily and indeed wholeheartedly consent to a marriage offer from Ted, even though I have no other offers, and continued bachelorhood would be, for me, an utter disaster. In this situation, Ted might drive a hard bargain, but his own aims and values, or cultural norms, or legal regulation of marriage contracts might inhibit him from doing that.

Along similar lines, I would urge that where informed consent really is beyond reach, because subjects cannot comprehend the contract that is being offered, nothing inherently precludes proxy consent from working effectively to safeguard the interests of these subjects. In my example above, the political system with its checks and balances operating in the village, or the virtue and wisdom of the chieftain, may well bring it about that she acts effectively as a trustee, and that this is manifest to the agents of the company conducting the research, so the study can be done without wrongfully exploiting participants.

The claim I am making is that voluntary informed consent can be given when the person consenting lacks other options, and anyway voluntary informed consent is not a necessary condition for the moral acceptability of conducting medical research. But neither is voluntary informed consent to an interaction a sufficient condition of its moral acceptability.

2. One can give voluntary informed consent to a wrongfully exploitative deal. The consent neither extinguishes the exploitation nor renders it morally acceptable. There can be mutually beneficial exploitation where the victim voluntarily consents to the deal. Assume, as is plausible, that when large medical corporations undertake medical experiments on willing research subjects in poor countries, the deals struck will not take place in a competitive market setting, with many buyers and many sellers of the service being sold. The large corporation will have considerable bargaining power. On this setting, is an unfair deal in which the large company gouges the poor individuals who serve as its research subjects virtually inevitable?

No. Without relying on the conscience of profit-maximizing corporations, one can locate and seek to enhance other mechanisms of restraint. Customers of the medical firm can threaten to boycott its products if it engages in sleazy deals that take milk from the mouths of hungry babes in third-world countries. International ethical guidelines can be promulgated and enforced by treaty or international regulatory bodies or aggressive jawboning by nongovernmental organizations such as Doctors Without Borders. Media campaigns in host countries can target abusers of the weak and vulnerable. Governments in poor countries can establish regulations that offset the undeniable bargaining advantages of powerful corporations. Nothing guarantees that any such mechanism or combination of them will succeed, but nothing guarantees failure either. It all depends.

The remainder of this chapter does not pursue the question, what are the best mechanisms of restraint of exploitative gouging, and how can they be strengthened? The focus instead is on how to characterize exploitation and how to draw the line between morally acceptable and unacceptable deals. Mutually beneficial exploitation raises special concern. A transaction can be mutually beneficial but unfair and hence morally condemnable. Surely, one morally ought not to engage in exploitive transactions. Surely one ought not to be an exploiter.

Three Puzzles

There is a puzzle lying just around the corner, the puzzle of *discouraging exploitation*. To keep things simple, let us confine our attention to cases of mutually beneficial exploitation in which all participating parties actually benefit *ex post* from the arrangement. All benefit, but some gain far less than others, and are unfairly treated. Suppose we condemn the exploitive behavior and try to discourage people from engaging in such interactions. We might enforce this condemnation by making transactions of this type illegal and imposing criminal law penalties on exploiters. We might also enforce this condemnation by peer pressure, avoidance of interaction with the exploiter, shunning, shaming, and so on. These efforts might be successful or unsuccessful at reducing the incidence of the targeted exploitive transactions: Let us suppose they are successful. This might occur by inducing some who were inclined to engage in exploitive transactions to interact with the same partners but on terms more favorable to those who would have been getting the short end of the stick.

But the reduction in incidence of exploitation might occur by inducing those inclined to exploit to leave the market altogether or cease to interact on any terms with the potential targets of exploitation. As described, this outcome would seem to be in an obvious way morally desirable: we have achieved a reduction of mutually beneficial exploitation. But how can this be morally desirable? Absent our introduction of norms and rules against exploitation of this type, people would have made mutually beneficial deals, voluntary on the part of all participants. Some of these deals might have been to the enormous advantage of those getting the short end of the stick. The gains to the potential victims of exploitation that are forgone by our decision to undertake a campaign against exploitation might be literally matters of life and death for these people. How can we thump our chests and take pride in our success in reducing the incidence of exploitation if we are thereby bringing about a state of affairs from which a change could be made that renders some significantly better off without making anyone at all worse off? Call this the significant Pareto improvement norm. (Formulating the requirement as triggered by *significant* Pareto improvement blocks it from being deployed to criticize a practice that leads to a state of affairs that is trivially worse than an alternative practice would bring about.) A very plausible view maintains that while this Pareto norm is a very weak fairness constraint, it is nonetheless a fairness constraint. It is unfair to embrace and implement policies that bring about outcomes that are vulnerable to the significant Pareto norm criticism. Such policies are unfair to those who might have been made better off without making anyone else worse off. Countenancing and accepting mutually beneficial exploitation thus appears to be both condemned by fairness norms and required by fairness norms.

There is another puzzle that lurks in discussions of the topic of exploitation. What exactly are we talking about? As is often noted, *exploitation* when used in a pejorative sense is a moralized notion. To exploit a person is to take unfair advantage of another person. In other words, the exploiter seeks to advance her aims by using another person in a way that is unfair to that person. To understand how to abide by a norm against exploiting people, it would seem that one needs a conception of unfairness that enables one to determine whether any given instance of interaction with other persons crosses the boundary into unfairness. One needs a standard that tells what constitutes fair treatment. Lacking such a standard, the person seeking to understand the nature of exploitation finds herself, so to speak, with a big hole at the center of the doughnut. But as Alan Wertheimer (1999), perhaps the preeminent contemporary theorist of exploitation, observes, "Unfortunately, there is no nonproblematic account of fair transactions." He does not make this observation as a prelude to proposing a definitive account. In the same essay from which the quotation just introduced was taken, Wertheimer observes, "Although I cannot produce a nonproblematic theory of fair transactions, I remain convinced that some mutually advantageous transactions are quite unfair and exploitative." Now, one can see how it might be useful for a language to contain terms that allow people with entirely opposed convictions and judgments to express judgments of approbation and disapprobation in some domain. Such terms are handy devices. I do not need a theory of beauty to call a painting or a scene beautiful, and you can understand my meaning even if you find the same scene revolting or obscenely ugly. The same goes with claims of exploitation. Nonetheless, it is disturbing that philosophical attempts to specify standards of fairness for determining when transactions are exploitative seem to have come up with empty pockets. Call this the *no standards* puzzle.

Another puzzle about exploitation that involves interaction between an agency based in an affluent nation and poor people in poor countries might be called the *irrelevant beneficiaries* problem. In discussions of international clinical trials, the idea surfaces that a highly relevant consideration in determining whether proposed research in a poor country is exploitative or not is whether any medical treatment shown to be successful in the experiment will be made available at affordable rates to present or future members of the host country in which the experiment is conducted. The puzzle is this: If we are deciding whether A's treatment of B is exploitative or not, how can whether or not benefits accrue to some third party C have any bearing on the question? Alan Wertheimer (1999) sensibly observes, "if the principles of medical ethics are primarily interested in the way in which patients or subjects are treated, I do not see why the availability of drugs to *other* persons has much bearing on the ethical status of a study."

In this chapter, I shall propose a solution to the three puzzles about exploitation just characterized. The account I propose delivers the result that international clinical trials such as the examples described at the outset of this chapter have no inherent tendency to be exploitative. They might be, but need not be. Moreover, there is a general issue here. When a person in an affluent developed nation buys prescription drugs that have come to market through international clinical trials, she may be complicit in exploitive practices, just as when a person in an affluent country buys cheap good-quality cars or clothes or computers manufactured abroad under conditions of labor that would not be tolerable in the affluent country itself. My account delivers a principled way of deciding whether fair labor standards or international regulations fixing standards of fairness for clinical trials in poor countries are morally acceptable or not.

Act Consequentialism and Priority

This chapter approaches the topic from a resolutely act-consequentialist standpoint. The act consequentialist holds that one morally ought always to choose the act or policy of those available that would bring about the best outcome. There are many varieties of act consequentialism—as many as there are different possible standards of outcome assessment. To give the act-consequentialist idea a fair hearing, one must couple it to the most plausible standard of outcome assessment we can identify. Searching for the best outcome standard is not a task this chapter can undertake. I shall simply adopt what strikes me as the most plausible standard and go from there. The standard relied on here is individualist and welfarist. What matters ultimately from the moral standpoint is the well-being of the complete lives of individual persons (Arneson, 1999, 2000). Good or bad that accrues to a collective such as a family or clan or race or nation does not have any intrinsic moral significance and matters only insofar as gains or losses to collectives are instrumental for achieving gains and avoiding losses that accrue to individual persons. What matters ultimately from the moral point of view is entirely a function of good lives for people, fairly distributed across people. The idea of fair distribution that figures in the standard to be employed is a simple prioritarianism: benefits matter more, the worse off in lifetime well-being is the person who would get the benefits (see Parfit, 1997; Holtug, 2010; and for the first statement of the prioritarian idea known to me, Scheffler, 1982). The characterization so far yields a family of views. To obtain a specific standard for outcome assessment, one would need to determine a priority weighting, a specification of how exactly the moral value of obtaining a benefit or obtaining a loss varies with the size of the benefit, the number of people who would obtain it, and the lifetime well-being these people are headed toward (apart from receipt of the benefit in question).

Multi-Level Consequentialism

It might seem obvious that a welfarist act consequentialism of the sort just sketched must bite the bullet in response to the puzzle of discouraging exploitation.

More well-being for a person is always better than none, so the prioritarian act consequentialist must embrace the Pareto norm and reject any principle that condemns mutually beneficial exploitation and thus runs afoul of the Pareto norm. For any variety of act consequentialism, half a loaf is better than none, and a crumb is better than no bread.

Not so, I say. The reasoning in the preceding paragraph gallops too fast. We need to take proper account of levels of moral reasoning. A plausible act consequentialism must be a multi-level doctrine (see Hare, 1981; Railton, 1988). Humans have limited cognitive abilities, tend to favor themselves and those near and dear to them in their choices, tend to choose near-term rewards over greater later gains, tend to be ignorant or have false beliefs concerning matters germane to their choices, and generally have limited ability to integrate the facts they do know into their deliberations of what to do. Given these facts, humans will do better in choice-making and choice execution as assessed by the act-consequentialist standard if they do not use act consequentialism standardly as a guide to choice but instead guide their decision-making by fairly simple rules that do not make excessive demands on their deliberative capacities and on their capacity for making impartial choices.

This point applies when the issue is selection of legal rules. The same point applies when what is at issue is selection (more plausibly, influencing the content) of social norms (norms enforced by informal social sanctions rather than by legal procedures and penalties). I would contend that the same point applies when the issue is selection or alteration of a public morality, a set of moral norms specifying moral rights and duties and obligations that is to be promulgated as in some sense the official morality of the society. At all of these derived levels, the norms ideally should be selected according to the act-consequentialist standard. The optimal set of norms is the one the introduction of which in the actual circumstances would do best in terms of promoting good consequences.

What one should do, according to act consequentialism, is whatever would bring about best consequences, and the norms in place will have an impact in determining that—more so, the better the norms (assessed by the consequences of having them in place).

Exploitation

This familiar account of multi-level act consequentialism has implications for the consequentialist treatment of issues of exploitation. Norms against exploitation are a good idea from the act-consequentialist standpoint. Enforcing them reduces gouging of excessively large profits in beneficial interactions and cooperative schemes. Deals recognized as exploitive will rankle and create resentment in those who get the short end of the stick, especially if they reliably get the worse of such deals. The resentment frays cooperation, from which we all benefit. Exploitive deals will also tend to score badly according to prioritarian assessment. Those who are headed for low lifetime well-being are more likely than others to be the exploited parties in these transactions. Actions and policies that improve the deals they are likely to get make the world morally better by prioritarian standards.

A hypothetical example may serve to illustrate the points just made. Suppose that Medical, Inc. is willing to undertake a clinical trial of a product it wishes to test in a certain poor country on certain terms. The terms violate international standards covering such trials propounded by bodies including agencies of the United Nations, and following the lead of these international guidelines, the would-be host-country government declares the proposed arrangement with Medical, Inc. to be exploitative and denies legal permission for the clinical trial to be conducted as proposed. Medical, Inc. decides it is unwilling to offer better terms and scraps the proposed study altogether. The clinical trial as proposed would have benefited the volunteer participants, but only slightly.

Priority is likely to condemn the behavior of Medical, Inc. as just described. Suppose that the company is breaking off negotiations to send a message. The company's action is aimed to induce terms more favorable to it in future similar negotiations. Let us suppose this is a rational profit-maximizing choice on its part. But this does not show that the action is acceptable on prioritarian grounds. The company surely could have pursued a different course of action that yields less profit for its well-off managers, workers, and shareholders, and creates greater gains for poor people such as those who will be volunteer participants in its study. According to this version of act consequentialism, it is roughly the case that what the company morally ought to do is whatever would maximize priority-weighted aggregate well-being, which would surely be miles apart from the profit-maximizing strategy we are supposing it follows. This is "roughly the case," because the question becomes, what each of the individuals who wield influence on company affairs ought to do. One might suspect that in a competitive business environment, if the company ceases to follow the path that yields it highest expected profits, it will make zero sales and immediately go bankrupt. Not so! Without raising the price it charges to consumers above the competitive price, the firm CEO could take a big pay cut and give more to volunteer medical-trial participants, and what the CEO could do, each person connected with the firm including shareholders could do, and according to priority calculation, likely ought to do.

Notice that showing that the members of Medical Inc. behave wrongly by the act-consequentialist standard does not show that they are being exploitative or that the company policy is exploitative. Whether a policy is exploitative depends on whether it violates anti-exploitation social obligations that apply to it. The character of such obligations depends on what social norms are actually in place and accepted in the society. Even in a society that is ideally run according to act-consequentialist standards, for familiar reasons, the legal rules and social norms and public morality enforced will consist of rules that are less demanding and more administrable than the abstract prioritarian principle. So, even in a society that was ideally run according to act-consequentialist principles, not every act or policy that fails to bring about the best attainable outcome (and so is wrong according to act consequentialism) will qualify as exploitative. It is of course also the case that not every act that violates extant norms against exploitation will be wrong according to act-consequentialist principles. Assessments of acts at different levels of moral thinking can differ. (So, sometimes what one morally ought to do merits condemnation and punishment.)

In commonsense thinking, exploitation wrongs the person who is unfairly used, and is morally unacceptable on the ground of this unfair treatment of a particular victim. In contrast, in the consequentialist perspective, whether an act is right or wrong depends on its overall long-term consequences, including its impact on those remote in time or space who are affected, and importantly the effects it might have had on uninvolved persons who would have enjoyed gain or suffered loss had a different action been done instead. So, consequentialist thinking seems just ill-suited to explaining and justifying norms against exploitation, which are part of a different conceptual framework (see Arneson, 2008).

I resist the skepticism voiced in the preceding paragraph. To my mind, it just begs the question against the project of multi-level consequentialism. For starters, notice that any remotely credible view about deontological rules will have to allow that when the consequences of abiding by the rule are sufficiently bad, the rules should give way. So, for example, when it comes to exploitation, if the overall long-term consequences of what in a narrow view looks to be Tom's unfairly taking advantage of Randy are good enough, the presumption that what Tom is doing is morally wrong is overturned. Any sensible view will accept this idea. The question then arises, how do we decide when the offsetting good consequences are sufficient to remove an initial presumption of unfair wrongdoing? The consequentialist takes a plausible stance on this: we count effects on the well-being of all affected and possibly affected parties of any act one might do as having exactly the same weight, taking account of proper prioritarian adjustments to weight. This is of course a contestable position but not one that floats in the sky with no footing in commonsense conviction. (In passing, I note that perhaps there is a double priority: benefits are morally more valuable, the worse off in lifetime welfare the person to whom they accrue, and morally more valuable, the more deserving this person is (see Arneson, 2006).)

Suppose that I am in the back of a crowd with my young child trying to get a view of a passing parade. Seeing that you are wearing sturdy boots, I step on your toes and place my child on my shoulders to get a better view for my child. (I borrow this example from Darwall, 2006.) Or I murmur an apology and plop my child on your sturdy shoulders for the same purpose. You have a presumptive complaint against me—in the familiar idiom, I am using you unfairly to advance my ends, imposing costs on you by unilateral fiat. "Be reasonable," I might say to your complaint. Given the sturdiness of your boots and shoulders, any discomfort I impose on you is trivial, despite its being, strictly speaking, an assault, and my child will get enormous pleasure from seeing the (to him) wondrous passing show. You might still object that I should first ask your permission, but we can imagine that had I initiated negotiations of that sort, the parade would have passed before negotiations would have been completed and your fully voluntary consent forthcoming. And perhaps you are in a grouchy mood and would have refused consent.

The multi-level consequentialist assessment of this type of incident is complex. Establishing and sustaining norms against assaulting persons (touching them without their consent) are surely justified by act utilitarian calculation. The same is true of norms against unilaterally imposing costs on another person in the course of advancing one's projects. Internalizing these norms oneself and training one's children and associates to internalize them are also likely justified acts from the act-consequentialist perspective. Having done that, we then find ourselves disposed to react negatively when people violate these norms, especially when we are in the victim role, and disposed to react negatively to the prospect of violating these norms ourselves. When this is so, these reactions and their likely consequences are part of the input to act-consequentialist reasoning about what to do in the passing parade situation. In the actual situation, one will have uncertain information: How do I know your toes are not afflicted with painful gout? How do I know I am not inadvertently training my son to antisocial me-first habits of thought? There are strong reasons, weighty in act-consequentialist calculation, for abiding by useful social rules that tend to promote fair resolution of conflicts of interest and help sustain habits of mutually respectful cooperation in people generally. Nonetheless, all of that can be true, yet in the actual situation, taking all these considerations on board at their true weight, it still remains the case that the thing to do, the act that brings about the best outcome, is the exploitative act of stepping on your toes.

Exploitation and the Three Puzzles

Adoption of the prioritarian principle enables us to resolve the puzzles about exploitation introduced at the start of this chapter and tells us how to resolve questions about whether particular international clinical trials are exploitative and, if so, whether it would be morally desirable to prevent their occurrence.

Consider, for illustrative purposes, a very simple set of ethical guidelines forbidding exploitation in international clinical trials:

1. If a rich-country business firm or nonprofit agency conducts medical experiments on people in poor countries, special standards apply. A sliding scale applies: the more impoverished the country, and the more impoverished particular persons who are to be research subjects, the more concern must be shown for the welfare of the particular research subjects and the broader community in the host country.
2. Medical experiments governed by these guidelines are not to be conducted except on persons who give voluntary informed consent to the procedures in which they are to be involved, unless there are intractable barriers to enabling the potential research subjects to achieve sufficient comprehension of the undertaking, in which case proxy consent by parents or guardians of children or accountable political leaders of adult citizens may suffice, these consenting individuals to be trustees representing the interests of those on whose behalf they tender consent.
3. In no case may research go forward unless there is clear substantial ex ante overall benefit for each participant, and no uncompensated losses ex post.
4. The research being conducted must provide substantial benefits to the local community and the wider community of the host country in which the research is conducted. If the outcome of the research itself does not promise such benefit, some form of substantial side payment or compensation must be made via individual payments or provision of collective benefit, with special concern to benefit especially badly off members of the local and wider communities.

(These rules as stated are too vague to be administrable, but we can imagine specifications of them that would be administrable, and that are altered to suit changing conditions.) We can imagine the rules as enforced by international treaties and international law, or instead as mandated as parts of human rights codes promoted by international bodies such as the United Nations.

I shall suppose that some such guidelines in a given state of the world would yield sufficient benefit that it would be morally right to campaign for them and bring about their acceptance in the international community. Now, imagine a business firm that is willing to undertake medical research in a poor country on terms that would elicit voluntary informed consent of all research subjects but that would fail to satisfy the ethical guidelines just stated. First, we can see that *irrelevant beneficiaries* is not a puzzle at all. Whether an act that impinges on person A should be regarded as unfair to A all things considered depends on the overall mix of benefits and losses the act generates. A bombing that kills some innocent bystanders is not unfair to those bystanders if the bombing is required to achieve a substantial objective in a just war, and the damage done to the bystanders is not disproportionate to the gains for the just-war cause that the bombing achieves. Whether a medical experiment that involves A as a research subject is fair to A all things considered can depend on the mix of benefits and losses the act achieves taking into account all of its effects and the effects of what might have been done instead.

Second, the puzzle of *discouraging exploitation* also loses its sting when seen in the framework of multi-level consequentialism. We need to distinguish assessments of different types at different levels of moral thinking. The act of conducting a medical experiment in an impoverished country, achieving huge profit for the medical company and its well-off customers and hardly any benefit that to its research subjects or to the wider community, is sure to be terribly wrong according to the priority principle. We are also supposing that the act of carrying forward this research as proposed also violates the stipulated ethical guidelines (as made more specific for the times). So, conducting this research would be exploitative and should be condemned. Note that simply doing a wrong act does not render one blameworthy or apt for condemnation (the shortfall between what one does and the best one might have done might be trivial). But doing an act with great shortfall from the best one might have done merits condemnation. Moreover, violating the extant accepted ethical guidelines (provided they are "good enough" as assessed by the prioritarian principle) is violating a social obligation and rendering oneself apt for blame and punishment.

But why forbid the exploitative act, given that, as described, allowing it makes some better off and no one worse off? Answer: we should consider not only the consequences of doing the act but the consequences of not forbidding it. If the ethical guidelines are good according to prioritarian assessment, then accepting and supporting them, and enforcing them, are very likely to be morally right acts. Discouraging mutually beneficial exploitation is morally right to do just in case it brings about better consequences by the priority standard than anything else one might instead have done. This condition can be met. So, there is nothing puzzling from an act-consequentialist standpoint, as to why we should sometimes act to discourage or squash mutually beneficial exploitation. Discouraging exploitation by following priority-approved norms against exploitation either (1) actually works to bring about the best attainable outcomes in the long run or (2) in some cases is itself morally wrong but an unavoidable side effect of pursuing the best-available strategy for bringing about the best-attainable outcomes.

If one asks how we can sensibly deploy norms against exploitation without being able to articulate a clear and compelling standard of fairness that fixes the content of those norms, priority has a ready and plausible answer. There are ideas of fairness that partially determine the act-consequentialist best-outcome standard. (In particular, priority to the worse off is a fairness idea.) Beyond that, given unavoidable features of the world we inhabit, the project of trying to live according to act consequentialism requires working with others to establish and sustain and improve legal rules, social norms, and a public morality of constraints and options. A general deference on our part to such rules, checked by background allegiance to priority itself as fundamental, is the best we can do. These secondary norms and rules are not fixed once and for all time; they surely should vary with changes in circumstances. What should strike hunter gatherers as fair and reasonable is different from what should strike twenty-first-century participants in democratic market societies as fair and reasonable. But within the idiom of fairness and justice itself, there will be no determinate answer to the question, what is really fair, and hence the *no standards puzzle* is only superficially puzzling.

Summary

Our ethical concerns about fairness should sweep widely. All effects of what we do and omit doing and might have done instead are relevant to determining whether an action or practice is exploitative. Norms against exploitation should be crafted, and revised with changing circumstances, so that their operation brings about outcomes as morally good as we can obtain, with our fairness concerns incorporated in the standards for outcome assessment. In the regulation of dealings between rich countries and poor countries, long-term benefit to people whose lives will be going badly is a paramount concern. When interaction produces a large surplus to be divided between wealthy-country company and poor-country people, we should aim to craft rules that channel as much of the surplus as can be squeezed to poor people. But we must avoid killing the geese that lay golden eggs, the geese here being mutually beneficial interaction between people in rich and poor countries. Our ethical principles should not be leading us to discourage wealthy corporations from setting up factories in poor countries that boost the economic development of poor countries, and for exactly the same reasons, we should eschew principles that would condemn international clinical trials as inherently unjust or tending to injustice.

Proposed fundamental ethical principles that sound high-minded but that would lead us to condemn policies that would produce better outcomes in the long run are a trap for the unwary. Prioritarian act consequentialism avoids the trap. This is a big point in its favor.

References

Arneson, R. (1999). Human flourishing versus desire satisfaction. *Social Philosophy and Policy, 16*, 113–142.

Arneson, R. (2000). Welfare should be the currency of justice. *Canadian Journal of Philosophy, 30*, 477–524.

Arneson, R. (2006). Desert and equality. In N. Holtug & K. Lippert-Rasmussen (Eds.), *Egalitarianism: New essays on the nature and value of equality* (pp. 262–294). Oxford: Oxford University Press.

Arneson, R. (2008). Broadly utilitarian theories of exploitation and multinational clinical research. In J. Hawkins & E. Emanuel (Eds.), *Exploitation and developing countries: The ethics of clinical research* (pp. 142–174). Princeton, NJ: Princeton University Press.

Darwall, S. (2006). *The second-person standpoint: Morality, respect, and accountability*. Cambridge, MA: Harvard University Press.

Hare, R. M. (1981). *Moral thinking: Its levels, method, and point*. Oxford: Oxford University Press, 1981.

Hawkins, J., & Emanuel, E. (Eds.). (2008). *Exploitation and developing countries: The ethics of clinical research*. Princeton, NJ: Princeton University Press.

Holtug, N. (2010). *Persons, interests, and justice*. Oxford: Oxford University Press.

Parfit, D. (1997). Equality and priority. *Ratio, 10*, 202–211.

Railton, P. (1988). Alienation, consequentialism, and the demands of morality. In S. Scheffler (Ed.), *Consequentialism and its critics* (pp. 93–133). Oxford: Oxford University Press.

Scheffler, S. (1982). *The rejection of consequentialism*. Oxford: Oxford University Press.

Wertheimer, A. (1999). *Exploitation*. Princeton, NJ: Princeton University Press.

Reply to Arneson

Jamie Carlin Watson

Happily, there are a few points on which Richard Arneson and I agree. First, we agree that international clinical trials are not *inherently* wrongfully exploitative. Arneson argues that, if researchers follow an act consequentialist decision-making process guided by a prioritarian standard of fairness, any resulting decision will not be immoral and, therefore, not wrongfully exploitative. I agree such trials are not inherently wrongfully exploitative, though for different reasons. Alternatively, I argue that, so long as the obstacles to informed consent are reasonably overcome, and researchers do not place a subject in circumstances in which the subject stands an unreasonable risk of losing something of fundamental value, then the trial is not wrongfully exploitative. On both accounts, those making a decision to conduct a clinical trial in a country other than their homes of origin must gather an extensive amount of information about the culture where the proposed trial is to take place and the potential test subjects. In some cases, the obstacles to gathering this sort of information are insurmountable, and the spectre of wrongful exploitation looms. We also agree that a plausible account of wrongful exploitation and decision procedure guided by this account could guide behavior in a way that avoids wrongfully exploitative acts. I, of course, conclude that the obstacles to employing such a decision procedure make it highly likely that any particular international clinical trial is wrongfully exploitative.

Second, we agree that a subject can give voluntary, informed consent to a wrongfully exploitative act. He explains that "one can voluntarily consent to an offer that one cannot reasonably refuse. I can voluntarily and indeed wholeheartedly consent to a marriage offer from Ted, even though I have no other offers, and continued bachelorhood would be, for me, an utter disaster." This seems right; in Valdman's snakebite case, *B* may willingly and happily pay $20,000 for the antivenin, even if it means his financial ruin. He may even admit that he is being exploited and respond, "But at least I'm alive."

Arneson goes on to argue that such consent is not a necessary condition for avoiding wrongful exploitation. Here, our agreement is less clear. I argue that informed consent is at least necessary because the potential exploitee's evaluations of reasonable risk and fundamental value are essentially subjective. Arneson does not quite disagree with the point, since he allows that certain types of proxies may make informed decisions for others. I accept the right of proxies to make decisions on behalf of others in cases where their own cognitive faculties are undeveloped (children, mentally handicapped) or compromised (brain damage). It is not obvious that Arneson would agree to limit the scope of proxies this much, but we agree that informed consent on the part of the test subject is necessary at least at some point along the decision chain.

Contemporary Debates in Bioethics, First Edition. Edited by Arthur L. Caplan and Robert Arp.

Despite our agreement, there are a number of points on which Arneson and I disagree. Before I highlight these points, though, I feel I need to clarify the relationship between our two projects. It seems that Arneson and I are not quite answering the same question. I argued that, while international clinical trials are not inherently wrongfully exploitative, there are strong reasons for thinking that any particular international clinical trial is likely to be wrongfully exploitative. Arneson does not disagree. Instead, he defends a particular framework for moral decision-making that, if followed by clinical researchers, would ameliorate concerns that international clinical trials are wrongfully exploitative. Since I agree with Arneson that international clinical trials are not inherently wrongfully exploitative, I agree that it is possible to employ a decision procedure that would allow clinical researchers to engage in international clinical trials without wrongfully exploiting test subjects. Thus, the primary source of our disagreement centers on the decision procedure that Arneson suggests is sufficient for avoiding wrongful exploitation.

I find Arneson's suggested decision procedure problematic for three reasons, and given space constraints, I will simply mention two and explain the third. First, he allows that "fairness" and "wrongful exploitation" are socially conditioned concepts, and that the latter must be "crafted, and revised with changing circumstances." The problem here is that there are no noncontroversial grounds on which to craft and revise them, since legal and cultural norms are not plausibly identified with moral norms and appeal to additional moral norms simply assumes what we need to prove.

A second reason I find Arneson's case uncompelling is that his concept of "wrongful exploitation" seems to come apart from his conception of a "wrongful act." In one place, he claims, "Surely, one morally ought not to engage in exploitative transactions," while in another he explains that, "Discouraging mutually beneficial exploitation is morally right to do just in case it brings about better consequences by the priority standard than anything else one might instead have done." This suggests that the priority principle may regard some acts as exploitative (even *wrongfully* exploitative, according to my analysis) but morally justifiable.

A third reason I find Arneson's case uncompelling is grounded in the (admitted!) difficulty of conducting a rule consequentialist cost/benefit analysis. Arneson argues that, if a rule consequentialist calculation guided by a prioritarian standard of fairness is used to guide decisions, then those decisions will not be immoral. But as I noted in my chapter, very few medical professionals are introduced to sophisticated moral theories like act consequentialism, much less prioritarian standards, and much, much less taught how to employ these effectively. Further, even sophisticated consequentialists disagree about how to weight certain consequences. Consider, again, the case I introduced from Torbjörn Tännsjö (1994). Tännsjö and his fellow consequentialists disagreed on the appropriate utility calculus to employ in evaluating the benefits of the clinical trials of ddI.

Arneson offers prioritarianism as a means of mitigating such disagreement. But this only raises another problem. According to Derek Parfit (1997) and others, the Priority View is the consequentialist view that "Benefiting people matters more the worse off these people are," such that "benefits to the worse off should be given more weight," morally speaking, than benefits to those who are better off (p. 213). In light of certain counterexamples, Parfit allows that priority for the worse off is not absolute, and that a significant enough benefit to those better off could outweigh the moral significance of benefit to those worse off. Nevertheless, this view faces a serious obstacle, namely, it is not clear how we could justify an *objective* standard of "worse off."

As I pointed out in my chapter, the value of a person's life, the risks they are willing to take, and the consequences they are willing to endure are subjective facts about the person. One person may be willing to pay what I regard as an exorbitant price for a piece of sci-fi memorabilia, another person may be willing to pay $20,000 for snake antivenin, and still another may be willing to endure the loss of eyesight as a possible side-effect of an experimental drug that has the potential to save his life. Further, prioritarians reject the idea that "worse off" is a function of the relative benefits of individuals, so one person cannot be regarded as worse off simply because she has fewer benefits than another. Instead, "worse off" is determined by an objective standard. But what could this standard be? The standard of living of a moral philosopher prefers? That of a Fortune 500 CEO? Presumably, neither is sufficient for all (or even moderately sized groups of) valuers. Thus, prioritarianism faces a serious measurement problem.

Although my account does derive from a complex deontological moral theory, its application requires no appeal to that theory or any calculation of values. Neither does its application require a heavy-handed governmental infrastructure of laws and prosecuting bodies. Regulation serves mostly to incentivize those clever enough to conduct business under restrictive conditions, and moral behavior is best motivated and checked by a reasonable and vocal community of morally educated individuals. Thus, my account requires only a conscientious application of the moral concepts already employed in international clinical trials: informed consent, individual rights, and the subjective nature of valuing. If the relationships among these concepts are understood even at an unsophisticated level, a medical researcher has a chance, though small, of conducting an international clinical trial that is not wrongfully exploitative.

References

Parfit, D. (1997). Equality and priority. *Ratio, 3*, 202–221.

Tännsjö, T. (1994). The morality of clinical research: A case study. *Journal of Medicine and Philosophy, 19*, 7–21.

Reply to Watson

Richard J. Arneson

In the generic circumstances of international clinical trials, opportunities for exploitation are easy to see. A large pharmaceutical corporation negotiates with poor people in a poor country regarding their possible participation in medical experiments from which the corporation might gain big bucks. The poor people, let us imagine, are suffering from serious disease (the disease whose treatment is the object of study) and have no healthcare options. They are desperate, and also ignorant about medical practices, the nature of experimental medical research, and other relevant facts. The large corporation may hold lopsided bargaining power. Those who become experimental subjects may choose to participate in desperation and without clearly understanding the terms of the contract.

The circumstances just described may often occur and, for all I know, may often result in exploitation or unfair treatment. However, these facts alone do not make a deal exploitative. Whether a deal is exploitative depends on its content—the distribution of costs and benefits among the contracting parties. For all that has been said, it might be that the officials negotiating on behalf of the corporation do not use their bargaining advantages to wrest an unfair share of benefits. For all that has been said, the corporation, in sympathy for the plight of the experimental subjects, might present a contract according to which all benefits from the transaction go to the experimental subjects.

So, nothing in the generic situation guarantees that international clinical trials will be exploitative. And if, assessed against some specific conception of exploitation, many actual trials were found to be wrongfully exploitative, either suitable coercively enforced regulation or alterations in the culture and motivation of pharmaceutical companies would suffice to right the wrong. We should not be disposed to do away with mutually beneficial transactions that do not impose wrongful harm on third parties, though we might do well to look for ways of rendering their terms more fair.

Here is another example that shows that defects in consent to a transaction do not by themselves render it exploitative. Suppose I am selling my car to a used-car dealer. I desperately need some cash now, so I must accept virtually any deal offered. I lack knowledge of the recent purchase price of cars like mine, and I am drunk and unable to bargain effectively to advance my interests. Seeing all that, the used-car dealer could gouge me, but does not. He offers me an extremely generous deal, and I accept. Despite the defects in my consent, this deal is not reasonably regarded as exploitative.

Professor Watson hews to the position that what renders a transaction exploitative is some defect in the quality of the consent that the exploited participant gives to what is going on. I have doubts about this entire class of views. The problem is that however

Contemporary Debates in Bioethics, First Edition. Edited by Arthur L. Caplan and Robert Arp.

faulty my consent to a transaction, it remains possible that the division of benefits and burdens generated by the transaction is impeccably fair. If I am duped or tricked into accepting a transaction that generously benefits me, and does not yield disproportionate benefit to other participants, I am not exploited. This judgment stands even if one were to hold that the duping or manipulation is unfair in itself.

Professor Watson goes astray at the outset by supposing that since agents decide whether or not to make exchanges based on their subjective sense of whether what they are getting from the exchange is worth more to them than what they are giving up, there can be no sense in assessing exchanges by some measure of fairness that is independent of the exchanging agents' subjective attitudes and opinions.

I do not deny that one might be a skeptic about objective value, objective standards of ethical assessment, including fairness. That is a possible position, with theoretical advantages and (to my mind, great) disadvantages. But Watson's reason for opting for skepticism is not persuasive.

From the fact that someone decides whether to say Yes to a proposed deal based on her subjective opinion as to whether she will gain from the transaction, nothing follows about the possibility of assessing the transaction as fair or unfair. This shows up immediately when one reflects that in an Easy Rescue case, where you are about to drown and I happen by and offer to save your life by reaching out my hand in exchange for your life savings, you can be both glad that I am on the scene and sure that you gain from the proposed exchange but also sure that this deal is exploitative and unfair.

Watson incorporates subjective assessment into his proposed test for the existence of exploitation: exploitation occurs via a contractual arrangement just in case "a responsible agent cannot reasonably reject a contract, where the inability to reasonably reject means that the agent perceives that he stands an unreasonable risk of losing something that he considers of fundamental value." The paradigm case of exploitation here is submission to an offer of easy rescue when the terms proposed involve giving up something the potential rescuee regards as fundamentally valuable. In the example just above, where the person at risk of death is asked to give up his entire life savings, he will see that whether he accepts or rejects the offer, he will lose something of fundamental value to him (his life, if he rejects the offer, and his life savings, if he accepts it).

But there are cases and cases. The incorporation of the agent's subjective attitudes into the test for exploitation sinks the proposal. Suppose I have suffered an accident and cannot mow my loan for a few weeks. Most of us would say this is no big deal, but suppose I have an egotistically inflated notion of the fundamental value of maintaining the front appearance of my house and lawn so it befits my inflated sense of my dignity. My neighbor offers to mow my lawn for the few weeks in which I am incapacitated for five dollars. Most of us would say this is a very generous offer, but I have an inflated sense of the fundamental value to me of maintaining as much cash on hand. Any loss of cash that is out of the ordinary strikes me as a disaster worse than the sinking of the *Titanic*. So, in this case, I face a subjectively horrible dilemma: Either I give up something of fundamental value (if I refuse the offer, my lawn becomes unkempt for a few weeks), or I lose something else of fundamental value to me ($5 of my precious cash on hand). Voila! My neighbor's offer, which had seemed generous, is revealed to be exploitative on Watson's account. Something has gone badly wrong here.

One might worry that the attitudes and opinions attributed to me in the lawn-mowing example mentioned previously are so bizarre as to call in question my sanity. Let us clarify that this is not the case. I am perfectly sane and rational, I just have a big ego and idiosyncratic preferences. My subjective attitudes and opinions do not have the power to transform a generous offer into an exploitative proposal.

Consider any customer of a public-utility company residing where the winters are severe. If I live in Minnesota, the utility company has me at its mercy. I need to keep the furnace fired up through the winter, because if I fail to do this, I stand an unreasonable risk of freezing to death on a cold night. I must pay virtually whatever the utility company charges for electricity and gas. None of this prevents the utility company from offering to sell its customers energy at an eminently reasonable price, and nothing prevents me from wholeheartedly voluntarily consenting to purchase energy from this company at this reasonable price. (My example is thinly described, and one could add further details to the case to render it the case that in this situation, I am not at unreasonable risk of losing something of fundamental value. I could survive through the winter in an unheated house if I wear warm clothing, and so on. This would lead to an unfruitful discussion. The misguided challenge just invites me to tighten up my description of the example to ensure that the crucial "unreasonable risk" condition obtains. This can be done.) One could say that my gladly paying a cheap price for goods I badly need is a paradigm case of *not* being exploited. Any theory of exploitation that conflicts with this judgment deserves to be rejected. Professor Watson's ingenious theory fails this test.

Another case to think about: windfall opportunities. Indulging in unreasonable optimism, I have planned my life around the expectation that sometime, somehow, I would become an invited regular member of an important first ascent climbing team, despite my weak physique and poor climbing abilities. Fulfilling this aim is of utmost importance to me. The strong likelihood is that no chance of fulfilling this extravagant aim would ever fall into my lap. However, I have publicized my great desire to be part of a significant first-ascent team on my popular sports blog, and by chance, the leader of a planned first-ascent trip to do new and immensely difficult routes in Patagonia reads my blog just as she realizes the finances of her planned trip are precarious. So, she offers me the opportunity to be a regular team member in exchange for a $20,000 contribution to the outstanding bills the preparations for the expedition have incurred. This is the chance of a lifetime, which I gladly accept. But according to the Watson account that we are here considering, not only is the expedition leader's reasonable offer to me an instance of wrongful exploitation, but also it is true that offering me the opportunity of a lifetime on even more favorable terms would also be exploitative, unless she offered me the opportunity at no cost to me whatsoever.

In these brief remarks I have raised some questions about some interesting features of Professor Watson's views. I have not offered further defense of my consequentialist approach to the analysis of exploitation issues. The reader will have to judge its plausibility. From a consequentialist standpoint, morality is a project of bringing about better lives for people, with good fairly distributed. Just in virtue of being a rational agent, each of us has a commitment to this project, even though as beings with human desires and traits and cognitive powers, we do not live up to it. The moral rules we should accept, as rational agents, are the rules that in given circumstances would help us come closer in our conduct to the conduct that would bring about best outcomes (better lives for people, fairly distributed). Rules against exploitatively taking advantage of others are in this respect on par with rules against lying, stealing, and murdering one's neighbors.

Index

Contemporary Debates in Bioethics, First Edition. Edited by Arthur L. Caplan and Robert Arp.

Printed in the United States
By Bookmasters